P9-APH-690

ACCORDING TO THE LATEST HEALTH SURVEYS, MORE THAN TWO-THIRDS OF AMERICANS EAT MORE FAT THAN IS GOOD FOR THEM.

Thirty-eight health organizations, ranging from the American Heart Association to the American Medical Association, recommend limiting the number of calories from fat to no more than 30 percent of the daily diet.

If you are among the 77 percent of Americans looking to do just that by choosing foods that are low in fat, you'll want to keep *THE FAT COUNTER* handy. Now in its fifth edition, and completely updated and revised with thousands of new entries, *THE FAT COUNTER* is unmatched in its quantity and range of listings. As in their entire bestselling Counter series, nutrition experts Annette Natow and Jo-Ann Heslin present cutting-edge dietary news, reliable counts, and helpful tips for healthy eating—all in one convenient, easy-to-use guide.

Annette B. Natow, Ph.D., R.D., and Jo-Ann Heslin, M.A., R.D., are the authors of twenty-six books on nutrition. Both are former faculty members of Adelphi University and the State University of New York, Downstate Medical Center. They are editors of the *Journal of Nutrition for the Elderly,* and serve as editorial board members for the *Environmental Nutrition Newsletter.*

Books by Annette B. Natow and Jo-Ann Heslin

The Antioxidant Vitamin Counter
Calcium Counts
Count On a Healthy Pregnancy
The Calorie Counter (Second Edition)
The Carbohydrate, Sugar and Fiber Counter
The Cholesterol Counter (Fifth Edition)
The Diabetes Carbohydrate and Calorie Counter
Eating Out Food Counter
The Fat Attack Plan
The Fat Counter (Fifth Edition)
The Food Shopping Counter
Megadoses
The Most Complete Food Counter
No-Nonsense Nutrition for Kids
The Pocket Encyclopedia of Nutrition
The Pocket Fat Counter (Second Edition)
The Pocket Protein Counter
The Pregnancy Nutrition Counter
The Protein Counter
The Sodium Counter

Published by POCKET BOOKS

THE
FAT
COUNTER

FIFTH EDITION
REVISED AND UPDATED

Annette B. Natow, Ph.D., R.D.
and
Jo-Ann Heslin, M.A., R.D.

POCKET BOOKS
New York   London   Toronto   Sydney   Singapore

POCKET BOOKS, a division of Simon & Schuster Inc.
1230 Avenue of the Americas, New York, NY 10020

Copyright © 1989, 1993, 1995, 1996, 2000 by Annette Natow and Jo-Ann Heslin

ISBN: 0-671-02565-1

First Pocket Books printing of this revised edition June 2000

10 9 8 7 6 5 4 3 2

POCKET and colophon are registered trademarks of
Simon & Schuster Inc.

Front cover photo © FoodPix

Printed in the U.S.A.

To our families, who support us through every project:
Harry, Allen, Irene, Sarah, Meryl, Laura, Marty,
George, Emily, Steven, Joe, Kristen, Brian and Karen

ACKNOWLEDGMENTS

Without the tireless cooperation of Steven Natow, MD, and Stephen Llano, *The Fat Counter* would never have been completed. Our thanks to all the food manufacturers and processors who shared product information. A special thanks to our most supportive agent, Nancy Trichter, and to our wonderfully perceptive editor, Jane Cavolina.

"Too much fat is a disadvantage . . . laying the foundation for troubles with the heart."

"Foods very high in fuel value, i.e. fats and dishes containing much fat, should be avoided."

Mary Swartz Rose, Ph.D.
Feeding the Family
The Macmillan Company, 1919

INTRODUCTION

Americans know that they eat more fat than is good for them and they want to do something about it. In fact, the American Dietetic Association's Center for Nutrition and Dietetics Consumer Hotline reports receiving more questions on fat than any other issue.

In spite of this we still eat too much fat. Thirty-three percent of total calories in the average American diet come from fat, down from 42 percent in the mid-sixties but still above the 30 percent goal. Current surveys show that only one third of Americans are meeting this goal. Saturated fat makes up 11 percent of calories, down from 16 percent in the mid-sixties but still nearly one and a half times the recommended level of 8 percent of calories.

Most experts agree, less fat is better. Thirty-eight health organizations ranging from the American Heart Association to the American Medical Association recommend limiting the number of calories from fat to no more than 30 percent of the daily diet.

> The American Heart Association recommends a decreased intake of fat, particularly saturated fat.
>
> Nutrition Committee of the
> American Heart Association, 1999

> Reduce dietary fat intake to an average of 30 percent of calories or less, and average saturated fat intake to less than 10 percent of calories among people aged 2 and older.
> Healthy People 2000
> Department of Health and Human Services

> Total fats and oils to provide 15 percent to no more than 30 percent total energy. Limit consumption of fatty foods, particularly those of animal origin. Choose modest amounts of appropriate vegetable oils.
> American Institute for Cancer Research, 1997

> The Women's Health Trial found that it's easier to meet health goals on a lowfat diet, than a low calorie diet.
> Fred Hutchinson Cancer Research Center

> Researchers have found that you can lose weight simply by reducing the amount of fat you eat.
> Division of Nutritional Sciences,
> Cornell University

And consumers are getting the message. In its 1999 Trends report, the Food Marketing Institute noted that the top nutritional concern of American consumers continues to be the amount of fat in their food. Fifty percent of consumers now focus on fat, and more than 77 percent have sought out and purchased products because of "lowfat" claims on the label. But even though the percentage of fat that Americans eat has gone down, the *total amount of fat eaten has not*. That is because we are now eating about 300 calories more a day than in the past.

TOO MUCH IS NOT SAFE

High fat diets are unhealthy. Almost three fourths of the two million Americans who die annually die from diseases linked to our high fat diet.

Eating too much fat increases the risk for:

HEART ATTACK—Each year Americans have more than one and a half million heart attacks resulting in more than half a million deaths.

STROKE—Americans have one half million each year, many result in death or disability.

CANCER—Studies suggest that high fat intake increases risk for breast, colon and prostate cancers.

OVERWEIGHT—Diets high in fat lead to overweight more easily than do diets high in protein or carbohydrate. Fat from your food is the main source of body fat. High fat diets make you fatter faster.

GALLBLADDER DISEASE—Overweight people with high fat diets have a greater risk of gallbladder trouble.

OSTEOARTHRITIS—High fat diets cause overweight, putting more strain on the joints.

GOUT—A high fat diet aggravates gout (joint inflammation).

HIGH BLOOD PRESSURE—Too much body fat puts you at greater risk for getting high blood pressure and also increases the amount of medication needed to control existing cases of high blood pressure.

DIABETES—High fat diets cause overweight, which increases the risk for diabetes. It also complicates treatment for existing cases.

FAT FACT

The amount of fat an average American eats in one week is equal to six sticks of butter.

FAT FACTS

Most foods contain fat. Some have more, some less, few have none. Some fat can be easily seen—butter, margarine, salad oils and the fat on your steak or chop. Much of the fat you eat can't be seen—invisible fat—in chips, milk, egg yolks, olives, walnuts, cakes, pies, cookies and candy. Whether you can see the fat or not, it adds up quickly.

FAT FACT: *Everyone should be eating less fat.* Americans eat too much fat. One third of all the calories we eat are from fat! Experts agree that we should be eating much less—no more than 30 percent of our calories should come from fat. Some experts state that less than 30 percent would be even better.

FAT FACT: *Fat makes you fatter faster.* The fat we eat gets turned into body fat much easier than the other things we eat. Fat calories make us fatter than calories from protein, sugar or starch. A lower fat diet is helpful in weight loss.

FAT FACT: *Fat comes in three forms*—saturated, polyunsaturated and monounsaturated.

There are different kinds of fats—saturated, polyunsaturated, monounsaturated—classified by the types of fatty acids they contain. Most foods contain all three of these fats. Some foods have more of one type than another. For example, beef has a lot more saturated fat, margarine a lot of polyunsaturated fat, and olive oil is high in monounsaturated fat.

Saturated Fat

If you leave a stick of butter on the kitchen counter all day it would soften but it won't melt. Butter is high in saturated fat, which is solid at room temperature. Research shows that eating a lot of saturated fats raises blood cholesterol levels. People with higher blood cholesterol levels are more likely to have a heart attack. It has been found that not all saturated fats raise cholesterol. Even though that is true, foods we eat never contain only one type of saturated fat. All fats in foods are mixtures of fats. Foods often contain some saturated fats that raise cholesterol and other saturated fats that may not. That makes it difficult to translate these studies into food recommendations. *The best advice: eat less total fat.*

FAT FACT

Saturated fat has been shown to be a factor in cancer of the ovaries. A recent study suggests that eating as little as 10 extra grams of saturated fat a day may raise a woman's risk of ovarian cancer by 20 percent. The good news is that lowering fat intake by 10 grams a day reduces risk by 20 percent.

FOODS HIGH IN SATURATED FATS

Bacon	Ice cream
Beef	Lamb
Butter	Palm kernel oil
Cheese	Palm oil
Chocolate	Pork
Coconut	Sausage
Coconut oil	Sour cream
Cream	Veal
Deli meats	Whipped cream
Half and half	Whole milk
Hot dogs	

Polyunsaturated Fat

Corn oil left out on the kitchen counter will not become solid. It doesn't even solidify in the refrigerator because it is high in polyunsaturated fats which are liquid at room temperature. These fats may help lower cholesterol levels in the blood.

Researchers report that eating fatty fish once or twice a week reduces the risk of death from heart attacks. It is believed the protective effect of fish is due to the type of polyunsaturated fats (omega-3) they contain. These are sometimes called fish oils and can be bought as supplements.

Two types of polyunsaturated fats are omega-6 and omega-3. These names describe the structure of the polyunsaturated fats. Omega-6 fats are found in seeds and plant oils. Omega-3 fats are in fish, leafy vegetables, soybeans, flaxseed and canola oil. These polyunsaturated fats are converted in the body to essential fatty acids needed for body's functions.

Research suggest that too much polyunsaturated fat may not be good. High intake may cause gallbladder disease, depress the immune system and put you at greater risk for some cancers. *The best advice: eat less total fat.*

FOODS HIGH IN POLYUNSATURATED FATS

Bluefish	Salmon
Corn oil	Sesame oil
Cottonseed oil	Soft margarine
Herring	Soybean oil
Mackerel	Sunflower oil
Mayonnaise	Tuna
Rainbow trout	Walnut oil
Sablefish	Walnuts
Safflower oil	Wheat germ
Salad dressing	Whitefish

Monounsaturated Fats

Olive oil left out on the kitchen counter never becomes solid. In the refrigerator olive oil gets cloudy as it becomes partly solid. Monounsaturated fat stays liquid at room temperature but becomes partly solid when chilled. You have been hearing more about monounsaturated fats lately as part of the Mediterranean diet. Research shows these fats may help lower blood cholesterol. New research suggests that high intakes of monounsaturated fats may help protect against memory loss as people age. This sounds good, but too much of any fat is not good for you. *The best advice: eat less total fat.*

FOODS HIGH IN MONOUNSATURATED FAT

Almonds	Peanut butter
Canola oil	Peanut oil
Cashews	Peanuts
Chicken fat	Pine nuts (pignolia)
Hazelnuts (filberts)	Pistachio nuts
Macadamia nuts	Sesame oil
Olive oil	Soybean oil
Olives	Soybean oil margarine

Trans Fatty Acids

When liquid oils are hardened to make margarine and solid shortenings, some of the unsaturated fats become trans fatty acids which, like saturated fat, can raise blood cholesterol. In the ingredient list on food labels these hardened oils are called "partially hydrogenated" or "hydrogenated vegetable oils." Research suggests that eating trans fatty acids increases risk of heart disease in the same way that saturated fat does. Margarine is a major source of trans fatty acids followed by cakes, cookies, pastries and restaurant french fries.

Choose tub margarines which have fewer trans fatty acids or those brands which advertise "no trans fat." If a food is low fat, there won't be enough trans fatty acids to worry about. So again, *the best advice is to use less of all fats because the less fat you eat, the fewer trans fatty acids you will eat.*

FAT FACT

As more research points to negative effects of trans fatty acids, manufacturers are limiting and eliminating them from their products.

CHOOSING LOWFAT FOODS

Choosing the Best Fats

Once in a while everyone feels like having some toast and butter or margarine. In most homes you find butter, margarine and some kind of cooking oil. Even lowfat recipes may call for some oil or shortening. There are things you should remember to help you choose the best fats.

When selecting a margarine, choose one with a liquid oil as the first ingredient. Soft tub margarines or liquid squeeze types are often highest in polyunsaturates. For example, if liquid sunflower oil is the first ingredient, this would be a highly polyunsaturated oil. Using moderate amounts of this or a similar margarine would be a good choice.

Butter blends are a combination of margarine and some butter. Blends have less saturated fat than butter but more saturated fat than margarines.

A good, all purpose cooking oil is tasteless and fries without smoking. Corn, safflower, sunflower, soybean and cottonseed are all highly polyunsaturated oils. Olive, canola and peanut oil are high in polyunsaturates and monounsaturates. All are good choices.

Choosing Lowfat Proteins

1. Choose "fat free" or "nonfat" (also labeled skim) or "reduced fat" (also labeled 2 percent fat) or lowfat (also labeled 1 percent fat) milk and lowfat or nonfat yogurt. Use skim milk cheese, reduced fat or fat free cheese. On occasions when you eat regular cheese, limit the portion.

2. Use lowfat or nonfat yogurt, reduced fat or fat free sour cream in place of regular sour cream.

3. Choose the leanest cuts of meat; remove all visible fat before cooking.

4. Choose lean or extra lean ground beef that has as little fat as possible. Supermarkets often label the ground beef with the percentage of fat; sometimes it is as low as 10 percent or less. Ground poultry is a good substitute for ground meat. It is usually, but not always, lower in fat. Check the label.

5. Roast, broil or grill meats on a rack so that fats drip off during cooking. When making soups, stews or sauces, skim fat off the top.

6. Avoid turkey and turkey breasts that are "self-basted." The basting usually adds more fat.

7. Poultry skin is high in fat. You can cook poultry with its skin on but remove it before eating.

8. All fish contains less fat than most cuts of meat. Very lean fish choices are: cod, scrod, flounder, halibut, pollock, sole and haddock. Shellfish, like shrimp, lobster, scallops, clams and crab, are low in fat too.

9. Choose tuna canned in water. Tuna is a lowfat fish but when it is canned in oil, this adds seven times more fat than tuna canned in water.

10. Choose poached, steamed, grilled or broiled fish instead of breaded, battered and fried.

11. Farmed fish tend to have more fat than fish grown wild. Farmed fish can sometimes have as much as twice the amount of fat.

Ten Steps to Lower Your Fat Intake

1. Choose fat free or nonfat (skim), lowfat or reduced fat milk, evaporated lowfat or fat free milk, lowfat or nonfat yogurt and reduced fat or fat free cheese. Look for the words: fat free, non-fat (skim), lowfat (1% fat), reduced fat (2%).

Beware: Cheeses labeled "made with partially skim milk" may contain almost as much fat as regular cheese. Even though there is only a one percent difference between 1 and 2 percent milk, 2 percent has almost double the amount of fat.

2. Choose lean meats trimmed of all visible fat and poultry without skin. Look for ground meat and poultry labeled "lean" or "extra lean" or lowfat ground beef. Vegetarian meat substitutes are another good choice but check the fat content on the label. Not all are lowfat.

Beware: Meat, poultry and fish contain invisible fat. Limit portion size to 3 ounces, about the size of a deck of cards or cassette case.

3. Choose lean fish like cod, scrod, haddock and halibut. When using fatty fish like salmon, bluefish or mackerel, remove the skin and all visible fat.

Beware: Canned fish packed in oil is high in fat. Choose fish canned in water, broth, mustard or tomato sauce.

4. Roast, broil, grill, bake or poach meat, poultry and fish so no extra fat is added. During cooking fat drips off; discard it.

Beware: When you add bread crumbs or cereal to ground meat or poultry for meat loaf or burgers, the crumbs act like a blotter soaking up fat instead of allowing it to drip off.

5. Use honey, all fruit preserves, jelly or jam as a spread on toast and bread instead of butter, margarine or regular cream cheese—good taste and no fat.

6. Sour cream as a topping for baked potatoes is a lower fat choice than butter, but nonfat plain sour cream, or lowfat or nonfat yogurt is even better. Try butter flavor sprinkles.

7. Use lowfat milk, lowfat or nonfat evaporated milk in tea or coffee instead of half and half, cream or nondairy creamers (whiteners). It gives beverages the same flavor but less fat.

8. Dress your salad with lemon juice, or flavored vinegar, or reduced fat and fat free dressings instead of regular oil-based salad dressings.

9. Sweet rolls, donuts and Danish pastries are high fat snacks. Try cinnamon raisin bread or bagels for a lowfat sweet treat.

10. Use cooking spray to oil pans and sauté foods.

These suggestions are just a beginning. To reduce the total amount of fat you eat you have to learn how to recognize fat when you see it and even when you don't see it. It's not always easy. *The Fat Counter* will help.

FAT FACT

To have healthy lowfat meals, fill three quarters of your plate with high complex carbohydrate foods like rice, bulgur and other grains, pasta, potatoes, vegetables, fruits and bread. Have lean meat, poultry, fish or beans on the other quarter of your plate .

FINDING FAT IN FOODS

Doesn't everybody need some fat?

Yes, you do need a small amount of fat. Fat is part of every cell in your body. It is used to make hormones, cushion bones and body organs and insulate the body to help maintain normal temperature. Food fats carry fat soluble vitamins, A, D, E and K.

Fats stay in the stomach longer, making you feel full so that you don't get hungry as quickly.

Most fruits and vegetables have little or no fat. There are a few exceptions like avocados and olives (see page 11 and page 352).

Dried peas and beans are all pretty low in fat. Soybeans have a little more fat than other beans (see pages 508 and 16). All nuts and seeds, including coconut and peanuts, have a lot of fat. All these are examples of hidden fat.

Grains like oats, rice, wheat, rye and barley contain little fat. Cereals, breads and pasta made from grains are usually low in fat. Exceptions are some regular granola-type cereals, cookies, pies, sweet rolls and cakes. You can tell how much fat is in a cookie by how soft it is. The softer the cookie, the more fat it has. Judge your cookies by breaking them in half; a cookie that bends instead of breaking is higher in fat. Place a croissant, muffin or Danish on a napkin for a few minutes. If a grease ring forms, it's high in fat.

People think of animal foods like meat, milk, cheese, eggs, poultry and fish as good protein foods. While this is true, it is also true that all animal foods contain fat. In fact, an ounce of lean meat has the same amount of calories from fat as from protein. In fatty meat like spare ribs, there may be twice as many calories from fat as from protein. Meats like bacon should really be thought of as fat not meat. The fat in one slice of bacon is equal to the fat in a pat of butter.

FAT FACT

The top ten sources of fat in our diets are margarine, whole milk, shortening, American cheese, ground beef, lowfat milk, eggs, butter, vanilla ice cream, mayonnaise and salad dressing.

Reading Labels

There's a lot of information on labels but sometimes it can be confusing. When you want to know more about a food, look at the list of ingredients. Packaged foods must have ingredient listings. The first ingredient listed is the main one in the food. If it is fat, this is a high fat food. But even if fat is the second or third ingredient listed, the food is fairly high in fat.

LABEL LINGO

Fat free: Less than ½ gram of fat in a serving

Lowfat: Three grams of fat or less in a serving

Lean: Meat, poultry, seafood or packaged meals with less than 10 grams of fat, less than 4 grams of saturated fat and less than 95 milligrams of cholesterol in a 3½ ounce serving

Extra lean: Meat, poultry, seafood or packaged meals with less than 5 grams of fat, 2 grams of saturated fat and 95 milligrams of cholesterol in a 3½ ounce serving

Light or Lite: One-third fewer calories or 50% less fat than in the original, higher calorie, higher fat version.

Fats on labels can appear as any of the following:

Animal fats	Margarine
(lard, suet, chicken fat)	Monoglycerides
Butter	Oil
Cocoa butter	Partially hydrogenated fat
Cream	Partially hydrogenated oil
Cheese	Shortening
Diglycerides	Vegetable fat
Fat	Vegetable oil
Hydrogenated fat	Whole milk
Hydrogenated oil	

When Is a Fat Not a Fat?

In spite of the fact that high fat foods make us fat and are not healthy, we love fatty foods. Fried foods, chips, cakes, pies, cookies, butter and ice cream are often named as favorites. This is where fat substitutes come in. They give reduced fat or fat free products the texture and mouth feel of higher fat foods with less fat and usually less calories. By replacing all or part of the fat in processed foods, they may offer us healthier choices.

You'll see fat substitutes as ingredients in frozen desserts, margarines, baked goods, puddings, salad dressings, sauces and other foods. Some that are commonly used are:

Carrageenan	Pectin
Cellulose	Polydextrose
Dextrins	Starch
Gelatin	Whey protein
Maltodextrin	Xanthum
Modified food starch	

Some ingredients that are used as fat substitutes also have other functions in food. Some of these have been used for years, others have been developed more recently. Many of these substitutes are natural like carrageenan which is found in seaweed. Others are synthetic, often made from ordinary foods like eggs, milk and corn. The synthetic fat substitutes require more testing than the natural substances before they are approved for use in food by the Food and Drug Administration (FDA).

Some fat replacers are made from fat. They provide less calories than the fat in foods. That is how they lower the calories in food. *Olestra* (Olean), an artificial fat, is made from sugar and oil. Because the molecule is too big to be digested, it passes through the body without being absorbed. Although found to be safe by the FDA after a nine-year review, Olestra has been criticized because it interferes with the absorption of carotenes (beneficial nutrients) and also causes cramping and diarrhea in some people. *Salatrim* (Benefat), another artificial fat, is made from soybean or canola oil. Processing rearranges the molecules so that only five of the original nine calories per gram of fat are absorbed while the other four pass out of the body. Used in cookies and chocolate chips, some people have reported nausea and bloating after eating large amounts of foods containing Salatrim.

Researchers at the U.S. Department of Agriculture (USDA) have developed *Z-Trim* made from the hulls of oats, soybeans, peas and rice, or bran from corn or wheat. The USDA claims that it won't upset the digestive system because it is made from natural fibers. Oatrim is a similar type of fat replacer.

Simplesse made from the protein of milk or eggs has no more than two calories a gram. It is often used in lowfat dairy foods, mayonnaise and salad dressings.

Because so many people want to avoid eating high fat foods, there is a ready market for fat substitutes. Many new ones are being developed and you'll be seeing them in more foods. Use these foods in moderation both because you may have trouble tolerating them and because even though the fat calories are reduced, some of these foods are still high in calories.

Food experts, including The American Dietetic Association, support the use of fat substitutes for some of the fat in foods when they are used as part of a healthy diet. While fat replacers can make lower-fat eating more enjoyable, they should not be used as an excuse for eating too many desserts or as a green light to eat more high fat foods because "you have saved so many calories with the fat replacers."

Finding Fat Calories in Food

Fat calories make you fatter faster. The food fat we eat is easily turned into body fat. You can limit fat calories by counting fat grams.

Nutrition labels can help you find out how much fat is in a food. Fat is listed in grams.

$$1 \text{ gram of fat} = 9 \text{ calories}$$

For example, 1 oz. of corn chips has 155 calories and 9 grams of fat. More than one half of the calories in corn chips come from fat.

$$9 \text{ grams of fat} \times 9 \text{ calories} = 81 \text{ fat calories}$$

Fat foods have a lot of calories. One teaspoon of fat has 45 calories. A teaspoon of protein, sugar or starch has only 20 calories.

For example, 1 oz. of pretzels has 120 calories and 1 gram of fat. Less than one tenth of the calories in pretzels come from fat. Pretzels are a good snack. Less fat, less fat calories, less fattening for you.

$$1 \text{ gram of fat} \times 9 \text{ calories} = 9 \text{ fat calories}$$

HOW MUCH FAT SHOULD YOU EAT?

Americans eat too much fat. Not too long ago, the average American got over 40 percent of his calories from fat. We now eat less. But still, we get a whopping 33 percent of our calories from fat. Experts agree we should be eating much less.

The American Heart Association, the American Cancer Society, the American Health Foundation and the National Institutes of Health all recommend lowering fat intake. Americans should eat no more than 30 percent of their calories as fat each day.

That's a good suggestion. How do you do it? The question is how many grams of fat can you eat and still limit your fat to no more than 30 percent of your calories? It's easy to find out.

STEP 1. *Find out how many calories you eat each day.* If you maintain the same weight, you are probably eating:

13 calories a pound, if you are not very active
15 calories a pound, if you are moderately active
17 calories a pound, if you are very active
20 calories a pound, if you are extremely active

For example, if you weigh 145 pounds and are moderately active you need 2175 calories a day. (145 pounds X 15 calories = 2175 calories a day.) Round that number to 2200 calories. You need 2200 calories a day to maintain your weight.

If you are overweight, estimate your best weight and multiply that by the appropriate number of calories per pound. For example if you would like to weigh 130 pounds and are not very active, estimate your calorie needs as follows:

130 pounds × 13 calories a pound = 1690 calories.

Round answer to 1700 calories.

STEP 2. *Find out how many of grams of fat you should be eating each day.* In Step 1 you found out how many calories you need each day. Find this number on the following list. Next to it is the maximum grams of fat allowed for the day. This amount will keep your fat intake to less than 30 percent of your total calories for the day.

For example, if you need 1800 calories a day, you should be eating no more than 60 grams of fat a day.

STEP 3. *Find out how many grams of saturated fat you should be eating each day.* In Step 1 you found out how many calories you need each day. Find the number of calories you need each day on the following list. On the same line is the upper limit of saturated fat for the day. This amount will keep your intake less than 10 percent of your total calories for the day.

UPPER LIMIT OF GRAMS OF FAT
AND SATURATED FAT EACH DAY

CALORIES	GRAMS OF FAT	GRAMS OF SATURATED FAT
1200	40	13
1300	43	14
1400	47	16
1500	50	17
1600	53	18
1700	57	19
1800	60	20
1900	63	21
2000	67	22
2100	70	23
2200	73	24
2300	77	26
2400	80	27
2500	83	28
2600	87	29
2700	90	30
2800	93	31
2900	97	32
3000	100	33

Now that you know how many grams of fat you should be eating each day, it's time to count up your fat.

Each day your target is:

_____calories
_____total fat grams
_____saturated fat grams

COUNTING UP YOUR FAT

We often eat on the run and pick foods high in fat. By the end of the day, we've eaten too much fat. You know you shouldn't be eating so much fat. You want to cut back. *The Fat Counter* will help you do it. Now it's simple to find out the amount of fat in all the foods you are eating.

Let's look at a typical day. Are the food choices familiar? Let's see how much fat this sample day has in it.

FAT COUNTING
SAMPLE DAY OF HIGH FAT FOOD CHOICES

FOOD	FAT GRAMS	SAT FAT GRAMS	TOTAL CALORIES
BREAKFAST			
Orange juice (1 cup)	tr	tr	111
French toast (1 slice)	7	2	151
Butter (1 pat)	4	3	36
Maple syrup (2 tbsp)	0	0	104
Pork sausage (1 link)	4	1	48
Coffee	0	0	4
Half & half (2 tbsp)	4	2	40
LUNCH			
Cheeseburger w/ bun	15	6	320
Ketchup (1 tbsp)	tr	tr	16
French fries (10 pieces)	4	2	111
Diet cola (12 oz)	0	0	2
SNACK			
Jelly doughnut	16	4	289
Coffee	0	0	4
Half & half (2 tbsp)	4	2	40
DINNER			
Flank steak, broiled (3 oz)	11	5	192
Mashed potato (1 cup)	tr	tr	198
Tossed salad (1½ cups)	tr	0	32
French dressing (1 tbsp)	6	1	67
Pound cake (1 slice)	6	3	117
Tea	0	0	2
Sugar (1 tsp)	0	0	15
TV SNACK			
Rich vanilla ice cream (½ cup)	12	7	178
TOTAL	**93**	**39**	**2077**

To determine your total fat calories for the day multiply the number of grams of fat by 9 (calories per gram of fat):

93 grams of fat × 9 calories = 837 fat calories

To determine the percentage of calories from fat, divide the total fat calories by the total calories for the day.

837 fat calories divided by 2077 = 40% fat (rounded)

To find the number of *saturated* fat calories, multiply the number of grams of saturated fat by 9 (calories per gram of fat). Saturated fat calories should be less than 10 percent of your total calories for the day. In the Sample Day of High-Fat Food Choices shown, there are 351 saturated fat calories. Ten percent of the total calories for this day would equal 208 calories of saturated fat.

39 grams of saturated fat × 9 calories = 351 saturated fat calories

This is too much fat and saturated fat for one day: 40 percent of the day's calories came from fat and well over 10 percent of the day's calories came from saturated fat. Now you can see how easy it is to eat too much fat.

TIME-SAVER: There's no need to count saturated fat every day. Keeping track of *total* fat is more important. Check your saturated fat intake once in a while. You'll find that when you eat less total fat, you automatically eat less saturated fat.

NOTE: In this and the following sample, as throughout *The Fat Counter*, the number of fat grams in each food has been rounded to the nearest whole number.

FAT COUNTING
SAMPLE DAY OF SMART FOOD CHOICES

FOOD	FAT GRAMS	SAT FAT GRAMS	TOTAL CALORIES
BREAKFAST			
Orange juice (1 cup)	tr	tr	111
Corn Flakes (1¼ cup)	tr	tr	110
Nonfat milk (1 cup)	tr	tr	86
Toast (1 slice)	1	tr	67
Strawberry jam (1 tbsp)	0	0	48
Coffee	0	0	4
Nonfat milk (2 tbsp)	0	0	11
LUNCH			
Hamburger with bun	12	4	275
Ketchup (1 tbsp)	tr	tr	16
Tossed salad (1½ cup)	tr	0	32
Reduced calorie Italian dressing (1 tbsp)	2	tr	16
Diet cola (12 oz)	0	0	2
SNACK			
Pear	1	tr	98
DINNER			
Flank steak, broiled (3 oz)	11	5	192
Mashed potato (1 cup)	tr	0	198
Peas and carrots (½ cup)	tr	tr	48
Dinner rolls (2)	4	tr	170
Angelfood cake (1 slice)	tr	tr	142
Tea	0	0	2
Sugar (1 tsp)	0	0	15
TV SNACK			
Light vanilla ice cream (½ cup)	3	2	92
TOTAL	34	11	1735

Now, determine the number of fat calories, the percentage of fat and the number of saturated fat calories in the sample day above.

34 grams of fat × 9 calories = 306 fat calories

Remember, the percentage of calories from fat is determined by dividing the calories from fat by the number of total calories.

306 fat calories divided by 1735 total calories =
18% fat (rounded)

Multiply the number of grams of saturated fat by 9 (calories per gram of fat) to determine the number of saturated fat calories, which should total no more than 10 percent of the total calories for the day. In this sample day that would be no more than 174 saturated fat calories. The actual figure is 99 saturated fat calories, far below 10 percent.

11 grams of saturated fat × 9 calories =
99 saturated fat calories

These smart food choices show a much healthier intake of fat for the day. When you cut down on grams of fat, you cut down on calories too. In this sample day fat calories are only 18 percent of the total.

TIME-SAVER: There's no need to count saturated fat every day. Keeping track of total fat is more important. Check your saturated fat intake once in a while. You'll find that when you eat less total fat, you automatically eat less saturated fat.

Now it's your turn to count your fat. Note everything you eat today, then look up the fat and saturated fat in each food and see how much fat you've eaten today. While you're at it, jot down the calories, too!

FAT COUNTING:
A SAMPLE WORKSHEET FOOD AMOUNT

FOOD	FAT GRAMS	SAT FAT GRAMS	TOTAL CALORIES
BREAKFAST			
SNACK			
LUNCH			
SNACK			
DINNER			
SNACK			
TOTAL			

Each day your target should be:

_____ calories
_____ fat grams
_____ saturated fat grams

Now it's time for the calculations.

_____ grams of fat × 9 calories = _____ fat calories

Calories from fat divided by total calories equals the percentage of calories from fat.

_____ fat calories divided by total calories = _____%

Grams of saturated fat times 9 calories (per gram) gives you saturated fat calories, which should total no more than 10 percent of total calories for the day.

___ grams of saturated fat × 9 calories = ___ saturated fat calories

10 percent of _____ (total calories) = _____

Did you eat more than 30 percent fat today? Did you eat more than 10 percent saturated fat? If you did, you're eating too much fat and saturated fat. Turn back to page XXX "Upper Limit of Grams of Fat and Saturated Fat Each Day."

Start right now to make lower fat food choices.

FAT FACT
___

If you are an average weight, moderately active adult and want a quick benchmark for total fat grams each day simply divide your weight in half.
___

USING YOUR FAT COUNTER

This book lists the fat, saturated fat and calorie content of over 22,000 foods. Now you can compare the fat values in your favorite foods and choose substitutes for them before you go out to shop or eat. This will help you save time while making smart food choices when you are deciding what to buy or eat.

The Fat Counter is divided into two parts, Part One: Brand Name, Nonbranded and Take-Out Foods, and Part Two: Restaurant Chains. All foods are listed alphabetically. For each category, you will find nonbranded (generic) foods are listed first in alphabetical order, followed by an alphabetical listing of brand name foods. The nonbranded listing will help you determine fat values for foods when you do not find your favorite brand listed. They also help you to evaluate store brands. Large categories are divided into subcategories such as canned, fresh, frozen, and ready-to-eat to make it easier to find what you are looking for. Many categories have take-out subcategories. Look there for foods you take-out or order in a store or restaurant because these foods are not nutrition labeled.

Most foods are listed alphabetically. But, in some cases, foods are grouped by category. For example, chow mein is found under the category ASIAN FOODS. Other group categories include:

ASIAN FOODS (Page 8): includes all types of Asian foods except egg rolls and sushi

DELI MEATS/COLD CUTS (Page 208): includes all sandwich meats except chicken, ham and turkey

DINNERS (Page 214): includes all frozen dinners by brand name

LIQUOR/LIQUEUR (Page 314): includes all alcoholic beverages except beer, champagne and wine

NUTRITION SUPPLEMENTS (Page 342): includes all meal replacers, diet bars and drinks, energy bars and drinks except sports drinks

SANDWICHES (Page 461): includes popular sandwich choices

SPANISH FOOD (Page 514): includes all types of Spanish and Mexican foods

DEFINITIONS

as prep (as prepared)—refers to food that has been prepared according to package directions

home recipe—describes homemade dishes; those included can be used as a guide to the fat values of similar products you may prepare, or take-out food you buy ready-to-eat

lean and fat—describes meat with some fat on its edges that is not cut away before cooking or poultry prepared with skin and fat as purchased

lean only—lean portion, trimmed of all visible fat

shelf stable—refers to prepared products found on the supermarket shelf that are ready-to-eat or to be heated, and do not require refrigeration

take-out—describes prepared dishes that you purchase ready-to-eat; those included serve as a guide to the fat values of similar products you may purchase

ABBREVIATIONS

avg	=	average
diam	=	diameter
fl	=	fluid
frzn	=	frozen
g	=	gram
in	=	inch
lb	=	pound
lg	=	large
med	=	medium
mg	=	milligram
oz	=	ounce
pkg	=	package
prep	=	prepared
pt	=	pint
qt	=	quart
reg	=	regular
sec	=	second
serv	=	serving
sm	=	small
sq	=	square
tbsp	=	tablespoon
tr	=	trace
tsp	=	teaspoon
w/	=	with
w/o	=	without
<	=	less than

EQUIVALENT MEASURES

1 tablespoon	=	3 teaspoons
4 tablespoons	=	¼ cup
8 tablespoons	=	½ cup
12 tablespoons	=	¾ cup
16 tablespoons	=	1 cup
1000 milligrams	=	1 gram
28 grams	=	1 ounce

LIQUID MEASUREMENTS

2 tablespoons	=	1 ounce
¼ cup	=	2 ounces
½ cup	=	4 ounces
¾ cup	=	6 ounces
1 cup	=	8 ounces
2 cups	=	1 pint
4 cups	=	1 quart

DRY MEASUREMENTS

4 ounces	=	¼ pound
8 ounces	=	½ pound
12 ounces	=	¾ pound
16 ounces	=	1 pound

NOTES

Fat and saturated fat values are given in grams (g).

A dash (—) indicates data not available.

tr (trace) = less than 1 gram of fat or less than 1 gram of saturated fat.

Discrepancies in figures are due to rounding, product reformulation and reevaluation. Labeling law allows rounding of values. Because most of the data is analysis data obtained directly from manufacturers, not from labels, in some cases our values may not be exactly the same as label information because they have not been rounded.

The values in this book are based on research conducted prior to 2000. Manufacture's ingredients are subject to change, so current values may vary from those listed in the book. If the serving size on the package label is different from that listed in this counter, use the nutrition information provided as a guide. If the nutrition information listed in the Nutrition Facts panel is different from the information in this counter, assume that the product has been recently reformulated.

NOTES

Research done at the Lipid Research Clinic of Methodist Hospital in
Houston showed that counting fat grams is easily taught to dieters and is
a simple and accurate...

PART • ONE

BRAND NAME,

NONBRANDED (GENERIC)

AND

TAKE-OUT FOODS

Research done at the Lipid Research Clinic of Methodist Hospital in Houston showed that counting fat grams is easily taught to dieters and is a simple and accurate way to monitor their fat intake.

FOOD	PORTION	CALS.	SAT. FAT	FAT
ABALONE				
fresh fried	3 oz	161	1	6
raw	3 oz	89	tr	1
ACEROLA				
fresh	1	2	—	tr
ACEROLA JUICE				
juice	1 cup	51	—	1
ADZUKI BEANS				
canned sweetened	1 cup	702	—	tr
dried cooked	1 cup	294	—	tr
yokan sliced	3¼ in slices	112	—	tr
Eden				
Organic	½ cup (4.6 oz)	110	0	0
ALE				
(see BEER AND ALE, MALT)				
ALFALFA				
(see also SPROUTS)				
sprouts	1 cup	40	tr	tr
sprouts	1 tbsp	1	tr	tr
ALLSPICE				
ground	1 tsp	5	tr	tr
ALMONDS				
almond butter honey & cinnamon	1 tbsp	96	1	8
almond butter w/ salt	1 tbsp	101	1	9
almond butter w/o salt	1 tbsp	101	1	10
almond meal	1 oz	116	tr	5
almond paste	1 oz	127	1	8
dried blanched	1 oz	166	1	15
dried unblanched	1 oz	167	1	15
dry roasted unblanched	1 oz	167	1	15
jordan almonds	10 (1.4 oz)	190	1	7
oil roasted blanched	1 oz	174	2	16
oil roasted blanched salted	1 oz	174	2	16
oil roasted unblanched	1 oz	176	2	16
toasted unblanched	1 oz	167	1	14
Beer Nuts				
Almonds	1 pkg (1 oz)	180	—	14
Dole				
Blanched Slivered	1 oz	170	—	14
Blanched Whole	1 oz	170	—	14
Chopped Natural	1 oz	170	—	14

FOOD	PORTION	CALS.	SAT. FAT	FAT
Dole (CONT.)				
Sliced Natural	1 oz	170	—	14
Whole Natural	1 oz	170	—	14
Hain				
Almond Butter Natural Raw	2 tbsp	190	2	18
Almond Butter Toasted	2 tbsp	220	2	19
Lance				
Smoked	1 pkg (0.8 oz)	130	1	10
Nutella				
Spread	1 tbsp (0.5 oz)	85	—	5
Planters				
Almonds	1 oz	170	1	15
Gold Measure Slivered	1 pkg (2 oz)	340	3	31
Honey Roasted	1 oz	160	1	14

AMARANTH
(see also CEREAL, COOKIES)

uncooked	1 cup (6.8 oz)	729	3	13
Arrowhead				
Seeds	¼ cup (1.6 oz)	170	1	2

ANASAZI BEANS
Arrowhead

Dried	¼ cup (1.5 oz)	150	0	1
Bean Cuisine				
Dried	½ cup	115	—	1

ANCHOVY
CANNED

in oil	5	42	tr	2
in oil	1 can (1.6 oz)	95	1	4
FRESH				
fillets	3 (0.4 oz)	21	—	1
raw	3 oz	62	1	4

ANISE

seed	1 tsp	7	—	tr

ANTELOPE

roasted	3 oz	127	1	2

APPLE
CANNED

sliced sweetened	1 cup	136	tr	1
Luck's				
Fried Apples	½ cup (4.7 oz)	130	0	0
DRIED				
cooked w/ sugar	½ cup	116	tr	tr

FOOD	PORTION	CALS.	SAT. FAT	FAT
cooked w/o sugar	½ cup	172	tr	tr
rings	10	155	tr	tr
Del Monte				
Sliced	⅓ cup (1.4 oz)	80	0	0
Mariani				
Apples	¼ cup	150	—	0
Sonoma				
Pieces	10–12 pieces (1.4 oz)	110	0	0
FRESH				
apple	1	81	tr	tr
w/o skin sliced	1 cup	62	tr	tr
w/o skin sliced & cooked	1 cup	91	tr	tr
w/o skin sliced & microwaved	1 cup	96	tr	tr
Cool Cut				
Apples & Caramel Dip	1 pkg (4.25 oz)	180	2	5
Dole				
Apple	1	80	—	1
Tastee				
Candy Apple	1 (3 oz)	160	2	5
Caramel Apple	1 (3 oz)	160	2	5
FROZEN				
sliced w/o sugar	½ cup	41	tr	tr
Stouffer's				
Escalloped	1 cup (6 oz)	180	0	3

APPLE JUICE

FOOD	PORTION	CALS.	SAT. FAT	FAT
frzn as prep	1 cup	111	tr	tr
frzn not prep	6 oz	349	tr	1
juice	1 cup	116	tr	tr
After The Fall				
Organic	1 bottle (10 oz)	110	0	0
Vermont Apple	1 bottle (10 oz)	110	0	0
Vermont Apple	1 bottle (8 oz)	90	0	0
Vermont Harvest Moon Sparkling Apple Cider	8 fl oz	110	0	0
Apple & Eve				
Cider	6 fl oz	80	0	0
Juice	6 fl oz	80	0	0
Nothin' But Juice	6 fl oz	78	0	0
Everfresh				
Apple Juice	1 can (8 oz)	110	0	0
Hi-C				
Jammin' Apple	8 fl oz	130	0	0
Hood				
Select Cider	1 cup (8 oz)	120	0	0

FOOD	PORTION	CALS.	SAT. FAT	FAT
Minute Maid				
Box	8.45 fl oz	120	0	0
Juices To Go	1 can (11.5 fl oz)	160	0	0
Juices To Go	1 bottle (10 fl oz)	140	0	0
Juices To Go	1 bottle (16 fl oz)	110	0	0
Naturals	8 fl oz	110	0	0
Mott's				
From Concentrate as prep	8 fl oz	120	0	0
Fruit Basket Cocktail as prep	8 fl oz	120	0	0
Natural	8 fl oz	120	0	0
Nantucket Nectars				
100% Pressed	8 oz	100	0	0
NutraBalance				
Plus Fibre	1 pkg (8 oz)	120	0	0
Ocean Spray				
100% Juice	8 oz	110	0	0
Odwalla				
Live Apple	8 fl oz	140	0	0
Red Cheek				
From Concentrate	8 fl oz	120	0	0
Natural	8 fl oz	120	0	0
Seneca				
Clarifed frzn, as prep	8 fl oz	120	0	0
Granny Smith frzn as prep	8 fl oz	120	0	0
Natural frzn as prep	8 fl oz	120	0	0
Sippin' Pak				
100% Pure	8.45 fl oz	110	0	0
Snapple				
Apple Crisp	10 fl oz	140	0	0
Tree Of Life				
East Coast Apple	8 fl oz	120	0	0
Tropicana				
Season's Best	8 oz	110	0	0
Veryfine				
100% Juice	1 bottle (10 oz)	150	0	0
Juice-Ups	8 fl oz	120	0	0
White House				
Juice	8 oz	120	0	0
APPLESAUCE				
sweetened	½ cup	97	tr	tr
unsweetened	½ cup	53	tr	tr
Mott's				
Chunky	5 oz	110	0	0
Cinnamon	5 oz	120	0	0

FOOD	PORTION	CALS.	SAT. FAT	FAT
Mott's (CONT.)				
Fruit Snacks Apple Spice	4 oz	70	0	0
Fruit Snacks Cinnamon	4 oz	90	0	0
Fruit Snacks Sweetened	4 oz	90	0	0
Sweetened	5 oz	110	0	0
Seneca				
Cinnamon	½ cup	100	0	0
Golden Delicious	½ cup	100	0	0
McIntosh	½ cup	100	0	0
Natural	½ cup	60	0	0
Regular	½ cup	100	0	0
Tree Of Life				
Applesauce	½ cup (4.3 oz)	50	0	0
White House				
Applesauce	½ cup (4.4 oz)	90	0	0
Chunky	½ cup (4.4 oz)	90	0	0
Cinnamon	½ cup (4.5 oz)	100	0	0
Natural Plus	½ cup (4.4 oz)	70	0	0

APRICOT JUICE

FOOD	PORTION	CALS.	SAT. FAT	FAT
nectar	1 cup	141	tr	tr
Del Monte				
Nectar	8 fl oz	140	0	0
Kern's				
Nectar	6 fl oz	110	0	0
Libby				
Nectar	1 can (11.5 fl oz)	220	0	0

APRICOTS
CANNED

FOOD	PORTION	CALS.	SAT. FAT	FAT
halves heavy syrup pack w/ skin	1 cup (9.1 oz)	214	tr	tr
halves water pack w/ skin	1 cup (8.5 oz)	65	tr	tr
halves water pack w/o skin	1 cup (8 oz)	51	tr	tr
heavy syrup w/ skin	3 halves	70	tr	tr
juice pack w/ skin	3 halves	40	tr	tr
light syrup w/ skin	3 halves	54	tr	tr
puree from heavy syrup pack w/ skin	¾ cup (9.1 oz)	214	tr	tr
puree from light pack w/ skin	¾ cup (8.9 oz)	160	tr	tr
puree from water pack w/ skin	¾ cup (8.5 oz)	65	tr	tr
puree juice pack w/ skin	1 cup (8.7 oz)	119	tr	tr
water pack w/ skin	3 halves	22	tr	tr
water pack w/o skin	4 halves	20	tr	tr
Del Monte				
Halves Unpeeled In Heavy Syrup	½ cup (4.5 oz)	100	0	0
Halves Unpeeled Lite	½ cup (4.3 oz)	60	0	0

FOOD	PORTION	CALS.	SAT. FAT	FAT
Libby				
Halves Unpeeled Lite	½ cup (4.4 oz)	60	0	0
DRIED				
halves	10	83	tr	tr
halves cooked w/o sugar	½ cup	106	tr	tr
Del Monte				
Sun Dried	⅓ cup (1.4 oz)	80	0	0
Mariani				
Apricots	¼ cup	140	—	0
Sonoma				
Dried	10 pieces (1.4 oz)	120	0	0
FRESH				
apricots	3	51	tr	tr
FROZEN				
sweetened	½ cup	119	tr	tr
ARROWHEAD				
fresh boiled	1 med (⅓ oz)	9	—	tr
ARROWROOT				
flour	1 cup (4.5 oz)	457	tr	tr
ARTICHOKE				
CANNED				
Progresso				
Hearts	2 pieces (2.9 oz)	35	0	0
Hearts Marinated	⅓ cup (3 oz)	160	2	14
FRESH				
boiled	1 med (4 oz)	60	tr	tr
hearts cooked	½ cup	42	tr	tr
Dole				
Large Whole	1	23	—	tr
FROZEN				
cooked	1 pkg (9 oz)	108	tr	1
ARUGULA				
raw	½ cup	2	—	tr
ASIAN FOOD				
(see also DINNER, EGG ROLLS, PASTA, SUSHI)				
CANNED				
chow mein chicken	1 cup	95	tr	tr
FRESH				
wonton wrappers	1	23	tr	tr
FROZEN				
Banquet				
Chow Mein Chicken	1 pkg (9 oz)	400	2	7

FOOD	PORTION	CALS.	SAT. FAT	FAT
Birds Eye				
Easy Recipe Meal Starter Oriental Stir Fry as prep	1 serv	280	2	8
Easy Recipe Meal Starter Spicy Asian	1 serv	280	2	8
Easy Recipe Meal Starter Teriyaki Stir Fry as prep	1 serv	280	2	8
Chun King				
Beef Pepper Steak	1 pkg (13 oz)	300	1	4
Chow Mein Chicken	1 pkg (13 oz)	370	5	14
Imperial Chicken	1 pkg (13 oz)	460	3	10
Sweet & Sour Pork	1 pkg (13 oz)	450	3	6
Walnut Chicken	1 pkg (13 oz)	460	5	19
Green Giant				
Create A Meal LoMein Stir Fry as prep	1¼ cups (10 oz)	320	2	70
Create A Meal Sweet & Sour Stir Fry as prep	1¼ cups (10 oz)	290	1	7
Create A Meal Szechuan Stir Fry as prep	1¼ cups (10 oz)	340	4	15
Create A Meal Teriyaki Stir Fry as prep	1¼ cups (10 oz)	240	1	6
Lean Cuisine				
Chicken Chow Mein With Rice	1 pkg (9 oz)	220	1	5
Chicken Oriental w/ Vegetables & Vermicelli	1 pkg (9 oz)	250	2	6
Oriental Style Dumplings	1 pkg (9 oz)	300	2	6
Teriyaki Stir Fry	1 pkg (10 oz)	290	1	4
Luigino's				
Chicken & Almonds With Rice	1 pkg (8 oz)	250	2	8
Chop Suey Pork With Rice	1 pkg (8.5 oz)	210	1	4
Lo Mein Chicken	1 pkg (8 oz)	320	2	5
Lo Mein Shrimp	1 pkg (8 oz)	190	1	3
Oriental Beef & Peppers With Rice	1 pkg (8 oz)	230	2	5
Pasta Favorites				
Chicken Lo Mein	1 pkg (10.5 oz)	270	1	6
Rice Gourmet				
Chicken Teriyaki Rice Bowl	1 bowl (10.9 oz)	430	1	6
Stouffer's				
Chicken Chow Mein w/ Rice	1 pkg (10.6 oz)	260	1	5
Tyson				
Chicken Fried Rice Kit w/ Sauce	1 pkg (14 oz)	440	2	6

FOOD	PORTION	CALS.	SAT. FAT	FAT
Weight Watchers				
Smart Ones Chicken Chow Mein	1 pkg (9 oz)	200	1	2
Smart Ones Hunan Style Rice & Vegetables	1 pkg (10.34 oz)	280	2	0
Smart Ones King Pao Noodles & Vegetables	1 pkg (10 oz)	250	1	8
Smart Ones Spicy Szechuan Style Vegetables & Chicken	1 pkg (9 oz)	220	1	2
MIX				
Kikkoman				
Chow Mein Seasoning	1.1 oz pkg	98	—	tr
READY-TO-EAT				
shrimp chips	1¼ cups (1 oz)	140	3	6
TAKE-OUT				
cha siu bao steamed buns w/ chicken filling	1 (2.3 oz)	160	1	3
chicken teriyaki w/ rice	1 serv (11 oz)	430	1	6
chop suey w/ beef & pork	1 cup	300	4	17
chow mein chicken	1 cup	255	4	10
chow mein vegetable	1 serv (8 oz)	90	0	3
sesame seed paste bun	1 (2.5 oz)	220	1	6
shu mai chicken & vegetable dumplings	6 (3.6 oz)	160	1	5
spring roll	1 (3.5 oz)	112	—	2
sweet & sour pork	1 serv (8 oz)	250	3	8
sweet red bean bun	1 (2.5 oz)	130	0	1
szechuan chicken w/ lo mein	1 cup (5.3 oz)	190	0	1

ASPARAGUS

FOOD	PORTION	CALS.	SAT. FAT	FAT
CANNED				
spears	½ cup	24	tr	1
Del Monte				
Salad Tips Tender Green	½ cup (4.4 oz)	20	0	0
Spears Cut Tender Green	½ cup (4.4 oz)	20	0	0
Spears Extra Long Tender Green	½ cup (4.4 oz)	20	0	0
Spears Tender Green	½ cup (4.4 oz)	20	0	0
Tips Tender Green	½ cup (4.4 oz)	20	0	0
Green Giant				
Cut Spears	½ cup (4.2 oz)	20	0	0
Cut Spears 50% Less Sodium	½ cup (4.2 oz)	20	0	0
Extra Long Spears	4.5 oz	20	0	0
Spears	4.5 oz	20	0	0
LeSueur				
Spears Extra Large	4.5 oz	20	0	0

FOOD	PORTION	CALS.	SAT. FAT	FAT
Owatonna				
Spears Cut	½ cup	20	—	0
Seneca				
Asparagus	½ cup	20	0	0
FRESH				
cooked	4 spears	14	tr	tr
cooked	½ cup	22	tr	tr
raw	½ cup	16	tr	tr
raw	4 spears	14	tr	tr
Dole				
Spears	5	18	—	0
FROZEN				
cooked	4 spears	17	tr	tr
cooked	1 pkg (10 oz)	82	tr	1
Big Valley				
Spears	5–6 (3 oz)	20	0	0
Green Giant				
Harvest Fresh Cuts	⅔ cup (3 oz)	25	0	0

ATEMOYA
fresh	½ cup	94	—	1

AVOCADO
fresh	1	324	5	31
mashed	1 cup	370	6	35

BACON
(see also BACON SUBSTITUTES)

breakfast strips cooked	3 strips	156	4	12
pan fried	3 strips	109	3	9
Armour				
Star cooked	1 strip	38	—	3
Black Label				
Center Cut cooked	3 slices (0.5 oz)	70	2	6
Cooked	2 slices (0.5 oz)	80	3	7
Low Salt cooked	2 slices (0.5 oz)	80	3	7
Hillshire				
Bacon	1 slice	120	—	12
Hormel				
Bacon Bits	1 tbsp (7 g)	30	1	2
Bacon Pieces	1 tbsp (7 g)	25	1	2
Microwave cooked	2 slices (0.5 oz)	70	2	5
Old Smokehouse				
Cooked	2 slices (0.5 oz)	80	3	7
Oscar Mayer				
Bacon Bits	1 tbsp (0.2 oz)	25	1	2

FOOD	PORTION	CALS.	SAT. FAT	FAT
Oscar Mayer (CONT.)				
Bacon Pieces	1 tbsp (0.2 oz)	25	1	2
Center Cut cooked	2 slices (0.4 oz)	70	2	5
Cooked	2 slices (0.5 oz)	70	2	6
Lower Sodium cooked	2 slices (0.5 oz)	70	2	5
Thick Cut cooked	1 slice (0.4 oz)	60	2	5
Range Brand				
Cooked	2 slices (0.7 oz)	100	4	9
Red Label				
Cooked	2 slices (0.5 oz)	80	3	7
Shannon				
Irish	1 oz	70	2	5
BACON SUBSTITUTES				
bacon substitute	1 strip	25	tr	2
Bac-Os				
Chips or Bits	1½ tbsp (7 g)	30	0	2
Harvest Direct				
Bacon Bits	3.5 oz	320	2	15
Lightlife				
Fakin' Bacon Bits	1 tsp	45	0	5
Louis Rich				
Turkey Bacon	1 slice (0.5 oz)	35	1	3
McCormick				
Bac'n Pieces	2 tsp	20	—	tr
Morningstar Farms				
Breakfast Strips	2 (0.5 oz)	60	1	5
Mr. Turkey				
Slice	1	25	—	2
Worthington				
Stripples	2 strips (0.5 oz)	60	1	5
BAGEL				
FRESH				
cinnamon raisin	1 (3½ in)	194	tr	1
cinnamon raisin toasted	1 (3½ in)	194	tr	1
egg	1 (3½ in)	197	tr	2
egg toasted	1 (3½ in)	197	tr	2
oat bran	1 (3½ in)	181	tr	1
oat bran toasted	1 (3½ in)	181	tr	1
onion	1 (3½ in)	195	tr	1
plain	1 (3½ in)	195	tr	1
plain toasted	1 (3½ in)	195	tr	1
poppy seed	1 (3½ in)	195	tr	1
Alvarado St. Bakery				
Sprouted Wheat	1 (3.3 oz)	260	0	1

FOOD	PORTION	CALS.	SAT. FAT	FAT
Alvarado St. Bakery (CONT.)				
Sprouted Wheat Cinnamon/Raisin	1 (3.3 oz)	280	0	1
Sprouted Wheat Onion/Poppyseed	1 (3.3 oz)	320	0	2
Sprouted Wheat Sesame	1 (3.3 oz)	320	1	4
Uncle B's				
Plain	1 (2.8 oz)	210	0	1
Wonder				
Blueberry	1 (3 oz)	210	1	1
Cinnamon Raisin	1 (3 oz)	210	0	1
Onion	1 (3 oz)	210	0	1
Plain	1 (3 oz)	210	0	1
Rye	1 (3 oz)	220	0	1
Wheat	1 (3 oz)	210	0	1
FROZEN				
Amy's Organic				
Cinnamon Raisin	1 (3.5 oz)	240	0	2
Plain	1 (3.5 oz)	230	0	2
Poppy Seed	1 (3.5 oz)	230	0	2
Sesame	1 (3.5 oz)	240	0	2
Otis Spunkmeyer				
Barnstormin' Blueberry	1 (3.6 oz)	250	0	3
Barnstormin' Cinnamon Raisin	1 (3.6 oz)	230	0	2
Barnstormin' Onion	1 (3.6 oz)	230	0	2
Barnstormin' Plain	1 (3.6 oz)	240	0	3
Sara Lee				
Blueberry	1 (2.8 oz)	210	1	1
Cinnamon Raisin	1 (2.8 oz)	220	0	1
Egg	1 (2.8 oz)	210	1	1
Oat Bran	1 (2.8 oz)	210	0	1
Onion	1 (2.8 oz)	210	0	0
Plain	1 (2.8 oz)	210	0	1
Poppy Seed	1 (2.8 oz)	210	0	1
Sesame Seed	1 (2.8 oz)	210	1	2
Tree Of Life				
Onion	1 (3 oz)	210	0	0
Plain	1 (3 oz)	210	0	0
Poppy	1 (3 oz)	210	0	0
Raisin	1 (3 oz)	210	0	0
Sesame	1 (3 oz)	210	0	0
BAKING POWDER				
baking powder	1 tsp	2	0	0
low sodium	1 tsp	5	0	0

FOOD	PORTION	CALS.	SAT. FAT	FAT
Calumet				
Baking Powder	¼ tsp (1 g)	0	0	0
Clabber Girl				
Baking Powder	1 tsp	0	0	0
Davis				
Baking Powder	1 tsp	6	0	0
Watkins				
Baking Powder	¼ tsp (1 g)	0	0	0
BAKING SODA				
baking soda	1 tsp	0	0	0
Arm & Hammer				
Baking Soda	1 tsp	0	0	0
BALSAM PEAR				
leafy tips cooked	½ cup	10	—	tr
leafy tips raw	½ cup	7	—	tr
pods cooked	½ cup	12	—	tr
BAMBOO SHOOTS				
CANNED				
sliced	1 cup	25	tr	1
FRESH				
cooked	½ cup	15	tr	tr
raw	½ cup	21	tr	tr
BANANA				
banana chips	1 oz	147	8	10
fresh	1	105	tr	tr
fresh mashed	1 cup	207	tr	1
powder	1 tbsp	21	tr	tr
Dole				
Fresh	1	120	—	1
Rainforest Farms				
Slices Dried	5 slices (1.3 oz)	60	0	0
BANANA JUICE				
Libby				
Nectar	1 can (11.5 fl oz)	190	0	0
BARBECUE SAUCE				
(see also SAUCE)				
barbecue	1 cup	188	1	5
Bull's Eye				
Original	2 tbsp	50	—	0
Hain				
Honey	1 tbsp	14	—	1

FOOD	PORTION	CALS.	SAT. FAT	FAT
Healthy Choice				
Hickory	2 tbsp (1.1 oz)	26	0	0
Hot & Spicy	2 tbsp (1.1 oz)	25	0	0
Original	2 tbsp (1.1 oz)	25	0	0
Heinz				
Select	1 oz	40	0	0
Select Hickory	1 oz	35	0	0
Thick & Rich Cajun Style	1 oz	35	0	0
Thick & Rich Chunky	1 oz	30	0	0
Thick & Rich Hawaiian Style	1 oz	40	0	0
Thick & Rich Hickory Smoke	1 oz	35	0	0
Thick & Rich Mesquite Smoke	1 oz	30	0	0
Thick & Rich Mushroom	1 oz	30	0	0
Thick & Rich Old Fashioned	1 oz	35	0	0
Thick & Rich Onion	1 oz	30	0	0
Thick & Rich Original	1 oz	35	0	0
Thick & Rich Texas Hot	1 oz	30	0	0
House Of Tsang				
Hong Kong	1 tbsp (0.6 oz)	10	0	0
Kraft				
Char-Grill	2 tbsp (1.3 oz)	60	0	0
Extra Rich Original	2 tbsp (1.2 oz)	50	0	0
Hickory Smoke	2 tbsp (1.2 oz)	40	0	0
Hickory Smoke Onion Bits	2 tbsp (1.2 oz)	45	0	0
Honey	2 tbsp (1.3 oz)	50	0	0
Honey Hickory	2 tbsp (1.3 oz)	60	0	0
Honey Mustard	2 tbsp (1.3 oz)	60	0	0
Hot	2 tbsp (1.2 oz)	40	0	0
Hot Hickory Smoke	2 tbsp (1.2 oz)	40	0	0
Kansas City Style	2 tbsp (1.2 oz)	50	0	0
Mesquite Smoke	2 tbsp (1.2 oz)	40	0	0
Molasses	2 tbsp (1.3 oz)	70	0	0
Onion Bits	2 tbsp (1.2 oz)	45	0	0
Original	2 tbsp (1.2 oz)	40	0	0
Roasted Garlic	2 tbsp (1.2 oz)	50	0	0
Spicy Honey	2 tbsp (1.3 oz)	60	0	0
Teriyaki	2 tbsp (1.3 oz)	60	0	0
Thick 'N Spicy Brown Sugar	2 tbsp (1.2 oz)	60	0	0
Thick 'N Spicy Hickory Bacon	2 tbsp (1.2 oz)	60	0	1
Thick 'N Spicy Hickory Smoke	2 tbsp (1.2 oz)	50	0	0
Thick 'N Spicy Honey	2 tbsp (1.3 oz)	60	0	0
Thick 'N Spicy Honey Mustard	2 tbsp (1.3 oz)	60	0	0
Thick'N Spicy Hickory Smoke	2 tbsp (1.2 oz)	60	0	0
Thick'N Spicy Honey	2 tbsp (1.2 oz)	60	0	0
Thick'N Spicy Kansas City Style	2 tbsp (1.3 oz)	60	0	0

FOOD	PORTION	CALS.	SAT. FAT	FAT
Kraft (CONT.)				
Thick'N Spicy Mesquite Smoke	2 tbsp (1.2 oz)	50	0	0
Thick'N Spicy Original	2 tbsp (1.2 oz)	50	0	0
Lawry's				
Dijon Honey	¼ cup	203	tr	1
McIlhenny				
Sauce	2 tbsp (1.1 oz)	70	1	5
Red Wing				
"K" Sauce	2 tbsp (1.2 oz)	45	0	0
Watkins				
Bold	2 tsp (0.4 oz)	25	0	0
Honey	2 tsp (0.4 oz)	25	0	0
Mesquite	2 tsp (0.4 oz)	25	0	0
Original	2 tsp (0.4 oz)	25	0	0
Smokehouse	2 tsp (0.4 oz)	25	0	0
BARLEY				
flour	1 cup (5.2 oz)	511	tr	2
malt flour	1 cup (5.7 oz)	585	1	3
pearled cooked	1 cup (5.5 oz)	193	tr	1
pearled uncooked	1 cup (7 oz)	704	tr	2
Arrowhead				
Barley	¼ cup (1.7 oz)	170	0	1
Hulless	¼ cup (1.6 oz)	140	0	1
BASIL				
fresh chopped	2 tbsp	1	tr	tr
ground	1 tsp	4	—	tr
leaves fresh	5	1	tr	tr
Watkins				
Liquid Spice	1 tbsp (0.5 oz)	120	2	14
BASS				
freshwater raw	3 oz	97	1	3
sea cooked	3 oz	105	1	2
sea raw	3 oz	82	tr	2
striped baked	3 oz	105	1	3
BAY LEAF				
crumbled	1 tsp	2	tr	tr
Watkins				
Bay Leaves	¼ tsp (0.5 g)	0	0	0

BEAN SPROUTS
(see ALFALFA, SPROUTS)

BEANS
(see also *individual names*)

FOOD	PORTION	CALS.	SAT. FAT	FAT
CANNED				
baked beans plain	½ cup	118	tr	1
baked beans vegetarian	½ cup	118	tr	1
baked beans w/ beef	½ cup	161	2	5
baked beans w/ franks	½ cup	182	3	8
baked beans w/ pork	½ cup	133	1	2
baked beans w/ pork & sweet sauce	½ cup	140	1	2
baked beans w/ pork & tomato sauce	½ cup	123	tr	1
refried beans	½ cup	134	1	1
Allen				
Baked	½ cup (4.5 oz)	150	1	1
B&M				
99% Fat Free Baked Beans	½ cup (4.6 oz)	160	0	1
Baked With Honey	½ cup (4.7 oz)	170	0	2
Barbeque Baked Beans	½ cup (4.7 oz)	170	1	2
Brick Oven Baked	½ cup (4.6 oz)	180	1	2
Extra Hearty Baked	½ cup (4.6 oz)	190	1	2
Brown Beauty				
Mexican Beans With Jalapeno	½ cup (4.5 oz)	120	0	1
Bush's				
Baked	½ cup (4.6 oz)	150	tr	1
Baked With Onions	½ cup (4.6 oz)	150	1	2
Homestyle Baked	½ cup (4.6 oz)	160	1	2
Vegetarian	½ cup (4.6 oz)	140	0	1
Campbell				
Barbecue Beans	½ can (7.9 oz)	210	—	4
Home Style Beans	½ can (8 oz)	220	—	4
Hot Chili Beans	½ can (7.75 oz)	180	—	4
Old Fashioned Beans In Molasses & Brown Sugar Sauce	½ can (8 oz)	230	—	3
Pork & Beans In Tomato Sauce	½ can (8 oz)	200	—	3
Vegetarian	½ can (7.75 oz)	170	—	1
Chi-Chi's				
Refried	½ cup (4.2 oz)	100	0	1
Refried Beans Fat Free	½ cup (4.2 oz)	120	0	0
Refried Beans Vegetarian	½ cup (4.2 oz)	100	0	1
Crest Top				
Pork And Beans	½ cup (4.5 oz)	130	1	1
Eden				
Organic Baked w/ Sweet Sorghum & Orangic Mustard	½ cup (4.6 oz)	150	0	0

FOOD	PORTION	CALS.	SAT. FAT	FAT
Friend's				
Maple Baked	8 oz	240	1	2
Original Baked	½ cup (4.6 oz)	170	0	1
Green Giant				
Pork And Beans w/ Tomato Sauce	½ cup (4.5 oz)	120	0	1
Spicy Chili	½ cup (4.5 oz)	110	0	1
Three Bean Salad	½ cup (4.2 oz)	90	0	0
Hanover				
Four Bean Salad	½ cup	80	—	0
Health Valley				
Honey Baked	½ cup	110	0	0
Honey Baked No Salt	½ cup	110	0	0
Heartland				
Iron Kettle Baked	½ cup (4.6 oz)	150	0	1
Hormel				
Beans & Wieners	1 can (7.5 oz)	290	4	12
Hunt's				
Big John's Beans & Fixin's	½ cup (4.7 oz)	127	1	4
Pork & Beans	½ cup (4.5 oz)	130	tr	1
Kid's Kitchen				
Microwave Meals Beans & Wieners	1 cup (7.5 oz)	310	5	13
Little Pancho				
Refried & Green Chili	½ cup	80	0	0
McIlhenny				
Spicy	1 oz	7	tr	tr
Old El Paso				
Mexe-Beans	½ cup (4.6 oz)	110	0	1
Refried	½ cup (4.2 oz)	110	1	2
Refried Fat Free	½ cup (4.4 oz)	110	0	0
Refried Spicy	½ cup (4.3 oz)	140	2	3
Refried Vegetarian	½ cup (4.1 oz)	100	0	1
Refried With Cheese	½ cup (4.2 oz)	130	2	4
Refried With Green Chilies	½ cup (4.3 oz)	110	0	1
Refried With Sausage	½ cup (4.1 oz)	200	5	13
S&W				
Barbecue Beans Ranch Recipe	½ cup (4.5 oz)	100	1	2
Taco Bell				
Home Originals Fat Free Refried Beans	½ cup (4.6 oz)	110	0	0
Home Originals Fat Free Refried Beans w/ Mild Chilies	½ cup (4.5 oz)	110	0	0
Home Originals Refried Beans	½ cup (4.7 oz)	140	1	3

FOOD	PORTION	CALS.	SAT. FAT	FAT
Trappey				
Mexi-Beans With Jalapeno	½ cup (4.5 oz)	130	1	2
Pork And Beans	½ cup (4.5 oz)	110	1	1
Pork And Beans With Jalapeno	½ cup (4.5 oz)	130	1	2
Van Camp's				
Baked Beans Fat Free	½ cup (4.6 oz)	130	0	0
Baked Beans Premium	½ cup (4.6 oz)	140	0	1
Beanee Weenee	1 cup (9 oz)	320	4	14
Beanee Weenee Baked Flavor	1 cup (9 oz)	410	4	14
Beanee Weenee Barbeque	1 cup (9 oz)	340	4	14
Brown Sugar Beans	½ cup (4.6 oz)	170	1	3
Mexican Style Chili Beans	½ cup (4.6 oz)	110	1	2
Pork And Beans	½ cup (4.6 oz)	110	1	2
Vegetarian In Tomato Sauce	½ cup (4.6 oz)	110	0	1
Wagon Master				
Pork And Beans	½ cup (4.5 oz)	110	1	1
FROZEN				
Hanover				
Romano Bean Medley	½ cup	25	—	0
Natural Touch				
Nine Bean Loaf	1 in slice (3 oz)	160	2	8
MIX				
Bean Cuisine				
Florentine Beans With Bow Ties	½ cup	199	2	7
Pasta & Beans Country French With Gemelli	½ cup	214	1	8
Melting Pot				
Terrazza Napoli Mixed Beans	1 cup	200	0	2
TAKE-OUT				
baked beans	½ cup	190	2	6
barbecue beans	3.5 oz	120	tr	tr
four bean salad	3.5 oz	100	tr	tr
BEAR				
simmered	3 oz	220	—	11
BEAVER				
roasted	3 oz	140	—	6
simmered	3 oz	141	—	5
BEECHNUTS				
dried	1 oz	164	2	14

BEEF

(see *also* BEEF DISHES, VEAL)

FOOD	PORTION	CALS.	SAT. FAT	FAT
CANNED				
corned beef	1 oz	71	—	4
corned beef	3 oz	85	4	5
Armour				
Chopped Beef	2 oz	170	7	15
Corned Beef	2 oz	120	3	7
Potted Meat	1 can (3 oz)	120	3	7
Tripe	3 oz	90	1	2
Hormel				
Corned Beef	2 oz	120	3	7
Cubed Beef	½ cup (4.9 oz)	130	1	3
Potted Meat	4 tbsp (2 oz)	100	4	8
Treet				
Luncheon Loaf	2 oz	130	4	11
Luncheon Loaf 50% Less Fat	2 oz	110	3	8
Underwood				
Roast Beef	2.08 oz	140	5	11
Roast Beef Mesquite Smoked	2.08 oz	126	5	11
Roast Beef Light	2.08 oz	90	2	6
DRIED				
Armour				
Sliced	7 slices (1 oz)	60	1	2
Hormel				
Pillow Pack	10 slices (1 oz)	45	tr	1
Oberto				
Beef Jerky	1 pkg (1.3 oz)	100	0	1
Rough Cut				
Beef Steak Hot	1 pkg (1 oz)	70	0	1
Beef Steak Original	1 pkg (1 oz)	60	0	1
Beef Steak Peppered	1 pkg (1 oz)	60	0	1
FRESH				
bottom round lean & fat trim 0 in Choice roasted	3 oz	172	3	8
bottom round lean & fat trim 0 in Select braised	3 oz	171	2	6
bottom round lean & fat trim 0 in Select roasted	3 oz	150	2	24
bottom round lean & fat trim 0 in braised	3 oz	193	3	26
bottom round lean & fat trim ¼ in Choice braised	3 oz	241	6	15
bottom round lean & fat trim ¼ in Choice roasted	3 oz	221	5	14
bottom round lean & fat trim ¼ in Select braised	3 oz	220	5	13

FOOD	PORTION	CALS.	SAT. FAT	FAT
bottom round lean & fat trim ¼ in Select roasted	3 oz	199	4	11
brisket flat half lean & fat trim 0 in braised	3 oz	183	3	8
brisket flat half lean & fat trim ¼ in braised	3 oz	309	9	24
brisket point half lean & fat trim 0 in braised	3 oz	304	10	24
brisket point half lean & fat trim ¼ in braised	3 oz	343	12	29
brisket whole lean & fat trim 0 in braised	3 oz	247	6	17
brisket whole lean & fat trim ¼ in braised	3 oz	327	11	27
chuck arm pot roast lean & fat trim 0 in braised	3 oz	238	6	14
chuck arm pot roast lean & fat trim ¼ in braised	3 oz	282	8	20
chuck blade roast lean & fat trim 0 in braised	3 oz	284	8	21
chuck blade roast lean & fat trim ¼ in braised	3 oz	293	9	22
corned beef brisket cooked	3 oz	213	5	16
eye of round lean & fat trim 0 in Choice roasted	3 oz	153	8	5
eye of round lean & fat trim 0 in Select roasted	3 oz	137	1	4
eye of round lean & fat trim ¼ in Choice roasted	3 oz	205	5	12
eye of round lean & fat trime ¼ in Select roasted	3 oz	184	4	10
flank lean & fat trim 0 in braised	3 oz	224	6	14
flank lean & fat trim 0 in broiled	3 oz	192	5	11
ground extra lean broiled medium	3 oz	217	5	14
ground extra lean broiled well done	3 oz	225	5	14
ground extra lean fried medium	3 oz	216	5	14
ground extra lean fried well done	3 oz	224	5	14
ground extra lean raw	4 oz	265	8	19
ground lean broiled medium	3 oz	231	6	16
ground lean broiled well done	3 oz	238	6	15
ground regular broiled medium	3 oz	246	7	18
ground regular broiled well done	3 oz	248	7	17
porterhouse steak lean & fat trim ¼ in Choice broiled	3 oz	260	8	19

FOOD	PORTION	CALS.	SAT. FAT	FAT
porterhouse steak lean only trim ¼ in Prime broiled	3 oz	185	4	9
rib eye small end lean & fat trim 0 in Choice broiled	3 oz	261	8	19
rib large end lean & fat trim 0 in roasted	3 oz	300	10	24
rib large end lean & fat trim ¼ in broiled	3 oz	295	10	24
rib large end lean & fat trim ¼ in roasted	3 oz	310	10	25
rib small end lean & fat trim 0 in broiled	3 oz	252	7	18
rib small end lean & fat trim ¼ in broiled	3 oz	285	9	22
rib small end lean & fat trim ¼ in roasted	3 oz	295	10	24
rib whole lean & fat trim ¼ in Choice broiled	3 oz	306	10	25
rib whole lean & fat trim ¼ in Choice roasted	3 oz	320	11	27
rib whole lean & fat trim ¼ in Prime roasted	3 oz	348	12	30
rib whole lean & fat trim ¼ in Select broiled	3 oz	274	9	21
rib whole lean & fat trim ¼ in Select roasted	3 oz	286	9	23
shank crosscut lean & fat trim ¼ in Choice simmered	3 oz	224	5	12
short loin top loin lean & fat trim 0 in Choice broiled	3 oz	193	4	10
short loin top loin lean & fat trim 0 in Choice broiled	1 steak (5.4 oz)	353	7	19
short loin top loin lean & fat trim 0 in Select broiled	1 steak (5.4 oz)	309	5	14
short loin top loin lean & fat trim ¼ in Choice braised	3 oz	253	7	18
short loin top loin lean & fat trim ¼ in Choice broiled	1 steak (6.3 oz)	536	15	38
short loin top loin lean & fat trim ¼ in Prime broiled	1 steak (6.3 oz)	582	17	43
short loin top loin lean & fat trim ¼ in Select broiled	1 steak (6.3 oz)	473	12	31
short loin top loin lean only trim 0 in Choice broiled	1 steak (5.2 oz)	311	5	14

FOOD	PORTION	CALS.	SAT. FAT	FAT
short loin top loin lean only trim ¼ in Choice broiled	1 steak (5.2 oz)	314	6	15
shortribs lean & fat Choice braised	3 oz	400	15	36
t-bone steak lean & fat trim ¼ in Choice broiled	3 oz	253	7	18
t-bone steak lean only trim ¼ in Choice broiled	3 oz	182	4	9
tenderloin lean & fat trim 0 in Select broiled	3 oz	194	4	11
tenderloin lean & fat trim ¼ in Choice broiled	3 oz	259	7	19
tenderloin lean & fat trim ¼ in Choice roasted	3 oz	288	9	22
tenderloin lean & fat trim ¼ in Choice broiled	3 oz	208	5	12
tenderloin lean & fat trim ¼ in Prime broiled	3 oz	270	8	20
tenderloin lean & fat trim ¼ in Select roasted	3 oz	275	8	21
tenderloin lean only trim 0 in Select broiled	3 oz	170	3	7
tenderloin lean only trim ¼ in Choice broiled	3 oz	188	4	10
tenderloin lean only trim ¼ in Select broiled	3 oz	169	3	7
tip round lean & fat trim 0 in Choice roasted	3 oz	170	3	8
tip round lean & fat trim 0 in Select roasted	3 oz	158	2	6
tip round lean & fat trim ¼ in Choice roasted	3 oz	210	5	13
tip round lean & fat trim ¼ in Prime roasted	3 oz	233	6	15
tip round lean & fat trim ¼ in Select roasted	3 oz	191	4	10
top round lean & fat trim 0 in Choice braised	3 oz	184	2	6
top round lean & fat trim 0 in Select braised	3 oz	170	2	5
top round lean & fat trim ¼ in Choice braised	3 oz	221	4	11
top round lean & fat trim ¼ in Choice broiled	3 oz	190	3	9

FOOD	PORTION	CALS.	SAT. FAT	FAT
top round lean & fat trim ¼ in Choice fried	3 oz	235	5	13
top round lean & fat trim ¼ in Prime broiled	3 oz	195	3	9
top round lean & fat trim ¼ in Select braised	3 oz	175	3	7
top round lean & fat trim ¼ in Select braised	3 oz	199	3	8
top sirloin lean & fat trim 0 in Choice broiled	3 oz	194	4	10
top sirloin lean & fat trim 0 in Select broiled	3 oz	166	3	6
top sirloin lean & fat trim ¼ in Choice broiled	3 oz	228	6	14
top sirloin lean & fat trim ¼ in Choice fried	3 oz	277	8	19
top sirloin lean & fat trim ¼ in Select broiled	3 oz	208	5	12
tripe raw	4 oz	111	2	4
Healthy Choice				
Ground Extra Lean	4 oz	130	2	4
Laura's Lean				
Eye Of Round	4 oz	140	2	4
Flank Steak	4 oz	140	2	5
Ground 92% Lean	4 oz	160	4	9
Ground Round 94% Lean	4 oz	140	2	5
Ribeye Steak	4 oz	140	2	5
Sirloin Tip Round	4 oz	120	2	3
Sirloin Top Butt	4 oz	140	2	5
Strip Steak	4 oz	140	2	4
Tenderloins	4 oz	140	2	6
Top Round	4 oz	130	1	3
Maverick Ranch				
Ground Round Extra Lean	4 oz	130	2	4
Organic Valley				
Extra Lean Ground	3 oz	130	3	6
Extra Lean Patties	1 (3.2 oz)	130	3	6
FROZEN				
patties broiled medium	3 oz	240	7	17
READY-TO-EAT				
Boar's Head				
Corned Beef Brisket	2 oz	80	2	3
Eye Round Pepper Seasoned	2 oz	90	2	3
Roast Beef Cajun	2 oz	80	2	3
Top Round Deluxe	2 oz	90	2	3

FOOD	PORTION	CALS.	SAT. FAT	FAT
Boar's Head (CONT.)				
Top Round Oven Roasted No Salt Added	2 oz	90	2	3
Healthy Choice				
Deli-Thin Roast Beef	6 slices (2 oz)	60	1	2
Fresh-Trak Roast Beef	1 slice (1 oz)	30	0	1
Jordan's				
Healthy Trim 97% Fat Free Roast Beef Medium	1 slice (1 oz)	30	1	1
Healthy Trim 97% Fat Free Roast Beef Rare	1 slice (1 oz)	30	1	1
Tyson				
Beef Strips Seasoned	1 serv (3 oz)	140	2	6
TAKE-OUT				
roast beef medium	2 oz	70	1	2
roast beef rare	2 oz	70	1	2
BEEF DISHES				
CANNED				
corned beef hash	3 oz	155	5	10
Armour				
Corned Beef Hash	1 cup (8.3 oz)	440	14	30
Corned Beef Hash w/ Peppers & Onions	1 cup (8.3 oz)	270	14	30
Roast Beef Hash	1 cup (8.4 oz)	400	12	25
Roast Beef In Gravy	½ cup (4.6 oz)	150	2	4
Stew	1 cup (8.6 oz)	220	5	12
Dinty Moore				
Meatball Stew	1 cup (8.4 oz)	250	7	15
Sliced Potatoes & Beef	1 can (7.5 oz)	230	4	9
Stew	1 cup (8.3 oz)	230	7	14
Stew	1 cup (8.2 oz)	230	7	14
Hormel				
Beef Goulash	1 can (7.5 oz)	230	5	11
Roast Beef With Gravy	2 oz	60	1	2
Mary Kitchen				
Corned Beef Hash	1 cup (8.3 oz)	410	10	27
Corned Beef Hash 50% Reduced Fat	1 cup (8.3 oz)	280	5	12
Roast Beef Hash	1 cup (8.3 oz)	390	10	24
Roast Turkey Hash	1 can (14.9 oz)	420	3	11
Sausage Hash	1 cup (8.3 oz)	410	9	27
FROZEN				
Hot Pocket				
Stuffed Sandwich Barbecue	1 (4.5 oz)	340	5	12

FOOD	PORTION	CALS.	SAT. FAT	FAT
Hot Pocket (CONT.)				
Stuffed Sandwich Beef & Cheddar	1 (4.5 oz)	360	9	18
Stuffed Sandwich Beef Fajita	1 (4.5 oz)	360	8	17
Lean Pockets				
Stuffed Sandwich Beef & Broccoli	1 (4.5 oz)	250	3	7
Luigino's				
Creamed Sauce Shaved Cured Beef With Croutons	1 pkg (8 oz)	360	6	20
Egg Noodles Rich Gravy Swedish Meatballs	1 cup (7.5 oz)	280	3	12
Egg Noodles Rich Gravy Swedish Meatballs	1 pkg (9 oz)	340	4	15
MIX				
Casbah				
Gyro as prep	1 patty (2 oz)	145	2	5
Hamburger Helper				
BBQ Beef as prep	1 cup	320	4	10
Beef Pasta as prep	1 cup	270	4	10
Beef Romanoff as prep	1 cup	280	4	10
Beef Stew as prep	1 cup	260	4	10
Beef Taco as prep	1 cup	280	4	10
Beef Teriyaki as prep	1 cup	290	4	10
Cheddar & Broccoli as prep	1 cup	350	6	15
Cheddar Melt as prep	1 cup	310	5	12
Cheddar'n Bacon as prep	1 cup	330	6	15
Cheeseburger Macaroni as prep	1 cup	360	6	16
Cheesy Hashbrowns as prep	1 cup	400	6	19
Cheesy Italian as prep	1 cup	320	6	14
Cheesy Shells as prep	1 cup	330	6	15
Chili Macaroni as prep	1 cup	290	4	10
Fettuccine Alfredo as prep	1 cup	300	5	13
Four Cheese Lasagne as prep	1 cup	330	5	14
Italian Parmesan w/ Rigatoni as prep	1 cup	300	4	11
Lasagne as prep	1 cup	270	4	10
Meat Loaf as prep	⅕ loaf	270	6	14
Meaty Spaghetti & Cheese as prep	1 cup	290	4	10
Mushroom & Wild Rice as prep	1 cup	310	5	12
Nacho Cheese as prep	1 cup	320	5	13
Pizza Pasta w/ Cheese Topping as pre	1 cup	280	4	10
Pizzabake as prep	⅙ pie	270	4	10

FOOD	PORTION	CALS.	SAT. FAT	FAT
Hamburger Helper (CONT.)				
Potatoes Au Gratin as prep	1 cup	280	5	13
Potatoes Stroganoff as prep	1 cup	250	5	11
Reduced Sodium Cheddar Spirals as prep	1 cup	300	5	13
Reduced Sodium Italian Herby as prep	1 cup	270	4	10
Reduced Sodium Southwestern Beef as prep	1 cup	300	4	10
Rice Oriental as prep	1 cup	280	4	10
Salisbury as prep	1 cup	270	4	10
Spaghetti as prep	1 cup	270	4	10
Stroganoff as prep	1 cup	320	5	13
Swedish Meatballs as prep	1 cup	290	5	14
Three Cheeses as prep	1 cup	340	5	15
Zesty Italian as prep	1 cup	300	4	10
Zesty Mexican as prep	1 cup	280	4	10
SHELF-STABLE				
Dinty Moore				
Microwave Cup Corned Beef Hash	1 pkg (7.5 oz)	350	9	22
Microwave Cup Hearty Burger Stew	1 pkg (7.5 oz)	240	5	13
Microwave Cup Stew	1 pkg (7.5 oz)	190	5	10
Hormel				
Microcup Meals Stew	1 cup (7.5 oz)	190	4	10
Lunch Bucket				
Beef Stew	1 pkg (7.5 oz)	170	4	9
TAKE-OUT				
bulgoghi korean grilled beef	1 serv (5.2 oz)	256	5	15
irish stew	1 cup (7 oz)	280	9	16
shepherds pie	1 serv (7 oz)	282	6	16
stew w/ vegetables	1 cup	220	4	11
BEEFALO				
roasted	3 oz	160	2	5
BEER AND ALE				
alcohol free beer	7 fl oz	50	—	tr
beer light	12 oz can	100	0	0
beer regular	12 oz can	146	0	0
pilsener lager beer	7 fl oz	85	—	tr
Amstel				
Light	12 oz	95	—	0
Anheuser Busch				
Natural Light	12 oz	110	—	0

FOOD	PORTION	CALS.	SAT. FAT	FAT
Bud				
Light	12 oz	108	—	0
Coors				
Beer	12 oz	132	0	0
Extra Gold	12 oz	147	0	0
Light	12 oz	101	0	0
Guinness				
Kaliber nonalcholic	12 oz	43	—	0
Killian's				
Beer	12 oz	212	0	0
Kingsbury				
Nonalcoholic	12 fl oz	60	—	0
Michelob				
Light	12 oz	134	—	0
Miller				
Lite	12 oz	96	—	0
Molson				
Light	12 oz	109	—	0
Piels				
Light	12 oz	136	—	0
Schmidts				
Light	12 oz	96	—	0
Winterfest				
Beer	12 oz	167	0	0

BEETS
CANNED
FOOD	PORTION	CALS.	SAT. FAT	FAT
harvard	½ cup	89	tr	tr
pickled	½ cup	75	tr	tr
sliced	½ cup	27	tr	tr
Del Monte				
Pickled Crinkle Style Sliced	½ cup (4.5 oz)	80	0	0
Sliced	½ cup (4.3 oz)	35	0	0
Whole	½ cup (4.3 oz)	35	0	0
Whole Tiny	½ cup (4.3 oz)	35	0	0
Green Giant				
Harvard	⅓ cup (3.1 oz)	60	0	0
Sliced	½ cup (4.2 oz)	35	0	0
Sliced No Salt Added	½ cup (4.2 oz)	35	0	0
Whole	½ cup (4.2 oz)	35	0	0
LeSueur				
Baby Whole	½ cup (4.3 oz)	35	0	0
Seneca				
Cut	½ cup	35	0	0
Diced	½ cup	35	0	0

FOOD	PORTION	CALS.	SAT. FAT	FAT
Seneca (CONT.)				
Harvard	½ cup	90	0	0
Pickled	2 tbsp	20	0	0
Pickled With Onions	2 tbsp	20	0	0
Sliced	½ cup	35	0	0
Whole	½ cup	35	0	0
FRESH				
greens cooked	½ cup	20	tr	tr
greens raw	½ cup	4	tr	tr
greens raw chopped	½ cup	4	tr	tr
raw sliced	½ cup (2.4 oz)	29	tr	tr
sliced cooked	½ cup (3 oz)	38	tr	tr
whole cooked	2 (3.5 oz)	44	tr	tr
whole raw	2 (5.7 oz)	70	tr	tr

BEVERAGES

(*see* BEER AND ALE, CHAMPAGNE, COFFEE, DRINK MIXERS, FRUIT DRINKS, ICED TEA, LIQUOR/LIQUEUR, MALT, MILKSHAKE, SODA, SPORTS DRINKS, TEA/HERBAL TEA, WATER, WINE, WINE COOLER)

BISCUIT

FOOD	PORTION	CALS.	SAT. FAT	FAT
FROZEN				
Jimmy Dean				
Chicken Twin	2 (3.2 oz)	280	4	13
Sausage Twin	2 (3.4 oz)	330	7	21
Steak Twin	2 (3.2 oz)	270	5	13
Rudy's Farm				
Ham Twin	2 (3 oz)	160	1	3
Sausage & Cheese Twin	2 (3 oz)	290	6	18
Sausage Twin	2 (2.7 oz)	296	6	18
MIX				
buttermilk	1 (2 oz)	191	2	7
plain	1 (2 oz)	191	2	7
Arrowhead				
Biscuit Mix	¼ cup (1.2 oz)	120	0	1
Bisquick				
Mix	⅓ cup (1.4 oz)	170	2	6
Reduced Fat	⅓ cup (1.4 oz)	150	1	3
Sweet	¼ cup (1.4 oz)	170	2	4
Gold Medal				
Biscuits	2	180	3	6
Jiffy				
As prep	1	150	3	7
Biscuit	¼ cup (1.1 oz)	130	1	5
Buttermilk as prep	1	170	2	4

FOOD	PORTION	CALS.	SAT. FAT	FAT
READY-TO-EAT				
Arnold				
Old Fashioned	1	60	—	3
REFRIGERATED				
buttermilk	1 (1 oz)	98	1	4
plain	1 (1 oz)	98	1	4
1869 Brand				
Buttermilk	1 (1.1 oz)	100	2	5
Hungry Jack				
Butter Tastin' Flaky	1 (1.2 oz)	100	1	5
Cinnamon & Sugar	1 (1.2 oz)	110	1	4
Flaky	1 (1.2 oz)	100	1	5
Flaky Buttermilk	1 (1.2 oz)	100	1	5
Pillsbury				
Big Country Butter Tastin'	1 (1.2 oz)	100	1	4
Big Country Buttermilk	1 (1.2 oz)	100	1	4
Big Country Southern Style	1 (1.2 oz)	100	1	4
Buttermilk	1 (2.2 oz)	150	0	2
Country	1 (2.2 oz)	150	0	2
Grands Blueberry	1 (2.1 oz)	210	3	9
Grands Butter Tastin'	1 (2.1 oz)	200	3	10
Grands Buttermilk	1 (2.1 oz)	200	3	10
Grands Buttermilk Reduced Fat	1 (2.1 oz)	190	2	7
Grands Extra Rich	1 (2.1 oz)	220	3	12
Grands Flaky	1 (2.1 oz)	200	2	9
Grands Golden Corn	1 (1.2 oz)	210	3	10
Grands HomeStyle	1 (2.1 oz)	210	3	10
Grands Southern Style	1 (2.1 oz)	200	3	10
Southern Style Flakey	1 (1.2 oz)	100	1	5
Tender Layer Buttermilk	1 (2.2 oz)	160	1	5
Roman Meal				
Biscuit	2 (2.4 oz)	180	1	4
Honey Nut Oat Bran	1 (1.5 oz)	131	1	5
TAKE-OUT				
buttermilk	1	127	1	6
plain	1 (35 g)	276	9	34
tea biscuit	1 (3 oz)	210	2	3
w/ egg	1 (4.8 oz)	316	6	20
w/ egg & bacon	1 (5.2 oz)	458	8	31
w/ egg & ham	1 (6.7 oz)	442	6	27
w/ egg & sausage	1 (6.3 oz)	581	15	39
w/ egg & steak	1 (5.2 oz)	410	9	28
w/ egg cheese & bacon	1 (5.1 oz)	477	11	31
w/ ham	1 (4 oz)	386	11	18

FOOD	PORTION	CALS.	SAT. FAT	FAT
w/ sausage	1 (4.4 oz)	485	14	32
w/ steak	1 (4.9 oz)	455	7	26
BISON				
roasted	3 oz	122	1	2
BLACK BEANS				
CANNED				
Allen				
Seasoned	½ cup (4.5 oz)	120	1	2
Eden				
Organic	½ cup (4.6 oz)	100	0	0
Organic w/ Ginger & Lemon	½ cup (4.6 oz)	120	0	0
Green Giant				
Black Beans	½ cup (4.5 oz)	50	0	0
Old El Paso				
Black Beans	½ cup (4.6 oz)	100	0	1
Refried	½ cup (4.2 oz)	120	0	2
Progresso				
Black Beans	½ cup (4.6 oz)	100	0	1
Trappey				
Seasoned	½ cup (4.5 oz)	120	1	2
DRIED				
cooked	1 cup	227	tr	1
MIX				
Bean Cuisine				
Black Turtle	½ cup	115	—	1
Pasta & Beans Black Beans With Fusilli	½ cup	174	1	4
Mahatma				
Black Beans & Rice	1 cup	200	0	2
BLACKBERRIES				
canned in heavy syrup	½ cup	118	—	tr
fresh	½ cup	37	—	tr
unsweetened frzn	1 cup	97	—	1
Allen-Wolco				
Canned	½ cup (5.3 oz)	60	0	1
Big Valley				
Frozen	⅔ cup (4.9 oz)	70	0	0
BLACKBERRY JUICE				
Kool-Aid				
Scary Blackberry Ghoul-Aid Drink as prep w/ sugar	1 serv (8 oz)	100	0	0

FOOD	PORTION	CALS.	SAT. FAT	FAT
BLACKEYE PEAS				
CANNED				
w/pork	½ cup	199	1	4
Allen				
Blackeye Peas	½ cup (4.5 oz)	110	1	1
Fresh Shell	½ cup (4.4 oz)	120	1	1
With Bacon	½ cup (4.5 oz)	105	1	2
With Snaps	½ cup (4.4 oz)	120	1	1
Dorman				
Fresh Shell	½ cup (4.4 oz)	120	1	1
East Texas Fair				
Blackeye Peas	½ cup (4.5 oz)	110	1	1
Fresh Shell	½ cup (4.4 oz)	120	1	1
With Snaps	½ cup (4.4 oz)	120	1	1
Green Giant				
Blackeye Peas	½ cup (4.4 oz)	90	0	0
Homefolks				
Fresh Shell	½ cup (4.4 oz)	120	1	1
With Jalapeno	½ cup (4.4 oz)	120	1	1
With Snaps	½ cup (4.4 oz)	120	1	1
Sunshine				
With Bacon	½ cup (4.5 oz)	105	1	2
Trappey				
With Bacon	½ cup (4.5 oz)	120	1	2
With Bacon & Jalapeno	½ cup (4.4 oz)	110	1	2
DRIED				
cooked	1 cup	198	tr	1
Hurst				
HamBeens California w/ Ham	1 serv	120	0	1
FROZEN				
Birds Eye				
Blackeye Peas	½ cup (2.8 oz)	110	0	1
Fresh Like				
Fresh Like	3.5 oz	138	—	1
BLINTZE				
Empire				
Apple	2 (4.4 oz)	220	2	6
Blueberry	2 (4.4 oz)	190	1	4
Cheese	2 (4.4 oz)	200	2	6
Cherry	2 (4.4 oz)	200	1	4
Potato	2 (4.4 oz)	190	2	6
Golden				
Apple Raisin	1 (2.25 oz)	80	0	2
Blueberry	1 (2.25 oz)	90	0	1

FOOD	PORTION	CALS.	SAT. FAT	FAT
Golden (cont.)				
Cheese	1 (2.25 oz)	80	1	2
Cherry	1 (2.25 oz)	95	0	1
Potato	1 (2.25 oz)	90	1	4
TAKE-OUT				
cheese	1 (2.7 oz)	160	4	9
BLUEBERRIES				
canned in heavy syrup	1 cup	225	—	1
fresh	1 cup	82	—	1
unsweetened frzn	1 cup	78	—	1
Big Valley				
Frozen	¾ cup (4.9 oz)	70	0	0
Sonoma				
Dried	¼ cup (1.3 oz)	140	0	0
BLUEBERRY JUICE				
After The Fall				
Maine Coast	1 cup (8 oz)	90	0	0
BLUEFIN				
fillet baked	4.1 oz	186	1	6
BLUEFISH				
fresh baked	3 oz	135	1	5
BOAR				
wild roasted	3 oz	136	1	4
BOK CHOY				
Dole				
Shredded	½ cup	5	—	tr
BONIATO				
fresh	½ cup	90	—	tr
BORAGE				
fresh chopped cooked	3½ oz	25	—	1
raw chopped	½ cup	9	—	tr
BOTTLED WATER				
(see WATER)				
BOYSENBERRIES				
in heavy sirup	1 cup	226	—	tr
unsweetened frzn	1 cup	66	—	tr
BRAINS				
beef pan-fried	3 oz	167	3	13
beef simmered	3 oz	136	2	11

FOOD	PORTION	CALS.	SAT. FAT	FAT
lamb braised	3 oz	124	2	9
lamb fried	3 oz	232	5	19
pork braised	3 oz	117	2	8
veal braised	3 oz	115	—	8
veal fried	3 oz	181	—	14
Armour				
Pork Brains In Milk Gravy	⅔ cup (5.5 oz)	150	3	5

BRAN

FOOD	PORTION	CALS.	SAT. FAT	FAT
corn	1 cup (2.7 oz)	170	tr	1
oat	½ cup (1.6 oz)	116	1	3
oat cooked	½ cup (3.8 oz)	44	tr	1
rice	½ cup (2.1 oz)	187	2	12
wheat	½ cup (2 oz)	63	tr	1
Arrowhead				
Oat Bran	⅓ cup (1.4 oz)	150	0	3
Wheat Bran	¼ cup (0.6 oz)	30	0	1
Good Shepherd				
Wheat Bran	1 oz	80	—	1
H-O				
Super Bran	⅓ cup	110	0	2
Hodgson Mill				
Oat	¼ cup (1.3 oz)	120	1	3
Wheat	¼ cup (0.5 oz)	30	0	1
Mother's				
Oat Bran	½ cup	150	1	3
Quaker				
Oat Bran	½ cup (1.4 oz)	150	1	3
Roman Meal				
Oat	1 oz	94	tr	3
Stone-Buhr				
Oat	⅓ cup (1 oz)	90	0	2

BRAZIL NUTS

FOOD	PORTION	CALS.	SAT. FAT	FAT
dried unblanched	1 oz	186	5	19

BREAD

(see also BAGEL, BISCUIT, BREADSTICK, CROISSANT, ENGLISH MUFFIN, MUFFIN, ROLL, SCONE)

CANNED

FOOD	PORTION	CALS.	SAT. FAT	FAT
B&M				
Brown Bread	½ in slice (2 oz)	130	0	1
Brown Bread Raisins	½ in slice (2 oz)	130	0	1
FROZEN				
Kineret				
Challah	⅛ loaf (2 oz)	150	1	4

FOOD	PORTION	CALS.	SAT. FAT	FAT
New York				
Garlic	1 slice (2 oz)	190	2	8
Garlic Reduced Fat	1 slice (2 oz)	160	1	4
Texas Garlic Toast	1 in slice (1.4 oz)	160	2	9
Pepperidge Farm				
Garlic	1 slice (1.8 oz)	170	3	10
Garlic Sourdough 30% Reduced Fat	1 slice (1.8 oz)	170	1	7
Monterey Jack Jalapeno Cheese	1 slice (2 oz)	145	4	11
Mozzeralla Garlic Cheese	1 slice (2 oz)	201	5	10
HOME RECIPE				
banana	1 slice (2 oz)	195	1	6
cornbread as prep w/ 2% milk	1 piece (2.3 oz)	173	1	5
cornbread as prep w/ whole milk	1 piece (2.3 oz)	176	1	5
datenut	½ in slice	92	—	3
irish soda bread	1 slice (2 oz)	174	1	3
MIX				
Aunt Jemima				
Corn Bread Easy Mix	⅓ cup (1.3 oz)	150	1	4
Natural Ovens				
Cracked Wheat	2 slices (2.4 oz)	140	0	1
English Muffin Bread	2 slices (2.4 oz)	140	0	1
Executive Fitness Sunny Millet	2 slices (2.6 oz)	160	0	2
Garden Bread	1 oz	50	0	1
Glorious Cinnamon & Raisin Fat Free	2 slices (2.1 oz)	110	0	1
Honey 'N Flax	2 slices (2.5 oz)	140	0	1
Hunger Filler Bread	2 slices (2.1 oz)	110	0	2
Light Wheat	2 slices (2.2 oz)	84	0	1
Nutty Natural Wheat Bread	2 slices (2.5 oz)	140	0	2
Seven Grain Herb	2 slices (2.5 oz)	140	0	1
Soft Hearth Whole Wheat	2 slices (2 oz)	100	0	2
Soft Sandwich Very Low Fat	2 slices (2.3 oz)	110	0	1
Stay Slim	2 slices (2 oz)	100	0	2
Zia Foods				
Cornbread Blue Cornmeal	1 piece (1.2 oz)	110	—	6
READY-TO-EAT				
baguette whole wheat	2 oz	140	0	0
cracked wheat	1 slice	65	tr	1
egg	1 slice (1.4 oz)	115	1	2
french	1 slice (1 oz)	78	tr	1
french	1 loaf (1 lb)	1270	4	18
gluten	1 slice	47	tr	tr

FOOD	PORTION	CALS.	SAT. FAT	FAT
italian	1 loaf (1 lb)	1255	1	4
italian	1 slice (1 oz)	81	tr	1
navajo fry	1 (10.5 in diam)	527	3	15
navajo fry	1 (5 in diam)	296	2	9
oat bran	1 slice	71	tr	1
oat bran reduced calorie	1 slice	46	tr	1
oatmeal	1 slice	73	tr	1
oatmeal reduced calorie	1 slice	48	tr	1
pita	1 reg (2 oz)	165	tr	1
pita	1 sm (1 oz)	78	tr	tr
pita whole wheat	1 sm (1 oz)	76	tr	1
pita whole wheat	1 reg (2 oz)	170	tr	2
protein	1 slice	47	tr	tr
pumpernickel	1 slice	80	tr	1
raisin	1 slice	71	tr	1
rice bran	1 slice	66	tr	1
rye	1 slice	83	tr	1
rye reduced calorie	1 slice	47	tr	1
seven grain	1 slice	65	tr	1
sourdough	1 slice (1 oz)	78	tr	1
vienna	1 slice (1 oz)	78	tr	1
wheat reduced calorie	1 slice	46	tr	1
wheat berry	1 slice	65	tr	1
wheat bran	1 slice	89	tr	1
wheat germ	1 slice	74	tr	1
white	1 slice	67	tr	1
white reduced calorie	1 slice	48	tr	1
white toasted	1 slice	67	tr	1
white cubed	1 cup	80	tr	1
whole wheat	1 slice	70	tr	1
Alvarado St. Bakery				
Barley	1 slice (1.2 oz)	70	0	1
California Style	1 slice (1.2 oz)	60	0	1
French	1 slice (1.2 oz)	80	0	1
Multi-Grain	1 slice (1.2 oz)	60	0	1
Multi-Grain No-Salt	1 slice (1.2 oz)	60	0	1
Oat Berry	1 slice (1.2 oz)	70	0	1
Raisin	1 slice (1.1 oz)	80	0	1
Rye Seed	1 slice (1.2 oz)	60	0	1
Sourdough	1 slice (1.2 oz)	80	0	1
Wheat	1 slice (1.3 oz)	90	0	1
Arnold				
12 Grain Natural	1 slice (0.8 oz)	60	0	0
Augusto Pan De Aqua	1 oz	80	—	1
Bran'nola Country Oat	1 slice (1.3 oz)	90	0	3

FOOD	PORTION	CALS.	SAT. FAT	FAT
Arnold (CONT.)				
Bran'nola Dark Wheat	1 slice (1.3 oz)	90	0	3
Bran'nola Hearty Wheat	1 slice (1.3 oz)	100	0	3
Bran'nola Nutty Grains	1 slice (1.3 oz)	90	0	2
Bran'nola Original	1 slice (1.3 oz)	90	0	2
Cinnamon Chip	1 slice	80	—	2
Cinnamon Raisin	1 slice (0.9 oz)	70	0	1
Country Bran Bakery Light	1 slice (0.8 oz)	40	0	tr
Cranberry	1 slice (0.9 oz)	70	0	1
French Twin Loaves Francisco	2 slices (2 oz)	150	—	2
French Stick Francisco	1 slice (1 oz)	70	—	2
French Stick Savoni	1 oz	80	—	tr
Italian Bakery Light	1 slice (0.7 oz)	40	0	tr
Italian Francisco	1 slice (1 oz)	70	—	1
Italian Stick Francisco	1 oz	90	—	1
Oatmeal Bakery	1 slice	60	—	1
Oatmeal Bakery Light	1 slice	40	0	tr
Oatmeal Raisin	1 slice (0.9 oz)	60	0	tr
Pita Wheat	½ pocket (1 oz)	71	—	0
Pita White	½ pocket (0.5 oz)	71	0	0
Pumpernickel	1 slice (1.1 oz)	70	0	1
Rye Bakery Soft Light	1 slice (1.1 oz)	40	0	tr
Rye Bakery Soft Seeded	1 slice (1.1 oz)	70	0	1
Rye Bakery Soft Unseeded	1 slice (1.1 oz)	70	0	1
Rye Dill	1 slice (1.1 oz)	60	0	1
Rye Real Jewish Dijon	1 slice	70	—	tr
Rye Real Jewish Melba Thin	1 slice (0.7 oz)	40	0	tr
Rye Real Jewish Unseeded	1 slice	80	—	tr
Rye Real Jewish With Caraway	1 slice	70	—	tr
Rye Real Jewish Without Seeds	1 slice (1.1 oz)	70	0	tr
Sourdough Francisco	1 slice	90	—	1
Wheat Brick Oven	1 slice (0.8 oz)	60	0	2
Wheat Golden Light	1 slice (0.8 oz)	40	0	tr
Wheat Natural	1 slice (1.3 oz)	80	0	1
Wheat Berry Honey	1 slice (1.1 oz)	80	0	2
White Brick Oven	1 slice (0.8 oz)	60	0	1
White Country	1 slice (1.3 oz)	100	tr	2
White Extra Fiber Brick Oven	1 slice (0.9 oz)	50	0	tr
White Light Brick Oven	1 slice (0.8 oz)	40	0	tr
White Premium Light	1 slice	40	0	tr
White Thin Sliced Brick Oven	1 slice	40	—	tr
Whole Wheat 100% Light Brick Oven	1 slice (0.8 oz)	40	—	tr
Whole Wheat 100% Stoneground	1 slice (0.8 oz)	50	0	1

FOOD	PORTION	CALS.	SAT. FAT	FAT
August Bros.				
Pumpernickel	1 slice	80	—	1
Rye Onion	1 slice	80	—	1
Rye With Seeds	1 slice (1 lb loaf)	80	—	1
Rye Without Seeds	1 slice	80	—	1
Rye N' Pump	1 slice	90	—	1
Beefsteak				
Pumpernickel	1 slice (1 oz)	70	0	1
Rye Hearty	1 slice (1 oz)	70	0	1
Rye Light	2 slices (1.6 oz)	70	0	1
Rye Mild	2 slices (1.4 oz)	90	0	1
Rye Soft	1 slice (1 oz)	70	0	1
Wheat Hearty	1 slice (1 oz)	70	0	1
Wheat Soft	1 slice (1 oz)	70	0	1
White Robust	1 slice (1 oz)	70	0	1
Bread Du Jour				
French	3 in slice (2 oz)	140	0	1
Cedar's				
Mountain Bread Six Grain	1 piece (2.4 oz)	200	0	4
Damascus				
Mountain Shepard Lahvash	⅓ loaf (2 oz)	135	0	0
Wraps Spinach	1 (2 oz)	280	0	0
Wraps Tomato	1 12–inch (4 oz)	240	0	0
Dicarlo's				
Foccaccia	⅓ bread (2 oz)	130	0	2
French Parisian	2 slices (1 oz)	70	0	1
Ensemble				
Split-Top Sandwich	2 slices (2.2 oz)	140	0	1
Stone Ground Wheat	2 slices (2.2 oz)	150	0	2
Freihofer's				
Country Potato	1 slice (1.3 oz)	100	0	1
Country White	1 slice (1.3 oz)	100	0	1
Wheat Light	1 slice (1.6 oz)	80	0	0
White Light	2 slices (1.6 oz)	80	0	1
Whole Wheat 100%	1 slice (1.3 oz)	90	0	2
Home Pride				
Hearty Buttermilk & Biscuit White	1 slice (1.3 oz)	100	0	2
Hearty Deli Rye	1 slice (2 oz)	140	0	2
Hearty Golden Honey Wheat	1 slice (1.3 oz)	90	0	2
Hearty Honey Oats & Cracked Wheat	1 slice (1.4 oz)	100	0	2
Hearty Seven Grain Multi Grain	1 slice (1.3 oz)	100	0	2
Honey Wheat	1 slice (1 oz)	70	0	1
Seven Grain	1 slice (0.9 oz)	60	0	1

FOOD	PORTION	CALS.	SAT. FAT	FAT
Home Pride (CONT.)				
Wheat	1 slice (0.9 oz)	70	0	1
Wheat Light	3 slices (2.1 oz)	110	0	2
White	1 slice (0.9 oz)	70	0	1
White Grain	1 slice (1 oz)	60	0	1
White Light	3 slices (0.9 oz)	110	0	2
Whole Wheat Hearty 100% Stoneground	1 slice (1.4 oz)	90	0	2
La Mexicana				
Wraps Chocolate	1 (1.3 oz)	120	1	3
Wraps Southwestern Mild Chili	1 (1.3 oz)	120	1	4
Wraps Spinach	1 (1.3 oz)	120	1	4
Wraps Tomato Basil	1 (1.3 oz)	120	1	4
Mediterranean Magic				
Focaccia	½ loaf (1.8 oz)	140	0	2
Milton's				
Healthy Multi-Grain	1 slice (1.4 oz)	110	0	1
Monks' Bread				
Hi-Fibre	1 slice	50	—	1
Raisin	1 slice	70	—	2
Sunflower & Bran	1 slice	70	—	1
White	1 slice	60	—	1
Whole Wheat 100% Stoneground	1 slice	70	—	1
Pepperidge Farm				
Deli Swirl Rye & Pump	1 slice (1.1 oz)	80	0	1
Sandwich Pocket Wheat	1 (2 oz)	160	1	1
Sandwich Pocket White	1 (2 oz)	150	0	1
Roman Meal				
Brown & Serve Mini Loaf	½ loaf (2 oz)	136	tr	2
Cracked Wheat	1 slice (1.4 oz)	92	tr	2
Hearty Wheat Light	1 slice (0.8 oz)	42	tr	tr
Honey Nut Oat Bran	1 slice (1 oz)	72	tr	2
Honey Oat Bran	1 slice (1 oz)	70	tr	1
Oat	1 slice (1 oz)	69	tr	1
Oat Bran	1 slice (1 oz)	68	tr	1
Oat Bran Light	1 slice (0.8 oz)	42	tr	tr
Round Top	1 slice (1 oz)	67	tr	1
Sandwich	1 slice (0.8 oz)	55	tr	1
Seven Grain	1 slice (1 oz)	67	tr	1
Seven Grain Light	1 slice (0.8 oz)	42	tr	1
Sourdough Light	1 slice (0.8 oz)	41	tr	tr
Sourdough Whole Grain Light	1 slice (0.8 oz)	40	tr	tr
Sun Grain	1 slice (1 oz)	70	tr	2
Twelve Grain	1 slice (1 oz)	70	tr	2

FOOD	PORTION	CALS.	SAT. FAT	FAT
Roman Meal (CONT.)				
Twelve Grain Light	1 slice (0.8 oz)	42	tr	tr
Wheat Light	1 slice (0.8 oz)	41	tr	tr
Wheatberry Honey	1 slice (1 oz)	67	tr	1
Wheatberry Light	1 slice (0.8 oz)	42	tr	tr
White Light	1 slice (0.8 oz)	41	tr	tr
Whole Grain 100%	1 slice (1.4 oz)	91	tr	1
Whole Grain Sourdough	1 slice (1 oz)	66	tr	1
Whole Wheat 100%	1 slice (1 oz)	64	tr	1
Whole Wheat 100% Light	1 slice (0.8 oz)	42	tr	tr
Stroehmann				
100% Whole Wheat	1 slice (1.3 oz)	90	0	1
D'Italiano Italian No Seeds	1 slice (1 oz)	80	0	1
D'Italiano Italian Seeded	1 slice (1 oz)	80	0	1
Family White	1 slice (0.8 oz)	65	0	1
Homestyle Split Top Wheat	1 slices (0.8 oz)	60	0	1
Homestyle Split Top White	1 slice (0.8 oz)	65	0	0
Honey Cracked Wheat	1 slice (1.2 oz)	80	0	1
King White	1 slice (0.8 oz)	65	0	1
Potato	1 slice (1.2 oz)	100	0	2
Ranch White	1 slice (0.8 oz)	65	0	1
Rye	1 slice (1.1 oz)	80	0	1
Rye w/ Caraway	1 slice (1.1 oz)	80	0	1
Twelve Grain	1 slice (1.2 oz)	90	0	1
Sunmaid				
Raisin	1 slice	70	tr	tr
Tree Of Life				
100% Spelt	1 slice (1.8 oz)	130	1	3
Millet	1 slice (1.8 oz)	130	0	2
Rye Sour Dough	1 slice (1.8 oz)	110	0	0
Sprouted Seven Grain	1 slice (1.8 oz)	110	0	2
Valley Lahvosh				
Valley Wraps	1 (1 oz)	100	0	1
ZA				
Pit-Za Hearty Multi-Grain	½ bread (2 oz)	130	0	2
Pit-Za Salt-Free Garlic Whole Wheat	½ bread (2 oz)	150	0	1
REFRIGERATED				
Pillsbury				
Crusty French Loaf	⅛ loaf (2.2 oz)	150	1	2
Grands Wheat	1 (2.1 oz)	200	2	8
Roman Meal				
Loaf	1 slice (1 oz)	85	1	3

FOOD	PORTION	CALS.	SAT. FAT	FAT
Stefano's				
Stuffed Bread Broccoli & Cheese	½ bread (6 oz)	450	6	17
TAKE-OUT				
chapatis as prep w/ fat	1 bread (1.6 oz)	95	1	2
focaccia onion	1 piece (4.6 oz)	282	1	10
focaccia rosemary	1 piece (3.5 oz)	251	1	7
focaccia tomato olive	1 piece (4.7 oz)	270	1	8
garlic bread	2 slices (2 oz)	190	2	8
naan	1 bread (3.5 oz)	286	5	9
paratha	1 bread (2.1 oz)	201	7	10

BREAD COATING

FOOD	PORTION	CALS.	SAT. FAT	FAT
Don's Chuck Wagon				
All Purpose Mix	¼ cup (1 oz)	100	0	0
Fish & Chips Mix	¼ cup (1 oz)	100	0	0
Fish Mix	¼ cup (1 oz)	95	0	0
Frying Mix Chicken	¼ cup (1 oz)	95	0	0
Frying Mix Seafood Seasoned	¼ cup (1 oz)	95	0	1
Mushroom Mix	¼ cup (1 oz)	95	0	0
Onion Ring Mix	¼ cup (1 oz)	100	0	0
Little Crow				
Fryin' Magic	0.5 oz	43	—	tr
Mrs. Dash				
Crispy Coating	2 tbsp (0.6 oz)	65	—	1
Oven Fry				
Extra Crispy For Chicken	⅛ pkg (0.5 oz)	60	0	1
Extra Crispy For Pork	⅛ pkg (0.5 oz)	60	0	2
Shake 'N Bake				
Buffalo Wings	⅒ pkg (0.4 oz)	40	0	1
Classic Italian Chicken or Pork	⅛ pkg (0.4 oz)	40	0	1
Country Mild Recipe	⅛ pkg (0.3 oz)	35	1	2
Glazes Barbecue Chicken Or Pork	⅛ pkg (0.4 oz)	45	0	1
Glazes Honey Mustard Chicken Or Pork	⅛ pkg (0.4 oz)	45	0	1
Glazes Tangy Honey Chicken Or Pork	⅛ pkg (0.4 oz)	45	0	1
Home Style Flour Recipe For Chicken	⅛ pkg (0.4 oz)	40	0	1
Hot & Spicy Chicken Or Pork	⅛ pkg (0.4 oz)	40	0	1
Original For Chicken	⅛ pkg (0.4 oz)	40	0	1
Original For Fish	¼ pkg (0.7 oz)	80	0	2
Original For Pork	⅛ pkg (0.4 oz)	45	0	1

FOOD	PORTION	CALS.	SAT. FAT	FAT

BREAD MACHINE MIX
Fleischmann's

FOOD	PORTION	CALS.	SAT. FAT	FAT
Apple Cinnamon	⅛ loaf	160	0	1
Cinnamon Raisin	⅛ loaf	160	0	1
Country White	⅛ loaf (1.6 oz)	170	1	3
Cranberry Orange	⅛ loaf	150	0	2
Honey Oatmeal	⅛ loaf	160	0	2
Italian Herb	⅛ loaf	160	1	2
Sourdough	⅛ loaf	150	1	2
Stoneground Wheat	⅛ loaf	160	0	1
Sassafras				
Apricot Oatmeal	1 slice (1.4 oz)	140	0	1
Wanda's				
Dried Tomato Cheddar	¼ cup mix per serv (1.2 oz)	140	0	0
European White	¼ cup mix per serv (1.2 oz)	130	0	0
Oatmeal	¼ cup mix per serv (1.2 oz)	120	0	0
Oatmeal Cinnamon	¼ cup mix per serv (1.2 oz)	120	0	0
Old World Rye	¼ cup mix per serv (1.9 oz)	90	0	0
Onion	¼ cup mix per serv (1.2 oz)	120	0	0
Orange Cinnamon	¼ cup mix per serv (1.3 oz)	130	0	0
Oregano Garlic	¼ cup mix per serv (1.2 oz)	130	0	1
Rosemary Basil	¼ cup mix per serv (1.2 oz)	130	0	0
Rye	¼ cup mix per serv (1.2 oz)	120	0	0
Rye Caraway	¼ cup mix per serv (1.2 oz)	120	0	0
Sourdough	¼ cup mix per serv (1.2 oz)	120	0	0
Sunflower Sesame Poppyseed	¼ cup mix per serv (1.2 oz)	120	0	0
Ten Grain	¼ cup mix per serv (1.4 oz)	140	0	0
Wheat	¼ cup mix per serv (1.2 oz)	130	0	0
White	¼ cup mix per serv (1.2 oz)	130	0	0

FOOD	PORTION	CALS.	SAT. FAT	FAT
Wanda's (CONT.)				
Whole Wheat	¼ cup mix per serv (1.3 oz)	130	0	0

BREADCRUMBS

FOOD	PORTION	CALS.	SAT. FAT	FAT
dry	1 cup	426	1	6
dry seasonsed	1 cup (4 oz)	441	1	3
fresh	⅔ cup	76	tr	1
Arnold				
Italian	½ oz	50	0	tr
Plain	½ oz	50	0	tr
Contadina				
Plain	⅓ cup	100	—	2
Progresso				
Italian Style	¼ cup (1 oz)	110	0	2
Lemon Herb	¼ cup (0.9 oz)	100	0	1
Plain	¼ cup (1 oz)	100	0	2
Tomato Basil	¼ cup (1.1 oz)	120	0	2

BREADFRUIT

FOOD	PORTION	CALS.	SAT. FAT	FAT
fresh	¼ small	99	—	tr
seeds cooked	1 oz	48	tr	1
seeds raw	1 oz	54	tr	2
seeds roasted	1 oz	59	tr	tr

BREADNUTTREE SEEDS

FOOD	PORTION	CALS.	SAT. FAT	FAT
dried	1 oz	104	tr	tr

BREADSTICKS

FOOD	PORTION	CALS.	SAT. FAT	FAT
plain	1 sm	25	tr	1
plain	1	41	tr	1
Angonoa				
Cheese	5 (1 oz)	120	1	3
Cheese Mini	16 (1 oz)	120	1	3
Garlic	6 (1 oz)	120	0	2
Italian Style Plain	5 (1 oz)	120	1	3
Low Sodium With Sesame Seed	6 (1 oz)	130	1	4
Onion	6 (1 oz)	120	1	2
Pizza Mini	26 (1 oz)	120	0	2
Sesame Mini	16 (1 oz)	130	1	4
Sesame Royale	6 (1 oz)	130	1	4
Whole Wheat Mini	14 (1 oz)	130	1	4
Bread Du Jour				
Original	1 (1.9 oz)	130	0	1
Sourdough	1 (1.9 oz)	130	0	1
J.J. Cassone				
Garlic	1 (1.6 oz)	150	0	3

FOOD	PORTION	CALS.	SAT. FAT	FAT
New York				
Garlic Soft	1 (1.5 oz)	140	1	4
Pillsbury				
Soft	1 (1.4 oz)	110	0	2
Soft Garlic & Herb	1 (2.1 oz)	180	2	7
Roman Meal				
Brown & Serve Soft	1 (2.7 oz)	181	tr	3
Refrigerated	1 (1.4 oz)	117	1	4
Stella D'Oro				
Deli Garlic Fat Free	5	60	0	0
Deli Original Fat Free	5	60	0	0
Garlic	1	35	—	1
Grissini Garlic Fat Free	3	60	—	0
Grissini Original Fat Free	3	60	—	0
Onion	1	40	—	1
Regular	1 (9 g)	40	0	1
Regular Sodium Free	2	80	—	2
Sesame Low Fat	2	70	—	1
Sesame Sodium Free	1	50	—	3
Traditional Garlic Fat Free	2	70	0	0
Traditional Original Fat Free	2	70	0	0
Wheat	1	40	—	1

BREAKFAST BAR
(*see also* CEREAL BARS, NUTRITION SUPPLEMENTS)

Carnation				
Chewy Chocolate Chip	1 (1.26 oz)	150	3	6
Nutri-Grain				
Apple Cinnamon	1 (1.3 oz)	140	1	3
Blueberry	1 (1.3 oz)	140	1	3
Peach	1 (1.3 oz)	140	1	3
Raspberry	1 (1.3 oz)	140	1	3
Strawberry	1 (1.3 oz)	140	1	3

BREAKFAST DRINKS
(*see also* NUTRITION SUPPLEMENTS)

orange drink powder	3 rounded tsp	93	0	0
orange drink powder as prep w/water	6 oz	86	0	0
Carnation				
Instant Breakfast Cafe Mocha	1 pkg	130	0	1
Instant Breakfast Cafe Mocha	1 pkg + skim milk (9 fl oz)	220	tr	1
Instant Breakfast Cafe Mocha	1 can (10 fl oz)	220	1	3
Instant Breakfast Classic Chocolate Malt	1 pkg + skim milk (9 fl oz)	220	1	1

FOOD	PORTION	CALS.	SAT. FAT	FAT
Carnation (CONT.)				
Instant Breakfast Classic Chocolate Malt	1 pkg	130	1	2
Instant Breakfast Creamy Milk Chocolate	1 pkg	130	1	1
Instant Breakfast Creamy Milk Chocolate	1 pkg + skim milk (9 fl oz)	220	1	1
Instant Breakfast Creamy Milk Chocolate	8 fl oz	220	2	3
Instant Breakfast Creamy Milk Chocolate	1 can (10 fl oz)	220	1	3
Instant Breakfast French Vanilla	1 pkg + skim milk	220	tr	1
Instant Breakfast French Vanilla	1 pkg	130	0	0
Instant Breakfast No Sugar Added Classic Chocolate	1 pkg + skim milk (9 fl oz)	160	1	2
Instant Breakfast No Sugar Added Classic Chocolate	1 pkg	70	1	2
Instant Breakfast No Sugar Added Creamy Milk Chocolate	1 pkg + skim milk (9 fl oz)	160	1	1
Instant Breakfast No Sugar Added Creamy Milk Chocolate	1 pkg	70	1	1
Instant Breakfast No Sugar Added French Vanilla	1 pkg + skim milk (9 fl oz)	150	tr	1
Instant Breakfast No Sugar Added French Vanilla	1 pkg	70	0	0
Instant Breakfast No Sugar Added Strawberry Creme	1 pkg + skim milk (9 fl oz)	150	tr	1
Instant Breakfast No Sugar Added Strawberry Creme	1 pkg	70	0	0
Instant Breakfast Strawberry Creme	1 pkg	130	0	0
Instant Breakfast Strawberry Creme	1 pkg + skim milk	220	tr	1
BROAD BEANS				
canned	1 cup	183	tr	1
dried cooked	1 cup	186	tr	1
fresh cooked	3.5 oz	56	tr	tr
BROCCOFLOWER				
fresh raw	½ cup (1.8 oz)	16	tr	tr
Dole				
Fresh	⅕ head	35	0	0

FOOD	PORTION	CALS.	SAT. FAT	FAT
BROCCOLI				
FRESH				
chinese broccoli (gai lan) cooked	1 cup (3.1 oz)	19	tr	1
chopped cooked	½ cup	22	tr	tr
raw chopped	½ cup	12	tr	tr
Dole				
Spear	1 med	40	—	1
FROZEN				
chopped cooked	½ cup	25	tr	tr
spears cooked	10 oz pkg	69	tr	tr
spears cooked	½ cup	25	tr	tr
Amy's Organic				
Pocket Sandwich Broccoli & Cheese	1 (4.5 oz)	270	4	10
Big Valley				
Chopped	¾ cup (3 oz)	25	0	0
Cuts	¾ cup (3 oz)	25	0	0
Birds Eye				
Baby Broccoli Blend	1 cup (3.4 oz)	70	0	2
Baby Florets	1 cup (3 oz)	25	0	0
In Cheese Sauce	½ cup (3.9 oz)	110	2	5
Fresh Like				
Spear	3.5 oz	26	—	tr
Green Giant				
Butter Sauce	4 oz	50	1	2
Cheese Sauce	⅔ cup (3.9 oz)	70	1	3
Chopped	¾ cup (2.8 oz)	25	0	0
Cuts	1 cup (2.9 oz)	25	0	0
Harvest Fresh Cut	⅔ cup (3.2 oz)	25	0	0
Harvest Fresh Spears	3.5 oz	25	0	0
Select Florets	1⅓ cups (2.9 oz)	25	0	0
Select Spears	3 oz	25	0	0
Hanover				
Cut	½ cup	25	—	0
Florets	½ cup	30	—	0
Stouffer's				
Au Gratin	1 serv (4 oz)	100	2	4
Tree Of Life				
Broccoli	1 cup (3.1 oz)	25	0	0
BROWNIE				
FROZEN				
Greenfield				
Fat Free Homestyle	1 (1.3 oz)	110	0	0

FOOD	PORTION	CALS.	SAT. FAT	FAT
Otis Spunkmeyer				
Blue Yonder w/ Walnuts	1 (2 oz)	230	3	10
Weight Watchers				
Brownie A La Mode	1 (3.14 oz)	190	2	4
Double Fudge Brownie Parfait	1 (5.3 oz)	190	2	3
HOME RECIPE				
plain	1 (0.8 oz)	112	2	7
w/nuts	1 (0.8 oz)	95	1	6
MIX				
plain	1 (1.2 oz)	139	1	7
plain low calorie	1 (0.8 oz)	84	1	2
Betty Crocker				
Caramel	1	190	2	9
Caramel No Cholesterol Recipe	1	170	1	5
Chocolate Chunk Supreme	1	180	3	9
Dark Chocolate Fudge	1	170	2	7
Dark Chocolate w/ Hershey Syrup	1	170	2	7
Frosted Supreme	1	210	2	9
Fudge	1	190	2	7
Fudge No Cholesterol Recipe	1	140	1	4
German Chocolate	1	220	2	8
Hot Fudge Supreme	1	170	2	8
Original Supreme	1	160	1	6
Peanut Butter Candies w/ Reese's Pieces	1	180	3	9
Pouch Dessert Fudge	1	190	2	8
Stir'n Bake w/ Mini Kisses	1 serv	220	3	8
T-Rex Fossils	1	180	2	8
T-Rex Fossils No Cholesterol Recipe	1	170	2	8
Turtle	1	170	2	8
Walnut Supreme	1	160	2	9
Estee				
Brownie Mix as prep	2	100	2	4
Jiffy				
Fudge as prep	1	160	1	4
Sweet Rewards				
Reduced Fat Fudge	1	140	1	4
Reduced Fat Fudge No Cholesterol Recipe	1	140	1	3
READY-TO-EAT				
plain	1 sm (1 oz)	115	1	5
plain	1 lg (2 oz)	227	2	9
w/ nuts	1 (1 oz)	100	2	4

FOOD	PORTION	CALS.	SAT. FAT	FAT
Dolly Madison				
Fudge	1 (3 oz)	330	4	11
Greenfield				
Blondie Fat Free Apple Spice	1 (1.3 oz)	110	0	0
Health Valley				
Bar w/ Fudge Filling	1 bar	110	0	0
Hostess				
Brownie Bites	3 (1.3 oz)	170	2	9
Fudge	1 (3 oz)	330	4	11
Light	1 (1.4 oz)	140	1	3
Lance				
Fudge Nut	1 (2.25 oz)	340	3	13
Little Debbie				
Brownie Lights	1 (2 oz)	190	0	3
Brownie Loaves	1 (2.1 oz)	260	3	15
Fudge	1 pkg (2.1 oz)	270	3	13
Sweet Rewards				
Low Fat Homestyle	1 (1.1 oz)	120	1	2
Tastykake				
Fudge Walnut	1 (3 oz)	370	4	17
TAKE-OUT				
plain	1 2 in sq (2.1 oz)	243	3	10

BRUSSELS SPROUTS

FOOD	PORTION	CALS.	SAT. FAT	FAT
FRESH				
cooked	½ cup	30	tr	tr
cooked	1 sprout	8	tr	tr
raw	½ cup	19	tr	tr
raw	1 sprout	8	tr	tr
Dole				
Sprouts	½ cup	19	—	tr
FROZEN				
cooked	½ cup	33	tr	tr
Big Valley				
Whole	5–8 pieces (3 oz)	35	0	0
Birds Eye				
Burssels Sprouts	6 (3 oz)	35	0	0
Fresh Like				
Sprouts	3.5 oz	37	—	tr
Green Giant				
Butter Sauce	⅔ cup (3.6 oz)	60	2	2
Hanover				
Brussels Sprouts	½ cup	40	—	0

BUCKWHEAT

FOOD	PORTION	CALS.	SAT. FAT	FAT
groats roasted cooked	1 cup (5.9 oz)	647	tr	1
groats roasted uncooked	1 cup (5.7 oz)	567	1	4

FOOD	PORTION	CALS.	SAT. FAT	FAT
Wolff's				
Brown Groats Roasted	1 cup (8 oz)	900	—	4
Flour	1 cup (8 oz)	860	—	5
Kasha Coarse cooked	¼ cup (1.6 oz)	170	0	2
Kasha Fine cooked	¼ cup (1.6 oz)	170	0	2
Kasha Medium cooked	¼ cup (1.6 oz)	170	0	2
Kasha Whole cooked	¼ cup (1.6 oz)	170	0	2
White Grits	1 cup (8 oz)	840	—	3

BUFFALO

water buffalo roasted	3 oz	111	1	2

BULGUR

cooked	1 cup (6.3 oz)	151	tr	tr
uncooked	1 cup (4.9 oz)	479	tr	2
Casbah				
Pilaf Mix as prep	1 cup	200	0	1
Salad Mix as prep	⅔ cup	90	0	tr
Good Shepherd				
Bulgur	¼ cup (43 g)	150	—	1
Hodgson Mill				
Bulgur	¼ cup (1.4 oz)	120	0	1

BURBOT (FISH)

fresh baked	3 oz	98	tr	1

BURDOCK ROOT

cooked	1 cup	110	—	tr
raw	1 cup	85	—	tr

BUTTER

(see also BUTTER BLENDS, BUTTER SUBSTITUTES, MARGARINE)

clarified butter	3½ oz	876	62	99
stick	1 pat (5 g)	36	3	4
stick	1 stick (4 oz)	813	57	92
whipped	4 oz	542	38	61
whipped	1 pat (4 g)	27	2	3
Cabot				
Stick	1 tsp	35	3	4
Unsalted Stick	1 tsp	35	3	4
Crystal				
Salted Stick	1 tbsp (0.5 oz)	102	7	11
Unsalted Stick	1 tbsp (0.5 oz)	102	7	11
Hotel Bar				
Stick	1 tsp	35	—	4
Keller's				
Stick	1 tsp	35	—	4

FOOD	PORTION	CALS.	SAT. FAT	FAT
Land O'Lakes				
Light Stick	1 tbsp	50	4	6
Light Unsalted Stick	1 tbsp	50	4	6
Stick	1 tbsp (0.5 oz)	100	7	11
Unsalted Stick	1 tbsp (0.5 oz)	100	7	11
Unsalted Tub	1 tbsp	60	5	7
Whipped	1 tbsp (0.3 oz)	70	5	7
Organic Valley				
Butter	1 tbsp (0.5 oz)	100	8	11
Unsalted	1 tbsp (0.5 oz)	110	8	12

BUTTER BEANS
CANNED
Allen

FOOD	PORTION	CALS.	SAT. FAT	FAT
Baby	½ cup (4.5 oz)	120	1	1
Large	½ cup (4.5 oz)	120	0	1
Green Giant				
Butter Beans	½ cup (4.5 oz)	90	0	0
Hanover				
Butter Beans	½ cup	80	—	0
In Sauce	½ cup	100	—	0
Sunshine				
Butter Beans	½ cup (4.5 oz)	120	0	1
Trappey				
Baby White With Bacon	½ cup (4.5 oz)	130	1	2
Large White With Bacon	½ cup (4.5 oz)	110	0	1
Van Camp's				
Butter Beans	½ cup	110	0	1
FROZEN				
Birds Eye				
Butter Beans	½ cup (2.7 oz)	100	0	0
Speckled	½ cup (2.7 oz)	100	0	0

BUTTER BLENDS
(see also BUTTER, BUTTER SUBSTITUTES, MARGARINE)
Brummel & Brown

FOOD	PORTION	CALS.	SAT. FAT	FAT
Spread Make With Yogurt	1 tbsp (0.5 oz)	50	1	5
Country Morning				
Blend Light Stick	1 tbsp (0.5 oz)	50	3	6
Blend Light Tub	1 tbsp (0.5 oz)	50	3	6
Blend Stick	1 tbsp	100	3	11
Blend Tub	1 tbsp	100	2	11
Blend Unsalted Stick	1 tbsp	100	3	11

BUTTER SUBSTITUTES
(see also BUTTER BLENDS, MARGARINE)

FOOD	PORTION	CALS.	SAT. FAT	FAT
Butter Buds				
Mix	1 tsp (2 g)	5	0	0
Sprinkles	1 tsp (2 g)	5	0	0
Molly McButter				
Cheese	1 tsp	5	0	0
Light Sodium	1 tsp	5	0	0
Natural Butter	1 tsp	5	0	0
Roasted Garlic	1 tsp	5	0	0
Morningstar Farms				
Roasted Soy Butter	2 tbsp (1.1 oz)	170	2	11
Mrs. Bateman's				
Butterlike Baking Butter	1 tbsp (0.5 oz)	36	tr	1
Butterlike Saute Butter	1 tbsp (0.5 oz)	40	1	2
Natural Touch				
Roasted Soy Butter	2 tbsp (1.1 oz)	170	2	11
Watkins				
Butter Sprinkles	1 tsp (2 g)	5	0	0
Imitation Butter Flavored Mist	1 tbsp (0.5 oz)	120	2	14
BUTTERBUR				
canned fuki chopped	1 cup	3	—	tr
fresh fuki raw	1 cup	13	—	tr
BUTTERFISH				
baked	3 oz	159	—	9
BUTTERNUTS				
dried	1 oz	174	tr	16
BUTTERSCOTCH				
(see also CANDY)				
Hershey				
Chips	1 tbsp (0.5 oz)	80	4	4
Nestle				
Morsels Butterscotch	1 tbsp	80	4	4
CABBAGE				
(see also COLESLAW)				
FRESH				
chinese pak-choi raw shredded	½ cup	5	tr	tr
chinese pak-choi shredded cooked	½ cup	10	tr	tr
chinese pe-tsai raw shredded	1 cup	12	tr	tr
chinese pe-tsai shredded cooked	1 cup	16	tr	tr
danish raw	1 head (2 lbs)	228	tr	2
danish raw shredded	½ cup (1.2 oz)	9	tr	tr
danish shredded cooked	½ cup (2.6 oz)	17	tr	tr

FOOD	PORTION	CALS.	SAT. FAT	FAT
green raw	1 head (2 lbs)	228	tr	2
green raw shredded	½ cup (1.2 oz)	9	tr	tr
green shredded cooked	½ cup (2.6 oz)	17	tr	tr
napa cooked	1 cup (3.8 oz)	13	0	tr
red raw shredded	½ cup	10	tr	tr
red shredded cooked	½ cup	16	tr	tr
savoy raw shredded	½ cup	10	tr	tr
savoy shredded cooked	½ cup	18	tr	tr
Dole				
Cabbage	1/12 med head	18	—	0
Napa shredded	½ cup	6	—	tr

CAKE

(see *also* BROWNIE, CAKE MIX, COOKIE, DANISH PASTRY, DOUGHNUT, PIE)

FOOD	PORTION	CALS.	SAT. FAT	FAT
angelfood	1 cake (11.9 oz)	876	tr	3
angelfood home recipe	1/12 cake (1.9 oz)	142	tr	tr
apple crisp home recipe	1 recipe 6 serv (29.6 oz)	1377	6	31
boston cream pie frzn	⅙ cake (3.2 oz)	232	2	8
carrot w/ cream cheese icing home recipe	1 cake 10 in diam	6175	66	328
cheesecake	⅙ cake (2.8 oz)	256	9	18
cheesecake	1 cake 9 in diam	3350	120	213
cheesecake home recipe	1/12 cake (4.5 oz)	456	18	9
cherry fudge w/ chocolate frosting	⅛ cake (2.5 oz)	187	3	9
chocolate cupcake creme filled w/ frosting home recipe	1 (1.8 oz)	188	2	7
chocolate w/o frosting home recipe	1/12 cake (3.3 oz)	340	5	14
chocolate w/o frosting home recipe	2 layers (39.9 oz)	4067	62	172
coffeecake creme-filled chocolate frosting home recipe	⅙ cake (3.2 oz)	298	3	10
coffeecake crumb topped cinnamon home recipe	1/12 cake (2.1 oz)	240	2	12
coffeecake fruit	⅛ cake (1.8 oz)	156	1	5
cream puff shell home recipe	1 (2.3 oz)	239	4	17
devil's food cupcake w/ chocolate frosting	1	120	4	4
devil's food w/ creme filling	1 (1 oz)	105	2	4
eclair home recipe	1 (3 oz)	262	4	16
fruitcake	1 piece (1.5 oz)	139	tr	4
fruitcake dark home recipe	1 cake 7½ in x 2¼ in	5185	48	228
jelly roll lemon filled	1 slice (3 oz)	210	1	2

FOOD	PORTION	CALS.	SAT. FAT	FAT
pound	1 cake (8½ x 3½ x 3 in	1935	52	94
pound	1/10 cake (1 oz)	117	3	6
pound fat free	1 cake (12 oz)	961	1	4
pound cake home recipe	1 loaf 8½ in x 3½ in	1935	21	94
sheet cake w/ white frosting home recipe	1 cake 9 in sq	4020	42	129
sheet cake w/o frosting home recipe	1/9 cake	315	3	12
sheet cake w/o frosting home recipe	1 cake 9 in sq	2830	30	108
shortcake home recipe	1 (2.3 oz)	225	2	9
sour cream pound	1/10 cake (1 oz)	117	1	5
sponge	1/12 cake (1.3 oz)	110	tr	1
sponge home recipe	1/12 cake (2.2 oz)	140	1	2
sponge cake dessert shell	1 (0.8 oz)	75	tr	1
sponge w/ creme filling	1 (1.5 oz)	155	1	5
tiramisu	1 cake (4.4 lbs)	5732	217	421
toaster pastry apple	1 (1.75 oz)	204	1	5
toaster pastry blueberry	1 (1.75 oz)	204	1	5
toaster pastry brown sugar cinnamon	1 (1.75 oz)	206	2	7
toaster pastry cherry	1 (1.75 oz)	204	1	5
toaster pastry strawberry	1 (1.75 oz)	204	1	5
white w/ coconut frosting home recipe	1/12 cake (3.9 oz)	399	4	12
white w/o frosting home recipe	1/12 cake (2.6 oz)	264	2	9
white w/ white frosting	1/9 cake	260	2	9
white w/ white frosting	1 cake 9 in diam	4170	33	148
yellow w/ chocolate frosting	1/9 cake (2.2 oz)	242	3	11
yellow w/ chocolate frosting	1 cake 9 in diam	3895	92	175
yellow w/o frosting home recipe	2 layers (28.7 oz)	2947	32	119
yellow w/o frosting home recipe	1/12 cake (2.4 oz)	245	3	10
Baby Watson				
Cheesecake	1 slice (3.8 oz)	390	18	30
Cheesecake Light	1/16 cake (3.9 oz)	280	9	16
Baker Maid				
Creole Royal Pineapple Apricot	3 slices (5 oz)	270	1	3
Creole Royal Pineapple Apricot	1 slice (1.7 oz)	90	0	1
Carousel				
New York Cheese Cake	1 cake (3 oz)	250	11	19
Dolly Madison				
Angel Food	1 slice (2.1 oz)	160	0	2
Apple Crumb	1 (1.6 oz)	160	2	5

FOOD	PORTION	CALS.	SAT. FAT	FAT
Dolly Madison (CONT.)				
Banana Dream Flip	1 (3.5 oz)	390	3	16
Bear Claw	1 (2.75 oz)	270	4	10
Carrot	1 (4 oz)	360	3	8
Chocolate Snack Squares	1 (1.6 oz)	210	6	10
Cinnamon Buttercrumb	1 (1.6 oz)	170	2	6
Cinnamon Buttercrumb Low Fat	1 (1.5 oz)	140	0	2
Cinnamon Stix	1 (1.3 oz)	170	4	9
Creme Cakes	2 (1.9 oz)	210	4	8
Cupcakes Chocolate	1 (2 oz)	210	3	7
Cupcakes Spice	1 (2 oz)	230	4	10
Dunkin' Stix	1 (1.3 oz)	170	4	9
Frosty Angel	1 (3.5 oz)	330	4	6
Holiday Cupcakes	1 (1.9 oz)	180	1	3
Honey Bun	1 (3.7 oz)	440	11	25
Koo Koos	1 (1.8 oz)	200	6	9
Mini Coconut Loaf	1 (3.5 oz)	350	2	10
Mini Pound Cake	1 (3.2 oz)	310	5	11
Raspberry Square	1 (1.8 oz)	190	4	8
Sweet Roll Apple	1 (2.2 oz)	200	2	6
Sweet Roll Cherry	1 (2.2 oz)	210	3	6
Sweet Roll Cinnamon	1 (2.2 oz)	230	3	7
Texas Cinnamon Bun	1 (4.2 oz)	440	6	15
Zingers Devil's Food	2 (2.6 oz)	270	4	8
Zingers Lemon	1 (1.4 oz)	150	3	6
Zingers Raspberry	1 (1.4 oz)	150	3	6
Zingers Yellow	2 (2.5 oz)	280	3	8
Drake's				
Coffee Cake Low Fat	1 (1.1 oz)	110	1	2
Light & Fruity Apple	1 (1.2 oz)	90	—	1
Light & Fruity Blueberry	1 (1.2 oz)	90	—	1
Light & Fruity Cinnamon Raisin	1 (1.2 oz)	90	—	1
Mini Coffee Cakes	4 (1.83 oz)	220	2	9
Yodel's	1 (1 oz)	150	—	9
Dutch Mill				
Dessert Shells Chocolate Covered	1 (0.5 oz)	80	2	5
Ensemble				
Carrot w/ Icing	1 (3 oz)	280	2	7
Mini-Loaves Apple Cinnamon	1 (3 oz)	230	0	3
Mini-Loaves Blueberry	1 (3 oz)	230	0	3
Mini-Loaves Lemon-Poppyseed	1 (3 oz)	240	1	3
Entenmann's				
Apple Puffs	1 (3 oz)	280	—	13

FOOD	PORTION	CALS.	SAT. FAT	FAT
Entenmann's (CONT.)				
Apple Strudel Old Fashioned	1 serv (1.5 oz)	120	—	5
Cheese Topped Buns	1 (2.3 oz)	240	—	12
Cinnamon Buns	1 (2.1 oz)	230	—	10
Cinnamon Filbert Ring	1 serv (1.5 oz)	190	—	12
Coffee Cake Cheese	1 serv (1.6 oz)	150	—	7
Coffee Cake Cheese Filled Crumb	1 serv (1.4 oz)	130	—	6
Coffee Cake Crumb	1 serv (1.3 oz)	160	—	7
Danish Ring	1 serv (1.5 oz)	180	—	10
Danish Ring Pecan	1 serv (1.5 oz)	190	—	12
Danish Ring Walnut	1 serv (1.5 oz)	190	—	12
Danish Twist Lemon	1 serv (1.2 oz)	140	—	7
Danish Twist Raspberry	1 serv (1.2 oz)	140	—	7
Devil's Food Cake Fudge Iced	1 serv (1.2 oz)	130	—	5
French Crumb Cake All Butter	1 serv (1.6 oz)	180	—	8
Hot Cross Buns	1 (2.3 oz)	230	2	7
Louisiana Crunch Cake	1 serv (1.7 oz)	180	—	8
Pound Loaf All Butter	1 serv (1 oz)	110	—	5
Pound Loaf Sour Cream	1 serv (1 oz)	120	—	7
Stollen Fruit	⅛ cake (2 oz)	210	2	7
Thick Fudge Golden Cake	1 serv (1.2 oz)	130	—	6
Freihofer's				
Angel Food	⅛ cake (2 oz)	150	0	0
Cinnamon Swirl Buns	1 (2.8 oz)	290	2	9
Coffee Cake Cinnamon Pecan	⅛ cake (2 oz)	220	2	9
Crumb	⅛ cake (2 oz)	240	2	11
Homestyle Golden Loaf	⅛ cake (1.8 oz)	200	2	9
Pound	⅛ cake (2.8 oz)	330	4	17
Greenfield				
Blondie Apple Spice	1 (1.4 oz)	120	0	0
Blondie Fat Free Chocolate Chip	1 (1.3 oz)	110	0	0
Hostess				
Angel Food	⅛ cake (2 oz)	160	0	2
Chocodiles	1 (1.6 oz)	240	8	11
Chocolicious	1 (1.6 oz)	190	3	7
Coffee Crumb	1 (1.1 oz)	130	2	5
Crumb Cake Light	1 (1 oz)	90	0	1
Cupcakes Chocolate	1 (1.8 oz)	180	3	6
Cupcakes Orange	1 (1.5 oz)	160	2	5
Cupcakes Light Chocolate	1 (1.6 oz)	140	1	2
Ding Dongs	2 (2.7 oz)	360	12	19
Ho Ho's	2 (2 oz)	250	8	12

FOOD	PORTION	CALS.	SAT. FAT	FAT
Hostess (CONT.)				
Honey Bun Glazed	1 (2.7 oz)	320	9	19
Honey Bun Iced	1 (3.4 oz)	410	11	24
Shortcake Dessert Cups	1 (1 oz)	100	1	2
Sno Balls	1 (1.8 oz)	180	3	5
Suzy Q's	1 (2 oz)	230	4	9
Sweet Roll Cherry	1 (2.2 oz)	210	3	6
Sweet Roll Cinnamon	1 (2.2 oz)	230	3	7
Twinkies	1 (1.5 oz)	150	2	5
Twinkies Light	1 (1.5 oz)	130	1	2
Jell-O				
Cheesecake Snack Original	1 (3.3 oz)	160	3	6
Cheesecake Snack Strawberry	1 (3.3 oz)	150	3	5
Kellogg's				
Pop-Tarts Apple Cinnamon	1 (1.8 oz)	210	1	6
Pop-Tarts Blueberry	1 (1.8 oz)	210	1	5
Pop-Tarts Brown Sugar Cinnamon	1 (1.8 oz)	210	1	6
Pop-Tarts Cherry	1 (1.8 oz)	200	1	5
Pop-Tarts Chocolate Graham	1 (1.8 oz)	210	2	6
Pop-Tarts Frosted Apple Cinnamon	1 (1.8 oz)	190	1	3
Pop-Tarts Frosted Blueberry	1 (1.8 oz)	200	1	5
Pop-Tarts Frosted Brown Sugar Cinnamon	1 (1.8 oz)	210	2	7
Pop-Tarts Frosted Cherry	1 (1.8 oz)	200	1	5
Pop-Tarts Frosted Chocolate Vanilla Creme	1 (1.8 oz)	200	1	5
Pop-Tarts Frosted Chocolate Fudge	1 (1.8 oz)	200	1	5
Pop-Tarts Frosted Grape	1 (1.8 oz)	200	1	5
Pop-Tarts Frosted Raspberry	1 (1.8 oz)	210	1	5
Pop-Tarts Frosted S'mores	1 (1.8 oz)	200	1	6
Pop-Tarts Frosted Strawberry	1 (1.8 oz)	200	1	5
Pop-Tarts Frosted Wild Berry	1 (2 oz)	210	1	5
Pop-Tarts Frosted Wild Watermelon	1 (2 oz)	210	1	5
Pop-Tarts Low Fat Blueberry	1 (1.8 oz)	190	1	3
Pop-Tarts Low Fat Cherry	1 (1.8 oz)	190	1	3
Pop-Tarts Low Fat Frosted Brown Sugar Cinnamon	1 (1.8 oz)	190	1	3
Pop-Tarts Low Fat Frosted Chocolate Fudge	1 (1.8 oz)	190	1	3

FOOD	PORTION	CALS.	SAT. FAT	FAT
Kellogg's (CONT.)				
Pop-Tarts Low Fat Frosted Strawberry	1 (1.8 oz)	190	1	3
Pop-Tarts Low Fat Strawberry	1 (1.8 oz)	190	1	3
Pop-Tarts Strawberry	1 (1.8 oz)	200	1	5
Lance				
Dunking Sticks	1 (2.75 oz)	180	3	10
Fig Cake	½ piece (2.1 oz)	110	5	2
Fig Cake Fat Free	½ piece (2.1 oz)	100	0	0
Honey Bun	1 (3 oz)	330	5	13
Pecan Twirls	1 pkg (2 oz)	220	4	9
Swiss Rolls	1 (2.5 oz)	170	5	9
Little Debbie				
Angel Cakes Lemon	1 (1.6 oz)	130	0	1
Angel Cakes Raspberry	1 (1.6 oz)	130	0	1
Banana Nut Loaves	1 (1.9 oz)	220	2	10
Banana Twins	1 (2.2 oz)	250	3	10
Be My Valentine Chocolate	1 (2.2 oz)	280	3	13
Be My Valentine Vanilla	1 (2.2 oz)	290	3	14
Blueberry Loaves	1 (2 oz)	220	2	10
Chocolate Chip	1 (2.4 oz)	310	4	15
Christmas Tree Cake	1 pkg (1.5 oz)	190	2	10
Coconut Creme	1 (1.7 oz)	210	3	10
Coffee Cake Apple	1 (2.1 oz)	230	2	7
Cupcake Creme Filled Chocolate	1 (1.6 oz)	180	2	9
Cupcake Creme Filled Orange	1 (1.7 oz)	210	3	10
Cupcake Creme Filled Strawberry	1 (1.7 oz)	210	3	10
Devil Cremes	1 (1.6 oz)	190	2	8
Devil Squares	1 (2.2 oz)	270	3	13
Easter Basket Cake Chocolate	1 (2.4 oz)	300	4	14
Easter Basket Cake Vanilla	1 (2.5 oz)	320	4	10
Fall Party Cake Chocolate	1 (2.4 oz)	290	3	14
Fall Party Cake Vanilla	1 (2.5 oz)	310	4	15
Fancy Cakes	1 (2.4 oz)	300	4	15
Frosted Fudge	1 (1.5 oz)	200	3	10
Golden Cremes	1 (1.5 oz)	150	2	5
Holiday Cake Roll Cherry Creme	1 (2.1 oz)	260	3	12
Holiday Snack Cake Chocolate	1 (2.4 oz)	300	3	14
Holiday Snack Cake Vanilla	1 (2.5 oz)	320	4	15
Honey Bun	1 (1.8 oz)	220	4	13
Pecan Spinwheels	1 (1 oz)	110	1	4

FOOD	PORTION	CALS.	SAT. FAT	FAT
Little Debbie (CONT.)				
Snack Cake Chocolate	1 (2.5 oz)	310	4	15
Strawberry Shortcake Roll	1 (2.1 oz)	230	2	8
Swiss Rolls	1 (2.1 oz)	270	3	12
Zebra Cakes	1 (2.6 oz)	330	4	16
Nabisco				
Frosted Strawberry	1 (1.7 oz)	190	2	5
Nature's Choice				
Toaster Pastries Fat Free Apple Cinnamon	1 (1.9 oz)	180	0	0
Toaster Pastries Fat Free Blueberry	1 (1.9 oz)	180	0	0
Toaster Pastries Fat Free Raspberry	1 (1.9 oz)	180	0	0
Toaster Pastries Fat Free Strawberry	1 (1.9 oz)	180	0	0
Toaster Pastries Low Fat Cherry	1 (1.9 oz)	180	0	3
Toaster Pastries Low Fat Frosted Blueberry	1 (1.9 oz)	190	0	2
Toaster Pastries Low Fat Frosted Chocolate	1 (1.9 oz)	200	0	3
Toaster Pastries Low Fat Frosted Cinnamon	1 (1.9 oz)	190	0	2
Toaster Pastries Low Fat Frosted Strawberry	1 (1.9 oz)	190	0	2
Toaster Pastries Low Fat Peach Apricot	1 (1.9 oz)	180	0	3
Pepperidge Farm				
Apple Turnover	1 (3.1 oz)	330	3	14
Blueberry Turnovers	1 (3.1 oz)	340	3	16
Cherry Turnover	1 (3.1 oz)	320	3	13
Large Layer Chocolate Fudge	⅛ cake (2.4 oz)	260	3	11
Large Layer Coconut	⅛ cake (2.4 oz)	260	3	11
Large Layer Vanilla	⅛ cake (2.4 oz)	250	3	11
Mini Turnover Apple	1 (1.4 oz)	140	2	8
Mini Turnover Cherry	1 (1.4 oz)	140	2	8
Mini Turnover Strawberry	1 (1.4 oz)	140	2	7
Peach Turnover	1 (3.1 oz)	340	3	15
Raspberry Turnovers	1 (3.1 oz)	330	3	14
Perugina				
Pannettone Au Beurre	⅛ cake (2.9 oz)	310	5	12
Pet-Ritz				
Cobbler Apple	⅙ cake (4.33 oz)	290	—	9

FOOD	PORTION	CALS.	SAT. FAT	FAT
Pet-Ritz (CONT.)				
Cobbler Blackberry	⅙ cake (4.33 oz)	250	—	10
Cobbler Blueberry	⅙ cake (4.33 oz)	270	—	12
Cobbler Cherry	⅙ cake (4.33 oz)	280	—	10
Cobbler Peach	⅙ cake (4.33 oz)	260	—	10
Cobbler Strawberry	⅙ cake (4.33 oz)	290	—	9
Pillsbury				
Apple Turnovers	1 (2 oz)	170	2	8
Cherry Turnovers	1 (2 oz)	180	2	8
Sara Lee				
Banana	⅛ cake (2.3 oz)	230	3	8
Banana Sundae	⅒ cake (2.8 oz)	270	10	14
Carrot	⅛ cake (3.2 oz)	320	4	17
Cheesecake Cherry	¼ cake (4.7 oz)	350	5	12
Cheesecake Chocolate Chip	¼ cake (4.2 oz)	410	14	21
Cheesecake Chocolate Mousse	⅕ cake	400	20	25
Cheesecake French	⅙ cake	350	13	21
Cheesecake Singles Fudge Brownie Crumble	1 slice (4 oz)	400	15	22
Cheesecake Singles Strawberry Drizzle	1 slice (4 oz)	380	13	20
Cheesecake Strawberry	¼ pie (4.7 oz)	330	5	12
Cheesecake Strawberry French	⅙ cake	320	9	14
Cheesecake Bars Chocolate Dipped Original	1 bar (2.7 oz)	190	11	14
Cheesecake Bites Chocolate Praline Pecan	1 piece (0.8 oz)	100	4	6
Cheesecake Bites Chocolate Dipped Original	1 piece (0.8 oz)	100	5	7
Cheesecake Bits Toasted Almond Crunch	1 (0.8 oz)	90	5	6
Coffee Cake Butter Streusel	⅙ cake (1.9 oz)	220	6	12
Coffee Cake Cheese	⅙ cake (1.9 oz)	180	2	6
Coffee Cake Crumb	⅛ cake (2 oz)	220	2	9
Coffee Cake Pecan	⅙ cake (1.9 oz)	230	5	12
Coffee Cake Raspberry	⅙ cake (1.9 oz)	200	3	8
Harvest Pumpkin Spice	⅛ cake (2.9 oz)	270	9	14
Layer Cake Coconut	⅛ cake (2.8 oz)	280	12	14
Layer Cake Double Chocolate	⅛ cake (2.8 oz)	260	11	13
Layer Cake Fudge Golden	⅛ cake (2.8 oz)	270	10	13
Layer Cake German Chocolate	⅛ cake (2.9 oz)	280	11	15
Layer Cake Vanilla	⅛ cake (2.8 oz)	250	10	13
Origial Cheesecake Reduced Fat	¼ cake (4.2 oz)	310	8	13

FOOD	PORTION	CALS.	SAT. FAT	FAT
Sara Lee (CONT.)				
Pound Cake	¼ cake (2.7 oz)	320	9	16
Pound Cake Chocolate Swirl	1 slice (1 oz)	110	3	5
Pound Cake Family Size	⅙ cake (2.7 oz)	310	9	177
Pound Cake Free & Light	¼ cake (2.5 oz)	200	1	4
Pound Cake Golden	1 slice (1 oz)	120	1	5
Pound Cake Reduced Fat	1 slice (1 oz)	100	1	4
Pound Cake Strawberry	¼ cake (2.9 oz)	290	3	11
Red White & Blueberry	⅒ cake (3 oz)	210	6	8
Slice Chocolate	1 (3 oz)	320	4	16
Strawberry Shortcake	⅛ cake (2.5 oz)	180	5	7
Sinbad				
Baklava	1 piece (2 oz)	337	4	20
Tastykake				
Banana Creamie	1 (1.5 oz)	170	1	7
Bear Claw Appled	1 (3 oz)	280	2	7
Bear Claw Cinnamon	1 (3 oz)	300	2	8
Big Texas	1 (3 oz)	300	2	9
Breakfast Bun Chocolate Raisin	1 (3.2 oz)	330	2	8
Bunny Trail Treats	1 (1.3 oz)	150	1	6
Chocolate Creamie	1 (1.5 oz)	180	1	8
Chocolate Krimpies	2 (2.2 oz)	240	2	10
Coffee Roll Glazed	1 (3 oz)	300	2	9
Coffee Roll Vanilla	1 (3.2 oz)	320	2	9
Cupcakes Butter Cream Cream Filled Iced	2 (2.2 oz)	240	2	8
Cupcakes Chocolate Cream Filled Iced	2 (2.2 oz)	230	1	8
Cupcakes Cupcake	2 (2.1 oz)	200	1	5
Cupcakes Low Fat Chocolate Cream Filled	2 (2.2 oz)	200	1	3
Cupcakes Low Fat Vanilla Cream Filled	2 (2.2 oz)	190	0	2
Cupid Kake	1 (1.3 oz)	150	1	6
Honey Bun Glazed	1 (3.2 oz)	350	4	17
Honey Bun Iced	1 (3.2 oz)	350	4	17
Junior Chocolate	1 (3.3 oz)	330	2	12
Junior Coconut	1 (3.3 oz)	310	4	8
Junior Koffee Kake	1 (2.5 oz)	270	2	9
Junior Pound Kake	1 (3 oz)	320	5	13
Kandy Kakes Chocolate	3 (2 oz)	250	8	13
Kandy Kakes Coconut	2 (2.7 oz)	330	13	18
Kandy Kakes Peanut Butter	2 (1.3 oz)	190	5	9
Koffee Kake Cream Filled	2 (2 oz)	240	2	10

FOOD	PORTION	CALS.	SAT. FAT	FAT
Tastykake (CONT.)				
Koffee Kake Low Fat Apple	2 (2 oz)	170	0	2
Koffee Kake Low Fat Lemon	2 (2 oz)	180	0	3
Koffee Kake Low Fat Raspberry	2 (2 oz)	170	0	2
Kreepy Kakes	2 (2.2 oz)	240	2	8
Kreme Krimpies	2 (2 oz)	230	1	9
Krimpets Butterscotch Iced	2 (2 oz)	210	1	5
Krimpets Jelly Filled	2 (2 oz)	190	1	3
Krimpets Strawberry	2 (2 oz)	210	1	5
Kringle Kake	1 (1.3 oz)	150	1	6
Santa Snacks	2 (2.2 oz)	240	2	8
Sparkle Kake	1 (1.3 oz)	150	1	6
Tasty Tweets	2 (2.2 oz)	240	2	8
Tropical Delight Coconut	2 (2 oz)	190	5	9
Tropical Delight Guava	2 (2 oz)	190	4	7
Tropical Delight Papaya	2 (2 oz)	200	4	7
Tropical Delight Pineapple	2 (2 oz)	200	4	7
Vanilla Creamie	1 (1.5 oz)	190	1	9
Witchy Treat	1 (1.3 oz)	150	1	6
Toastettes				
Frosted Blueberry	1 (1.7 oz)	190	2	5
Frosted Brown Sugar Cinnamon	1 (1.7 oz)	190	2	5
Frosted Cherry	1 (1.7 oz)	190	2	5
Frosted Fudge	1 (1.7 oz)	190	2	5
Strawberry	1 (1.7 oz)	190	2	5
Tortuga				
Cayman Island Rum Cake	1 piece (2 oz)	194	2	9
Weight Watchers				
Chocolate Raspberry Royale	1 (3.5 oz)	190	1	3
Chocolate Eclair	1 (2.1 oz)	150	1	4
Danish Coffee Cake Apple Cinnamon	1 piece (1.9 oz)	160	1	3
Danish Coffee Cake Cheese	1 piece (1.9 oz)	160	1	3
Danish Coffee Cake Raspberry	1 piece (1.9 oz)	160	1	3
Double Fudge	1 piece (2.75 oz)	190	2	4
French Style Cheesecake	1 piece (3.9 oz)	170	2	4
New York Style Cheesecake	1 piece (2.5 oz)	150	3	5
Strawberry Parfait Royale	1 (5.24 oz)	180	1	2
Triple Chocolate Eclair	1 (2.14 oz)	160	1	5
Well-Bred Loaf				
Banana Bread	1 slice (3.5 oz)	330	5	11
Banana Nut	1 slice (4.3 oz)	440	8	19
Blueberry	1 slice (4.3 oz)	440	10	16
Carrot	1 slice (4.3 oz)	480	11	24

FOOD	PORTION	CALS.	SAT. FAT	FAT
Well-Bred Loaf (CONT.)				
Carrot Traditional	1 slice (4.3 oz)	440	6	16
Chocolate Chip	1 slice (4.3 oz)	490	11	19
Cinnamon Walnut	1 slice (4.3 oz)	480	10	18
Coconut Rum	1 slice (4.3 oz)	490	13	23
Cranberry	1 slice (4.3 oz)	460	9	15
Marble	1 slice (4.3 oz)	530	11	18
Pound All Butter	1 slice (4.3 oz)	470	10	17
Pound Mandarin Orange	1 slice (4 oz)	460	5	18
Raisin	1 slice (4.3 oz)	460	9	15
TAKE-OUT				
angelfood	1/12 cake (1 oz)	73	tr	tr
apple crisp	½ cup (5 oz)	230	1	5
boston cream pie	1/6 cake (3.3 oz)	293	4	12
carrot w/ cream cheese icing	1/12 cake (3.9 oz)	484	5	29
cheesecake w/ cherry topping	1/12 cake (5 oz)	359	13	23
chocolate w/ chocolate frosting	1/8 cake (2.2 oz)	235	3	11
coffeecake cheese	1/6 cake (2.7 oz)	258	4	12
coffeecake crumb topped cheese	1/6 cake (2.7 oz)	258	4	12
coffeecake crumb topped cinnamon	1/9 cake (2.2 oz)	263	4	15
cream puff w/ custard filling	1 (4.6 oz)	336	5	20
eclair w/ chocolate icing & custard filling	1	205	—	10
french apple tart	1 (3.5 oz)	302	9	15
fruitcake	1/36 cake (2.9 oz)	302	1	10
gingerbread	1/9 cake (2.6 oz)	264	3	12
panettone dal forno	1/9 cake (1.9 oz)	212	4	8
petit fours	2 (0.9 oz)	120	3	7
pineapple upside down	1/9 cake (4 oz)	367	3	14
pound fat free	1 oz	80	tr	tr
pound cake	1 slice (1 oz)	120	1	5
sheet cake w/ white frosting	1/9 cake	445	5	14
strudel apple	1 piece (2½ oz)	195	2	8
tiramisu	1 piece (5.1 oz)	409	15	30
yellow w/ vanilla frosting	1/8 cake (2.2 oz)	239	2	9
CAKE ICING				
chocolate as prep w/ butter	1/12 box (1.5 oz)	161	—	6
chocolate as prep w/ butter	1 box (13.7 oz)	1908	—	65
chocolate as prep w/ butter home recipe	1/12 recipe (1.8 oz)	200	4	6
chocolate as prep w/ butter home recipe	1 recipe (21.1 oz)	2409	43	69
chocolate as prep w/ margarine	1 box (13.7 oz)	1909	—	65

FOOD	PORTION	CALS.	SAT. FAT	FAT
chocolate as prep w/ margarine	½ box (1.5 oz)	161	—	6
chocolate as prep w/ margarine home recipe	½ recipe (1.8 oz)	200	1	6
chocolate as prep w/ margarine home recipe	1 recipe (21.1 oz)	2411	16	69
chocolate ready-to-use	½ pkg (1.3 oz)	151	2	7
chocolate ready-to-use	1 pkg (16 oz)	1834	26	81
coconut ready-to-use	1 pkg (16 oz)	1903	32	111
coconut ready-to-use	½ pkg (1.3 oz)	157	3	9
cream cheese ready-to-use	1 pkg (16 oz)	1906	23	80
cream cheese ready-to-use	½ pkg (1.3 oz)	157	2	7
glaze home recipe	1 recipe (11.5 oz)	1173	6	26
glaze home recipe	½ recipe (1 oz)	97	tr	2
seven minute home recipe	1 recipe (13.6 oz)	1231	0	0
seven minute home recipe	½ recipe (1.1 oz)	102	0	0
sour cream ready-to-use	½ pkg (1.3 oz)	157	2	7
sour cream ready-to-use	1 pkg (16 oz)	1904	23	80
vanilla as prep w/ butter	½ pkg (1.5 oz)	182	—	7
vanilla as prep w/ butter	1 pkg (14.5 oz)	2188	—	86
vanilla as prep w/ butter home recipe	½ recipe (1.7 oz)	165	1	2
vanilla as prep w/ butter home recipe	1 recipe (20.1 oz)	1972	14	24
vanilla as prep w/ margarine	1 pkg (14.5 oz)	2190	—	86
vanilla as prep w/ margarine	½ pkg (1.5 oz)	182	—	7
vanilla as prep w/ margarine home recipe	½ recipe (1.7 oz)	195	1	5
vanilla as prep w/ margarine home recipe	1 recipe (20.1 oz)	2326	13	62
vanilla ready-to-use	½ pkg (1.3 oz)	159	2	6
vanilla ready-to-use	1 pkg (16 oz)	1936	23	78
white as prep w/ water	1 pkg (11.1 oz)	770	—	0
white as prep w/ water	½ pkg (0.9 oz)	64	—	0
Betty Crocker				
Mix Coconut Pecan as prep	2 tbsp	160	3	8
Mix White Fluffy as prep	6 tbsp	100	0	0
Ready-To-Spread Butter Cream	2 tbsp (1.3 oz)	150	2	6
Ready-To-Spread Cherry	2 tbsp (1.2 oz)	140	2	5
Ready-To-Spread Chocolate	2 tbsp (1.2 oz)	130	2	5
Ready-To-Spread Chocolate w/ Stars	2 tbsp (1.2 oz)	140	2	5
Ready-To-Spread Coconut Pecan	2 tbsp (1.2 oz)	140	3	8

FOOD	PORTION	CALS.	SAT. FAT	FAT
Betty Crocker (CONT.)				
Ready-To-Spread Cream Cheese	2 tbsp (1.2 oz)	140	2	5
Ready-To-Spread Dark Chocolate	2 tbsp (1.3 oz)	140	2	6
Ready-To-Spread French Vanilla	2 tbsp (1.2 oz)	140	2	5
Ready-To-Spread Lemon	2 tbsp (1.2 oz)	140	2	5
Ready-To-Spread Milk Chocolate	2 tbsp (1.3 oz)	150	2	6
Ready-To-Spread Rainbow Chip	2 tbsp (1.2 oz)	140	3	6
Ready-To-Spread Sour Cream Chocolate	2 tbsp (1.3 oz)	150	2	6
Ready-To-Spread Sour Cream White	2 tbsp (1.3 oz)	150	2	6
Ready-To-Spread Strawberry Cream Cheese	2 tbsp (1.3 oz)	150	2	6
Ready-To-Spread Vanilla	2 tbsp (1.2 oz)	140	2	5
Ready-To-Spread Vanilla w/ Stars	2 tbsp (1.2 oz)	140	2	5
Ready-To-Spread Whipped Deluxe Chocolate	2 tbsp (0.8 oz)	100	2	5
Ready-To-Spread Whipped Deluxe Cream Cheese	2 tbsp (0.8 oz)	100	2	5
Ready-To-Spread Whipped Deluxe Fluffy White	2 tbsp (0.8 oz)	100	2	4
Ready-To-Spread Whipped Deluxe Lemon	2 tbsp (0.8 oz)	100	2	5
Ready-To-Spread Whipped Deluxe Milk Chocolate	2 tbsp (0.8 oz)	100	2	5
Ready-To-Spread Whipped Deluxe Strawberry	2 tbsp (0.8 oz)	100	2	5
Ready-To-Spread Whipped Deluxe Vanilla	2 tbsp (0.8 oz)	100	2	5
Ready-To-Spread White Chocolate	2 tbsp (1.2 oz)	140	2	5
Duncan Hines				
Chocolate Creamy Homestyle	2 tbsp	130	2	5
Milk Chocolate Creamy Homestyle	2 tbsp	130	2	5
Vanilla Creamy Homestyle	2 tbsp	140	2	5
Estee				
Frosting as prep	⅓ pkg	100	0	0
Jiffy				
Fudge	¼ cup (1.2 oz)	150	2	4
White	¼ cup (1.2 oz)	150	1	5

FOOD	PORTION	CALS.	SAT. FAT	FAT
Sweet Rewards				
Ready-To-Spread Reduced Fat Chocolate	2 tbsp (1.2 oz)	120	1	3
Ready-To-Spread Reduced Fat Milk Chocolate	2 tbsp (1.2 oz)	120	1	3
Ready-To-Spread Reduced Fat Vanilla	2 tbsp (1.2 oz)	120	1	2
CAKE MIX				
(see *also* CAKE)				
angelfood	10 in cake (20.9 oz)	1535	tr	2
angelfood	1/12 cake (1.8 oz)	129	tr	tr
carrot w/o frosting	2 layers (29.6 oz)	2886	22	133
carrot w/o frosting	1/12 cake (2.5 oz)	239	2	11
cheesecake no-bake	1/8 cake (3.5 oz)	271	7	13
chocolate pudding type w/o frosting	2 layers (32.4 oz)	3234	35	172
chocolate pudding type w/o frosting	1/12 cake (2.7 oz)	270	3	14
chocolate w/o frosting	2 layers (26.8 oz)	2393	21	92
chocolate w/o frosting	1/12 cake (2.3 oz)	198	2	8
chocolate w/o frosting low sodium	1/10 cake (1.3 oz)	116	1	3
coffeecake crumb topped cinnamon	1/8 cake (2 oz)	178	1	5
devil's food w/o frosting	1/12 cake (2.3 oz)	198	2	8
devil's food w/ chocolate frosting	1/16 cake	235	4	8
devil's food w/ chocolate frosting	1 cake 9 in diam	3755	56	136
fudge w/o frosting	1/12 cake (2.3 oz)	198	2	8
german chocolate pudding type w/ coconut nut frosting	1/12 cake (3.9 oz)	404	5	21
gingerbread	1 cake 8 in sq	1575	10	39
gingerbread	1/9 5cake (2.4 oz)	207	2	7
lemon w/o frosting no sugar low sodium	1/10 cake (1.3 oz)	118	tr	3
marble pudding type w/o frosting	1/12 cake (2.6 oz)	253	2	12
marble pudding type w/o frosting	2 layers (30.6 oz)	3021	27	148
white pudding type w/o frosting	1/12 cake (2.4 oz)	244	2	10
white pudding type w/o frosting	2 layers (29 oz)	2915	23	123
white w/o frosting	2 layer cake (26 oz)	2265	9	57
white w/o frosting	1/12 cake (2.2 oz)	190	1	5
white w/o frosting no sugar low sodium	1/10 cake (1.3 oz)	118	tr	3
yellow pudding-type w/o frosting	1/12 cake (2.6 oz)	257	2	12
yellow pudding-type w/o frosting	2 layers (31 oz)	3084	28	139
yellow w/ chocolate frosting	1/16 cake	235	3	8
yellow w/o frosting	1/12 cake (2.2 oz)	202	1	6

FOOD	PORTION	CALS.	SAT. FAT	FAT
yellow w/o frosting	2 layers (26.5 oz)	2415	12	71
yellow w/ chocolate frosting	1 cake 9 in diam	3895	92	175
Aunt Jemima				
Coffee Cake Easy Mix	⅓ cup (1.4 oz)	170	1	5
Betty Crocker				
Angel Food Confetti	1/12 cake	150	0	0
Angel Food One-Step White	1/12 cake	140	0	0
Angel Food Swirl	1/12 cake	150	0	0
Angel Food Traditional	1/12 cake	130	0	0
Butter Chocolate	1/12 cake	270	7	13
Butter Pecan	1/12 cake	250	3	11
Butter Pecan No Cholesterol Recipe	1/12 cake	210	2	7
Butter Yellow	1/12 cake	260	6	11
Carrot	1/10 cake	320	2	15
Carrot No Cholesterol Recipe	1/10 cake	260	2	9
Cherry Chip	1/10 cake	280	3	11
Cherry Chip	1/10 cake	290	3	12
Chocolate Chip	1/12 cake	280	3	14
Chocolate Chip No Cholesterol Recipe	1/12 cake	210	2	7
Chocolate Fudge	1/12 cake	270	3	12
Coffee Cake Cinnamon Streusel	1/12 cake	170	2	7
Devils Food	1/12 cake	240	3	11
Devils Food No Cholesterol Recipe	1/12 cake	200	2	6
Double Chocolate Swirl	1/12 cake	250	3	11
Double Chocolate Swirl No Cholesterol Recipe	1/12 cake	230	2	9
Easy Angel Food	¼ cake	170	0	0
Fat Free Apple Cinnamon	⅛ cake	170	0	0
Fat Free Banana	⅛ cake	170	0	0
Fat Free Chocolate	⅛ cake	170	0	0
Fat Free Lemon	⅛ cake	170	0	0
French Vanilla	1/12 cake	250	3	10
French Vanilla No Cholesterol Recipe	1/12 cake	210	2	7
Fudge Marble	1/12 cake	250	3	11
Fudge Marble No Cholesterol Recipe	1/12 cake	220	2	7
German Chocolate	1/12 cake	250	3	11
German Chocolate No Cholesterol Recipe	1/12 cake	220	2	7

FOOD	PORTION	CALS.	SAT. FAT	FAT
Betty Crocker (CONT.)				
Gingerbread	1/8 cake	230	2	6
Gingerbread No Cholesterol Recipe	1/8 cake	220	2	6
Golden Vanilla	1/12 cake	280	3	14
Golden Vanilla No Cholesterol Recipe	1/12 cake	220	2	7
Lemon	1/12 cake	280	3	14
Lemon No Cholesterol Recipe	1/12 cake	230	2	8
Milk Chocolate	1/12 cake	240	3	10
Milk Chocolate No Cholesterol Recipe	1/12 cake	230	2	9
Party Swirl	1/12 cake	250	3	11
Party Swirl No Cholesterol Recipe	1/12 cake	220	2	7
Peanut Butter Chocolate Swirl	1/12 cake	240	3	10
Peanut Butter Chocolate Swirl No Cholesterol Recipe	1/12 cake	210	2	6
Pineapple Upside Down	1/6 cake	400	4	15
Pineapple Upside Down No Cholesterol Recipe	1/6 cake	390	4	14
Pound Cake	1/8 cake	260	3	8
Pound Cake No Cholesterol Recipe	1/8 cake	250	3	7
Rainbow Chip	1/12 cake	250	3	11
Reduced Fat White	1/12 cake	190	1	4
Sour Cream White	1/10 cake	280	3	12
Spice	1/12 cake	250	3	11
Spice No Cholesterol Recipe	1/12 cake	220	2	7
Stir'n Bake Carrot Cake w/ Cream Cheese	1 serv	250	2	7
Stir'n Bake Cinnamon Streusel Coffee Cake	1 serv	200	2	6
Stir'n Bake Devils Food w/ Chocolate	1 serv	240	2	7
Strawberry Swirl	1/10 cake	290	3	12
Strawberry Swirl No Cholesterol Recipe	1/10 cake	250	2	7
White No Cholesterol Recipe	1/12 cake	230	3	10
White Richer Recipe	1/12 cake	250	3	11
White Chocolate Swirl	1/12 cake	250	3	11
White Chocolate Swirl No Cholesterol Recipe	1/12 cake	210	2	7
White Olympic Party Cake	1/12 cake	240	3	11

FOOD	PORTION	CALS.	SAT. FAT	FAT
Betty Crocker (CONT.)				
White Olympic Party Cake Richer Recipe	1/12 cake	250	4	11
Yellow	1/12 cake	250	3	10
Yellow No Cholesterol Recipe	1/12 cake	230	2	9
Bisquick				
Mix	1/3 cup (1.4 oz)	170	2	6
Reduced Fat	1/3 cup (1.4 oz)	150	1	3
Dromedary				
Date Bread	1/11 cake (2 oz)	190	2	7
Date Nut Roll	½ in slice	80	—	2
Gingerbread	1 piece (2 in x 2 in)	100	—	2
Pound	½ in slice	150	—	6
Duncan Hines				
Angel Food as prep	1/12 pkg (1.3 oz)	140	0	0
Butter Recipe Golden as prep	1/12 cake	320	7	16
Cupcake Yellow as prep	1	180	2	0
Dark Chocolate Fudge as prep	1/12 cake	290	3	15
Devil's Food Moist Deluxe as prep	1/12 cake (1.5 oz)	290	3	15
French Vanilla	1/12 cake (1.5 oz)	250	2	11
Fudge Marble Moist Deluxe as prep	1/12 cake (1.5 oz)	250	2	17
Lemon Supreme Moist Deluxe	1/12 cake (1.5 oz)	250	2	17
White Moist Deluxe as prep	1/12 cake	190	1	6
Yellow Moist Deluxe as prep	1/12 cake (1.5 oz)	250	11	17
Yellow Moist Deluxe as prep	1/12 cake	250	2	11
Estee				
Chocolate as prep	1/5 cake	190	2	4
White as prep	1/5 cake	200	2	4
Hain				
Whole Wheat Baking Mix	1.5 oz	150	—	1
Jell-O				
No Bake Cherry Cheesecake as prep	1/8 cake (4.8 oz)	340	5	12
No Bake Double Layer Chocolate as prep	1/8 cake (4.4 oz)	260	5	12
No Bake Double Layer Cookies And Creme as prep	1/8 cake (4.5 oz)	390	7	19
No Bake Double Layer Lemon as prep	1/8 cake (4.4 oz)	260	4	12
No Bake Homestyle Cheesecake as prep	1/8 cake (4.6 oz)	360	4	15

FOOD	PORTION	CALS.	SAT. FAT	FAT
Jell-O (CONT.)				
No Bake Peanut Butter Cup as prep	⅛ cake (3.8 oz)	380	10	23
No Bake Reduced Fat Strawberry Swirl Cheesecake as prep	⅛ cake (4 oz)	250	2	6
No Bake Strawberry Cheesecake as prep	⅛ cake (4.8 oz)	340	5	12
Real Cheesecake as prep	⅛ cake (4.6 oz)	360	6	16
Jiffy				
Devil's Food as prep	⅕ cake	220	2	6
Golden Yellow as prep	⅕ cake	220	1	5
White as prep	⅕ cake	210	1	5
Pillsbury				
Strawberry	1/12 cake	260	—	11
Sweet Rewards				
Reduced Fat Devils Food	1/12 cake	200	2	5
Reduced Fat Devils Food No Cholesterol Recipe	1/12 cake	190	1	4
Reduced Fat White Whole Egg Recipe	1/12 cake	200	2	5
Reduced Fat Yellow	1/12 cake	200	1	5
Reduced Fat Yellow No Cholesterol Recipe	1/12 cake	190	1	4
Wanda's				
Double Chocolate	¼ cup mix per serv (1.4 oz)	170	1	2
CALABAZA				
fresh	½ cup	32	—	tr
CALZONE				
TAKE-OUT				
cheese	1 (12 oz)	1020	24	54
CANADIAN BACON				
grilled	1 pkg (6 oz)	257	4	12
Boar's Head				
Canadian Bacon	2 oz	70	1	3
Hormel				
Canadian Bacon	2 oz	70	2	3
Oscar Mayer				
Canandian Bacon	2 slices (1.6 oz)	50	1	2
Yorkshire Farms				
Uncured	3 oz	100	2	4

FOOD	PORTION	CALS.	SAT. FAT	FAT
CANDY				
(see also MARSHMALLOW)				
butterscotch	1 piece (6 g)	24	tr	tr
butterscotch	1 oz	112	tr	1
candy corn	1 oz	105	0	0
caramels	1 pkg (2.5 oz)	271	5	6
caramels	1 piece (8 g)	31	1	1
caramels chocolate	1 piece (6 g)	22	tr	tr
caramels chocolate	1 bar (2.3 oz)	231	tr	2
carob bar	1 (3.1 oz)	453	7	28
crisped rice bar almond	1 bar (1 oz)	130	1	6
crisped rice bar chocolate chip	1 bar (1 oz)	115	1	4
dark chocolate	1 oz	150	6	10
fondant chocolate coated	1 sm (0.4 oz)	40	1	1
fondant chocolate coated	1 lg (1.2 oz)	128	2	3
fondant mint	1 oz	105	0	0
gumdrops	10 sm (0.4 oz)	135	0	0
gumdrops	10 lg (3.8 oz)	420	0	0
hard candy	1 oz	106	0	0
jelly beans	10 sm (0.4 oz)	40	—	tr
jelly beans	10 lg (1 oz)	104	—	tr
lollipop	1 (6 g)	22	0	0
marzipan	1 oz	128	1	7
milk chocolate	1 bar (1.55 oz)	226	8	14
milk chocolate crisp	1 bar (1.45 oz)	203	7	11
milk chocolate w/ almonds	1 bar (1.45 oz)	215	7	14
peanut bar	1 (1.4 oz)	209	2	14
peanuts chocolate covered	10 (1.4 oz)	208	6	13
peanuts chocolate covered	1 cup (5.2 oz)	773	22	50
pretzels chocolate covered	1 oz	130	2	5
pretzels chocolate covered	1 (0.4 oz)	50	1	2
sesame crunch	1 oz	146	1	9
sesame crunch	20 pieces (1.2 oz)	181	2	12
sweet chocolate	1 bar (1.45 oz)	201	8	14
sweet chocolate	1 oz	143	6	10
100 Grand				
Bar	1 bar (1.5 oz)	200	5	8
3 Musketeers				
Bar	2 fun size (1.2 oz)	140	3	4
Bar	1 (2.1 oz)	260	4	8
5th Avenue				
Snack Size	1 bar (0.58)	80	2	4
Almond Joy				
Snack Size	1 (0.68 oz)	90	4	5

FOOD	PORTION	CALS.	SAT. FAT	FAT
Andes				
Chocolate Covered Mint Patties	1 (0.5 oz)	60	1	1
Baby Ruth				
Bar	1 (2.1 oz)	270	7	13
Fun Size	2 pieces	200	5	9
Barricini				
Dark Chocolate Raspberry Creme Shells	1 piece (0.3 oz)	47	1	3
Bits O Brickle				
Candy	1 tbsp (0.5 oz)	80	2	5
Bonus				
Bar	1 bar (2.1 oz)	290	7	16
Breath Savers				
Sugar Free Mint Cinnamon	1 piece (2 g)	10	0	0
Sugar Free Peppermint	1 piece (2 g)	10	0	0
Sugar Free Spearmint	1 piece (2 g)	10	—	0
Sugar Free Wintergreen	1 piece (2 g)	10	—	0
Brock				
Butterscotch Discs	3 pieces (0.6 oz)	70	0	0
Candy Corn	21 pieces (1.4 oz)	150	0	0
Candy Rolls	2 rolls (0.5 oz)	50	0	0
Caramel Dots	3 pieces (1.3 oz)	140	1	3
Cinnamon Discs	3 pieces (0.6 oz)	70	0	0
Circus Peanuts	11 pieces (2.5 oz)	260	0	0
Coconut Mountains	4 pieces (1.4 oz)	170	1	6
Fruit Basket	3 pieces (0.6 oz)	60	0	0
Fruit Kisses	3 pieces (0.6 oz)	70	0	0
Glitters	2 pieces (0.5 oz)	50	0	0
Gummy Bears	5 pieces (1.4 oz)	130	0	0
Gummy Squirms	5 pieces (1.3 oz)	120	0	0
Jelly Beans	12 pieces (1.4 oz)	140	0	0
Lemon Drops	3 pieces (0.5 oz)	60	0	0
Orange Slices	4 pieces (1.5 oz)	140	0	0
Party Mints	9 pieces (0.5 oz)	60	0	0
Peanut Butter Crunch	3 pieces (0.6 oz)	80	—	2
Pops Assorted	2 (0.5 oz)	60	0	0
Sour Balls	3 pieces (0.6 oz)	70	0	0
Sour Sharks	23 pieces (2.5 oz)	30	1	3
Spearmint Starlights	3 pieces (0.6 oz)	60	0	0
Spice Drops	12 pieces (1.4 oz)	130	0	0
Starlight Mints	3 pieces (0.6 oz)	60	0	0
Toffee	6 pieces (1.5 oz)	170	2	5
Butterfinger				
BB's	1 pkg (1.7 oz)	230	7	10
Bar	1 (2.1 oz)	280	6	11
Fun Size	2 bars (1.6 oz)	200	4	8

FOOD	PORTION	CALS.	SAT. FAT	FAT
Carmello				
Snack Size	1 (0.66 oz)	90	3	4
Cellas				
Chocolate Covered Cherries Dark Chocolate	2 pieces (1 oz)	100	3	4
Chocolate Covered Cherries Milk Chocolate	2 pieces (1 oz)	110	3	4
Certs				
Breath Mints	1 piece (1.67 g)	6	0	0
Mini Sugar Free	1 piece (0.365 g)	1	0	0
Sugar Free	1 piece (1.67 g)	7	0	0
Charleston Chew				
Candy	1 pkg (1.9 oz)	230	6	7
Chocolate	½ bar	120	—	3
Strawberry	½ bar	120	—	3
Vanilla	½ bar	120	—	3
Charms				
Blow Pop	1 (0.6 oz)	70	0	0
Lollipop Sour	1 (0.6 oz)	70	0	0
Lollipop Sweet	1 (0.6 oz)	70	0	0
Chuckles				
Candy	4 pieces (1.4 oz)	140	0	0
Chunky				
Bar	1 (1.4 oz)	200	6	11
Clorets				
Mints	1 piece (1.67 g)	6	0	0
Crunch				
Fun Size	4 bars (1.5 oz)	200	6	10
Del Monte				
Radical Raizins Cinnamon	1 pkg (0.7 oz)	70	0	0
Radical Raizins Rainbow	1 pkg (0.7 oz)	70	0	0
Dove				
Dark Chocolate	¼ bar (1.5 oz)	230	8	14
Dark Chocolate	1 bar (1.3 oz)	200	7	12
Dark Chocolate Minatures	7 (1.5 oz)	220	8	14
Milk Chocolate	1 bar (1.3 oz)	200	7	12
Milk Chocolate	¼ bar (1.5 oz)	230	8	13
Milk Chocolate Miniatures	7 (1.5 oz)	230	8	13
Truffles	3 (1.2 oz)	200	9	13
Dream				
Caramel & Nougat In Milk Chocolate	1 bar (1 oz)	90	2	3
Estee				
Caramels Vanilla & Chocolate	5	115	1	5
Dark Chocolate	½ bar (1.4 oz)	200	8	14

FOOD	PORTION	CALS.	SAT. FAT	FAT
Estee (CONT.)				
Milk Chocolate	½ bar (1.4 oz)	230	10	17
Milk Chocolate w/ Almonds	½ bar (1.4 oz)	230	9	17
Milk Chocolate w/ Crisp Rice	½ bar (1.2 oz)	370	15	26
Milk Chocolate w/ Fruit & Nuts	½ bar (1.4 oz)	220	9	16
Mint Chocolate	½ bar (1.4 oz)	200	8	14
Peanut Brittle	⅓ box (1.3 oz)	160	2	9
Peanut Butter Cups	5	200	7	12
Sugar Free Assorted Fruit	5	30	0	0
Sugar Free Assorted Mint	5	30	0	0
Sugar Free Butterscotch	2	25	0	0
Sugar Free Fruit Gum Drops	23	80	0	0
Sugar Free Gourmet Jelly Beans	26	70	0	0
Sugar Free Gummy Apple Rings	5	70	0	0
Sugar Free Gummy Bears Assorted Fruit	17	100	0	0
Sugar Free Licorice Gum Drops	11	90	0	0
Sugar Free Peppermint Swirl	3	30	0	0
Sugar Free Sour Citrus Slices	9	60	0	0
Sugar Free Toffee	5	30	0	0
Sugar Free Tropical Fruit	5	30	0	0
Favorite Brands				
Candy Corn	24 pieces (1.4 oz)	150	0	0
Cinnamon Imperials	52 (0.5 oz)	80	0	0
Circus Peanuts	5 pieces (1.6 oz)	160	0	0
Gummallo Apple Ring	5 pieces (1.4 oz)	120	0	0
Gummallo Peach Ring	5 pieces (1.4 oz)	120	0	0
Gummi Bears	18 pieces (1.4 oz)	130	0	0
Gummi Dinos	7 pieces (1.3 oz)	120	0	0
Gummi Worms	4 pieces (1.4 oz)	130	0	0
Jelly Beans	13 (1.4 oz)	150	0	0
Marshmallow Eggs	3 (1.3 oz)	140	0	0
Neon Worms	4 pieces (1.4 oz)	120	0	0
Sour Gummi Bears	16 pieces (1.4 oz)	110	0	0
Sour Gummi Worms	4 pieces (1.6 oz)	130	0	0
Ferrero Rocher				
Candy	2 pieces (0.9 oz)	150	3	10
Franklin				
Crunch 'N Munch Candied	1.25 oz	170	—	7
Crunch 'N Munch Caramel	1.25 oz	160	—	5
Crunch 'N Munch Maple Walnut	1.25 oz	160	—	6
Crunch 'N Munch Toffee	1.25 oz	160	—	5

FOOD	PORTION	CALS.	SAT. FAT	FAT
Godiva				
Almond Butter Dome	3 pieces (1.5 oz)	240	6	17
Bouchee Au Chocolat	1 piece (1.5 oz)	210	6	11
Bouchee Ivory Raspberry	1 pieces (1 oz)	160	3	9
Gold Ballotin	3 pieces (1.5 oz)	210	4	10
Truffle Amaretto Di Saronno	2 pieces (1.5 oz)	210	6	12
Truffle Deluxe Liqueur	2 pieces (1.5 oz)	210	6	13
Goldenberg's				
Peanut Chews	3 pieces (1.3 oz)	180	2	9
Goo Goo Supreme				
With Pecans	1 pkg (1.5 oz)	188	2	5
Goobers				
Peanuts	1 pkg (1.38 oz)	210	5	13
Good & Fruity				
Candy	1 box (1.8 oz)	140	—	1
Good & Plenty				
Snacksize	3 boxes (1.5 oz)	140	0	0
Haviland				
Chocolate Covered Thin Mints	6 (1.5 oz)	170	3	5
Heath				
Bar	1 (1.4 oz)	210	7	13
Hershey				
Amazin'Fruit Gummy Candy	1 snack pkg (0.7 oz)	60	0	0
Bar	1 (0.6 oz)	100	3	6
Candy-Coated Milk Chocolate Eggs	4 pieces	90	3	5
Cookies 'n' Mint	1 bar (0.6 oz)	90	2	5
Hugs	1 piece	25	1	2
Hugs w/ Almonds	1 piece	25	1	2
Kisses	1	25	1	2
Kisses w/ Almond	1	25	1	2
Milk Chocolate	1 bar (0.6 oz)	90	4	5
Milk Chocolate w/ Almonds	1 bar (0.6 oz)	100	3	6
Miniature Milk Chocolate	1 (0.3 oz)	45	2	3
Nuggets Cookies 'n' Creme	1 (0.35 oz)	50	2	3
Nuggets Cookies 'n' Mint	1 (0.35 oz)	50	2	3
Nuggets Milk Chocolate	1 (0.35 oz)	50	2	3
Nuggets Milk Chocolate w/ Almonds	1 (0.35 oz)	50	2	3
Pot Of Gold Solitaires	5 pieces	90	3	6
Special Dark Miniature	1 (0.3 oz)	45	0	2
Sweet Escapes Chocolate Toffee Crisp	1 bar (0.66 oz)	80	2	4
Sweet Escapes Peanut Butter Crispy	1 bar (0.7 oz)	70	1	3

FOOD	PORTION	CALS.	SAT. FAT	FAT
Hershey (CONT.)				
Sweet Escapes Triple Chocolate Wafer	1 bar (0.7 oz)	80	2	3
Tastetations Butterscotch	3 pieces (0.6 oz)	60	1	2
Tastetations Caramel	3 pieces (0.6 oz)	60	1	2
Tastetations Chocolate	3 pieces (0.6 oz)	60	1	1
Tastetations Chocolate Mint	3 pieces (0.6 oz)	60	1	2
Tastetations Peppermint	3 pieces (0.6 oz)	60	0	0
Jolly Rancher				
Candies	3 pieces (0.6 oz)	60	0	0
Joyva				
Halvah	1.5 oz	240	3	16
Halvah Chocolate Covered	1 bar (2 oz)	380	5	23
Jells Raspberry	3 pieces (1.6 oz)	200	2	3
Joys Raspberry	1 (1.6 oz)	200	2	3
Marshmallow Twists Chocolate Covered	2 (1.5 oz)	190	2	4
Rings Orange & Raspberry	3 pieces (1.5 oz)	190	2	3
Sesame Crunch	3 pieces (0.5)	80	1	4
Sticks Orange	3 pieces (1.6 oz)	200	2	3
Twists Vanilla & Cherry	2 (1.5 oz)	190	2	4
Juicefuls				
Candy	3 pieces (0.5 oz)	60	0	0
Junior Mints				
Candies	1 pkg (1.6 oz)	190	3	4
Snack Size	1 pkg (0.7 oz)	75	1	1
Just Born				
Hot Tamales	1 pkg (2.1 oz)	220	0	0
Mike and Ike Berry Fruits	1 pkg (2.1 oz)	220	0	0
Mike and Ike Cherry & Bubble Gum	1 pkg (2.1 oz)	220	0	0
Mike and Ike Chewy Grape	1 pkg (2.1 oz)	220	0	0
Mike and Ike Lemon Watermelon	1 pkg (2.1 oz)	220	0	0
Mike and Ike Original	1 pkg (1.2 oz)	220	0	0
Mike and Ike Strawberry & Banana	1 pkg (2.1 oz)	220	0	0
Mike and Ike Tropical Fruits	1 pkg (2.1 oz)	220	0	0
Super Hot Tamales	1 pkg (2.1 oz)	220	0	0
Teenee Beanee Assorted Fruits	36 pieces (1.4 oz)	150	0	0
Teenee Beanee Berry Berry	36 pieces (1.4 oz)	150	0	0
Teenee Beanee Tropical Mix	36 pieces (1.4 oz)	150	0	0
Kit Kat				
Bar	1 (0.56 oz)	80	3	4

FOOD	PORTION	CALS.	SAT. FAT	FAT
Krackel				
Bar	1 (0.6 oz)	90	3	5
Miniature	1 (0.3 oz)	45	2	3
Lance				
Chocolaty Peanut Bar	1 (2 oz)	290	4	15
Cinnamon Chews	1 pkg (1.06 oz)	120	0	1
Fruit Chews	1 pkg (1.06 oz)	120	0	1
Gum Ball Pops	1 (0.45 oz)	45	0	0
K-Nuts	4 pieces (1.5 oz)	240	5	15
Mint Chews	1 pkg (1.06 oz)	120	0	1
Peanut Bar	1 (1.75 oz)	270	3	15
Pop-A-Lance	1 piece (0.42 oz)	45	0	0
Popcorn'n'Carmel	1 bar (0.75 oz)	90	0	0
Starlight Mints	3 pieces (1 oz)	60	0	0
Strawberry Chews	1 pkg (1.06 oz)	120	0	1
Suckers	3 pieces (0.5 oz)	50	0	0
Whistle Pop	1 (0.67 oz)	70	0	0
Lifesavers				
Big Tablet Candy Cane	4 pieces (0.5 oz)	60	0	0
Cards 'N Candy	4 pieces (0.4 oz)	40	0	0
Christmas Tin	4 pieces (0.5 oz)	60	0	0
Egg-Sortment	1 roll (0.4 oz)	40	0	0
Gummi Bunnies	3 pkg (1.6 oz)	140	0	0
Gummi Savers Five Flavor	1 roll (1.5 oz)	130	0	0
Gummi Savers Five Flavor	1 pkg (1.8 oz)	160	0	0
Gummi Savers Mixed Berry	1 roll (1.5 oz)	130	0	0
Gummi Savers Mixed Berry	1 pkg (1.8 oz)	160	0	0
Gummi Savers Tangy Fruits	1 pkg (1.8 oz)	160	0	0
Gummi Savers Tangy Fruits	1 roll (1.5 oz)	130	0	0
Gummi Savers Variety	2 pkg (1.3 oz)	120	0	0
Gummi Savers Wacky Frootz	1 roll (1.5 oz)	130	0	0
Gummi Savers Wacky Frootz	1 pkg (1.8 oz)	160	0	0
Gummi Shapes Barnum's Animals	1 pkg (0.8 oz)	70	0	0
Holes Five Flavor	20 pieces (5 g)	20	0	0
Holes Island Fruit	20 pieces (5 g)	20	0	0
Holes Sour 'N Sweet	16 pieces (5 g)	20	0	0
Holes Sunshine Fruits	20 pieces (0.2 oz)	20	0	0
Holes Super Tart	20 pieces (5 g)	20	0	0
Holes Wild Fruits	20 pieces (5 g)	20	—	0
Lollipops Candy Cane	1 (0.4 oz)	40	0	0
Lollipops Christmas	1 (0.4 oz)	40	0	0
Lollipops Easter	1 (0.4 oz)	40	0	0
Lollipops Fruit Flavors	1 (0.4 oz)	45	0	0
Lollipops Swirled Flavors	1 (0.4 oz)	40	0	0

FOOD	PORTION	CALS.	SAT. FAT	FAT
Lifesavers (CONT.)				
Lollipops Valentine	1 (0.4 oz)	40	0	0
Roll Butter Rum	2 pieces (5 g)	20	0	0
Roll Candy Cane	4 pieces (0.4 oz)	40	0	0
Roll Cryst-O-Mint	2 pieces (5 g)	20	0	0
Roll Five Flavor	2 pieces (5 g)	20	0	0
Roll Fruits On Fire	2 pieces (5 g)	20	0	0
Roll Pep-O-Mint	3 pieces (5 g)	20	0	0
Roll Spear-O-Mint	3 pieces (5 g)	20	0	0
Roll Sunshine Fruits	2 pieces (5 g)	20	0	0
Roll Tangy Fruit Swirl	2 pieces (5 g)	20	0	0
Roll Tangy Fruit Watermelon	1 pieces (5 g)	20	0	0
Roll Tangy Fruits	2 pieces (5 g)	20	0	0
Roll Tropical Fruits	2 pieces (5 g)	20	0	0
Roll Wild Cherry	1 pieces (5 g)	20	0	0
Roll Wild Flavors	2 pieces (5 g)	20	0	0
Roll Wild Sour Berries	2 pieces (5 g)	20	0	0
Roll Wint-O-Green	3 pieces (5 g)	20	0	0
Sack'it Butter Rum	4 pieces (0.5 oz)	60	0	0
Sack'it Five Flavor	4 pieces (0.5 oz)	60	0	0
Sack'it Holiday Tin	4 pieces (0.5 oz)	60	0	0
Sack'it Pep-O-Mint	4 pieces (0.5 oz)	60	0	0
Sack'it Tangy Fruits	4 pieces (0.5 oz)	60	0	0
Sack'it Wild Cherry	4 pieces (0.5 oz)	60	0	0
Sack'it Wint-O-Green	4 pieces (0.5 oz)	60	0	0
Sugar Free Iced Mint	1 pieces (2 g)	10	0	0
Sugar Free Vanilla Mint	1 pieces (2 g)	10	0	0
Valentine Book	2 pieces (5 g)	20	0	0
Lindt				
Truffles Milk Chocolate	3 pieces (1.3 oz)	210	12	17
M&M's				
Almond	1.5 oz	220	4	12
Almond	1 pkg (1.3 oz)	200	4	11
Mint	1 pkg (1.7 oz)	230	6	10
Mint	1.5 oz	200	5	9
Peanut	½ bag king size (1.6 oz)	240	5	12
Peanut	1 fun size (0.7 oz)	110	2	5
Peanut	1 pkg (1.7 oz)	250	5	13
Peanut	1.5 oz	220	5	11
Peanut Butter	1 fun size (0.7 oz)	110	4	6
Peanut Butter	1.5 oz	220	8	12
Peanut Butter	1 pkg (1.6 oz)	240	8	13
Plain	1 pkg fun size (0.7 oz)	100	3	4

FOOD	PORTION	CALS.	SAT. FAT	FAT
M&M's (CONT.)				
Plain	½ pkg king size (1.6 oz)	220	6	9
Plain	1 pkg (1.7 oz)	230	10	10
Plain	1.5 oz	200	5	9
Mars				
Almond Bar	2 fun size (1.3 oz)	190	3	10
Almond Bar	1 bar (1.8 oz)	240	4	13
Mayfair				
Mints	5 pieces (1.3 oz)	180	5	9
Milk Duds				
Pieces	1 box (1.8 oz)	230	6	8
Snack Size	4 boxes (1.3 oz)	160	4	5
Milkshake				
Bar	1 bar (1.8 oz)	220	4	7
Milky Way				
Bar	2 fun size (1.4 oz)	180	4	7
Bar	1 (2.1 oz)	280	5	11
Bar	½ king size (1.2 oz)	160	3	6
Dark	1 fun size (0.7 oz)	90	2	3
Dark	1 bar (1.8 oz)	220	5	8
Miniature	5 (1.5 oz)	190	4	7
Mounds				
Bar	1 (0.68 oz)	90	4	5
Mr. Goodbar				
Miniature	1 (0.3 oz)	45	1	3
NECCO				
Mint	1 piece	12	—	tr
Nestle				
Areo Bar	1 bar (1.45 oz)	210	7	13
Buncha Crunch	1 pkg (1.4 oz)	90	5	10
Crunch	1 bar (1.55 oz)	230	7	12
Milk Chocolate	1 bar (1.45 oz)	220	7	13
Treasures Crunch	4 pieces (1.4 oz)	210	7	11
Turtles Bite Size	1 piece (0.4 oz)	50	1	2
Turtles Pecan Caramel Candy	2 pieces (1.2 oz)	160	3	9
Newman's Own				
Organics Espresso Sweet Dark Chocolate	1 bar (1.2 oz)	190	7	12
Nibs				
Cherry	1 pkg (0.49 oz)	45	0	0
Licorice	1 pkg (0.49 oz)	40	0	0
Nips				
Butter Rum	2 pieces (0.5 oz)	60	2	2
Caramel	2 pieces (0.5 oz)	60	2	2

FOOD	PORTION	CALS.	SAT. FAT	FAT
Nips (CONT.)				
Chocolate Mint	2 pieces (0.5 oz)	60	2	2
Chocolate Parfait	2 pieces (0.5 oz)	60	2	2
Peanut Butter Parfait	2 pieces (0.5 oz)	60	2	2
Oh Henry!				
Bar	1 (1.8 oz)	230	4	9
Palmer				
Milk Chocolate Lollipop	1 (0.9 oz)	130	4	7
PayDay				
Bar	1 (1.85 oz)	240	2	12
Pearson's				
Licorice	2 pieces (0.5 oz)	60	2	2
Mint Patties	5 (1.3 oz)	150	2	3
Pez				
Candy	1 roll (0.3 oz)	30	0	0
Sugar Free	1 roll (0.3 oz)	30	0	0
Planters				
Original Peanut Bar	1 pkg (1.6 oz)	230	2	14
Pom Pom				
Candies	1 pkg (1.6 oz)	200	5	6
Raisinets				
Candy	1 pkg (1.58 oz)	200	4	8
Fun Size	3 pkg (1.7 oz)	210	5	8
Reese's				
Eggs	1 (0.6 oz)	90	2	5
Nutrageous	1 (0.6 oz)	90	2	5
Peanut Butter Cups	1 (0.28 oz)	40	1	3
Pieces	25 (0.7 oz)	100	4	4
Riesen				
Candy	5 pieces (1.4 oz)	180	3	7
Rokeach				
Cotton Candy	2 cups (1 oz)	110	0	0
Rolo				
Caramels In Milk Chocolate	3 pieces (0.64 oz)	90	2	4
Russell Stover				
Assorted Creams	3 pieces (1.4 oz)	180	4	7
Looney Tunes Peanut Butter Nougat w/ Peanuts in Milk Chocolate	1 snack size (0.7 oz)	90	2	5
Peanut Butter & Grape Jelly	1 piece (0.8 oz)	100	2	6
Peanut Butter & Red Raspberry Cups	1 (0.8 oz)	100	2	6
Pecan Roll	1 (2 oz)	300	3	20
See's				
Lollypop Butterscotch	1	90	2	3

FOOD	PORTION	CALS.	SAT. FAT	FAT
See's (CONT.)				
Lollypop Cafe Latte	1	90	2	3
Lollypop Chocolate	1	90	3	5
Lollypop Peanut Butter	1	90	1	4
Simply Lite				
Sugar Free Lil'l Bits Chocolately	36 pieces (1.4 oz)	130	5	5
Sugar Free Lil'l Bits Peanut Buttery	36 pieces (1.4 oz)	140	5	5
Sugar Free Patteez	5 pieces (1.3 oz)	110	2	3
Skittles				
Original	2 pkg fun size (1.6 oz)	180	0	2
Original	1 pkg (2.8 oz)	250	1	3
Original	½ king size (1.3 oz)	150	0	2
Original	1.5 oz	170	0	2
Tropical	2 bags fun size (1.4 oz)	160	0	2
Tropical	1.5 oz	170	0	2
Tropical	1 bag (2.2 oz)	250	1	3
Wild Berry	1 bag (2.2 oz)	250	1	3
Wild Berry	2 bags fun size (1.4 oz)	160	0	2
Wild Berry	1.5 oz	170	0	2
Smucker's				
Fruit Fillers Strawberry	1 pkg (0.9 oz)	80	0	0
Jelly Beans	1 pkg (0.7 oz)	70	0	0
Snickers				
Bar	2 bars fun size (1.4 oz)	190	4	9
Bar	1 bar (2.1 oz)	280	5	14
Bar	⅓ king size (1.2 oz)	170	3	8
Miniatures	4 (1.3 oz)	170	3	8
Munch Bar	1 (1.4 oz)	230	4	15
Peanut Butter	1 bar (2 oz)	310	7	20
Sno-Caps				
Candies	1 pkg (2.3 oz)	300	8	13
Sour Punch				
Candy Straws Sour Apple	6 pieces (1.4 oz)	130	—	1
Spice Stix				
And Drops	14 pieces (1.6 oz)	140	0	0
Starburst				
California Fruits	8 pieces (1.4 oz)	160	1	3
California Fruits	1 stick (2.1 oz)	240	1	5
Original Fruits	⅓ king size (1.2 oz)	140	1	3

FOOD	PORTION	CALS.	SAT. FAT	FAT
Starburst (CONT.)				
Original Fruits	8 pieces (1.4 oz)	160	1	3
Original Fruits	1 stick (2.1 oz)	240	1	5
Strawberry Fruits	8 pieces (1.4 oz)	160	1	3
Strawberry Fruits	1 stick (2.1 oz)	240	1	5
Tropical Fruits	1 stick (2.1 oz)	240	1	5
Tropical Fruits	8 pieces (1.4 oz)	160	1	3
Sugar Babies				
Candies	1 pkg (1.7 oz)	190	2	2
Tidbits	1 pkg	180	—	2
Sugar Daddy				
Candies	1 pkg (1.7 oz)	200	3	3
Swedish Fish				
Original	19 pieces (1.4 oz)	160	0	0
Sweet'N Low				
Sugar Free Butter Toffee	4 pieces (0.5 oz)	30	1	1
Sugar Free Butterscotch	1 piece	7	0	0
Sugar Free Cinnamon	1 piece	7	0	0
Sugar Free Fancy Fruit	1 piece	7	0	0
Sugar Free Fruit Flavors	1 piece	7	0	0
Sugar Free Hard Candy Coffee	4 pieces (0.5 oz)	30	0	0
Sugar Free Peppermint	1 piece	7	0	0
Sugar Free Soft Candy Fruitie Flavors	1 piece	11	—	tr
Sugar Free Soft Candy Tropical Flavors	1 piece	11	—	tr
Sugar Free Watermelon	1 piece	7	0	0
Sugar Free Wild Cherry	1 piece	7	0	0
Switzer				
Cherry Bites	12 pieces (1.6 oz)	50	0	0
Licorice Bites	12 pieces (1.6 oz)	46	0	0
Symphony				
Bar	1 (0.6 oz)	100	4	6
W/ Almonds & Chocolate Chips	1 bar (0.6 oz)	90	4	6
Terry's				
Orange Milk Chocolate	5 pieces (1.5 oz)	240	9	14
Tootsie Roll				
Candy	1 (1 oz)	110	0	2
Dots	12 (1.5 oz)	160	0	0
Midgees	6 (1.4 oz)	160	1	3
Pop	1 (0.6 oz)	60	0	0
Twix				
Caramel	1 pkg (2 oz)	280	5	14
Caramel	1 (1 oz)	140	3	7

FOOD	PORTION	CALS.	SAT. FAT	FAT
Twix (CONT.)				
Caramel	1 fun size (0.5 oz)	80	2	4
Caramel	1 king size (0.8 oz)	120	2	6
Peanut Butter	1 (0.9 oz)	130	3	8
Twizzlers				
Cherry	1 pieces	35	0	0
Chocolate	1 piece	30	0	0
Licorice	1 piece	35	0	0
Pull'n'Peel Cherry	1 piece (1 oz)	90	0	0
Strawberry	1 piece	35	0	0
Velamints				
Cocoamint	1 piece (1.7 g)	5	0	0
Peppermint	1 piece (1.7 g)	5	0	0
Spearmint	1 piece (1.7 g)	5	0	0
Wintergreen	1 piece (1.7 g)	5	0	0
Very Special				
Chocolate Bottles Liquor Filled	3 pieces (1 oz)	150	4	6
Whatchamacallit				
Bar	1 (0.58 oz)	80	2	4
Whitman's				
Assorted	3 pieces (1.4 oz)	190	5	8
Dark Chocolate	3 pieces (1.4 oz)	200	6	10
Little Ambassadors	7 pieces (1.4 oz)	190	5	9
Pecan Delight	1 bar (2 oz)	310	7	20
Pecan Roll	1 bar (2 oz)	300	3	20
Sampler	3 pieces (1.4 oz)	200	6	11
Snoopy Treats Caramel Peanuts Milk Chocolate	1 snack size (1.4 oz)	80	3	5
Whoppers				
Candy	1 pkg (1.8 oz)	230	8	10
York				
Peppermint Patty	1 (0.49 oz)	50	1	1
Zero				
Bar	2 pieces (1.4 oz)	170	3	6
HOME RECIPE				
divinity	1 recipe 48 pieces (19 oz)	1891	—	tr
divinity	1 (11 g)	38	0	0
fondant	1 recipe 60 pieces (32.6 oz)	3327	—	tr
fondant	1 piece (0.6 oz)	57	—	0
fudge brown sugar w/ nuts	1 piece (0.5 oz)	56	tr	1
fudge brown sugar w/ nuts	1 recipe 60 pieces (30.7 oz)	3453	15	88

FOOD	PORTION	CALS.	SAT. FAT	FAT
fudge chocolate	1 piece (0.6 oz)	65	1	1
fudge chocolate	1 recipe 48 pieces (29 oz)	3161	43	70
fudge chocolate marshmallow	1 recipe (43.1 oz)	5182	125	207
fudge chocolate marshmallow	1 piece (0.7 oz)	84	2	3
fudge chocolate marshmallow w/ nuts	1 piece (0.8 oz)	96	2	4
fudge chocolate marshmallow w/ nuts	1 recipe 60 pieces (43.1 oz)	5182	125	207
fudge chocolate marshmallow w/ nuts	1 recipe 60 pieces (46.1 oz)	5742	127	258
fudge chocolate w/ nuts	1 recipe 48 pieces (32.7 oz)	3967	52	150
fudge chocolate w/ nuts	1 piece (0.7 oz)	81	1	3
fudge peanut butter	1 piece (0.6 oz)	59	tr	1
fudge peanut butter	1 recipe 36 pieces (20.4 oz)	2161	9	38
fudge vanilla	1 piece (0.6 oz)	59	1	1
fudge vanilla	1 recipe 48 pieces (27.5 oz)	2893	26	42
fudge vanilla w/ nuts	1 recipe 60 pieces (31 oz)	3666	33	117
fudge vanilla w/ nuts	1 piece (0.5 oz)	62	1	2
peanut brittle	1 recipe (17.6 oz)	2288	25	95
peanut brittle	1 oz	128	1	5
praline	1 recipe 23 pieces (31.8 oz)	4116	17	220
praline	1 piece (1.4 oz)	177	1	10
taffy	1 piece (0.5 oz)	56	tr	1
taffy	1 recipe 48 pieces (25 oz)	2677	15	24
toffee	1 piece (0.4 oz)	65	2	4
toffee	1 recipe 48 pieces (19.4 oz)	2997	113	182
truffles	1 piece (0.4 oz)	59	3	4
truffles	1 recipe 49 pieces (21.5 oz)	2985	132	210

CANTALOUPE

FOOD	PORTION	CALS.	SAT. FAT	FAT
dried	3.5 pieces (1.4 oz)	140	0	0
fresh	½	94	—	1
fresh cubed	1 cup	57	—	tr
Big Valley				
Balls frzn	¾ cup (4.9 oz)	40	0	0

FOOD	PORTION	CALS.	SAT. FAT	FAT
Dole				
Fresh	¼	50	—	0
CAPERS				
Progresso				
Capers	1 tsp (5 g)	0	0	0
Reese				
Capers	1 tsp (5 g)	0	0	0
CARAWAY				
seed	1 tsp	7	tr	tr
CARDAMON				
ground	1 tsp	6	tr	tr
CARDOON				
fresh cooked	3.5 oz	22	tr	tr
raw shredded	½ cup	36	tr	tr
CARIBOU				
roasted	3 oz	142	1	4
CARISSA				
fresh	1	12	—	tr
CAROB				
carob mix	3 tsp	45	0	0
carob mix as prep w/ whole milk	9 oz	195	5	8
flour	1 tbsp	14	tr	tr
flour	1 cup	185	tr	1
CARP				
fresh cooked	3 oz	138	1	6
fresh cooked	1 fillet (6 oz)	276	2	12
raw	3 oz	108	1	5
roe raw	3.5 oz	130	—	2
CARROT JUICE				
canned	6 oz	73	tr	tr
Hain				
Juice	6 fl oz	80	0	0
Hollywood				
Juice	6 fl oz	80	0	0
Odwalla				
Juice	8 fl oz	70	0	0
CARROTS				
CANNED				
slices	½ cup	17	tr	tr
slices low sodium	½ cup	17	tr	tr

FOOD	PORTION	CALS.	SAT. FAT	FAT
Allen				
Sliced	½ cup (4.5 oz)	35	0	1
Crest Top				
Sliced	½ cup (4.5 oz)	35	0	1
Del Monte				
Cut	½ cup (4.3 oz)	35	0	0
Sliced	½ cup (4.3 oz)	35	0	0
Green Giant				
Sliced	½ cup (4.2 oz)	25	0	0
LeSueur				
Baby Whole	½ cup (4.2 oz)	35	0	0
Seneca				
Diced	½ cup	30	0	0
Sliced	½ cup	30	0	0
FRESH				
baby raw	1 (½ oz)	6	tr	tr
raw	1 (2.5 oz)	31	tr	tr
raw shredded	½ cup	24	tr	tr
slices cooked	½ cup	35	tr	tr
Dole				
Shredded	1 cups (3 oz)	40	0	0
FROZEN				
slices cooked	½ cup	26	tr	tr
Big Valley				
Carrots	½ cup (3 oz)	35	0	0
Birds Eye				
Baby Whole	⅔ cup (3 oz)	35	0	0
Fresh Like				
Carrots	3.5 oz	42	—	tr
Green Giant				
Harvest Fresh Baby	⅔ cup (3 oz)	20	0	0
Select Baby Cut	¾ cup (2.8 oz)	30	0	0
Hanover				
Crinkle Sliced	½ cup	35	—	0
CASABA				
cubed	1 cup	45	—	tr
fresh	⅒	43	—	tr
CASHEWS				
cashew butter w/o salt	1 tbsp	94	2	8
dry roasted	1 oz	163	3	13
dry roasted salted	1 oz	163	3	13
oil roasted	1 oz	163	3	14
oil roasted salted	1 oz	163	3	14

FOOD	PORTION	CALS.	SAT. FAT	FAT
Beer Nuts				
Cashews	1 pkg (1 oz)	170	—	13
Fisher				
Honey Roasted Halves	1 oz	150	3	13
Honey Roasted Whole	1 oz	150	3	13
Oil Roasted Halves	1 oz	170	3	15
Oil Roasted Whole	1 oz	170	3	15
Frito Lay				
Salted	1 oz	180	3	15
Guy's				
Whole Salted	1 oz	170	—	14
Hain				
Cashew Butter Raw	2 tbsp	190	3	15
Cashew Butter Raw Unsalted	2 tbsp	210	3	19
Cashew Butter Toasted	2 tbsp	210	3	17
Lance				
Cashews	1 pkg (1⅛ oz)	200	3	16
Planters				
Fancy Oil Roasted	1 oz	170	3	14
Fancy Oil Roasted	1 pkg (2 oz)	340	6	29
Halves Lightly Salted Oil Roasted	1 oz	160	3	13
Halves Oil Roasted	1 oz	170	3	14
Honey Roasted	1 oz	150	2	12
Honey Roasted	1 pkg (2 oz)	310	4	24
Munch'N Go Honey Roasted	1 pkg (2 oz)	310	4	24
Munch'N Go Singles Oil Roasted	1 pkg (2 oz)	330	6	28
Oil Roasted	1 pkg (1 oz)	160	3	14
Oil Roasted	1 pkg (1.5 oz)	250	4	21
CASSAVA				
raw	3½ oz	120	tr	tr
CATFISH				
channel breaded & fried	3 oz	194	3	11
channel raw	3 oz	99	1	4
CATSUP				
(see KETCHUP)				
CAULIFLOWER				
FRESH				
cooked	½ cup (2.2 oz)	14	tr	tr
flowerets cooked	3 (2 oz)	12	tr	tr
flowerets raw	3 (2 oz)	14	tr	tr

FOOD	PORTION	CALS.	SAT. FAT	FAT
green cooked	1½ cup (3.2 oz)	29	tr	tr
green raw	1 head 7 in diam (18 oz)	158	tr	2
green raw	1 cup (2.2 oz)	20	tr	tr
green raw floweret	1 (0.9 oz)	8	tr	tr
raw	½ cup (1.8 oz)	13	tr	tr
Dole				
Cauliflower	⅙ med head	18	—	0
FROZEN				
cooked	½ cup	17	tr	tr
Big Valley				
Florets	¾ cup (3 oz)	25	0	0
Birds Eye				
Frzn	⅔ cup	25	0	0
In Cheese Sauce	½ cup (4.1 oz)	80	2	5
Fresh Like				
Cauliflower	3.5 oz	26	—	tr
Green Giant				
Cheese Sauce	½ cup (3.5 oz)	60	1	3
Florets	1 cup (2.8 oz)	25	0	0
Hanover				
Cauliflower	½ cup	20	—	0
Florets	½ cup	20	—	0
CAVIAR				
black	1 oz	71	—	5
black	1 tbsp	40	—	3
red	1 tbsp	40	—	3
red	1 oz	71	—	5
CELERIAC				
fresh cooked	3.5 oz	25	—	tr
raw	½ cup	31	—	tr
CELERY				
diced cooked	½ cup	13	tr	tr
fresh	1 stalk (1.3 oz)	6	tr	tr
raw diced	½ cup	10	tr	tr
seed	1 tsp	8	tr	tr
Dole				
Stalks	2 med	20	—	0
Fresh Like				
Frozen	3.5 oz	14	—	tr
CELTUCE				
raw	3.5 oz	22	—	tr

FOOD	PORTION	CALS.	SAT. FAT	FAT
CEREAL				
bran flakes	¾ cup (1 oz)	90	tr	1
corn flakes	1¼ cup (1 oz)	110	tr	tr
corn flakes low sodium	1 cup (0.9 oz)	100	tr	tr
corn grits white regular & quick as prep w/ water & salt	¾ cup (6.4 oz)	109	tr	tr
corn grits white regular or quick as prep	¾ cup (6.4 oz)	109	tr	tr
corn grits yellow regular & quick as prep w/ water & salt	¾ cup (6.4 oz)	109	tr	tr
corn grits yellow regular & quick not prep	1 cup (5.5 oz)	579	tr	2
crispy rice	1 cup (1 oz)	111	tr	tr
crispy rice low sodium	1 cup (0.9 oz)	105	tr	tr
farina as prep w/ water	¾ cup (6.1 oz)	88	tr	tr
farina not prep	1 tbsp (0.4 oz)	40	0	tr
granola	½ cup (2.1 oz)	285	3	15
oatmeal instant as prep w/ water	1 cup (8.2 oz)	138	tr	2
oatmeal instant cooked w/o salt	1 cup	145	tr	2
oatmeal instant w/ bran & raisins as prep w/ water	1 pkg (6.8 oz)	158	tr	2
oatmeal instant w/ cinnamon & spice as prep w/ water	1 pkg (5.6 oz)	177	tr	2
oatmeal instant w/ raisins & spice as prep w/ water	1 cup (5.5 oz)	161	tr	2
oatmeal quick cooked w/o salt	1 cup	145	tr	2
oatmeal regular & quick as prep w/ water	¾ cup (6.1 oz)	149	tr	2
oatmeal regular & quick not prep	⅓ cup (0.9 oz)	104	tr	2
oatmeal regular cooked w/o salt	1 cup	145	tr	2
puffed rice	1 cup (0.5 oz)	56	tr	tr
puffed wheat	1 cup (0.4 oz)	44	tr	tr
shredded mini wheats	1 cup (1.1 oz)	107	tr	1
shredded wheat rectangular	1 biscuit (0.8 oz)	85	tr	tr
shredded wheat round	2 biscuits (1.3 oz)	136	tr	1
sugar-coated corn flakes	¾ cup (1 oz)	110	tr	1
whole wheat hot natural as prep w/ water	¾ cup (6.4 oz)	113	tr	1
Albers				
Hominy Quick Grits uncooked	¼ cup	140	—	1
Arrowhead				
4 Grain + Flax	¼ cup (1.6 oz)	150	0	2
7 Grain	⅓ cup (1.4 oz)	140	0	2
Amaranth Flakes	1 cup (1.2 oz)	130	0	2
Apple Corns	1 cup (1.5 oz)	150	0	2

FOOD	PORTION	CALS.	SAT. FAT	FAT
Arrowhead (CONT.)				
Bear Mush	¼ cup (1.6 oz)	160	0	1
Bran Flakes	1 cup (1 oz)	100	0	1
Kamut Flakes	1 cup (1.1 oz)	120	0	1
Maple Corns	1 cup (1.9 oz)	190	1	3
Multi Grain Flakes	1 cup (1.2 oz)	140	0	2
Nature O's	1 cup (1.1 oz)	130	1	2
Oat Bran Flakes	1 cup (1.2 oz)	110	1	2
Oat Flakes Rolled	⅓ cup (1.2 oz)	130	1	3
Oat Groats	¼ cup (1.5 oz)	160	1	3
Oatmeal Instant Original	1 oz	100	—	0
Puffed Corn	1 cup (0.8 oz)	80	0	0
Puffed Kamut	1 cup (0.6 oz)	50	0	0
Puffed Millet	1 cup (0.9 oz)	90	0	1
Puffed Rice	1 cup (0.8 oz)	90	0	0
Puffed Wheat	1 cup (0.9)	90	0	1
Rice & Shine	¼ cup (1.5 oz)	150	0	1
Spelt Flakes	1 cup (1.1 oz)	100	0	1
Wheat Flakes Rolled	⅓ cup (1.2 oz)	110	0	1
Barbara's				
Apple Cinnamon Toasted O's	¾ cup	110	0	1
Bite Size Shredded Oats	1¼ cups (2 oz)	220	1	3
Breakfast O's	1 cup (1 oz)	120	0	2
Brown Rice Crisps	1 cup (1 oz)	120	0	1
Cocoa Crunch Stars	1 cup (1 oz)	110	0	1
Corn Flakes	1 cup (1 oz)	110	0	0
Frosted Corn Flakes	1 cup (1 oz)	110	0	0
Honey Crunch Stars	1 cup (1 oz)	110	0	0
Honey Nut Toasted O's	¾ cup	120	1	2
Organic Ultra Minis Frosted	¾ cup (1.9 oz)	190	0	1
Organic Ultra Minis Original	¾ cup (1.9 oz)	190	0	1
Organic Fruity Punch	1 cup (1 oz)	110	0	1
Puffins	¾ cup (0.9 oz)	90	0	1
Shredded Spoonfuls	¾ cup (1.1 oz)	120	0	2
Shredded Wheat	2 biscuits (1.4 oz)	140	0	1
Betty Crocker				
Dutch Apple	1 cup (1.9 oz)	220	0	2
Streusel	¾ cup (1 oz)	120	0	2
Ensemble				
Apple Cinnamon	1 cup (1.2 oz)	120	0	2
Honey Nut	1 cup (1.2 oz)	120	0	2
Multi-Grain	1 cup (1.2 oz)	110	0	1
General Mills				
Apple Cinnamon Cheerios	¾ cup (1 oz)	120	0	2
Basic 4	1 cup (1.9 oz)	200	0	2

FOOD	PORTION	CALS.	SAT. FAT	FAT
General Mills (CONT.)				
Berry Berry Kix	¾ cup (1 oz)	120	0	2
Body Buddies Natural Fruit	1 cup (1 oz)	120	0	2
Boo Berry	1 cup (1 oz)	120	0	1
Cheerios	1 cup (1 oz)	110	0	2
Cinnamon Grahams	¾ cup (1 oz)	120	0	1
Cinnamon Toast Crunch	¾ cup (1 oz)	130	1	4
Cocoa Puffs	1 cup (1 oz)	120	0	1
Cookie Crisp	1 cup (1 oz)	120	0	2
Corn Chex	1 cup (1 oz)	110	0	0
Count Chocula	1 cup (1 oz)	120	0	1
Country Corn Flakes	1 cup (1 oz)	120	0	1
Crispy Wheaties 'n Raisins	1 cup (1.9 oz)	190	0	1
Fiber One	½ cup (1 oz)	60	0	1
Frankenberry	1 cup (1 oz)	120	0	1
French Toast Crunch	¾ cup (1 oz)	120	0	2
Frosted Cheerios	1 cup (1 oz)	120	0	1
Golden Grahams	¾ cup (1 oz)	120	0	1
Grand Slams Major League	1 cup (1 oz)	120	0	1
Honey Frosted Wheaties	¾ cup (1 oz)	110	0	1
Honey Nut Cheerios	1 cup (1 oz)	120	0	2
Honey Nut Clusters	1 cup (1.9 oz)	210	0	3
Honey Nut Chex	¾ cup (1 oz)	120	0	1
Jurassic Park Crunch	1 cup (1 oz)	120	0	1
Kaboom	1¼ cup (1 oz)	120	0	2
Kix	1⅓ cup (1 oz)	120	0	1
Lucky Charms	1 cup (1 oz)	120	0	1
Multi-Bran Chex	1 cup (2 oz)	200	0	2
Multi-Grain Cheerios Plus	1 cup (1 oz)	110	0	1
Oatmeal Crisp Almond	1 cup (1.9 oz)	220	1	5
Oatmeal Crisp Apple Cinnamon	1 cup (1.9 oz)	210	0	2
Oatmeal Crisp Raisin	1 cup (1.9 oz)	210	0	3
Raisin Nut Bran	¾ cup (1.9 oz)	200	1	4
Reese's Peanut Butter Puffs	¾ cup (1 oz)	130	1	3
Rice Chex	1¼ cup (1.1 oz)	120	0	0
Sunrise Organic	¾ cup (1 oz)	110	0	1
Team Cheerios	1 cup (1 oz)	120	0	1
Total Corn Flakes	1⅓ cup (1 oz)	110	0	1
Total Raisin Bran	1 cup (1.9 oz)	180	0	1
Total Whole Grain	¾ cup (1 oz)	110	0	1
Trix	1 cup (1 oz)	120	0	2
USA Olympic Crunch	1 cup (1 oz)	120	0	1
Wheat Chex	1 cup (1.9 oz)	180	0	1
Wheat Hearts	¼ cup (1.3 oz)	130	0	1
Wheaties	1 cup (1 oz)	110	0	1

FOOD	PORTION	CALS.	SAT. FAT	FAT
Good Shepherd				
Granola Crunchy	1 oz	130	—	5
Granola Honey Almond	1 oz	120	—	4
Millet Rice Flakes Wheat Free	1 oz	95	—	1
Organic Granola 5 Grain Muesli	1 oz	160	—	3
Organic Granola Brown Rice	1 oz	130	—	4
Organic Granola Wheat Free	1 oz	90	—	3
Organic Granola Wheat Free Apple Cinnamon	1 oz	125	—	4
Organic Granola Wheat Free Blueberry Amaranth	1 oz	110	—	1
Organic Granola Wheat Free Strawberry Amaranth	1 oz	110	—	1
Spelt	1 oz	90	—	tr
Spelt Flakes	1 oz	100	—	6
Grist Mill				
Apple Cinnamon Natural	½ cup (1.9 oz)	260	2	10
Bran	½ cup (1.9 oz)	250	6	8
Granola Low Fat w/ Raisins	⅔ cup (1.9 oz)	220	1	3
Oat & Honey Natural	½ cup (1.9 oz)	270	3	12
Oat Honey & Raisin Natural	½ cup (1.9 oz)	260	2	10
H-O				
Farina Instant	1 pkg	110	0	0
Farina not prep	3 tbsp	120	0	0
Oatmeal Instant	½ cup	130	0	2
Oatmeal Instant	1 pkg	110	0	2
Oatmeal Instant Apple Cinnamon	1 pkg	130	0	2
Oatmeal Instant Maple Brown Sugar	1 pkg	160	0	2
Oatmeal Instant Raisin & Spice	1 pkg	150	0	2
Health Valley				
10 Bran O's Apple Cinnamon	¾ cup	100	0	0
Bran w/ Apples & Cinnamon	¾ cup	160	0	0
Golden Flax	½ cup	190	—	3
Granola 98% Fat Free Date Almond	⅔ cup	180	—	1
Healthy Crunches & Flakes Almond	¾ cup	130	0	0
Healthy Crunches & Flakes Apple Cinnamon	¾ cup	130	0	0
Healthy Crunches & Flakes Honey Crunch	¾ cup	130	0	0
Hot Cereal Cups Amazing Apple!	1 pkg	220	—	2

FOOD	PORTION	CALS.	SAT. FAT	FAT
Health Valley (CONT.)				
Hot Cereal Cups Banana Gone Nuts	1 pkg	240	—	3
Hot Cereal Cups Maple Madness!	1 pkg	240	—	2
Hot Cereal Cups Terrific 10 Grain!	1 pkg	220	—	3
Oat Bran O'S	¾ cup	100	0	0
Organic Amaranth Flakes	¾ cup	100	0	0
Organic Blue Corn Bran Flakes	¾ cup	100	0	0
Organic Bran w/ Raisin	¾ cup	160	0	0
Organic Fiber 7 Flakes	¾ cup	100	0	0
Organic Healthy Fiber Flakes	¾ cup	100	0	0
Organic Oat Bran Flakes	¾ cup	100	0	0
Organic Oat Bran Flakes w/ Raisins	¾ cup	110	0	0
Puffed Honey Sweetened Corn	1 cup	110	0	0
Puffed Honey Sweetened Crisp Brown Rice	1 cup	110	0	0
Raisin Bran Flakes	1¼ cup	190	0	0
Real Oat Bran	½ cup	200	—	3
Healthy Choice				
Almond Crunch With Raisins	1 cup (2 oz)	210	0	3
Golden Multi-Grain Flakes	¾ cup (1.1 oz)	110	0	0
Toasted Brown Sugar Squares	1 cup (2 oz)	190	0	1
Heartland				
Coconut	1 oz	130	—	5
Plain	1 oz	130	—	4
Raisin	1 oz	130	—	4
Kashi				
Go Berry Tart	½ cup (4.9 oz)	260	0	3
Kellogg's				
All-Bran	½ cup (1.1 oz)	80	0	1
All-Bran Bran Buds	⅓ cup (1 oz)	80	0	1
All-Bran Extra Fiber	½ cup (0.9 oz)	50	0	1
Apple Jacks	1 cup (1.2 oz)	120	0	0
Cocoa Frosted Flakes	¾ cup (1.1 oz)	120	0	0
Cocoa Krispies	¾ cup (1.1 oz)	120	0	1
Complete Oat Bran Flakes	¾ cup (1 oz)	110	1	1
Complete Wheat Bran Flakes	¾ cup (1 oz)	90	0	1
Corn Flakes	1 cup (1 oz)	100	0	0
Corn Pops K-Sentials	1 oz	100	0	0
Country Inn Greyfield Blend	¾ cup (2 oz)	320	1	6
Country Inn Greyfield Inn Blend	¾ cup (2 oz)	320	1	6
Cracklin' Oat Bran	¾ cup (1.7 oz)	190	2	7

FOOD	PORTION	CALS.	SAT. FAT	FAT
Kellogg's (CONT.)				
Crispix	1 cup (1 oz)	110	0	0
Froot Loops k-Sentials	1 oz	100	0	1
Frosted Flakes	¾ cup (1.1 oz)	120	0	0
Granola Low Fat	½ cup (1.7 oz)	190	1	3
Honey Crunch Corn Flakes	¾ cup (1.1 oz)	120	0	1
Just Right Crunchy Nuggets	1 cup (2 oz)	210	0	2
Just Right Fruit & Nut	1 cup (2.1 oz)	220	0	2
Low Fat With Raisins	⅔ cup (2.1 oz)	220	1	3
Mini-Wheat Frosted	1 cup (1.8 oz)	180	0	1
Mini-Wheat Strawberry Squares	¾ cup (1.8 oz)	170	0	1
Mini-Wheats Apple Cinnamon Squares	¾ cup (1.9 oz)	180	0	1
Mini-Wheats Blueberry Squares	¾ cup (1.9 oz)	180	0	1
Mini-Wheats Frosted Bite Size	24 pieces (2.1 oz)	200	0	1
Mini-Wheats Raisin Squares	¾ cup (1.9 oz)	180	0	1
Mueslix Apple & Almond Crunch	¾ cups (1.9 oz)	200	1	5
Mueslix Raisin & Almond	⅔ cup (1.9 oz)	200	0	3
Nutri-Grain Almond Raisin	1¼ cup (1.7 oz)	180	0	3
Nutri-Grain Golden Wheat	¾ cup (1 oz)	100	0	1
Product 19	1 cup (1 oz)	100	0	0
Raisin Bran	1 cup (2.1 oz)	200	0	2
Rice Krispies	1¼ cup (1.2 oz)	120	0	0
Rice Krispies Razzle Dazzle	¾ cup (1 oz)	110	0	0
Rice Krispies Treats	¾ cup (1 oz)	120	0	2
Smacks	¾ cup (1 oz)	100	0	1
Smart Start	1 cup (1.8 oz)	180	0	1
Special K	1 cup (1.1 oz)	110	0	0
Kolln				
Crispy Oats	1 cup (1.8 oz)	190	1	3
Oat Bran Crunch	⅔ cup (2.1 oz)	220	1	5
Oat Muesli Fruit	¾ cup (2 oz)	200	1	5
Maltex				
Cereal	1 oz	105	tr	1
Maypo				
30 Second	1 oz	100	tr	1
Vermont Style	1 oz	105	tr	1
With Oat Bran	1 oz	130	tr	2
McCann's				
Irish Oatmeal	1 oz	110	—	2
Morning Traditions				
Blueberry Morning	1¼ cup (1.9 oz)	220	1	3
Cranberry Almond Crunch	1 cup (1.9 oz)	220	0	3
Great Grains Crunchy Pecan	⅔ cup (1.9 oz)	220	1	6

FOOD	PORTION	CALS.	SAT. FAT	FAT
Morning Traditions (CONT.)				
Great Grains Raisins Dates & Pecans	⅔ cup (1.9 oz)	210	1	5
Morning Tradtions				
Banana Nut Crunch	1 cup (2 oz)	250	1	6
Mother's				
Oatmeal Instant	½ cup (1.4 oz)	150	1	3
Whole Wheat Natural	½ cup (1.4 oz)	130	0	1
Mueslix				
Crispy Blend	⅔ cup (1.9 oz)	200	0	2
Nabisco				
100% Bran	⅓ cup (1 oz)	80	0	1
Cream Of Wheat Instant as prep	1 cup	120	—	0
Cream Of Wheat Quick as prep	1 cup	120	—	0
Cream Of Wheat Regular as prep	1 cup	120	—	0
Frosted Shredded Wheat Bite Size	1 cup (1.8 oz)	190	0	1
Honey Nut Shredded Wheat Bite Size	1 cup (1.8 oz)	200	0	2
Original Shredded Wheat	2 biscuits (1.6 oz)	160	0	1
Original Shredded Wheat 'N Bran	1¼ cup (2.1 oz)	200	0	1
Original Shredded Wheat Spoon Size	1 cup (1.7 oz)	170	0	1
Nature Valley				
Granola Low Fat Fruit	⅔ cup (1.9 oz)	210	0	3
Nutri-Grain				
Almond Raisin	1¼ cup (2 oz)	200	0	3
Golden Wheat	¾ cup (1.1 oz)	100	0	1
Post				
Alpha-Bits	1 cup (1 oz)	130	0	2
Alpha-Bits Marshmallow	1 cup (1 oz)	120	0	1
Bran Flakes	¾ cup (1 oz)	100	0	1
Cocoa Pebbles	¾ cup (1 oz)	120	1	1
Fruit & Fibre Dates Raisins & Walnuts	1 cup (1.9 oz)	210	1	3
Fruit & Fibre Peaches Raisins & Almonds	1 cup (1.9 oz)	210	1	3
Fruity Pebbles	¾ cup (1 oz)	110	0	1
Golden Crisp	¾ cup (1 oz)	110	0	0
Grape-Nuts	¾ cup (1 oz)	100	0	1
Grape-Nuts Flakes	¾ cup (1 oz)	100	0	1

FOOD	PORTION	CALS.	SAT. FAT	FAT
Post (CONT.)				
Honey Bunches Of Oats	¾ cup (1 oz)	120	1	2
Honey Bunches Of Oats With Almonds	¾ cup (1.1 oz)	130	1	3
Honeycomb	1⅓ cups (1 oz)	110	0	1
Post Toasties	1 cup (1 oz)	100	0	0
Raisin Bran	1 cup (2 oz)	190	0	1
Waffle Crisp	1 cup (1 oz)	130	0	3
Pritikin				
Apple Raisin Spice	1 pkg (1.6 oz)	170	1	3
Multigrain	1 pkg	160	0	2
Quaker				
Instant Grits Original	1 pkg (1 oz)	100	0	0
Multigrain	½ cup (1.4 oz)	130	0	2
Oatmeal Instant	1 pkg (1 oz)	100	0	2
Oatmeal Instant Apples & Cinnamon	1 pkg (1.2 oz)	130	1	2
Oatmeal Instant Bananas & Cream	1 pkg (1.2 oz)	130	1	3
Oatmeal Instant Blueberries & Cream	1 pkg (1.2 oz)	130	1	3
Oatmeal Instant Cinnamon & Spice	1 pkg (1.6 oz)	170	0	2
Oatmeal Instant Kid's Choice Chocolate Chip Cookie	1 pkg (1.5 oz)	160	1	3
Oatmeal Instant Kid's Choice Cookie'n Cream	1 pkg (1.5 oz)	160	1	3
Oatmeal Instant Kid's Choice Fruity Marshmallow	1 pkg (1.4 oz)	150	1	2
Oatmeal Instant Kid's Choice Oatmeal Raisin Cookie	1 pkg (1.5 oz)	160	1	2
Oatmeal Instant Kid's Choice Radical Raspberry	1 pkg (1.4 oz)	150	1	3
Oatmeal Instant Kid's Choice S'mores	1 pkg (1.5 oz)	160	1	3
Oatmeal Instant Kid's Choice Strawberries'n Stuff	1 pkg (1.4 oz)	150	1	2
Oatmeal Instant Kid's Choice Twisted Strawberry Banana	1 pkg (1.4 oz)	150	1	2
Oatmeal Instant Maple & Brown Sugar	1 pkg (1.5 oz)	160	0	2
Oatmeal Instant Peaches & Cream	1 pkg (1.2 oz)	140	1	3

FOOD	PORTION	CALS.	SAT. FAT	FAT
Quaker (cont.)				
Oatmeal Instant Raisin & Spice	1 pkg (1.5 oz)	150	1	2
Oatmeal Instant Raisin Date & Walnut	1 pkg (1.3 oz)	140	1	3
Oatmeal Instant Strawberries & Cream	1 pkg (1.2 oz)	140	1	3
Oatmeal Quick'n Hearty Microwave	1 pkg (1 oz)	110	1	2
Oatmeal Quick'n Hearty Microwave Apple Spice	1 pkg (1.6 oz)	170	1	2
Oatmeal Quick'n Hearty Microwave Brown Sugar Cinnamon	1 pkg (1.5 oz)	150	1	2
Oatmeal Quick'n Hearty Microwave Cinnamon Double Raisin	1 pkg (1.6 oz)	170	1	2
Oatmeal Quick'n Hearty Microwave Honey Bran	1 pkg (1.4 oz)	150	1	2
Oats Old Fashion	½ cup (1.4 oz)	150	1	3
Oats Quick	½ cup (1.4 oz)	150	1	3
Oats Steel Cut	½ cup (1.4 oz)	150	1	3
Whole Wheat Hot Natural	½ cup (1.4 oz)	130	0	1
Ralston				
Almond Delight	1 cup (1.8 oz)	210	0	3
Bran Flakes	¾ cup (1.1 oz)	110	0	1
Chex Multi-Bran	1¼ cup (2 oz)	220	0	2
Cocoa Crispy Rice	1 cup (1.8 oz)	200	0	1
Cocoa Crunchies	¾ cup (1.1 oz)	120	0	1
Cookie Crisp	1 cup (1 oz)	120	0	2
Corn Flakes	1¼ cup (1.1 oz)	120	0	0
Crisp Crunch	¾ cup (1.1 oz)	120	0	1
Crisp Rice	1¼ cup (1.2 oz)	130	0	0
Frosted Flakes	¾ cup (1.1 oz)	120	0	0
Fruit Rings	¾ cup (0.9 oz)	100	0	1
Magic Stair	¾ cup (1.1 oz)	120	0	1
Muesli Blueberry	1 cup (1.9 oz)	200	2	3
Muesli Cranberry	¾ cup (1.9 oz)	200	0	3
Muesli Peach	¾ cup (1.9 oz)	200	0	3
Muesli Raspberry	¾ cup (2 oz)	220	0	3
Muesli Strawberry	1 cup (1.9 oz)	210	2	3
Multi Vitamin Whole Grain Flakes	1 cup (1.1 oz)	120	0	1
Nutty Nuggets	½ cup (1.7 oz)	180	0	2
Raisin Bran	¾ cup (1.9 oz)	190	0	1

FOOD	PORTION	CALS.	SAT. FAT	FAT
Ralston (CONT.)				
Tasteeos	1¼ cup (1.1 oz)	130	0	3
Tasteeos Apple Cinnamon	1 cup (1.2 oz)	130	0	2
Tasteeos Honey Nut	1 cup (1.2 oz)	130	0	2
Roman Meal				
Apple Cinnamon	1.2 oz	105	tr	2
Cream Of Rye	1.3 oz	111	tr	1
Oats Wheat Dates Raisins Almonds	1.3 oz	129	tr	2
Oats Wheat Honey Coconuts Almonds	1.3 oz	155	3	5
Original	1 oz	83	tr	1
Original With Oats	1.2 oz	108	tr	1
Stone-Buhr				
4 Grain	⅓ cup (1.6 oz)	140	0	2
7 Grain	⅓ cup (1.6 oz)	140	0	2
Bran Flakes	¼ cup (0.6 oz)	64	0	0
Cracked Wheat	¼ cup (2.4 oz)	210	0	1
Granola Hot Apple	⅓ cup (1.6 oz)	153	0	1
Manna Golden	6 tsp (1.6 oz)	160	0	0
Rolled Oats Old Fashion	6 tsp (1.6 oz)	150	1	3
Scotch Oats	¼ cup (1.6 oz)	150	1	4
Sunbelt				
Berry Basic	½ cup (1.9 oz)	220	2	6
Granola Banana Nut	½ cup (1.9 oz)	250	4	9
Granola Cinnamon Raisins	½ cup (1.9 oz)	200	1	3
Granola Fruit & Nut	½ cup (1.9 oz)	240	2	7
Muesli 5 Whole Grains	½ cup (1.9 oz)	210	1	2
Uncle Roy's				
Granola Cashew Raisin	½ cup (1.6 oz)	180	1	6
Granola Fruit & Nut	½ cup (1.6 oz)	175	1	5
Granola Maple Date Nut	½ cup (1.6 oz)	180	1	6
Granola Nut Butter & Almonds	½ cup (1.6 oz)	195	1	8
Granola Fat Free Apple Cinnamon	½ cup (1.6 oz)	175	tr	1
Granola Fat Free Wild Cherry	½ cup (1.6 oz)	175	tr	1
Granola Low Fat Berries Jubilee	½ cup (1.6 oz)	175	1	3
Granola Low Fat Crispy	½ cup (1.4 oz)	160	1	3
Granola Low Fat Luscious Raspberry	½ cup (1.6 oz)	175	1	3
Granola Low Fat True Blueberry	½ cup (1.6 oz)	175	1	3
Granola Organic Golden Honey	½ cup (1.6 oz)	190	1	6
Granola Organic Maple Nut'N Rice	½ cup (1.4 oz)	170	1	6

FOOD	PORTION	CALS.	SAT. FAT	FAT
Uncle Roy's (CONT.)				
Granola Organic Maple Raisin	½ cup (1.6 oz)	190	1	6
Muesli Swiss Style	½ cup (1.6 oz)	170	1	5
Wheatena				
Cereal	⅓ cup (1.4 oz)	150	0	1

CEREAL BARS

(see also NUTRITION SUPPLEMENTS)

FOOD	PORTION	CALS.	SAT. FAT	FAT
chewy raisin	1 (1 oz)	127	3	5
granola	1 (1 oz)	134	1	7
granola almond	1 (1 oz)	140	4	7
granola chocolate chip	1 (1 oz)	124	3	5
granola peanut	1 (1 oz)	136	1	6
granola peanut butter	1 (1 oz)	137	1	7
granola chewy	1 (1 oz)	126	2	5
granola chewy chocolate chip	1 (1 oz)	119	3	5
granola chewy chocolate chip graham & marshmallow	1 (1 oz)	121	3	4
granola chewy chocolate coated chocolate chip	1 (1 oz)	132	4	7
granola chewy chocolate coated peanut butter	1 (1 oz)	144	5	9
granola chewy nut & raisin	1 (1 oz)	129	3	6
granola chewy peanut butter	1 (1 oz)	121	1	5
granola chewy peanut butter & chocolate chip	1 (1 oz)	122	2	6
Cap'n Crunch				
Bar	1 (0.8 oz)	90	1	2
Berries Bar	1 (0.8 oz)	90	—	2
Carnation				
Chewy Peanut Butter Chocolate Chip	1 (1.26 oz)	140	2	5
Chocolate Chunk	1 (1.26 oz)	140	2	5
Honey & Oats	1 (1.26 oz)	130	2	4
Dolly Madison				
Apple	1 (1.3 oz)	120	0	2
Blueberry	1 (1.3 oz)	120	0	2
Raspberry	1 (1.3 oz)	120	0	2
Strawberry	1 (1.3 oz)	120	0	2
Estee				
Rice Crunchie Chocolate	1 (0.7 oz)	50	0	0
Rice Crunchie Chocolate Chip	1 (0.7 oz)	50	0	0
Rice Crunchie Peanut Butter	1 (0.7 oz)	60	0	1
Rice Crunchie Vanilla	1 (0.7 oz)	60	0	0

FOOD	PORTION	CALS.	SAT. FAT	FAT
Fi-Bar				
Coconut	1	120	1	4
Peanut Butter	1	130	1	4
Glenny's				
Chocolate Crunch Creamy Low Fat	1 bar (1.75 oz)	190	1	3
Chocolate Crunch Roasted Peanut	1 bar (1.75 oz)	200	1	4
Chocolate Crunch Toasted Almond	1 bar (1.75 oz)	200	0	4
Grist Mill				
Chewy Apple Cinnamon	1 (1 oz)	120	1	4
Chewy Chocolate Chip	1 (1 oz)	130	1	4
Chewy Chunky Nut & Raisin	1 (1 oz)	130	2	6
Chewy Peanut Butter	1 (1 oz)	130	1	5
Chewy Peanut Butter Chocolate	1 (1 oz)	130	1	4
Chocolate Snack Chocolate Chip	1 (1.2 oz)	180	5	10
Chocolate Snack Nutty Fudge	1 (1.3 oz)	190	5	11
Crunchy Cinnamon	1 (0.8 oz)	110	1	5
Crunchy Oats 'N Honey	1 (0.8 oz)	110	1	5
Health Valley				
98% Fat Free Raisin Cinnamon	⅔ cup	180	—	1
98% Fat Free Tropical	⅔ cup	180	—	1
Blueberry	1	140	0	0
Breakfast Bakes Apple Cinnamon	1 bar	110	0	0
Breakfast Bakes Mountain Blueberry	1 bar	110	0	0
Breakfast Bakes Red Raspberry	1 bar	110	0	0
Chocolate Chip	1	140	0	0
Crisp Rice Bars Apple Cinnamon	1	110	0	0
Crisp Rice Bars Orange Date	1	110	0	0
Crisp Rice Bars Tropical Fruit	1	110	0	0
Date Almond	1	140	0	0
Fiber 7 Flakes w/ Strawberry	1 bar	110	0	0
O's Almond	¾ cup	120	0	0
O's Apple Cinnamon	¾ cup	120	0	0
O's Honey Crunch	¾ cup	120	0	0
Oat Bran Flakes w/ Blueberry	1 bar	110	0	0
Raisin	1	140	0	0

FOOD	PORTION	CALS.	SAT. FAT	FAT
Health Valley (CONT.)				
Raisin Bran Flakes w/ Apple Raisin	1 bar	110	0	0
Raspberry	1	140	0	0
Strawberry	1	140	0	0
Hostess				
Apple	1 (1.3 oz)	120	0	2
Banana Nut	1 (1.3 oz)	120	0	2
Blueberry	1 (1.3 oz)	120	0	2
Raspberry	1 (1.3 oz)	120	0	2
Strawberry	1 (1.3 oz)	120	0	2
Kellogg's				
Nutri-Grain Apple Cinnamon	1 (1.3 oz)	140	1	3
Nutri-Grain Blueberry	1 (1.3 oz)	140	1	3
Nutri-Grain Cherry	1 (1.3 oz)	140	1	3
Nutri-Grain Mixed Berry	1 (1.3 oz)	140	1	3
Nutri-Grain Peach	1 (1.3 oz)	140	1	3
Nutri-Grain Raspberry	1 (1.3 oz)	140	1	3
Nutri-Grain Strawberry	1 (1.3 oz)	140	1	3
Rice Krispies Treats	1 (0.8 oz)	90	1	2
Rice Krispies Treats Chocolate Chip Squares	1 (0.8 oz)	90	1	3
Kudos				
Chocolate Chunk	1 (0.7 oz)	90	1	3
Chocolate Coated Chocolate Chip	1 (1 oz)	120	3	5
Chocolate Coated Milk & Cookies	1 (1 oz)	130	3	5
Chocolate Coated Nutty Fudge	1 (1 oz)	130	3	5
Chocolate Coated Peanut Butter	1 (1 oz)	130	3	5
Low Fat Blueberry	1 (0.7 oz)	90	0	2
Low Fat Strawberry	1 (0.7 oz)	80	0	2
Little Debbie				
Raspberry	1 (1.3 oz)	130	0	3
S'mores Granola Treats	1 (1 oz)	130	2	5
Strawberry	1 (1.3 oz)	130	0	3
Nature Valley				
Crunchy Cinnamon	2 bars (1.6 oz)	200	1	6
Crunchy Oats'n Honey	2 bars (1.6 oz)	200	1	6
Crunchy Peanut Butter	2 bars (1.6 oz)	200	1	6
Low Fat Chewy Apple Brown Sugar	1 bar (1 oz)	110	0	2
Low Fat Chewy Chocolate Chip	1 bar (1 oz)	110	1	2
Low Fat Chewy Honey Nut	1 bar (1 oz)	110	0	2

FOOD	PORTION	CALS.	SAT. FAT	FAT
Nature Valley (CONT.)				
Low Fat Chewy Oatmeal Raisin	1 bar (1 oz)	110	0	2
Low Fat Chewy Orchard Blend	1 bar (1 oz)	110	0	2
Low Fat Chewy Triple Berry	1 bar (1 oz)	110	0	2
Nature's Choice				
Carob Chip	1 bar (0.7 oz)	80	0	3
Cinnamon & Raisin	1 bar (0.7 oz)	80	0	2
Fat Free Apple	1 bar (1.3 oz)	110	0	0
Fat Free Blueberry	1 bar (1.3 oz)	110	0	0
Fat Free Cranberry	1 bar (1.3 oz)	110	0	0
Fat Free Peach	1 bar (1.3 oz)	110	0	0
Fat Free Raspberry	1 bar (1.3 oz)	110	0	0
Fat Free Strawberry	1 bar (1.3 oz)	110	0	0
Low Fat Triple Berry	1 bar (1.3 oz)	130	0	2
Low Fat Very Cherry	1 bar (1.3 oz)	130	0	2
Oats 'n Honey	1 bar (0.7 oz)	80	0	2
Peanut Butter	1 bar (0.7 oz)	80	0	3
Quaker				
Dipps Rocky Road	1	140	—	7
Sunbelt				
Apple	1 (1.3 oz)	130	0	3
Blueberry	1 (1.3 oz)	130	0	3
Chewy Granola Almond	1 (1 oz)	130	2	7
Chewy Granola Apple Cinnamon	1 (1.2 oz)	140	0	3
Chewy Granola Chocolate Chip	1 (1.2 oz)	160	3	7
Chewy Granola Oatmeal Raisin	1 (1.2 oz)	130	0	3
Chewy Granola Oats & Honey	1 (1 oz)	120	2	5
Granola Fudge Dipped Chocolate Chip	1 (1.5 oz)	200	4	10
Granola Fudge Dipped Macaroon	1 (1.4 oz)	190	4	10
Weight Watchers				
Apple Cinnamon	1 (1 oz)	100	1	2
Blueberry	1 (1 oz)	100	1	2
Raspberry	1 (1 oz)	100	1	2

CHAMPAGNE

FOOD	PORTION	CALS.	SAT. FAT	FAT
sekt german champagne	3.5 fl oz	84		0
Andre				
Blush	1 fl oz	22	0	0
Brut	1 fl oz	21	0	0
Cold Duck	1 fl oz	25	0	0
Extra Dry	1 fl oz	23	0	0
Ballatore				
Spumante	1 fl oz	23	0	0

FOOD	PORTION	CALS.	SAT. FAT	FAT
Eden Roc				
Brut	1 fl oz	21	0	0
Brut Rose'	1 fl oz	22	0	0
Extra Dry	1 fl oz	21	0	0
Tott's				
Blanc de Noir	1 fl oz	22	0	0
Brut	1 fl oz	20	0	0
Extra Dry	1 fl oz	21	0	0
CHAYOTE				
fresh cooked	1 cup	38	—	1
raw	1 (7 oz)	49	—	1
raw cut up	1 cup	32	—	tr
CHEESE				
(see also CHEESE DISHES, CHEESE SUBSTITUTES, COTTAGE CHEESE, CREAM CHEESE)				
american	1 oz	93	4	7
american cheese food	1 pkg (8 oz)	745	35	56
american cheese spread	1 jar (5 oz)	412	19	30
american cold pack	1 pkg (8 oz)	752	35	56
american cheese spread	1 oz	82	4	6
beaufort	1 oz	115	6	9
blue	1 oz	100	6	8
blue crumbled	1 cup (4.7 oz)	477	25	39
brick	1 oz	105	5	8
brie	1 oz	95	—	8
cacio di roma sheep's milk cheese	1 oz	130	6	10
camembert	1 oz	85	4	7
camembert	1 wedge (1.3 oz)	114	6	9
cantal	1 oz	105	6	9
caraway	1 oz	107	—	8
chabichou	1 oz	95	5	8
chaource	1 oz	83	4	7
cheddar	1 oz	114	6	9
cheddar low fat	1 oz	49	1	2
cheddar low sodium	1 oz	113	6	9
cheddar shredded	1 cup	455	24	37
cheshire	1 oz	110	—	9
colby	1 oz	112	6	9
colby low fat	1 oz	49	1	2
colby low sodium	1 oz	113	6	9
comte	1 oz	114	5	9
coulommiers	1 oz	88	5	7
crottin	1 oz	105	6	9
edam	1 oz	101	5	8
feta	1 oz	75	4	6

FOOD	PORTION	CALS.	SAT. FAT	FAT
fontina	1 oz	110	5	9
gjetost	1 oz	132	5	8
goat fresh	1 oz	23	1	2
goat hard	1 oz	128	7	10
goat semisoft	1 oz	103	6	8
goat soft	1 oz	76	4	6
gorgonzola	3.5 oz	376	—	31
gouda	1 oz	101	5	8
gruyere	1 oz	117	5	9
limburger	1 oz	93	5	8
maroilles	1 oz	97	5	8
monterey	1 oz	106	—	9
morbier	1 oz	99	5	8
mozzarella	1 oz	80	4	6
mozzarella	1 lb	1276	60	98
mozzarella low moisture	1 oz	90	4	7
mozzarella low moisture part skim	1 oz	79	3	5
mozzarella part skim	1 oz	72	3	5
muenster	1 oz	104	5	9
parmesan grated	1 oz	129	5	9
parmesan grated	1 tbsp (5 g)	23	1	2
parmesan hard	1 oz	111	5	7
picodon	1 oz	99	5	8
pimento	1 oz	106	6	9
pont l'eveque	1 oz	86	4	7
port du salut	1 oz	100	5	8
provolone	1 oz	100	5	8
pyrenees	1 oz	101	5	8
queso anego	1 oz	106	5	9
queso asadero	1 oz	101	5	8
queso chichuahua	1 oz	106	5	8
raclette	1 oz	102	5	8
reblochon	1 oz	88	5	7
ricotta part skim	½ cup (4.4 oz)	171	6	10
ricotta part skim	1 cup (8.6 oz)	340	12	19
ricotta whole milk	½ cup (4.4 oz)	216	10	16
ricotta whole milk	1 cup (8.6 oz)	428	20	32
romano	1 oz	110	—	8
roquefort	1 oz	105	5	9
rouy	1 oz	95	5	8
saint marcellin	1 oz	94	5	8
saint nectaire	1 oz	97	5	8
saint paulin	1 oz	85	4	6
sainte maure	1 oz	99	5	8
selles sur cher	1 oz	93	5	8

FOOD	PORTION	CALS.	SAT. FAT	FAT
swiss	1 oz	107	5	8
swiss cheese food	1 pkg (8 oz)	734	—	55
swiss processed	1 oz	95	5	7
tilsit	1 oz	96	5	7
tome	1 oz	92	5	7
triple creme	1 oz	113	7	11
vacherin	1 oz	92	5	8
whey cheese	3.5 oz	440	18	27
yogurt cheese	1 oz	20	—	0
yogurt cheese	1 oz	80	3	7
Alouette				
Brie Baby	1 oz	110	5	9
Brie Baby With Herbs	1 oz	110	5	9
French Onion	2 tbsp (0.8 oz)	70	5	7
Garlic	2 tbsp (0.8 oz)	70	5	7
Light Dill	2 tbsp (0.8 oz)	50	3	4
Light Garlic	2 tbsp (0.8 oz)	50	3	4
Light Herb	2 tbsp (0.8 oz)	50	3	4
Light Herbs & Garlic	2 tbsp (0.8 oz)	50	3	4
Light Spring Vegetable	2 tbsp (0.8 oz)	50	3	4
Salmon	2 tbsp (0.8 oz)	60	3	5
Scallions	2 tbsp (0.8 oz)	70	5	7
Spinach	2 tbsp (0.8 oz)	60	4	6
Alpine Lace				
American	1 slice (0.66 oz)	50	2	3
American Fat Free	1 piece (1 oz)	45	tr	tr
American Hot Pepper Less Fat Less Sodium	1 piece (1 oz)	80	4	20
American Less Fat Less Sodium	1 piece (1 oz)	80	4	6
Cheddar Fat Free	1 piece (1 oz)	45	tr	tr
Cheddar Reduced Fat	1 piece (1 oz)	80	3	5
Colby Reduced Fat	1 piece (1 oz)	80	3	5
Fat Free For Parmesan Lovers	2 tsp (5 g)	10	0	0
Fat Free Mexican Macho	2 tbsp (1 oz)	30	tr	tr
Fat Free Singles	1 slice (0.66 oz)	25	0	0
Feta Reduced Fat	1 piece (1 oz)	60	3	4
Goat	1 oz	40	2	3
Mozzarella Fat Free	1 piece (1 oz)	45	tr	tr
Mozzarella Reduced Sodium Part Skim	1 piece (1 oz)	70	3	5
Muenster Reduced Sodium	1 piece (1 oz)	100	5	9
Provolone Smoked Reduced Fat	1 piece (1 oz)	70	3	5
Swiss Reduced Fat	1 piece (1 oz)	90	4	6

FOOD	PORTION	CALS.	SAT. FAT	FAT
Boar's Head				
American	1 oz	100	6	9
Baby Swiss	1 oz	110	6	9
Canadian Cheddar	1 oz	110	6	10
Double Glouster White	1 oz	110	6	10
Double Glouster Yellow	1 oz	110	6	10
Havarti	1 oz	110	7	10
Havarti w/ Dill	1 oz	110	7	10
Havarti w/ Jalapeno	1 oz	110	7	10
Longhorn Colby	1 oz	110	5	9
Monerey Jack	1 oz	100	6	9
Monerey Jack w/ Jalapeno	1 oz	100	6	9
Mozzarella	1 oz	90	4	7
Muenster	1 oz	100	5	8
Muenster Low Sodium	1 oz	100	5	8
Provolone Picante Sharp	1 oz	100	5	8
Swiss	1 oz	110	5	8
Swiss No Salt Added	1 oz	110	5	8
Bongrain				
Chavrie	2 tbsp (0.8 oz)	40	2	3
Montrachet	1 oz	70	4	6
Montrachet Chive	1 oz	70	4	6
Montrachet Classic	1 oz	70	4	6
Montrachet Classic Herb	1 oz	70	4	6
Montrachet Herbs & Garlic	1 oz	70	4	6
Montrachet In Oil drained	1 oz	70	4	6
Montrachet With Ash	1 oz	70	4	6
Breakstone's				
Ricotta	¼ cup (2.2 oz)	110	5	8
Bresse				
Brie	1 oz	110	5	9
Brie Light	1 oz	70	3	4
Brie With Herbs	1 oz	110	5	9
Creme De Brie	2 tbsp (1 oz)	90	5	8
Creme De Brie Herb	2 tbsp (1 oz)	90	5	8
Brier Run				
Cherve	1 oz	61	—	5
Quark	1 oz	34	—	3
Bristol Gold				
Cheddar Light	1 oz	70	—	4
French Onion Light	1 oz	70	—	4
Garlic & Herb Light	1 oz	70	—	4
Horseradish Light	1 oz	70	—	4
Smoke Light	1 oz	70	—	4
Wine Light	1 oz	70	—	4

FOOD	PORTION	CALS.	SAT. FAT	FAT
Cabot				
Cheddar	1 oz	110	6	9
Mediterranean Cheddar	1 oz	110	5	9
Monterey Jack	1 oz	80	5	5
Vermont Cheddar 50% Light	1 oz	70	3	5
Vitalait	1 oz	70	2	4
Vitalait Jalapeno	1 oz	70	2	4
Cheez Whiz				
Light	2 tbsp (1.2 oz)	80	2	3
Churney				
Diet Snack Cheddar Flavored	1 oz	70	—	3
Diet Snack Port Wine Flavored	1 oz	70	—	3
Feta	1 oz	80	4	6
Cracker Barrel				
Baby Swiss	1 oz	110	6	9
Cheddar Extra Sharp	1 oz	120	7	10
Cheddar Marbled Sharp	1 oz	110	6	9
Cheddar New York Aged	1 oz	120	7	10
Cheddar Sharp	1 oz	120	7	10
Cheddar Vermont Sharp	1 oz	110	6	9
Reduced Fat Cheddar Extra Sharp	1 oz	90	4	6
Reduced Fat Cheddar Sharp	1 oz	90	4	6
Reduced Fat Cheddar Vermont Sharp	1 oz	90	4	6
Whipped Spreadable Cream Cheese & Extra Sharp Cheddar	2 tbsp (0.9 oz)	80	5	8
Whipped Spreadable Cream Cheese & Sharp Cheddar	2 tbsp (0.9 oz)	80	5	8
Whipped Spreadable Cream Cheese & Sharp Cheddar w/ Herbs	2 tbsp (0.9 oz)	80	5	8
Delice De France				
Cheese	1 oz	110	5	9
With Herbs	1 oz	110	5	9
Delico				
Alouette Cajun	2 tbsp (0.8 oz)	70	5	7
Alouette French Onion	2 tbsp (0.8 oz)	70	5	7
Alouette Garden Vegetable	2 tbsp (0.8 oz)	60	4	6
Alouette Garlic	2 tbsp (0.8 oz)	70	5	7
Alouette Horseradish & Chive	2 tbsp (0.8 oz)	60	4	7
Alouette Spinach	2 tbsp (0.8 oz)	60	4	6
Di Giorno				
Parmesan Grated	2 tsp (5 g)	25	1	2

FOOD	PORTION	CALS.	SAT. FAT	FAT
Di Giorno (CONT.)				
Parmesan Shredded	2 tsp (5 g)	20	1	2
Parmesan Shredded	2 tsp (5 g)	20	1	2
Romano Grated	2 tsp (5 g)	25	1	2
Romano Shredded	2 tsp (5 g)	20	1	2
Easy Cheese				
Spread American	2 tbsp (1.2 oz)	100	4	7
Spread Cheddar	2 tbsp (1.2 oz)	100	4	7
Spread Cheddar'n Bacon	2 tbsp (1.2 oz)	100	4	7
Spread Nacho	2 tbsp (1.2 oz)	100	4	7
Spread Sharp Cheddar	2 tbsp (1.2 oz)	100	4	7
Father Time				
Cheddar Extra-Sharp Premium	1 oz	110	5	9
Formagg				
Formaggio D'Oro	1 oz	70	3	5
Friendship				
Farmer	2 tbsp (1 oz)	50	2	3
Farmer No Salt Added	2 tbsp (1 oz)	50	2	3
Hoop	2 tbsp (1 oz)	20	0	0
Frigo				
Asiago	1 oz	110	—	9
Blue	1 oz	100	—	8
Cheddar	1 oz	110	6	9
Cheddar Lite	1 oz	80	3	5
Feta	1 oz	100	—	8
Impastata	1 oz	60	—	5
Mozzarella Part Skim Low Moisture	1 oz	80	3	5
Mozzarella Whole Milk Low Moisture	1 oz	90	4	7
Mozzarella Lite Whole Milk Low Moisture	1 oz	60	2	2
Parmazest	1 oz	120	—	7
Parmesan & Romano Dry Grated	1 oz	130	—	9
Parmesan & Romano Grated	1 oz	110	—	7
Parmesan Dry Grated	1 oz	130	—	9
Parmesan Grated	1 oz	110	—	7
Parmesan Whole	1 oz	110	—	7
Pizza Shredded	1 oz	65	—	3
Provolone	1 oz	100	5	7
Provolone Lite	1 oz	70	2	4
Ricotta Low Fat Low Salt	1 oz	30	—	1
Ricotta Part Skim	1 oz	40	—	3
Ricotta Whole Milk	1 oz	60	—	5

FOOD	PORTION	CALS.	SAT. FAT	FAT
Frigo (CONT.)				
Romano Dry Grated	1 oz	130	—	9
Romano Grated	1 oz	110	—	8
Romano Whole	1 oz	110	—	8
String	1 oz	80	—	5
String Lite	1 oz	60	—	2
Swiss	1 oz	110	—	8
Taco Shredded	1 oz	110	—	9
Gerard				
Brie	1 oz	90	5	7
Handi-Snacks				
Cheez'n Breadsticks	1 pkg (1.1 oz)	120	3	6
Cheez'n Crackers	1 pkg (1.1 oz)	110	3	7
Cheez'n Pretzels	1 pkg (1 oz)	100	3	5
Mozzarella String Cheese	1 piece (1 oz)	80	4	6
Nacho Stix'n Cheez	1 pkg (1.1 oz)	110	3	6
Healthy Choice				
American Singles White	1 slice (0.7 oz)	30	0	0
American Singles Yellow	1 slice (0.7 oz)	30	0	0
Cheddar Fancy Shreds	¼ cup (1 oz)	45	0	0
Cheddar Shreds	¼ cup (1 oz)	45	0	0
Loaf	1 in cube (1 oz)	35	0	0
Mexican Shreds	¼ cup (1 oz)	45	0	0
Mozzarella	1 oz	45	0	0
Mozzarella Fancy Shreds	¼ cup (1 oz)	45	0	0
Mozzarella Shreds	¼ cup (1 oz)	45	0	0
Mozzarella String Cheese	1 stick (1 oz)	45	0	0
Pizza Fancy Shreds	¼ cup (1 oz)	45	0	0
Pizza String	1 stick (1 oz)	45	0	0
Heluva Good Cheese				
American	1 slice (0.7)	45	3	5
Cheddar Curds Snack	1 oz	113	5	9
Cheddar Extra-Sharp	1 oz	110	5	9
Cheddar Mild	1 oz	110	5	9
Cheddar Mild Reduced Fat	1 oz	80	4	6
Cheddar Mild White	1 oz	110	5	9
Cheddar Sharp	1 oz	110	5	9
Cheddar Sharp White	1 oz	110	5	9
Cheddar Shredded	¼ cup (1 oz)	110	5	9
Cheddar Very Low Sodium	1 oz	110	6	9
Cheddar White Extra-Sharp	1 oz	110	5	9
Cheddar White Very Low Sodium	1 oz	110	6	9
Cheddar White Shredded	¼ cup (1 oz)	110	5	9
Colby	1 oz	117	6	9

FOOD	PORTION	CALS.	SAT. FAT	FAT
Heluva Good Cheese (CONT.)				
Colby-Jack	1 oz	110	6	9
Cold Pack Cheddar Sharp	2 tbsp (1 oz)	90	3	7
Cold Pack Cheddar Sharp With Bacon	2 tbsp (1 oz)	90	3	7
Cold Pack Cheddar Sharp With Horseradish	2 tbsp (1 oz)	90	3	7
Cold Pack Cheddar Sharp With Jalapenos	2 tbsp (1 oz)	90	3	7
Cold Pack Cheddar Sharp With Port Wine	2 tbsp (1 oz)	90	3	7
Monterey Jack	1 oz	100	6	8
Monterey Jack Shredded	¼ cup (1 oz)	100	5	8
Monterey Jack With Jalapenos	1 oz	100	6	8
Mozzarella Part Skim Low Moisture Shredded	¼ cup (1 oz)	80	3	5
Mozzarella Whole Milk	1 oz	80	4	6
Muenster	1 oz	100	6	8
Swiss	1 oz	112	5	8
Washed Curd Cheese	1 oz	110	5	9
Hoffman				
American Yellow	1 oz	110	6	9
Hot Pepper	1 oz	90	5	7
Super Sharp	1 oz	110	6	9
Holland Farm				
Edam	1 oz	97	—	8
Farmer	1 oz	102	—	8
Gouda	1 oz	103	—	8
Monterey Jack	1 oz	102	—	9
Muenster	1 oz	102	—	9
Hollow Road Farms				
Sheep's Milk	1 oz	45	—	3
Keller's				
Chub	2 tbsp (1 oz)	100	6	10
Kraft				
Cheddar Extra Sharp	1 oz	120	7	10
Cheddar Medium	1 oz	110	6	9
Cheddar Mild	1 oz	110	6	9
Cheddar Sharp	1 oz	120	7	10
Cheddary Melts Medium Cheddar	1 oz	110	6	9
Cheddary Melts Mild Cheddar	1 oz	110	6	9
Cheddary Melts Shreds Medium Cheddar	¼ cup (1.1 oz)	120	6	9

FOOD	PORTION	CALS.	SAT. FAT	FAT
Kraft (CONT.)				
Cheddary Melts Shreds Mild Cheddar	¼ cup (1.1 oz)	120	6	9
Cheese Food w/ Garlic	1 oz	90	5	7
Cheese Food w/ Jalapeno Peppers	1 oz	90	5	7
Colby	1 oz	110	6	9
Colby Monterey Jack	1 oz	110	6	9
Deluxe American	1 oz	100	6	9
Deluxe American White	1 oz	100	6	9
Deluxe Singles American	1 (1 oz)	110	6	9
Deluxe Singles American	1 (0.7 oz)	70	4	6
Deluxe Singles Pimento	1 (1 oz)	100	6	8
Deluxe Singles Swiss	1 (1 oz)	90	5	7
Deluxe Singles Swiss	1 slice (0.7 oz)	70	4	5
Free Grated	2 tsp (5 g)	15	0	0
Free Shredded Cheddar	¼ cup (0.9 oz)	40	0	0
Free Shredded Mozzarella	¼ cup (1 oz)	45	0	0
Grated Parm Plus! Garlic Herb	2 tsp (5 g)	15	0	0
Grated Parm Plus! Zesty Red Pepper	2 tsp (5 g)	15	0	0
Grated Parmesan	2 tsp (5 g)	20	1	2
Grated Romano	2 tsp (5 g)	20	1	2
Marbled Cheddar Mild	1 oz	110	6	9
Marbled Cheddar & Monterey Jack	1 oz	110	6	9
Marbled Cheddar & Whole Milk Mozzarella	1 oz	100	5	8
Marbled Colby Monterey Jack	1 oz	110	6	9
Monterey Jack	1 oz	110	6	9
Monterey Jack w/ Jalapeno Peppers	1 oz	110	6	9
Mozzarella Part Skim Low Moisture	1 oz	80	4	5
Mozzarella String Cheese Low Moisture Part Skim	1 piece (1 oz)	80	4	6
Pizza Shredded Four Cheese	¼ cup (0.9 oz)	90	5	7
Pizza Shredded Mozzarella & Cheddar	⅓ cup (1.1 oz)	120	6	9
Pizza Shredded Mozzarella & Provolone w/ Smoke Flavor	¼ cup (0.9 oz)	90	5	7
Reduced Fat Cheddar Mild	1 oz	90	4	6
Reduced Fat Cheddar Sharp	1 oz	90	4	6
Reduced Fat Colby	1 oz	80	4	6
Reduced Fat Monterey Jack	1 oz	80	4	6

FOOD	PORTION	CALS.	SAT. FAT	FAT
Kraft (CONT.)				
Shredded Cheddar Medium	¼ cup (0.9 oz)	100	6	8
Shredded Cheddar Mild	¼ cup (0.9 oz)	100	6	8
Shredded Cheddar Sharp	1 oz (0.9 oz)	110	6	9
Shredded Cheddar & Monterey Jack	¼ cup (0.9 oz)	100	6	8
Shredded Colby & Monterey Jack	¼ cup (0.9 oz)	100	6	8
Shredded Hearty Italian	⅓ cup (1.1 oz)	100	5	8
Shredded Italian Style Classic Garlic	⅓ cup (1.1 oz)	100	5	8
Shredded Italian Style Mozzarelle & Parmesan	⅓ cup (1.1 oz)	100	5	8
Shredded Lower Fat Cheddar Mild	¼ cup (0.9 oz)	80	4	6
Shredded Lower Fat Cheddar Sharp	¼ cup (0.9 oz)	80	4	6
Shredded Lower Fat Colby & Monterey Jack	¼ cup (0.9 oz)	80	4	5
Shredded Lower Fat Mozzarella	⅓ cup (1.1 oz)	80	3	5
Shredded Lower Fat Pizza Cheese	⅓ cup (1.1 oz)	90	4	6
Shredded Mexican Style Cheddar & Monterey Jack	⅓ cup (1.1 oz)	120	7	10
Shredded Mexican Style Cheddar & Monterey Jack w/ Jalapeno Peppers	⅓ cup (1.1 oz)	120	6	10
Shredded Mexican Style Four Cheese	⅓ cup (1.1 oz)	120	7	10
Shredded Mexican Style Taco Cheese	⅓ cup (1.1 oz)	120	7	10
Shredded Monterey Jack	¼ cup (0.9 oz)	100	6	8
Shredded Parmesan	2 tsp (5 g)	20	1	2
Shredded Part Skim Mozzarella	¼ cup (1.1 oz)	90	4	6
Shredded Swiss	¼ cup (0.9 oz)	100	5	8
Shredded Whole Milk Mozzarella	¼ cup (1.1 oz)	100	5	8
Shredded Finely Cheddar Mild	¼ cup (1.1 oz)	120	6	10
Shredded Finely Cheddar Sharp	¼ cup (1.1 oz)	120	7	10
Shredded Finely Colby & Monterey Jack	¼ cup (1 oz)	110	6	9
Shredded Finely Lower Fat Cheddar Mild	⅓ cup (1.1 oz)	100	5	7
Shredded Finely Lower Fat Cheddar Sharp	⅓ cup (1.1 oz)	100	5	7

FOOD	PORTION	CALS.	SAT. FAT	FAT
Kraft (CONT.)				
Shredded Finely Part Skim Mozzarella	¼ cup (1.1 oz)	90	4	6
Shredded Finely Swiss	¼ cup (0.9 oz)	110	6	8
Singles American	1 (1.2 oz)	110	6	8
Singles American	1 (0.7 oz)	60	3	5
Singles American	1 (0.6 oz)	60	3	5
Singles Mild Mexican	1 (0.7 oz)	70	4	5
Singles Monterey	1 slice (0.7 oz)	70	4	5
Singles Pimento	1 (0.7 oz)	60	3	5
Singles Reduced Fat American	1 (0.7 oz)	50	2	3
Singles Reduced Fat American White	1 (0.7 oz)	50	2	3
Singles Sharp	1 slice (0.7 oz)	70	4	6
Singles Swiss	1 slice (0.7 oz)	70	4	5
Singles Nonfat American	1 (0.7 oz)	30	0	0
Singles Nonfat American White	1 (0.7 oz)	30	0	0
Singles Nonfat Sharp Cheddar	1 (0.7 oz)	35	0	0
Singles Nonfat Swiss	1 slice (0.7 oz)	30	0	0
Slices Cheddar Mild	1 (1 oz)	110	6	9
Slices Colby	1 (1.6 oz)	180	10	14
Slices Part Skim Mozzarella	1 (1.6 oz)	130	6	8
Slices Part Skim Mozzarella	1 (1.5 oz)	120	5	8
Slices Provolone Smoke Flavor	1 (1.5 oz)	150	8	11
Slices Swiss	1 (1.5 oz)	170	9	13
Slices Swiss	1 (1.3 oz)	150	8	12
Slices Swiss	1 (0.8 oz)	90	5	7
Slices Swiss	1 (1.6 oz)	180	9	14
Slices Swiss Aged	1 (1.5 oz)	170	9	13
Slices Deli-Thin Part Skim Mozzarella	1 (1 oz)	80	4	5
Slices Deli-Thin Swiss	1 (0.8 oz)	90	5	7
Slices Deli-Thin Swiss Aged	1 (0.8 oz)	90	5	7
Slices Reduced Fat Swiss	1 (1.3 oz)	130	6	9
Spread Bacon	2 tbsp (1.1 oz)	90	5	8
Spread Olive & Pimento	2 tbsp (1.1 oz)	70	4	6
Spread Pimento	2 tbsp (1.1 oz)	80	4	6
Spread Pineapple	2 tbsp (1.1 oz)	70	4	5
Spread Pineapple	2 tbsp (1.1 oz)	70	4	5
Spread Roka Brand Blue	2 tbsp (1.1 oz)	90	5	8
Swiss	1 oz	110	6	9
Lactaid				
American	3.5 oz	328	15	25
Land O'Lakes				
American	1 slice (0.75 oz)	80	5	6

FOOD	PORTION	CALS.	SAT. FAT	FAT
Land O'Lakes (CONT.)				
American	2 slices (1 oz)	100	6	9
American	1 oz	110	6	9
American Less Salt	1 oz	110	6	9
American Light	1 oz	70	3	5
American Sharp	1 oz	110	6	9
American & Swiss	1 oz	100	6	8
Baby Swiss	1 oz	110	5	8
Brick	1 oz	100	5	8
Chedarella	1 oz	100	5	8
Cheddar Light	1 oz	70	3	4
Gouda	1 oz	110	5	8
Jalapeno Light	1 oz	70	3	4
Monterey Jack	1 oz	110	5	9
Mozzarella	1 oz	80	4	6
Muenster	1 oz	100	5	8
Provolone	1 oz	100	5	8
Swiss	1 oz	110	6	8
Swiss Light	1 oz	80	3	4
Laughing Cow				
Assorted Wedge	1 (1 oz)	70	4	6
Babybel	1 oz	90	5	7
Babybel Mini	1 (0.7 oz)	70	4	6
Bonbel	1 oz	100	5	8
Bonbel Mini	1 (0.7 oz)	70	4	6
Cheesebits	6 pieces (1 oz)	70	4	6
Gouda Mini	1 (0.7 oz)	80	4	6
Original Wedge	1 (1 oz)	70	4	6
Wedge Light	1 (1 oz)	50	2	3
Lifetime				
Cheddar Fat Free	1 oz	40	0	0
Cheddar Fat Free Lactose Free	1 oz	40	0	0
Garden Vegetable Fat Free	1 oz	40	0	0
Jalapeno Jack Fat Free	1 oz	40	0	0
Jalapeno Jack Fat Free Lactose Free	1 oz	40	0	0
Mild Mexican Fat Free	1 oz	40	0	0
Monterey Jack Fat Free	1 oz	40	0	0
Mozzarella Fat Free	1 oz	40	0	0
Mozzarella Fat Free Lactose Free	1 oz	40	0	0
Onions & Chives Fat Free	1 oz	40	0	0
Sharp Cheddar Fat Free	1 oz	40	0	0
Smoked Cheddar Fat Free	1 oz	40	0	0
Swiss Fat Free	1 oz	40	0	0

FOOD	PORTION	CALS.	SAT. FAT	FAT
Light N'Lively				
Singles American	1 (0.7 oz)	45	2	3
MayBud				
Edam	1 oz	100	6	8
Gouda	1 oz	100	6	8
Gouda Round	1 oz	100	6	8
New Holland				
Cheese	1 oz	90	5	7
Garlic	1 oz	90	5	7
Havarti Lower Fat Garden Vegetable	1 oz	80	4	6
Jalapeno	1 oz	80	4	6
Natural Vegetable	1 oz	80	4	6
Northfield				
Naturally Slender	1 oz	90	—	7
Old English				
American Sharp	1 slice (1 oz)	100	6	9
Organic Valley				
Aged Swiss Unpasteurized	1 oz	100	5	8
Cheddar Reduced Fat Low Sodium	1 oz	90	4	6
Cheddar Sharp & Mild	1 oz	110	6	9
Cheddar Sharp & Mild Unpasteurized	1 oz	110	6	9
Colby	1 oz	110	5	9
Colby Unpasteurized	1 oz	110	5	9
Farmer Reduced Fat	1 oz	90	4	6
Feta	1 oz	90	5	7
Monterey Jack	1 oz	100	6	8
Monterey Jack Reduced Fat	1 oz	80	3	5
Mozzarella Part Skim	1 oz	80	3	5
Muenster	1 oz	100	5	8
Pepper Jack	1 oz	110	6	9
Provolone	1 oz	100	4	8
String Part Skim	1 oz	80	3	5
Wisconsin Raw Milk Cheese	1 oz	100	6	8
Polly-O				
Mozzarella Free	1 oz	35	0	0
Mozzarella Lite	1 oz	60	2	3
Mozzarella Part Skim	1 oz	70	3	5
Mozzarella Part Skim Shredded	¼ cup	80	4	5
Mozzarella Shredded Free	¼ cup	45	0	0
Mozzarella Shredded Lite	¼ cup	60	2	3
Mozzarella Whole Milk	1 oz	80	4	6

FOOD	PORTION	CALS.	SAT. FAT	FAT
Polly-O (CONT.)				
Mozzarella Whole Milk Shredded	¼ cup	90	5	7
Ricotta Free	¼ cup	50	0	0
Ricotta Lite	¼ cup	70	2	3
Ricotta Part Skim	¼ cup	90	4	6
Ricotta Whole Milk	¼ cup	110	5	8
String	1 oz	80	—	6
String Lite	1 piece (1 oz)	60	2	3
President				
Feta Fat Free	1 oz	30	0	0
Price's				
Cheese & Bacon Spread	2 tbsp (1.1 oz)	90	3	7
Jalapeno Nacho Dip Hot	2 tbsp (1.1 oz)	80	3	7
Jalapeno Nacho Dip Mild	2 tbsp (1.1 oz)	80	3	7
Pimento Cheese Spread	2 tbsp (1.1 oz)	80	3	7
Pimento Cheese Spread Light	2 tbsp (1.1 oz)	60	1	4
Vegetable Garden	2 tbsp (1.1 oz)	70	2	5
Quaker				
Chub	2 tbsp (1 oz)	100	6	10
Rondele				
Light Soft Spreadable Garlic & Herb	2 tbsp (0.9 oz)	60	3	4
Soft Spreadable Garlic & Herbs	2 tbsp (1 oz)	100	6	9
Sargento				
Blue Crumbled	¼ cup (1 oz)	100	5	8
Cheddar	1 slice (1 oz)	110	6	9
Cheddar Shredded	¼ cup (1 oz)	110	6	9
Cheese For Nachos & Tacos Shredded	¼ cup (1 oz)	110	5	9
Cheese For Pizza Shredded	¼ cup (1 oz)	90	4	6
Cheese For Tacos Shredded	¼ cup (1 oz)	110	6	9
Colby	1 slice (1 oz)	110	6	9
Colby-Jack Shredded	¼ cup (1 oz)	110	6	9
Jarlsberg	1 slice (1.2 oz)	120	5	9
Monterey Jack	1 slice (1 oz)	100	5	9
Monterey Jack Shredded	¼ cup (1 oz)	100	6	9
MooTown Snackers Cheddar	1 piece (0.8 oz)	100	5	8
MooTown Snackers Cheddar Mild Light	1 piece (0.8 oz)	60	3	4
MooTown Snackers Cheese & Pretzels	1 pkg (0.9 oz)	90	2	3
MooTown Snackers Colby-Jack	1 piece (0.8 oz)	90	5	8

FOOD	PORTION	CALS.	SAT. FAT	FAT
Sargento (CONT.)				
MooTown Snackers Pizza Cheese & Sticks	1 pkg (1 oz)	100	3	4
MooTown Snackers String	1 piece (0.8 oz)	70	3	5
MooTown Snackers String Light	1 piece (0.8 oz)	60	2	3
Mozzarella	1 slice (1.5 oz)	130	6	9
Mozzarella Shredded	¼ cup (1 oz)	80	4	6
Muenster	1 slice (1 oz)	100	6	9
Parmesan Grated	1 tbsp (5 g)	25	1	2
Parmesan Shredded	¼ cup (1 oz)	110	5	7
Parmesan & Romano Shredded	¼ cup (1 oz)	110	5	7
Parmesan & Romano Grated	1 tbsp (5 g)	25	1	2
Pizza Double Cheese Shredded	¼ cup (1 oz)	90	5	6
Preferred Light Cheddar Mild Shredded	¼ cup (1 oz)	70	3	5
Preferred Light Cheese For Tacos Shredded	¼ cup (1 oz)	70	3	5
Preferred Light Mozzarella	1 slice (1.5 oz)	90	3	5
Preferred Light Mozzarella Shredded	¼ cup (1 oz)	70	2	3
Preferred Light Swiss	1 slice (1 oz)	80	3	4
Provolone	1 slice (1 oz)	100	5	8
Recipe Blend 4 Cheese Mexican Shredded	¼ cup (1 oz)	110	6	9
Recipe Blend 6 Cheese Italian Shredded	¼ cup (1 oz)	90	4	7
Ricotta Light	¼ cup (2.2 oz)	60	2	3
Ricotta Old Fashioned	¼ cup (2.2 oz)	90	4	6
Ricotta Part-Skim	¼ cup (2.2 oz)	80	3	5
Swiss	1 slice (0.7 oz)	80	4	6
Swiss Shredded	¼ cup (1 oz)	110	5	8
Swiss Wafer Thin	2 slices (1 oz)	110	5	9
Smart Beat				
American Fat Free	1 slice (0.6 oz)	25	0	0
Lactose Free Fat Free	1 slice (0.6 oz)	25	0	0
Mellow Cheddar Fat Free	1 slice (0.6 oz)	25	0	0
Sharp Cheddar Fat Free	1 slice (0.6 oz)	25	0	0
Treasure Cave				
Blue Crumbled	1 oz	110	6	9
Feta Crumbled	1 oz	80	4	6
Tree Of Life				
Cheddar 33% Reduced Fat Organic Milk	1 oz	90	4	6
Cheddar Low Sodium Raw Milk	1 oz	110	6	9
Cheddar Mild Organic Milk	1 oz	110	6	9

FOOD	PORTION	CALS.	SAT. FAT	FAT
Tree Of Life (CONT.)				
Cheddar Mild Raw Milk	1 oz	110	6	9
Cheddar Razor Sharp Raw Milk	1 oz	110	6	9
Cheddar Sharp Organic Milk	1 oz	110	6	9
Cheddar Sharp Raw Milk	1 oz	110	6	9
Colby Organic Milk	1 oz	120	6	10
Colby Raw Milk	1 oz	110	6	9
Farmer Part-Skim Organic Milk	1 oz	90	4	6
Jalapeno Jack Organic Milk	1 oz	110	6	9
Jalapeno Jack Semi-Soft Organic Milk	1 oz	110	6	9
Monterey Jack 35% Reduced Fat Organic Milk	1 oz	80	3	5
Monterey Jack Organic Milk	1 oz	100	6	8
Monterey Jack Semi-Soft Raw Milk	1 oz	110	6	9
Mozzarella Low Moisture Part Skim	1 oz	80	3	5
Mozzarella Low Moisture Part Skim Organic Milk	1 oz	80	3	5
Muenster Organic Milk	1 oz	100	5	8
Muenster Semi-Soft Raw Milk	1 oz	100	5	9
Provolone	1 oz	100	5	8
Swiss Raw Milk	1 oz	110	5	8
Velveeta				
Light	1 oz	60	2	3
Shredded	¼ cup (1.3 oz)	130	6	9
Shredded Mild Mexican w/ Jalapeno Pepper	¼ cup (1.3 oz)	120	6	9
Spread	1 oz	90	4	6
Spread Hot Mexican	1 oz	90	4	6
Spread Mild Mexican	1 oz	90	4	6
Weight Watchers				
Cheddar Mild Yellow	1 oz	80	3	5
Cheddar Sharp Yellow	1 oz	80	3	5
Fat Free Grated Italian Topping	1 tbsp	20	0	0
Fat Free Reduced Sodium Yellow	2 slices (0.75 oz)	30	0	0
Fat Free Sharp Cheddar	2 slices (0.75 oz)	30	0	0
Fat Free Swiss	2 slices (0.75 oz)	30	0	0
Fat Free White	2 slices (0.75 oz)	30	0	0
Fat Free Yellow	2 slices (0.75 oz)	30	0	0
Wholesome Valley				
Organic American Reduced Fat	1 slice (0.7 oz)	50	2	3

FOOD	PORTION	CALS.	SAT. FAT	FAT
WisPride				
Chunk	1 oz	110	3	8
Garlic & Herb Cup	2 tbsp (1.1 oz)	100	4	7
Hickory Smoked Cup	2 tbsp (1.1 oz)	100	4	7
Port Wine Ball	2 tbsp (1.1 oz)	100	4	8
Port Wine Cup	2 tbsp (1.1 oz)	100	4	7
Port Wine Light Cup	2 tbsp (1.1 oz)	80	2	3
Sharp Ball	2 tbsp (1.1 oz)	100	4	8
Sharp Cheddar Ball	2 tbsp (1.1 oz)	100	4	8
Sharp Cup	2 tbsp (1.1 oz)	100	4	7
Sharp Light Cup	2 tbsp (1.1 oz)	80	2	3
Swiss Ball	2 tbsp (1.1 oz)	110	3	8

CHEESE DISHES
FROZEN
Stouffer's

FOOD	PORTION	CALS.	SAT. FAT	FAT
Welsh Rarebit	½ cup (2.5 oz)	120	4	9

TAKE-OUT

FOOD	PORTION	CALS.	SAT. FAT	FAT
fondue	½ cup (3.8 oz)	247	9	15
souffle	1 serv (7 oz)	504	17	38

CHEESE SUBSTITUTES
Formagg

FOOD	PORTION	CALS.	SAT. FAT	FAT
American White	1 slice (0.66 oz)	60	1	4
American Yellow	1 slice (0.66 oz)	60	1	4
Caesar's Italian Garden American	1 oz	60	0	3
Cheddar	1 slice (0.66 oz)	60	tr	4
Cheddar Shredded	1 oz	60	0	3
Classic American	1 oz	60	0	3
Macaroni And Cheese Sauce	⅔ cup (5 oz)	190	0	2
Mozzarella Shredded	1 oz	60	0	3
Old World Mozzarella	1 oz	60	0	3
Parmesan Grated	2 tsp (5 g)	15	0	1
Swiss	1 oz	60	0	3
Swiss White	1 slice (0.66 oz)	60	1	4
Vintage Provolone	1 oz	60	0	3
Zesty Jalapeno American	1 oz	60	0	3
Frigo				
Imitation Cheddar	1 oz	90	1	7
Imitation Mozzarella	1 oz	90	1	7
Georgio's				
Imitation Cheddar Shredded	¼ cup (1 oz)	90	1	7
Imitation Mozzarella Shredded	¼ cup (1 oz)	90	1	7
Sargento				
Cheddar Shredded	¼ cup (1 oz)	90	2	7
Mozzarella Shredded	¼ cup (1 oz)	80	1	6

FOOD	PORTION	CALS.	SAT. FAT	FAT
White Wave				
Soy A Melt Cheddar	1 oz	80	1	5
Soy A Melt Fat Free Cheddar	1 oz	40	—	tr
Soy A Melt Fat Free Mozzarella	1 oz	40	—	tr
Soy A Melt Garlic Herb	1 oz	80	1	5
Soy A Melt Jalapeno Jack	1 oz	80	1	5
Soy A Melt Monterey Jack	1 oz	80	1	5
Soy A Melt Mozzarella	1 oz	80	1	5
Soy A Melt Singles American	1 slice (¾ oz)	60	1	4
Soy A Melt Singles Mozzarella	1 slice (¾ oz)	60	1	4

CHERIMOYA
fresh	1	515	—	2

CHERRIES
CANNED
sour in heavy syrup	½ cup	232	tr	tr
sour in light syrup	½ cup	189	tr	tr
sour water packed	1 cup	87	tr	tr
sweet in heavy sirup	½ cup	107	tr	tr
sweet in light syrup	½ cup	85	tr	tr
sweet juice pack	½ cup	68	tr	tr
sweet water pack	½ cup	57	tr	tr
Del Monte				
Dark Pitted In Heavy Syrup	½ cup (4.2 oz)	120	0	0
Sweet Dark Whole Unpitted In Heavy Syrup	½ cup (4.2 oz)	120	0	0

DRIED
Sonoma				
Pitted	¼ cup (1.4 oz)	140	0	0

FRESH
sour	1 cup	51	tr	tr
sweet	10	49	tr	1
Dole				
Cherries	1 cup	90	—	1

FROZEN
sour unsweetened	1 cup	72	tr	1
sweet sweetened	1 cup	232	tr	tr
Big Valley				
Dark Sweet	¾ cup (4.9 oz)	90	0	0

CHERRY JUICE
After The Fall				
Black Cherry	1 can (12 oz)	170	0	0
Capri Sun				
Wild Cherry Drink	1 pkg (7 oz)	100	0	0

FOOD	PORTION	CALS.	SAT. FAT	FAT
Hi-C				
Box	8.45 fl oz	140	0	0
Drink	8 fl oz	130	0	0
Juicy Juice				
Drink	1 box (8.45 fl oz)	130	0	0
Drink	1 bottle (6 fl oz)	90	0	0
Kool-Aid				
Black Cherry Drink as prep w/ sugar	1 serv (8 oz)	100	0	0
Bursts Cherry Drink	1 (7 oz)	100	0	0
Splash Drink	1 serv (8 oz)	110	0	0
Sugar Free Drink Mix as prep	1 serv (8 oz)	5	0	0
Ocean Spray				
Black Cherry Blast	8 oz	140	0	0
Tree Of Life				
Concentrate	8 tsp (1.4 oz)	110	0	0
Veryfine				
Juice-Ups	8 fl oz	130	0	0
CHERVIL				
seed	1 tsp	1	—	tr
CHESTNUTS				
chinese cooked	1 oz	44	tr	tr
chinese dried	1 oz	103	tr	tr
chinese raw	1 oz	64	tr	tr
chinese roasted	1 oz	68	tr	tr
cooked	1 oz	37	tr	tr
creme de marrons	1 oz	73	tr	tr
dried peeled	1 oz	105	tr	1
japanese cooked	1 oz	16	tr	tr
japanese dried	1 oz	102	tr	tr
japanese raw	1 oz	44	tr	tr
japanese roasted	1 oz	57	tr	tr
raw peeled	1 oz	56	tr	tr
roasted	2 to 3 (1 oz)	70	tr	1
roasted	1 cup	350	1	3
CHEWING GUM				
bubble gum	1 block (8 g)	27	0	0
stick	1 (3 g)	10	0	0
Arm & Hammer				
Dental Care Spearmint or Peppermint	2 pieces (2.5 g)	5	0	0
Bazooka				
Fruit Chunk	1 piece (6 g)	25	0	0

FOOD	PORTION	CALS.	SAT. FAT	FAT
Bazooka (CONT.)				
Fruit Soft	1 piece (6 g)	25	0	0
Gum	1 piece (4 g)	15	0	0
Gum	1 piece (6 g)	25	0	0
Beech-Nut				
Peppermint	1 stick (3 g)	10	0	0
Spearmint	1 stick (3 g)	10	0	0
Big Red				
Stick	1	10	—	tr
Brock				
Bubble Gum	1 piece (0.2 oz)	20	0	0
Bubble Yum				
Bananaberry Split	1 piece (0.3 oz)	25	0	0
Cotton Candy	1 piece (0.3 oz)	25	0	0
Grape	1 piece (0.3 oz)	25	0	0
Luscious Lime	1 piece (0.3 oz)	25	0	0
Regular	1 piece (0.3 oz)	25	0	0
Sour Apple	1 piece (0.3 oz)	25	0	0
Sour Cherry	1 piece (0.3 oz)	25	0	0
Sugarless	1 piece (0.2 oz)	15	—	0
Sugarless Grape	1 piece (0.2 oz)	15	—	0
Sugarless Peppermint	1 piece (0.2 oz)	15	—	0
Sugarless Strawberry	1 piece (0.2 oz)	15	—	0
Sugarless Variety	1 piece (0.2 oz)	15	—	0
Variety Pack	1 piece (0.3 oz)	25	0	0
Watermelon	1 piece (0.3 oz)	25	0	0
Wild Strawberry	1 piece (0.3 oz)	25	0	0
Bubblicious				
Gum	1 piece (7.9 g)	25	0	0
*Care*Free*				
Sugarless Bubble Gum	1 stick (3 g)	10	—	0
Sugarless Cinnamon	1 piece (3 g)	5	—	0
Sugarless Peppermint	1 piece (3 g)	5	—	0
Sugarless Spearmint	1 piece (3 g)	5	—	0
Sugarless Wild Cherry	1 stick (3 g)	10	0	0
Chiclets				
Original	1 piece (1.59 g)	6	0	0
Tiny Size	8 pieces (0.13 g)	tr	0	0
Clorets				
Clorets	1 piece (1.59 g)	6	0	0
Dentyne				
Cinn-A-Burst	1 piece (3.2 g)	9	0	0
Gum	1 piece (1.88 g)	6	0	0
Sugar Free	1 piece (1.88 g)	5	0	0

FOOD	PORTION	CALS.	SAT. FAT	FAT
Doublemint				
Chewing Gum	1 piece	10	—	tr
Extra Sugar Free				
Cinnamon	1 piece	8	—	tr
Spearmint & Peppermint	1 stick	8	—	tr
Winter Fresh	1 piece	8	—	tr
Freedent				
Spearmint Peppermint & Cinnamon	1 stick	10	—	tr
Freshen-Up				
Gum	1 piece (4.2 g)	13	0	0
Fruit Stripe				
Bubble Gum Jumbo Pack	1 stick (3 g)	10	0	0
Variety Pack Chewing & Bubble Gum	1 stick (3 g)	10	0	0
Hubba Bubba				
Bubble Gum Cola	1 piece	23	—	tr
Bubble Gum Sugarfree Grape	1 piece	13	—	tr
Bubble Gum Sugarfree Original	1 piece	14	—	tr
Original	1 piece	23	—	tr
Strawberry Grape Raspberry	1 piece	23	—	tr
Juicy Fruit				
Stick	1	10	—	tr
Lance				
Big Red Cinnamon	1 piece (3 g)	10	0	0
Double Bubble	1 piece (7 g)	25	0	0
Double Mint	1 piece (3 g)	10	0	0
Rain-Blo				
Bubble Gum Balls	1 piece (2 g)	5	0	0
*Stick*Free*				
Sugarless Peppermint	1 stick (3 g)	10	—	0
Sugarless Spearmint	1 stick (3 g)	10	—	0
Swell				
Bubble Gum	1 piece (3 g)	10	—	0
Trident				
Gum	1 piece (1.88 g)	5	0	0
Soft Bubble Gum	1 piece (3.3 g)	9	0	0
Winterfresh				
Stick	1 stick (3 g)	10	0	0
Wrigley's				
Spearmint	1 stick	10	—	tr
CHIA SEEDS				
dried	1 oz	134	3	7

FOOD	PORTION	CALS.	SAT. FAT	FAT

CHICKEN

(see also CHICKEN DISHES, CHICKEN SUBSTITUTES, DINNER, HOT DOG)

CANNED

FOOD	PORTION	CALS.	SAT. FAT	FAT
chicken spread	1 oz	55	—	3
chicken spread	1 tbsp	25	—	2
chicken spread barbeque flavored	1 oz	55	—	3
w/ broth	½ can (2.5 oz)	117	2	6
w/ broth	1 can (5 oz)	234	3	11
Swanson				
Chunk Style Mixin' Chicken	2.5 oz	130	—	8
White	2.5 oz	100	—	4
White & Dark	2.5 oz	100	—	4
Underwood				
Chunky	2.08 oz	150	3	9
Chunky Light	2.08 oz	80	1	3
Smoky	2.08 oz	150	2	8
FRESH				
broiler/fryer back w/ skin batter dipped & fried	½ back (2.5 oz)	238	4	16
broiler/fryer back w/ skin floured & fried	1.5 oz	146	2	9
broiler/fryer back w/ skin roasted	1 oz	96	2	7
broiler/fryer back w/ skin stewed	½ back (2.1 oz)	158	3	11
broiler/fryer back w/o skin fried	½ back (2 oz)	167	2	9
broiler/fryer breast w/ skin batter dipped & fried	½ breast (4.9 oz)	364	5	18
broiler/fryer breast w/ skin batter dipped & fried	2.9 oz	218	3	11
broiler/fryer breast w/ skin roasted	2 oz	115	1	5
broiler/fryer breast w/ skin roasted	½ breast (3.4 oz)	193	2	8
broiler/fryer breast w/ skin stewed	½ breast (3.9 oz)	202	2	8
broiler/fryer breast w/o skin fried	½ breast (3 oz)	161	1	4
broiler/fryer breast w/o skin roasted	½ breast (3 oz)	142	1	3
broiler/fryer breast w/o skin stewed	2 oz	86	tr	2
broiler/fryer dark meat w/ skin batter dipped & fried	5.9 oz	497	8	31
broiler/fryer dark meat w/ skin floured & fried	3.9 oz	313	5	19

FOOD	PORTION	CALS.	SAT. FAT	FAT
broiler/fryer dark meat w/ skin roasted	3.5 oz	256	4	16
broiler/fryer dark meat w/ skin stewed	3.9 oz	256	4	16
broiler/fryer dark meat w/o skin fried	1 cup (5 oz)	334	4	16
broiler/fryer dark meat w/o skin roasted	1 cup (5 oz)	286	4	14
broiler/fryer dark meat w/o skin stewed	1 cup (5 oz)	269	3	13
broiler/fryer dark meat w/o skin stewed	3 oz	165	2	8
broiler/fryer drumstick w/ skin batter dipped & fried	1 (2.6 oz)	193	3	11
broiler/fryer drumstick w/ skin floured & fried	1 (1.7 oz)	120	2	7
broiler/fryer drumstick w/ skin roasted	1 (1.8 oz)	112	2	6
broiler/fryer drumstick w/ skin stewed	1 (2 oz)	116	2	6
broiler/fryer drumstick w/o skin fried	1 (1.5 oz)	82	1	3
broiler/fryer drumstick w/o skin roasted	1 (1.5 oz)	76	1	2
broiler/fryer drumstick w/o skin stewed	1 (1.6 oz)	78	1	3
broiler/fryer leg w/ skin batter dipped & fried	1 (5.5 oz)	431	7	26
broiler/fryer leg w/ skin floured & fried	1 (3.9 oz)	285	4	16
broiler/fryer leg w/ skin roasted	1 (4 oz)	265	4	15
broiler/fryer leg w/ skin stewed	1 (4.4 oz)	275	4	16
broiler/fryer leg w/o skin fried	1 (3.3 oz)	195	2	9
broiler/fryer leg w/o skin roasted	1 (3.3 oz)	182	2	8
broiler/fryer leg w/o skin stewed	1 (3.5 oz)	187	2	8
broiler/fryer light meat w/ skin batter dipped & fried	4 oz	312	5	17
broiler/fryer light meat w/ skin floured & fried	2.7 oz	192	3	9
broiler/fryer light meat w/ skin roasted	2.8 oz	175	2	9
broiler/fryer light meat w/ skin stewed	3.2 oz	181	3	9

FOOD	PORTION	CALS.	SAT. FAT	FAT
broiler/fryer light meat w/o skin fried	1 cup (5 oz)	268	2	8
broiler/fryer light meat w/o skin roasted	1 cup (5 oz)	242	2	6
broiler/fryer light meat w/o skin stewed	1 cup (5 oz)	223	2	6
broiler/fryer neck w/ skin stewed	1 (1.3 oz)	94	2	7
broiler/fryer neck w/o skin stewed	1 (.6 oz)	32	tr	1
broiler/fryer skin batter dipped & fried	from ½ chicken (6.7 oz)	748	14	55
broiler/fryer skin batter dipped & fried	4 oz	449	9	33
broiler/fryer skin floured & fried	from ½ chicken (2 oz)	281	7	24
broiler/fryer skin floured & fried	1 oz	166	4	14
broiler/fryer skin roasted	from ½ chicken (2 oz)	254	6	23
broiler/fryer skin stewed	from ½ chicken (2.5 oz)	261	7	24
broiler/fryer thigh w/ skin batter dipped & fried	1 (3 oz)	238	4	14
broiler/fryer thigh w/ skin floured & fried	1 (2.2 oz)	162	3	9
broiler/fryer thigh w/ skin roasted	1 (2.2 oz)	153	3	10
broiler/fryer thigh w/ skin stewed	1 (2.4 oz)	158	3	10
broiler/fryer thigh w/o skin fried	1 (1.8 oz)	113	1	5
broiler/fryer thigh w/o skin roasted	1 (1.8 oz)	109	2	6
broiler/fryer thigh w/o skin stewed	1 (1.9 oz)	107	1	5
broiler/fryer w/ skin floured & fried	½ chicken (11 oz)	844	13	47
broiler/fryer w/ skin floured & fried	½ breast (3.4 oz)	218	2	9
broiler/fryer w/ skin fried	½ chicken (16.4 oz)	1347	22	81
broiler/fryer w/ skin roasted	½ chicken (10.5 oz)	715	11	41
broiler/fryer w/ skin stewed	½ chicken (11.7 oz)	730	12	42
broiler/fryer w/ skin neck & giblets batter dipped & fried	1 chicken (2.3 lbs)	2987	48	180
broiler/fryer w/ skin neck & giblets roasted	1 chicken (1.5 lbs)	1598	25	90
broiler/fryer w/ skin neck & giblets stewed	1 chicken (1.6 lbs)	1625	26	93
broiler/fryer w/o skin fried	1 cup	307	3	13
broiler/fryer w/o skin roasted	1 cup (5 oz)	266	3	10
broiler/fryer w/o skin stewed	1 oz	54	1	3
broiler/fryer w/o skin stewed	1 cup (5 oz)	248	3	9

FOOD	PORTION	CALS.	SAT. FAT	FAT
broiler/fryer wing w/ skin batter dipped & fried	1 (1.7 oz)	159	3	11
broiler/fryer wing w/ skin floured & fried	1 (1.1 oz)	103	2	7
broiler/fryer wing w/ skin roasted	1 (1.2 oz)	99	2	7
broiler/fryer wing w/ skin stewed	1 (1.4 oz)	100	2	7
capon w/ skin neck & giblets roasted	1 chicken (3.1 lbs)	3211	46	165
cornish hen w/ skin roasted	1 hen (8 oz)	595	12	42
cornish hen w/o skin & bone roasted	1 hen (3.8 oz)	144	1	4
cornish hen w/o skin & bone roasted	½ hen (2 oz)	72	1	2
cornish hen w/skin roasted	½ hen (4 oz)	296	6	21
roaster dark meat w/o skin roasted	1 cup (5 oz)	250	3	12
roaster light meat w/o skin roasted	1 cup (5 oz)	214	2	6
roaster w/ skin neck & giblets roasted	1 chicken (2.4 lbs)	2363	39	140
roaster w/ skin roasted	½ chicken (1.1 lbs)	1071	18	64
roaster w/o skin roasted	1 cup (5 oz)	469	3	28
stewing dark meat w/o skin stewed	1 cup (5 oz)	361	6	21
stewing w/ skin neck & giblets stewed	1 chicken (1.3 lbs)	1636	29	107
stewing w/ skin stewed	½ chicken (9.2 oz)	744	13	49
stewing w/ skin stewed	6.2 oz	507	9	34
Perdue				
Boneless Breasts Cooked	3 oz	120	1	2
Boneless Breast Tenderloins Cooked	3 oz	100	1	1
Boneless Thighs Roasted	2 (3.5 oz)	200	3	11
Breast Quarters Cooked	3 oz	180	3	10
Burger Cooked	1 (3 oz)	170	3	11
Chicken Breast Seasoned Barbecue Cooked	3 oz	110	1	1
Chicken Breast Seasoned Italian Cooked	3 oz	100	1	1
Chicken Breast Seasoned Lemon Pepper Cooked	3 oz	90	1	1
Chicken Breast Seasoned Oriental Cooked	3 oz	100	1	1
Cornish Hen Split Dark Meat Roasted	1 half (6.5 oz)	210	5	15

FOOD	PORTION	CALS.	SAT. FAT	FAT
Perdue (CONT.)				
Cornish Hen White Meat Cooked	3 oz	170	3	9
Drumsticks Roasted	1 (2 oz)	110	2	6
Drumsticks Skinless Roasted	2 (3.5 oz)	150	2	6
Ground Cooked	3 oz	180	4	12
Jumbo Drumsticks Roasted	1 (2 oz)	110	2	6
Jumbo Split Breast Roasted	1 (7 oz)	370	6	20
Jumbo Thighs Roasted	1 (3 oz)	240	5	18
Jumbo Whole Leg Roasted	2 (5.5 oz)	360	7	25
Jumbo Wings Roasted	2 (3 oz)	210	5	15
Leg Quarters Cooked	3 oz	210	5	16
Oven Stuffer Boneless Breast Cooked	3 oz	120	1	2
Oven Stuffer Boneless Breast Thin Sliced Cooked	1 slice (2 oz)	80	1	1
Oven Stuffer Boneless Thighs Roasted	1 (3.5 oz)	170	3	8
Oven Stuffer Dark Meat Roasted	3 oz	200	4	14
Oven Stuffer Drumbstick Roasted	1 (3.5 oz)	190	3	11
Oven Stuffer White Meat Roasted	3 oz	160	3	8
Oven Stuffer Whole Breast Cooked	3 oz	150	2	7
Oven Stuffer Wing Drummettes Roasted	2 (2.5 oz)	170	4	11
Split Breast Skinless Roasted	1 (6 oz)	250	3	8
Split Breasts Roasted	1 (7 oz)	370	6	20
Thighs Roasted	1 (3 oz)	240	5	18
Thighs Skinless Roasted	1 (2.5 oz)	160	3	9
Whole White Meat Cooked	3 oz	160	3	9
Whole Leg Roasted	1 (5.5 oz)	360	7	25
Wingettes Roasted	3 (3 oz)	200	4	14
Wings Roasted	2 (3 oz)	210	5	15
Tyson				
Broth Marinated Breast Filet	1 (4.7 oz)	140	1	4
Broth Marinated Drums	2 (4 oz)	140	2	7
Broth Marinated Thighs	1 (4.9 oz)	380	10	34
Broth Marinated Wings	4 pieces (4.2 oz)	240	5	18
Chicken Broccoli & Cheese	1 piece (5.9 oz)	320	5	16
Chicken Stuffed w/ Wild Rice & Mushroom	1 piece (5.9 oz)	300	3	12
Cordon Bleu	1 piece (5.9 oz)	350	6	17

FOOD	PORTION	CALS.	SAT. FAT	FAT
Tyson (CONT.)				
Cornish Hen	1 serv (4 oz)	180	4	12
Kiev	1 piece (5.9 oz)	460	16	32
Wampler				
Breast Tenders	4 oz	130	1	2
FROZEN				
Banquet				
Country Fried	1 serv (3 oz)	270	5	18
Drum Snackers	2.25 oz	190	3	13
Fried Breast	1 piece (4.45 oz)	240	13	26
Fried Hot & Spicy	1 serv (3 oz)	260	5	18
Fried Original	1 serv (3 oz)	270	5	18
Fried Thigh & Drumsticks	1 serv (3 oz)	260	5	18
Hot & Spicy Nuggets	2.5 oz	230	4	17
Hot Popcorn Chicken	1 pkg (3 oz)	290	4	19
Nuggets	3 oz	240	3	15
Nuggets Chicken & Cheddar	2.7 oz	280	6	19
Nuggets Chicken & Mozzarella	6 (2.8 oz)	210	4	11
Nuggets Southern Fried	6 (4.5 oz)	340	4	20
Nuggets Sweet & Sour	6 (4.5 oz)	320	4	18
Patties	1 (2.5 oz)	180	3	11
Patties Southern Fried	1 (2.5 oz)	190	3	12
Skinless Fried	1 serv (3 oz)	210	3	13
Skinless Fried Honey BBQ	1 serv (3 oz)	210	3	13
Southern Fried	1 serv (3 oz)	270	5	18
Tenders	3 pieces (3 oz)	260	4	16
Tenders Southern Fried	3 pieces (3 oz)	260	4	16
Wings Hot & Spicy	4 pieces (5 oz)	230	5	16
Country Skillet				
Chicken Chunks	5 (3.1 oz)	270	3	17
Chicken Nuggets	10 (3.3 oz)	280	4	18
Chicken Patties	2.5 oz	190	3	12
Southern Fried Chicken Chunks	5 (3.1 oz)	250	3	15
Southern Fried Chicken Patties	1 (2.5 oz)	190	3	12
Empire				
Nuggets	5 (3 oz)	180	2	9
Stix	4 (3.1 oz)	180	2	9
Ozark Valley				
Nuggets	4 (2.9 oz)	210	2	10
Patties	1 (3 oz)	210	3	11
Sensible Chef				
Fried Breast	1 (3 oz)	200	3	10
Swanson				
Chicken Nibbles	3¼ oz	300	—	19
Chicken Nuggets	3 oz	230	—	14

FOOD	PORTION	CALS.	SAT. FAT	FAT
Swanson (CONT.)				
Fried Chicken Breast Portion	4½ oz	360	—	20
Pre-Fried Chicken Parts	3¼ oz	270	—	16
Thighs & Drumsticks	3¼ oz	290	—	18
Weaver				
Breast Strips	3 pieces (3.3 oz)	210	2	11
Breast Tenders	5 pieces (3 oz)	220	3	15
Croquettes	1 serv (3.5 oz)	290	5	18
Dutch Frye Nuggets	5 pieces (3.3 oz)	280	5	20
Honey Battered Tenders	5 pieces (2.9 oz)	230	3	15
Hot Wings Buffalo Style	3 pieces (2.7 oz)	190	4	13
Mini Drums Crispy	5 pieces (3.3 oz)	250	3	16
Nuggets	4 pieces (2.7 oz)	210	4	15
Patties	1 (2.6 oz)	180	3	11
Rondelet	1 (2.6 oz)	170	3	10
Rondelet Dutch Frye	1 (2.6 oz)	230	4	16
Rondelet Italian	1 (2.6 oz)	210	3	14
READY-TO-EAT				
chicken roll light meat	2 oz	90	1	4
chicken roll light meat	1 pkg (6 oz)	271	3	13
poultry salad sandwich spread	1 tbsp (13 g)	109	tr	2
poultry salad sandwich spread	1 oz	238	1	4
Banquet				
Breast Tenders Fat Free	3 (3.2 oz)	130	0	0
Boar's Head				
Breast Hickory Smoked	2 oz	60	0	1
Breast Oven Roasted	2 oz	50	0	1
Carl Buddig				
Chicken Sliced	1 pkg (2.5 oz)	110	2	7
Lean Slices Honey Smoked Breast	1 pkg (2.5 oz)	70	1	1
Lean Slices Roasted Breast	1 pkg (2.5 oz)	60	1	1
Chicken By George				
Cajun	1 breast (4 oz)	130	1	4
Caribbean Grill	1 breast (4 oz)	150	1	4
Garlic & Herb	1 breast (4 oz)	120	1	3
Italian Bleu Cheese	1 breast (4 oz)	130	1	5
Lemon Herb	1 breast (4 oz)	120	1	3
Lemon Oregano	1 breast (4 oz)	130	1	4
Mesquite Barbecue	1 breast (4 oz)	130	1	3
Mustard Dill	1 breast (4 oz)	140	1	5
Roasted	1 breast (4 oz)	110	1	3
Teriyaki	1 breast (4 oz)	130	1	3
Tomato Herb With Basil	1 breast (4 oz)	140	1	5

FOOD	PORTION	CALS.	SAT. FAT	FAT
Empire				
Barbarcue Whole	5 oz	280	5	17
Battered & Breaded Cutlets	1 (3.3 oz)	200	2	9
Battered & Breaded Fried Breasts	3 oz	170	2	8
Battered & Breaded Nuggets	5 (3 oz)	200	3	13
Bologna	3 slices (1.8 oz)	200	2	7
Fried Drum & Thigh	3 oz	240	4	16
Falls				
BBQ	3 oz	150	—	8
Healthy Choice				
Deli-Thin Oven Roasted Breast	6 slices (2 oz)	45	0	0
Deli-Thin Smoked Breast	6 slices (2 oz)	60	1	2
Fresh-Trak Oven Roasted Breast	1 slice (1 oz)	30	0	1
Oven Roasted Breast	1 slice (1 oz)	25	0	0
Smoked Breast	1 slice (1 oz)	35	0	1
Hebrew National				
Deli Thin Oven Roasted	1.8 oz	45	—	1
Hillshire				
Deli Select Oven Roasted Breast	1 slice	10	—	tr
Deli Select Smoked Breast	1 slice	10	—	tr
Flavor Pack 90–99% Fat Free Smoked Breast	1 slice (0.75 oz)	20	—	tr
Lunch 'N Munch Smoked Chicken/ Monterey Jack	1 pkg (4.5 oz)	350	—	20
Lunch 'N Munch Smoked Chicken/ Monterey/ Snickers	1 pkg (4.25 oz)	400	—	23
Louis Rich				
Carving Board Classic Baked	2 slices (1.6 oz)	45	0	1
Carving Board Grilled	2 slices (1.6 oz)	45	0	1
Deli-Thin Oven Roasted Breast	4 slices (1.8 oz)	50	1	1
Oven Roasted Deluxe Breast	1 slice (1 oz)	30	0	1
Mr. Turkey				
Deli Cuts Hardwood Smoked	3 slices	30	—	tr
Deli Cuts Oven Roasted	3 slices	25	—	0
Oscar Mayer				
Free Oven Roasted Breast	4 slices (1.8 oz)	45	0	0
Lunchables Chicken/Monterey Jack	1 pkg (4.5 oz)	350	10	21
Lunchables Deluxe Chicken/Turkey	1 pkg (5.1 oz)	380	11	22
Lunchables Dessert Chocolate Pudding/Chicken/ Jack	1 pkg (6.2 oz)	370	9	18

FOOD	PORTION	CALS.	SAT. FAT	FAT
Perdue				
Cafe Meal Kit Stir Fry	1 serv (8.2 oz)	360	—	2
Cornish Hen Dark Meat Cooked	3 oz	200	5	15
Cornish Hen Split White Meat Roasted	½ hen (6.5 oz)	200	4	11
Nuggets Chicken & Cheese	5 (3 oz)	220	4	15
Nuggets Chik-Tac-Toe Cooked	5 (3 oz)	200	3	12
Nuggets Football Basketball Baseball	4 (3 oz)	230	4	15
Nuggets Original	5 (3 oz)	200	3	12
Nuggets Star & Drumstick	4 (3 oz)	200	3	12
Original Tenderloins Cooked	3 oz	160	3	7
Original Cutlets Cooked	1 (3.5 oz)	230	4	13
Oven Roasted Breast	1 (5 oz)	190	2	6
Oven Roasted Drumsticks	2 (2.5 oz)	100	1	4
Oven Roasted Half Dark Meat	3 oz	170	3	11
Oven Roasted Half White Meat	3 oz	140	2	7
Oven Roasted Thighs	1 (3 oz)	170	4	12
Oven Roasted Whole Chicken Dark Meat	3 oz	170	3	11
Oven Roasted Whole Chicken White Meat	3 oz	140	2	7
Seasoned Whole Chicken Dark Meat	3 oz	190	4	14
Seasoned Whole Chicken White Meat	3 oz	160	3	9
Short Cuts Italian	3 oz	110	1	2
Short Cuts Lemon Pepper	½ cup (2.5 oz)	90	1	2
Short Cuts Mesquite	3 oz	110	1	2
Short Cuts Oven Roasted	3 oz	110	1	2
Wings Barbecued	3 oz	200	4	13
Wings Hot & Spicy	3 oz	190	4	13
Shady Brook				
Slow Roasted Breast	2 oz	60	0	1
Tyson				
Breaded Breast Chunks	6 pieces (2.9 oz)	230	5	16
Breaded Breast Fillet	2 pieces (2.8 oz)	180	2	8
Breaded Breast Pattie	1 (2.6 oz)	190	3	12
Breaded Breast Tenders	5 pieces (3 oz)	220	3	15
Breaded Chicken Chunks	6 pieces (3 oz)	220	3	14
Chick'n Quick Chick'n Cheddar	1 patty (2.6 oz)	220	4	14
Chicken Bits Southern Fried	6 pieces (2.9 oz)	260	5	19
Chicken Strips	1 serv (3 oz)	90	0	1
Chicken Strips Southwestern	1 serv (3 oz)	110	1	3
Country Fried Chicken Fritter	5 pieces (2.9 oz)	260	4	18

FOOD	PORTION	CALS.	SAT. FAT	FAT
Tyson (CONT.)				
Drumsticks Hot BBQ Style	2 (3.5 oz)	160	2	7
Glazed Grilled Breast Pattie	1 (2.7 oz)	120	2	7
Grilled Chicken Pattie	1 (2.9 oz)	170	4	12
Nuggets Breaded White Meat	6 pieces (2.9 oz)	250	5	18
Patties Southern Fried	1 (2.9 oz)	260	5	19
Roasted Drumsticks	3 (5.6 oz)	320	5	15
Roasted Drumsticks w/o Skin	2 (3.3 oz)	140	2	5
Roasted Half Chicken	1 serv (3 oz)	160	4	11
Roasted Whole Chicken	1 serv (3 oz)	160	4	11
Roasted Breast Boneless w/o Skin	1 (3.7 oz)	130	1	3
Roasted Breast Half w/o Skin	1 (4.3 oz)	150	1	3
Roasted Half Breast w/ Skin	1 (5.1 oz)	260	4	13
Roasted Half Chicken w/o Skin	1 serv (3 oz)	120	2	6
Roasted Tabasco Wings	3 (3 oz)	190	4	13
Roasted Thigh w/ Skin	1 (3.6 oz)	270	7	21
Roasted Thighs w/o Skin	1 (2.9 oz)	150	3	8
Roll White Meat	2 oz	90	2	6
Southern Fried Breaded Breast Pattie	1 (2.6 oz)	180	3	12
Southern Fried Breast Fillets	2 pieces (3.4 oz)	210	2	11
Southern Fried Chunks	6 pieces (2.9 oz)	260	5	19
Tenders Breaded Honey Battered	5 pieces (2.9 oz)	230	3	15
Tenders Breaded Pattie	3 pieces (3.2 oz)	100	0	0
Thick'n Crispy Pattie	1 (2.6 oz)	200	3	14
Wings BBQ	3 pieces (3.2 oz)	200	4	13
Wings Hot N'Spicy	4 (3.2 oz)	210	4	14
Wings Teriyaki	4 pieces (3.4 oz)	190	3	12
Wings Of Fire	4 pieces (3.4 oz)	220	4	15
TAKE-OUT				
oven roasted breast of chicken	2 oz	60	0	1

CHICKEN DISHES

(see also CHICKEN SUBSTITUTES, DINNER)

CANNED

FOOD	PORTION	CALS.	SAT. FAT	FAT
Dinty Moore				
Noodles & Chicken	1 can (7.5 oz)	180	2	8
Stew	1 cup (8.5 oz)	220	3	11
Swanson				
Chicken & Dumplings	7½ oz	220	—	11
Chicken Ala King	5¼ oz	190	—	12
Chicken Stew	7⅝ oz	160	—	7

FOOD	PORTION	CALS.	SAT. FAT	FAT
FROZEN				
Croissant Pocket				
Stuffed Sandwich Chicken Broccoli & Cheddar	1 piece (4.5 oz)	300	4	11
Hot Pocket				
Stuffed Sandwich Chicken & Cheddar With Broccoli	1 (4.5 oz)	300	5	12
Jimmy Dean				
Grilled Breast Sandwich	1 (5.5 oz)	330	4	11
Lean Pockets				
Stuffed Sandwich Chicken Fajita	1 (4.5 oz)	260	3	8
Stuffed Sandwich Chicken Parmesan	1 (4.5 oz)	260	3	8
Stuffed Sandwich Glazed Chicken Supreme	1 (4.5 oz)	240	3	7
White Castle				
Grilled Chicken Sandwich	2 (4 oz)	250	3	9
Grilled Chicken Sandwich w/ Sauce	2 (4.8 oz)	290	3	9
MIX				
Chicken Skillet Helper				
Stir-Fried Chicken as prep	1 cup	270	2	9
Hamburger Helper				
Reduced Sodium Cheddar Spirals Chicken Recipe as prep	1 cup	240	2	6
Reduced Sodium Italian Herb Chicken Recipe as prep	1 cup	200	1	2
Reduced Sodium Southwestern Beef Chicken Recipe as prep	1 cup	220	1	3
Tyson				
Mandarin Wrap Kit	1½ wraps (14.6 oz)	630	4	15
READY-TO-EAT				
Shady Brook				
Chicken Breast w/ Rice Pilaf	1 serv (12 oz)	350	4	13
Teriyaki Breast	1 serv (12 oz)	490	1	3
Wampler				
Salad	⅓ cup	200	—	14
Salad Lite	⅓ cup	130	—	7
Salad Low Fat	⅓ cup	90	—	2
SHELF-STABLE				
Dinty Moore				
Microwave Cup Chicken & Dumpling	1 pkg (7.5 oz)	200	2	6
Microwave Cup Stew	1 pkg (7.5 oz)	180	2	8

FOOD	PORTION	CALS.	SAT. FAT	FAT
Lunch Bucket				
Chicken Fiesta	1 pkg (7.5 oz)	160	1	2
Dumplings'n Chicken	1 pkg (7.5 oz)	140	2	5
TAKE-OUT				
boneless breaded & fried w/ barbecue sauce	6 pieces (4.6 oz)	330	6	18
boneless breaded & fried w/ honey	6 pieces (4 oz)	339	5	18
boneless breaded & fried w/ mustard sauce	6 pieces (4.6 oz)	323	6	17
boneless breaded & fried w/ sweet & sour sauce	6 pieces (4.6 oz)	346	6	18
breast & wing breaded & fried	2 pieces (5.7 oz)	494	8	30
chicken & noodles	1 cup	365	5	18
chicken a la king	1 cup	470	13	34
chicken paprikash	1½ cups	296	—	10
drumstick breaded & fried	2 pieces (5.2 oz)	430	7	27
jamaican jerk wings	4 wings (9.9 oz)	709	14	51
thigh breaded & fried	2 pieces (5.2 oz)	430	7	27

CHICKEN SUBSTITUTES

FOOD	PORTION	CALS.	SAT. FAT	FAT
Harvest Direct				
TVP Poultry Chunks	3.5 oz	280	tr	1
TVP Poultry Ground	3.5 oz	280	tr	1
Knox Mountain Farm				
Chick'N Wheat Mix	1 serv (⅙ pkg)	110	—	1
Loma Linda				
Chicken Supreme Mix not prep	⅓ cup (0.9 oz)	90	0	1
Chik Nuggets	5 pieces (3 oz)	240	3	16
Fried Chik'n w/ Gravy	2 pieces (2.8 oz)	210	3	17
Morningstar Farms				
Chik Nuggets	4 pieces (3 oz)	160	1	4
Chik Patties	1 (2.5 oz)	150	1	6
Soy Is Us				
Chicken Not!	½ cup (1.75 oz)	140	1	2
White Wave				
Meatless Sandwich Slices	2 slices (1.6 oz)	80	0	0
Worthington				
Chic-Ketts	2 slices (1.9 oz)	120	1	7
Chicken Sliced	2 slices (2 oz)	80	1	5
ChikStiks	1 (1.6 oz)	110	1	7
CrispyChik Patties	1 (2.5 oz)	170	2	9
Cutlets	1 slice (2.1 oz)	70	0	1
Diced Chik	¼ cup (1.9 oz)	40	0	0
FriChik	2 pieces (3.2 oz)	120	1	8

FOOD	PORTION	CALS.	SAT. FAT	FAT
Worthington (CONT.)				
FriChik Low Fat	2 pieces (3 oz)	80	0	3
Golden Croquettes	4 pieces (3 oz)	210	2	10
Sliced Chik	3 slices (3.2 oz)	70	0	1
CHICKPEAS				
CANNED				
chickpeas	1 cup	285	tr	3
Allen				
Garbanzo	½ cup (4.4 oz)	120	1	3
East Texas Fair				
Garbanzo	½ cup (4.4 oz)	120	1	3
Eden				
Organic	½ cup (4.6 oz)	120	—	2
Goya				
Spanish Style	7.5 oz	150	—	2
Green Giant				
Garbanzo	½ cup (4.4 oz)	110	0	2
Hanover				
Chickpeas	½ cup	100	—	1
Old El Paso				
Garbanzo	½ cup (4.6 oz)	120	0	3
Progresso				
Chick Peas	½ cup (4.6 oz)	120	0	3
DRIED				
cooked	1 cup	269	tr	4
Bean Cuisine				
Garbanzo	½ cup	115	—	1
CHICORY				
greens raw chopped	½ cup	21	tr	tr
root raw	1 (2.1 oz)	44	tr	tr
roots raw cut up	½ cup (1.6 oz)	33	tr	tr
witloof head raw	1 (1.9 oz)	9	tr	tr
witloof raw	½ cup (1.6 oz)	8	tr	tr
CHILI				
chili w/ beans	1 cup	286	6	14
powder	1 tsp	8	—	tr
Allen				
Mexican w/ Beans	½ cup (4.5 oz)	120	0	1
Amy's Organic				
Whole Meals Chili & Cornbread	1 pkg (10.5 oz)	320	2	6
Armour				
Chili No Beans	1 cup (8.7 oz)	390	13	29
Chili W/ Beans Westren Style	1 cup (8.8 oz)	370	10	22

FOOD	PORTION	CALS.	SAT. FAT	FAT
Armour (CONT.)				
Chili w/ Beans	1 cup (8.9 oz)	370	9	21
Chili w/ Beans Hot	1 cup (8.9 oz)	370	9	21
Vienna Sausage & Chili	1 cup (8.7 oz)	410	11	27
Brown Beauty				
Mexican Chili Beans	½ cup (4.5 oz)	120	0	1
Chili Man				
Seasoning Mix	1 tbsp (7 g)	25	—	1
Del Monte				
Sauce	1 tbsp (0.6 oz)	20	0	0
Dennison's				
Chili Beans In Chili Gravy	7.5 oz	180	—	1
Chili Con Carne w/ Beans	7.5 oz	300	—	19
Chili Con Carne w/ Beans	7.5 oz	310	—	15
Chunky Chili w/ Beans	7.5 oz	310	—	14
Cook-off Chili w/ Beans	7.5 oz	340	—	19
Hot Chili Con Carne w/ Beans	7.5 oz	310	—	16
Eden				
Organic Chili Beans w/ Jalapeno & Red Peppers	½ cup (4.6 oz)	130	0	0
Gebhardt				
Chili Powder	1 tsp	15	—	tr
Chili Quik Seasoning	1 tsp	10	—	tr
Hot With Beans	1 cup	470	10	27
Plain	1 cup	530	16	43
With Beans	1 cup	495	10	28
Hain				
Hot	¼ pkg	30	—	1
Medium	¼ pkg	30	—	1
Mild	¼ pkg	30	—	1
Spicy Tempeh	7½ oz	160	—	4
Spicy Vegetarian	7½ oz	160	—	1
Spicy Vegetarian Reduced Sodium	7½ oz	170	—	1
Spicy With Chicken	7½ oz	130	—	2
Health Valley				
Burrito	1 cup	160	—	1
Enchilada	1 cup	160	—	1
Fajita	1 cup	80	0	0
In A Cup Black Bean Mild	¾ cup	120	—	1
In A Cup Texas Style Spicy	¾ cup	120	—	1
Vegetarian Lentil Mild	1 cup	160	—	1
Vegetarian Lentil No Salt	1 cup	80	0	0
Vegetarian Mild	1 cup	160	—	1
Vegetarian Mild No Salt	1 cup	160	—	1

FOOD	PORTION	CALS.	SAT. FAT	FAT
Health Valley (CONT.)				
Vegetarian Spicy	1 cup	160	—	1
Vegetarian Spicy No Salt	1 cup	160	—	1
Vegetarian w/ 3 Beans Mild	1 cup	160	—	1
Vegetarian w/ Black Beans Mild	1 cup	160	—	1
Vegetarian w/ Black Beans Spicy	1 cup	160	—	1
Hormel				
Chunky w/ Beans	1 cup (8.7 oz)	270	3	7
Hot No Beans	1 cup (8.3 oz)	210	3	9
Hot With Beans	1 cup (8.7 oz)	270	3	7
Microcup Meals Chili Mac	1 cup (7.5 oz)	200	4	9
Microcup Meals Hot With Beans	1 cup (7.3 oz)	220	3	6
Microcup Meals No Beans	1 cup (7.3 oz)	190	3	8
Microcup Meals With Beans	1 cup (7.3 oz)	220	3	6
No Beans	1 cup (8.3 oz)	210	3	9
Turkey No Beans	1 cup (8.3 oz)	190	1	3
Turkey w/ Beans	1 cup (8.7 oz)	210	1	3
Vegetarian	1 cup (8.7 oz)	200	0	1
With Beans	1 cup (8.7 oz)	270	3	7
With Beans	1 cup (8.7 oz)	270	3	7
Hunt's				
Chili Beans	½ cup (4.5 oz)	87	0	1
Hurst				
HamBeens Chili Beans	1 serv	130	0	1
Just Rite				
Hot With Beans	4 oz	195	4	10
With Beans	4 oz	200	4	11
Without Beans	4 oz	180	4	11
Lean Cuisine				
Three Bean w/ Rice	1 pkg (10 oz)	250	2	6
Luigino's				
Chili-Mac	1 pkg (8 oz)	230	3	7
Lunch Bucket				
Chili With Beans	1 pkg (7.5 oz)	260	5	12
Natural Choice				
Organic Vegan Three Bean	½ cup (4.6 oz)	140	0	1
Natural Touch				
Vegetarian	1 cup (8.1 oz)	170	0	1
Nile Spice				
Chili'n Beans Original	1 pkg	150	0	2
Chili'n Beans Spicy	1 pkg	150	0	2
Old El Paso				
Chili Seasoning Mix	1 tbsp (0.3 oz)	25	—	1
Chili With Beans	1 cup (8 oz)	200	2	7

FOOD	PORTION	CALS.	SAT. FAT	FAT
Stouffer's				
With Beans	1 pkg (8.75 oz)	270	4	10
Swanson				
Homestyle Chili Con Carne	8¼ oz	270	—	10
Tabatchnick				
Vegetarian	7.5 oz	210	1	6
Ultimate				
No Beans Hot	1 cup (8.7 oz)	420	13	30
Turkey w/ Beans	1 cup (8.7 oz)	260	3	9
W/ Beans	1 cup (8.7 oz)	320	7	16
W/ Beans Hot	1 cup (8.7 oz)	320	7	16
Van Camp's				
Chilee Beanee Weenee	1 can (8 oz)	240	3	12
Chili With Beans	1 cup (8.9 oz)	350	8	21
Watkins				
Powder	¼ tsp (0.5 g)	0	0	0
Seasoning	1¼ tsp (4 g)	15	0	0
Wolf Brand				
Plain	7.5 oz	330	—	22
Worthington				
Chili	1 cup (8.1 oz)	290	3	15
Low Fat	1 cup (8.1 oz)	170	0	1
TAKE-OUT				
con carne w/ beans	8.9 oz	254	3	8

CHINESE CABBAGE
(see CABBAGE)

CHINESE FOOD
(see ASIAN FOOD)

CHINESE PRESERVING MELON

cooked	½ cup	11	tr	tr

CHIPS
(see *also* POPCORN, PRETZELS, SNACKS)

barbecue	1 oz	139	2	9
barbecue	1 bag (7 oz)	971	16	64
corn	1 oz	153	1	10
corn	1 bag (7 oz)	1067	9	66
corn barbecue	1 bag (7 oz)	1036	9	65
corn barbecue	1 oz	148	1	9
corn cones	1 oz	145	6	8
corn cones nacho	1 oz	152	8	9
corn onion	1 oz	142	1	6
potato	1 oz	152	3	10

FOOD	PORTION	CALS.	SAT. FAT	FAT
potato	1 bag (8 oz)	1217	25	79
potato cheese	1 oz	140	2	8
potato cheese	1 bag (6 oz)	842	15	46
potato light	1 oz	134	1	6
potato light	1 bag (6 oz)	801	7	35
potato sour cream & onion	1 oz	150	3	10
potato sour cream & onion	1 bag (7 oz)	1051	18	67
potato sticks	1 oz	148	3	10
potato sticks	½ cup (0.6 oz)	94	2	6
potato sticks	1 pkg (1 oz)	148	3	10
taco	1 bag (8 oz)	1089	11	55
taco	1 oz	136	1	7
taro	1 oz	141	2	7
taro	10 (0.8 oz)	115	1	6
tortilla	1 bag (7.5 oz)	1067	11	56
tortilla	1 oz	142	1	7
tortilla nacho	1 bag (8 oz)	1131	11	58
tortilla nacho	1 oz	141	1	7
tortilla nacho light	1 bag (6 oz)	757	5	26
tortilla nacho light	1 oz	126	1	4
tortilla ranch	1 oz	139	1	7
tortilla ranch	1 bag (7 oz)	969	9	47
Barbara's				
No Salt Added	1¼ cups (1 oz)	150	1	10
Pinta Chips	13 (1 oz)	130	2	6
Pinta Chips Salsa	12 (1 oz)	130	1	6
Potato	1¼ cups (1 oz)	150	1	10
Ripple	1¼ cups (1 oz)	150	1	10
Tortilla Blue Corn	15 (1 oz)	140	tr	7
Yogurt & Green Onion	1¼ cups (1 oz)	150	1	9
Barrel O' Fun				
Barbeque	1 oz	145	2	9
Potato	1 oz	150	2	9
Sour Cream & Onion	1 oz	150	2	9
Tortilla Nacho	1 oz	140	2	6
Tortilla White	1 oz	140	2	6
Tostada Yellow	1 oz	140	2	6
Bruno & Luigi's				
Pasta Chips Garlic & Herb	1 oz	117	0	1
Butterfield				
Potato Sticks	1 pkg (1.7 oz)	250	5	15
Potato Sticks	⅔ cup (1 oz)	150	3	9
Cape Cod				
Potato	19 chips (1 oz)	150	2	8

FOOD	PORTION	CALS.	SAT. FAT	FAT
Chester's				
Flamin' Hot	1 oz	140	2	8
Salsa	1 oz	140	2	7
Cottage Fries				
No Salt Added	1 oz	160	—	11
Doritos				
3D's Cooler Ranch	27 (1 oz)	140	2	6
3D's Nacho Cheesier	27 (1 oz)	140	2	7
Cooler Ranch	12 (1 oz)	140	2	7
Flamin' Hot	11 (1 oz)	140	2	7
Nacho Cheesier	11 (1 oz)	140	1	7
Salsa Verde	12 (1 oz)	150	2	7
Smokey Red	12 (1 oz)	150	2	7
Spicy Nacho	12 (1 oz)	140	2	6
Toasted Corn	13 (1 oz)	140	2	7
Wow Nacho Cheesier	1 pkg (0.75 oz)	70	0	1
Durangos				
Tortilla	15 (1 oz)	150	1	7
Eden				
Vegetable Chips	50 (1 oz)	130	2	4
Wasabi Chip Hot & Spicy	50 (1 oz)	130	2	4
Energy Food Factory				
Corn Pops Fat Free	½ oz	50	0	0
Corn Pops Nacho	½ oz	50	0	1
Corn Pops Original	½ oz	50	0	1
Potato Pops Au Gratin	½ oz	60	1	2
Potato Pops Fat Free	½ oz	50	0	0
Potato Pops Herb & Garlic	½ oz	50	0	1
Potato Pops Mesquite	½ oz	50	0	1
Potato Pops Original	½ oz	50	0	1
Potato Pops Salt N' Vinegar	½ oz	50	0	1
Ensemble				
Potato Baked Barbecue	12 (1 oz)	110	1	3
Potato Baked Cheddar	12 (1 oz)	110	1	3
Potato Baked Sour Cream & Onion	12 (1 oz)	110	1	3
Fritos				
Chili Cheese	31 (1 oz)	160	2	10
Corn Chips BBQ	29 (1 oz)	150	1	9
Corn Chips King Size	12 (1 oz)	150	2	10
Corn Chips Sabrositas Flamin' Hot	30 (1 oz)	150	2	9
Corn Chips Sabrositas Lime'N Chile	28 (1 oz)	150	2	9
Corn Chips Wild N'Mild Ranch	28 (1 oz)	160	2	10

FOOD	PORTION	CALS.	SAT. FAT	FAT
Fritos (CONT.)				
Original	32 (1 oz)	160	2	10
Scoops	11 (1 oz)	160	1	10
Texas Grill Honey BBQ	15 (1 oz)	150	2	9
Guiltless Gourmet				
Tortilla Baked Chili Lime	18 (1 oz)	110	0	2
Tortilla Baked Mucho Nacho	18 (1 oz)	110	0	2
Tortilla Baked Organic Blue Corn	18 (1 oz)	110	0	2
Tortilla Baked Picante Ranch	18 (1 oz)	110	0	2
Tortilla Baked Red Corn	18 (1 oz)	110	0	2
Tortilla Baked Spicy Black Bean	18 (1 oz)	110	0	2
Tortilla Baked Sweet White Corn	18 (1 oz)	110	0	2
Tortilla Baked Yellow Corn	18 (1 oz)	110	0	2
Tortilla Baked Yellow Corn Unsalted	18 (1 oz)	110	0	1
Hain				
Carrot Chips	1 oz	150	—	9
Carrot Chips Barbecue	1 oz	140	—	8
Carrot Chips No Salt Added	1 oz	150	—	7
Tortilla Sesame	1 oz	140	—	7
Tortilla Sesame Cheese	1 oz	160	—	8
Tortilla Sesame No Salt Added	1 oz	140	—	7
Tortilla Taco Style	1 oz	160	—	11
Herr's				
Potato	1 oz	140	2	8
Tortilla Restaurant Style White Corn	10 chips (1 oz)	140	1	6
La FAMOUS				
Tortilla	1 oz	140	—	7
Tortilla No Salt Added	1 oz	140	—	7
Lance				
BBQ	22 (1 oz)	160	3	10
Cajun	15 (1 oz)	150	3	10
Corn Chips	39 (1.25 oz)	200	3	11
Corn Chips Hot BBQ	35 (1.25 oz)	210	4	13
Hot Fries	1 pkg (0.9 oz)	140	3	10
Mesquite BBQ	22 (1 oz)	150	3	10
Potato	23 (1 oz)	160	3	10
Ripple	15 (1 oz)	160	3	11
Salt & Vinegar	22 (1 oz)	160	3	10
Sour Cream & Onion	22 (1 oz)	160	3	10
Tortilla Fiesta Salsa Triangles	16 (1 oz)	140	2	7

FOOD	PORTION	CALS.	SAT. FAT	FAT
Lance (CONT.)				
Tortilla Nacho Mini Round	46 (1.25 oz)	180	3	9
Tortilla Nacho Triangles	15 (1 oz)	140	4	14
Lay's				
Adobadas	16 (1 oz)	170	3	10
Baked KC Masterpiece BBQ	11 (1 oz)	120	0	3
Baked Original	11 (1 oz)	110	0	2
Baked Roasted Herb	12 (1 oz)	130	1	3
Baked Sour Cream & Onion	12 (1 oz)	120	0	2
Classic	20 (1 oz)	150	3	10
Deli Style Hot N'Tangy BBQ	18 (1 oz)	150	3	10
Deli Style Jalapeno	17 (1 oz)	150	3	10
Deli Style Original	17 (1 oz)	140	3	10
Deli Style Salt & Vinegar	16 (1 oz)	90	3	10
Flamin' Hot	17 pieces (1 oz)	150	3	10
KC Masterpiece BBQ	15 (1 oz)	150	3	10
Onion & Garlic	19 (1 oz)	150	3	9
Salt & Vinegar	17 pieces (1 oz)	150	3	10
Sour Cream & Onion	17 pieces (1 oz)	160	3	11
Toasted Onion & Cheese	17 pieces (1 oz)	160	3	10
Wavy Au Gratin	13 (1 oz)	150	3	10
Wavy Original	11 pieces (1 oz)	160	3	10
Wavy Ranch	11 (1 oz)	160	3	11
Wow Mesquite BBQ	20 (1 oz)	75	0	0
Wow Mesquite BBQ	20 (1 oz)	75	0	0
Wow Original	20 (1 oz)	75	0	0
Wow Original	1 pkg (0.75 oz)	55	0	0
Wow Sour Cream & Chive	19 (1 oz)	80	0	0
Wow Sour Cream & Chive	19 (1 oz)	80	0	0
Louise's				
"1g" Mesquite BBQ	1 oz	110	—	1
"1g" Original	1 oz	110	—	1
70% Less Fat Mesquite BBQ	1 oz	110	—	3
70% Less Fat Original	1 oz	110	—	3
95% Fat-Free Tortilla	1 oz	120	—	2
Fat-Free Maui Onion	1 oz	110	0	0
Fat-Free Mesquite BBQ	1 oz	110	0	0
Fat-Free No Salt	1 oz	110	0	0
Fat-Free Original	1 oz	110	0	0
Fat-Free Vinegar & Salt	1 oz	110	0	0
Mr. Phipps				
Tater Crisps Bar-B-Que	21 (1 oz)	130	1	4
Tater Crisps Original	23 (1 oz)	120	1	7
Tater Crisps Sour Cream 'n Onion	22 (1 oz)	130	1	4

FOOD	PORTION	CALS.	SAT. FAT	FAT
Mr. Phipps (CONT.)				
Tortilla	28 (1 oz)	130	1	4
Tortilla Nacho	28 (1 oz)	130	1	4
New York Deli				
Chips	1 oz	160	—	11
Old Dutch Foods				
Augratin	1 oz	150	—	8
BBQ	1 oz	140	—	8
Dill Flavored	1 oz	150	—	8
Onion & Garlic	1 oz	150	—	9
Potato	1 oz	150	—	9
Ripple	1 oz	150	—	9
Sour Cream & Onion	1 oz	150	—	10
Old El Paso				
Tortilla NACHIPS	9 chips (1 oz)	150	2	8
Tortilla White Corn	11 chips (1 oz)	140	1	8
Planters				
Corn Chips	34 chips (1 oz)	170	2	10
Corn Chips King Size	17 chips (1 oz)	160	2	10
Corn Chips Snacks To Go	1 pkg (1.5 oz)	240	2	15
Pringles				
BBQ	14 chips (1 oz)	150	3	6
Cheez-ums	14 chips (1 oz)	150	3	10
Fat Free	15 chips (1 oz)	75	0	0
Original	14 chips (1 oz)	160	3	11
Ranch	14 chips (1 oz)	150	3	10
Ridges Cheddar & Sour Cream	12 chips (1 oz)	150	3	10
Ridges Mesquite BBQ	12 chips (1 oz)	150	3	10
Ridges Original	12 chips (1 oz)	150	3	10
Right BBQ	16 chips (1 oz)	140	2	7
Right Original	16 chips (1 oz)	140	2	7
Right Ranch	16 chips (1 oz)	140	2	7
Right Sour Cream 'N Onion	16 chips (1 oz)	140	2	7
Rippled Original	10 chips (1 oz)	160	3	11
Sour Cream N'Onion	14 chips (1 oz)	160	3	10
Robert's American Gourmet				
Spirulina Spirals	1 oz	120	0	2
Ruffles				
Baked	10 (1 oz)	110	0	2
Baked Cheddar & Sour Cream	9 (1 oz)	120	0	3
Buffalo Style	11 chips (1 oz)	160	3	10
Cheddar & Sour Cream	11 chips (1 oz)	160	3	10
French Onion	11 (1 oz)	150	3	10
MC Masterpiece Mesquite BBQ	11 (1 oz)	150	3	10
Original	12 chips (1 oz)	150	3	10

FOOD	PORTION	CALS.	SAT. FAT	FAT
Ruffles (CONT.)				
Ranch	13 (1 oz)	150	3	9
Reduced Fat	16 (1 oz)	130	1	7
The Works	12 (1 oz)	160	3	11
Wow Cheddar & Sour Cream	15 (1 oz)	75	0	0
Wow Cheddar & Sour Cream	15 (1 oz)	75	0	0
Wow Original	17 (1 oz)	75	0	0
Wow Original	17 (1 oz)	75	0	0
Santitas				
100% White Corn	6 (1 oz)	130	1	6
Restaurant Style Chips	7 (1 oz)	130	1	6
Restaurant Style Strips	10 (1 oz)	130	1	6
Snyder's of Hanover				
BBQ	1 oz	150	—	10
Cheddar Bacon	1 oz	150	—	10
Coney Island	1 oz	150	—	10
Corn BBQ	1 oz	160	—	11
Corn Chips	1 oz	160	—	11
Grilled Steak & Onion	1 oz	150	—	10
Hot Buffalo Wings	1 oz	150	—	10
Kosher Dill	1 oz	150	—	10
No Salt	1 oz	150	—	10
Potato	1 oz	150	—	10
Salt & Vinegar	1 oz	150	—	10
Sausage Pizza	1 oz	150	—	10
Sour Cream & Onion	1 oz	150	—	10
Sour Cream & Onion Unsalted	1 oz	150	—	10
Tortilla	1 oz	140	—	7
Tortilla Enchilada	1 oz	140	—	7
Tortilla Nacho Cheese	1 oz	140	—	7
Tortilla No Salt	1 oz	140	—	7
Tortilla Ranch	1 oz	140	—	7
Soya King				
Soy	1 pkg (0.75 oz)	110	1	5
State Line				
Chips	1 pkg (0.5 oz)	80	1	5
Sunchips				
French Onion	13 (1 oz)	140	1	7
Harvest Cheddar	13 (1 oz)	140	1	6
Original	14 (1 oz)	140	1	6
Terra Chips				
Sweet Potato	1 oz	140	1	7
Sweet Potato Spiced	1 oz	140	1	7
Taro Spiced	1 oz	130	1	5
Vegetable	1 oz	140	1	7

FOOD	PORTION	CALS.	SAT. FAT	FAT
Top Banana				
Plantain Chips	1 oz	150	—	8
Tostitos				
Baked Bite Size	20 (1 oz)	110	0	1
Baked Bite Size Salsa & Cream Cheese	16 (1 oz)	120	1	3
Baked Original	13 (1 oz)	110	0	1
Bite Size	15 (1 oz)	140	1	8
Crispy Rounds	13 (1 oz)	150	1	8
Nacho Style	6 (1 oz)	140	1	6
Restaurant Style	7 (1 oz)	140	1	6
Restaurant Style Hint Of Lime	6 (1 oz)	140	1	6
Santa Fe Gold	7 (1 oz)	140	1	6
Wow Original	6 (1 oz)	90	0	1
Wow Original	6 (1 oz)	90	0	1
Tyson				
Tortilla Salted	13 (1 oz)	150	1	7
Tortilla Yellow Corn Salted	13 (1 oz)	150	1	7
Utz				
Baked Crisps	12 (1 oz)	110	0	2
Carolina Barbeque	20 (1 oz)	150	2	9
Cheddar & Sour Cream	20 (1 oz)	160	3	10
Corn Chips	24 (1 oz)	160	2	10
Corn Chips Barbecue	24 (1 oz)	160	2	10
Grandma	20 (1 oz)	140	3	8
Grandma BBQ	20 (1 oz)	140	3	8
Home Style Kettle	20 (1 oz)	140	2	8
Home Style Kettle BBQ	20 (1 oz)	140	2	8
Kettle Classics Crunchy	20 (1 oz)	150	2	9
Kettle Classics Crunchy Mesquite BBQ	20 (1 oz)	150	2	9
No Salt Added	20 (1 oz)	150	2	9
Onion & Garlic	20 (1 oz)	150	2	9
Potato	20 (1 oz)	150	2	9
Reduced Fat BBQ	22 (1 oz)	140	2	6
Reducted Fat Ripple	24 (1 oz)	140	2	7
Ripple	20 (1 oz)	150	3	10
Ripple Sour Cream & Onion	20 (1 oz)	160	3	10
Ripple Barbeque	20 (1 oz)	150	3	10
Salt'N Vinegar	20 (1 oz)	150	2	9
The Crab Chip	20 (1 oz)	150	2	9
Tortilla Black Bean & Salsa	13 (1 oz)	150	1	7
Tortilla Low Fat Baked	10 (1 oz)	120	0	2
Tortilla Nacho	13 (1 oz)	150	1	8
Tortilla Restaurant Style	6 (1 oz)	140	1	7

FOOD	PORTION	CALS.	SAT. FAT	FAT
Utz (CONT.)				
Tortilla Spicy Nacho	13 (1 oz)	150	1	8
Tortilla White Corn	12 (1 oz)	140	1	7
Wavy	20 chips (1 oz)	150	2	9
Yes! Fat Free	20 (1 oz)	75	0	0
Yes! Fat Free Barbeque	20 (1 oz)	75	0	0
Yes! Fat Free Ripple	20 (1 oz)	75	0	0
Wise				
Corn Crunchies	1 oz	160	—	10
Crispy Corn	1 oz	160	—	10
Crispy Corn Nacho Cheese	1 oz	160	—	10
Dipsy Doodles	1 pkg (1.5 oz)	240	3	15
Natural	1 oz	160	—	11
Ridgies Barbecue	1 oz	150	—	10
Tortilla Bravos	1 oz	150	—	8
Wow				
Tortilla Nacho Cheese	11 (1 oz)	90	0	1

CHITTERLINGS

FOOD	PORTION	CALS.	SAT. FAT	FAT
pork cooked	3 oz	258	9	24

CHIVES

FOOD	PORTION	CALS.	SAT. FAT	FAT
freeze-dried	1 tbsp	1	tr	tr
fresh chopped	1 tbsp	1	tr	tr
fresh chopped	1 tsp	0	tr	tr

CHOCOLATE

(see also CANDY, CAROB, COCOA, ICE CREAM TOPPINGS, MILK DRINKS)

FOOD	PORTION	CALS.	SAT. FAT	FAT
BAKING				
baking	1 oz	145	9	15
grated unsweetened	1 cup (4.6 oz)	690	43	73
liquid unsweetened	1 oz	134	7	14
squares unsweetened	1 square (1 oz)	148	9	16
Baker's				
Bittersweet	½ square (0.5 oz)	70	3	6
German's Sweet	2 squares (0.5 oz)	60	2	4
Semi-Sweet	½ square (0.5 oz)	70	3	5
Unsweetened	½ square (0.5 oz)	70	5	7
White	½ square (0.5 oz)	80	3	5
Nestle				
Choco Bake	½ oz	80	5	8
Premier White	½ oz	80	3	5
Semi-Sweet	½ oz	70	3	4
Unsweetened	½ oz	80	2	7
CHIPS				
milk chocolate	1 cup (6 oz)	862	31	52

FOOD	PORTION	CALS.	SAT. FAT	FAT
semisweet	1 cup (6 oz)	804	30	50
semisweet	60 pieces (1 oz)	136	5	9
Baker's				
Chips	1 oz	143	—	8
Real Milk Chocolate	½ oz	70	2	4
Real Semi-Sweet	½ oz	60	2	4
Semi-Sweet	½ oz	70	3	4
Hershey				
Almond Joy Bits	1 tbsp (0.5 oz)	60	2	4
Chocolate & Peanut Butter Chips	1 tbsp (0.5 oz)	70	2	3
Holiday Baking Bits	1 tbsp (0.5 oz)	70	2	3
Milk Chocolate	1 tbsp (0.5 oz)	80	3	5
Mini Kisses For Baking	11 pieces (0.5 oz)	80	3	5
Mint Chocolate	1 tbsp (0.5 oz)	80	3	4
Premier White Milk Chips	1 tbsp (0.5 oz)	80	3	4
Raspberry Chips	1 tbsp (0.5 oz)	80	3	4
Semi-Sweet	1 tbsp (0.5 oz)	80	3	4
Semi-Sweet Mini	1 tbsp (0.5 oz)	80	3	4
Skor English Toffee Baking Bits	1 tbsp (0.5 oz)	70	3	5
M&M's				
Baking Bits Milk Chocolate	0.5 oz	70	2	3
Baking Bits Semi-Sweet	0.5 oz	70	2	4
Nestle				
Morsels Milk Chocolate	1 tbsp	70	—	4
Morsels Mint Chocolate	1 tbsp	70	2	4
Morsels Rainbow	1 tbsp	70	2	3
Morsels Mini Semi-Sweet	1 tbsp	70	—	4
Semi-Sweet Morsels	1 tbsp	40	—	4
Tollhouse				
Mint-Chocolate	2 tbsp (1.5 oz)	130	2	3
Semi-Sweet	2 tbsp (1.5 oz)	130	2	4
MIX				
powder	2–3 heaping tsp	75	tr	1
powder as prep w/ whole milk	9 oz	226	5	9
Quik				
Chocolate Powder	2 tbsp (0.8 oz)	90	1	1
Chocolate Powder No Sugar Added	2 tbsp (0.4 oz)	40	1	1

CHOCOLATE MILK

(see CHOCOLATE, COCOA, MILK DRINKS, MILKSHAKE)

CHOCOLATE SYRUP

chocolate fudge	1 tbsp (0.7 oz)	73	1	3
chocolate fudge	1 cup (11.9 oz)	1176	19	46

FOOD	PORTION	CALS.	SAT. FAT	FAT
syrup	1 cup	653	2	3
syrup	2 tbsp	82	tr	tr
syrup as prep w/ whole milk	9 oz	232	5	9
Estee				
Chocolate	2 tbsp	15	0	0
Hershey				
Chocolate Fudge (canned)	1 tbsp (0.7 oz)	70	2	3
Chocolate Malt	2 tbsp (1.4 oz)	100	0	0
Lite	2 tbsp (1.2 oz)	50	0	0
Syrup	2 tbsp (1.4 oz)	100	0	0
Marzetti				
Syrup	2 tbsp	40	1	4
Quik				
Chocolate	2 tbsp (1.3 oz)	100	0	1
Red Wing				
Syrup	2 tbsp (1.4 oz)	110	1	1
CHUTNEY				
coconut	¼ cup	74	6	7
Sonoma				
Dried Tomato	1 tbsp (0.7 g)	35	0	0
CILANTRO				
fresh	1 tsp (2 g)	tr	0	tr
fresh	1 cup (1.6 oz)	11	tr	tr
Watkins				
Dried	¼ tsp (0.5 oz)	0	0	0
CINNAMON				
ground	1 tsp	6	tr	tr
sticks	0.5 oz	39	tr	tr
Watkins				
Ground	¼ tsp (0.5 g)	0	0	0
CISCO				
raw	3 oz	84	tr	2
smoked	3 oz	151	1	10
smoked	1 oz	50	tr	3
CLAM JUICE				
Doxsee				
Canned	3 fl oz	4	0	0
CLAMS				
CANNED				
liquid only	3 oz	2	—	tr
liquid only	1 cup	6	—	tr

FOOD	PORTION	CALS.	SAT. FAT	FAT
meat only	3 oz	126	tr	2
meat only	1 cup	236	tr	3
Doxsee				
Chopped	6.5 oz	90	—	tr
Gorton's				
Minced & Chopped	½ can	70	—	1
Progresso				
Creamy Clam	½ cup (4.2 oz)	100	2	6
Minced	¼ cup (2 oz)	25	0	0
Red Clam	½ cup (4.4 oz)	80	1	3
White Clam Sauce	½ cup (4.4 oz)	120	2	9
Snow's				
Minced	6.5 oz	90	—	tr
FRESH				
cooked	20 sm	133	tr	2
cooked	3 oz	126	tr	2
raw	9 lg (180 g)	133	tr	2
raw	3 oz	63	tr	1
raw	20 sm (180 g)	133	tr	2
FROZEN				
Gorton's				
Microwave Crunchy Clam Strips	3.5 oz	330	6	22
Mrs. Paul's				
Fried	2½ oz	200	—	9
Microwave Fried Clams	2.5 oz	260	—	15
TAKE-OUT				
breaded & fried	20 sm	379	5	21
CLOVES				
ground	1 tsp	7	tr	tr
COCOA				
(see also CHOCOLATE)				
hot cocoa	1 cup	218	6	9
mix as prep w/ water	7 oz	103	1	1
mix w/ equal as prep w/ water	7 oz	48	tr	tr
powder unsweetened	1 tbsp (5 g)	11	tr	1
powder unsweetened	1 cup (3 oz)	197	7	12
Carnation				
Hot Cocoa 70 Calorie	3 tsp (21 g)	70	—	tr
Hot Cocoa Milk Chocolate	1 pkg or 4 heaping tsp (1 oz)	110	—	1
Hot Cocoa Natural Mint	1 pkg or 4 heaping tsp (1 oz)	110	—	1

FOOD	PORTION	CALS.	SAT. FAT	FAT
Carnation (CONT.)				
Hot Cocoa Rich Chocolate	1 pkg or 4 heaping tsp (1 oz)	110	—	1
Hot Cocoa Rich Chocolate w/ Marshmallows	1 pkg or 4 heaping tsp (1 oz)	110	—	1
Hot Cocoa Sugar Free Mint	1 pkg or 4 heaping tsp (15 g)	50	—	tr
Hot Cocoa Sugar Free Rich Chocolate	1 pkg or 4 heaping tsp (15 g)	50	—	tr
Hershey				
Cocoa	1 tbsp (5 g)	20	0	1
European Cocoa	1 tbsp (5 g)	20	0	1
Nestle				
Cocoa	1 tbsp	15	0	1
Swiss Miss				
Cocoa Diet	6 oz	20	—	tr
Hot Cocoa Bavarian Chocolate	6 oz	110	1	3
Hot Cocoa Double Rich	6 oz	110	1	1
Hot Cocoa Milk Chocolate	6 oz	110	tr	1
Hot Cocoa Milk Chocolate	1 serv	110	tr	1
Hot Cocoa Mini-Marshmallow	1 serv	109	tr	1
Hot Cocoa Rich Chocolate	1 serv	110	tr	1
Hot Cocoa Sugar Free	1 serv	67	tr	tr
Hot Cocoa Sugar Free Milk Chocolate	1 serv	49	tr	tr
Hot Cocoa Sugar Free Mini-Marshmallow	1 serv	51	tr	1
Hot Cocoa White Chocolate	1 serv	109	tr	1
Hot Cocoa With Mini Marshmallows	6 oz	110	tr	1
Hot Cocoa Lite	1 serv	74	tr	tr
Lite as prep	6 oz	70	—	tr
Sugar Free With Sugar Free Marshmallows as prep	6 oz	50	—	tr
Sugar Free as prep	6 oz	60	—	tr
Ultra Slim-Fast				
Hot Cocoa as prep w/ water	8 oz	190	—	tr
Weight Watchers				
Hot Cocoa Mix as prep	1 pkg	70	0	0
COCONUT				
coconut water	1 tbsp	3	tr	tr
coconut water	1 cup	46	tr	tr
cream canned	1 cup	568	47	52
cream canned	1 tbsp	36	3	3
dried sweetened flaked	7 oz pkg	944	57	64

FOOD	PORTION	CALS.	SAT. FAT	FAT
dried sweetened flaked	1 cup	351	21	24
dried sweetened flaked canned	1 cup	341	22	24
dried sweetened shredded	7 oz pkg	997	63	71
dried sweetened shredded	1 cup	466	29	33
dried toasted	1 oz	168	12	13
dried unsweetened	1 oz	187	16	18
fresh	1 piece (1.5 oz)	159	13	15
fresh shredded	1 cup	283	24	27
milk canned	1 tbsp	30	3	3
milk canned	1 cup	445	43	48
milk frozen	1 tbsp	30	3	3
milk frozen	1 cup	486	44	50
Baker's				
Angel Flake	1 tbsp (0.5 oz)	70	5	5
Angel Flake (canned)	2 tbsp (0.5 oz)	70	5	6
Premium Shred	2 tbsp (0.5 oz)	70	5	5
Coco Lopez				
Cream Of Coconut	2 tbsp	120	—	5
COD				
CANNED				
atlantic	3 oz	89	tr	1
atlantic	1 can (11 oz)	327	1	3
roe	3.5 oz	118	—	3
DRIED				
atlantic	3 oz	246	tr	2
FRESH				
atlantic cooked	1 fillet (6.3 oz)	189	tr	2
atlantic cooked	3 oz	89	tr	1
atlantic raw	3 oz	70	tr	1
pacific baked	3 oz	95	tr	1
roe baked w/ butter & lemon juice	3.5 oz	126	—	3
roe raw	3½ oz	130	—	2
tarama	3.5 oz	547	—	55
FROZEN				
Gorton's				
Fishmarket Fresh	5 oz	110	—	1
Mrs. Paul's				
Light Fillets	1 fillet	240	—	11
Van De Kamp's				
Lightly Breaded Fillets	1 (4 oz)	220	2	10
COFFEE				
(see also COFFEE BEVERAGES, COFFEE SUBSTITUTES)				
INSTANT				
decaffeinated	1 rounded tsp (1.8 g)	4	0	0

FOOD	PORTION	CALS.	SAT. FAT	FAT
decaffeinated as prep	6 oz	4	0	0
regular	1 rounded tsp	4	0	0
regular as prep	6 oz	4	0	0
regular w/ chicory	1 rounded tsp	6	0	0
regular w/ chicory as prep	6 oz	6	0	0
REGULAR				
brewed	6 oz	4	0	0
Folgers				
Colombian Supreme	1 tbsp	16	—	tr
Custom Roast	1 tbsp	16	—	tr
Decaffeinated	1 tbsp	17	—	tr
French Roast	1 tbsp	16	—	tr
Gourmet Supreme	1 tbsp	16	—	tr
Instant	1 tsp	8	—	tr
Instant Decaffeinated	1 tsp	8	—	tr
Singles	1 bag	21	—	tr
Singles Decaffeinated	1 bag	21	—	tr
Special Roast	1 tbsp	16	—	tr
Vacuum Pack	1 tbsp	16	—	tr
Maryland Club				
Ground	1 tbsp	16	—	tr
TAKE-OUT				
cafe au lait	1 cup (8 fl oz)	77	3	4
cafe brulot	1 cup (4.8 fl oz)	48	0	2
cappuccino	1 cup (8 fl oz)	77	3	4
coffee con leche	1 cup (8 fl oz)	77	3	4
espresso	1 cup (3 fl oz)	2	0	0
irish coffee	1 serv (9 fl oz)	107	2	3
latte w/ skim milk	13 oz	88	tr	tr
latte w/ whole milk	13 oz	152	5	8
mocha	1 mug (9.6 fl oz)	202	9	15

COFFEE BEVERAGES

(see also COFFEE SUBSTITUTES)

cappuccino mix as prep	7 oz	62	2	2
french mix as prep	7 oz	57	3	3
mocha mix as prep	7 oz	51	2	2
Arizona				
Iced Latte Supreme	8 oz	110	1	2
Iced Mocha Latte	8 oz	110	1	2
Gehl's				
Iced Cappuccino	1 can (11 oz)	190	1	2
General Foods				
Cappuccino Coolers French Vanilla as prep w/ 2% milk	1 serv	180	3	5

FOOD	PORTION	CALS.	SAT. FAT	FAT
General Foods (CONT.)				
International Coffee Sugar Free Cafe Vienna as prep	1 serv (8 oz)	30	1	2
International Coffee Sugar Free Fat Free Suisse Mocha as prep	1 serv (8 oz)	25	0	0
International Coffees Cafe Francais as prep	1 serv (8 oz)	60	1	4
International Coffees Cafe Vienna as prep	1 serv (8 oz)	70	1	3
International Coffees Decaffeinated French Vanilla Cafe as prep	1 serv (8 oz)	60	1	3
International Coffees Decaffeinated Suisse Mocha as prep	1 serv (8 oz)	60	1	2
International Coffees French Vanilla Cafe as prep	1 serv (8 oz)	60	1	3
International Coffees Hazelnut Belgain Cafe as prep	1 serv (8 oz)	70	1	2
International Coffees Irish Creme Cafe as prep	1 serv (8 oz)	60	1	2
International Coffees Italian Cappuccino as prep	1 serv (8 oz)	60	1	2
International Coffees Kahlua Cafe as prep	1 serv (8 oz)	60	1	2
International Coffees Orange Cappuccino as prep	1 serv (8 oz)	70	1	2
International Coffees Suisse Mocha as prep	1 serv (8 oz)	60	1	2
International Coffees Viennese Chocolate Cafe as prep	1 serv (8 oz)	50	1	2
International Coffees Sugar Free Fat Free Decaffeinated French Vanilla	1 serv (8 oz)	25	0	0
International Coffees Sugar Free Fat Free Decaffeinated Suisse Mocha	1 serv (8 oz)	25	0	0
International Coffees Sugar Free Fat Free French Vanilla Cafe as prep	1 serv (8 oz)	25	0	0
Maxwell House				
Cafe Cappuccino Amaretto as prep	1 serv (8 oz)	90	0	1

FOOD	PORTION	CALS.	SAT. FAT	FAT
Maxwell House (CONT.)				
Cafe Cappuccino Decaffeinated Mocha as prep	1 serv (8 oz)	100	1	3
Cafe Cappuccino Decaffeinated Vanilla as prep	1 serv (8 oz)	90	0	1
Cafe Cappuccino Irish Cream as prep	1 serv (8 oz)	90	0	1
Cafe Cappuccino Mocha as prep	1 serv (8 oz)	100	1	3
Cafe Cappuccino Sugar Free Mocha as prep	1 serv (8 oz)	60	1	3
Cafe Cappuccino Sugar Free Vanilla as prep	1 serv (8 oz)	60	1	3
Cafe Cappuccino Vanilla as prep	1 serv (8 oz)	90	0	1
Iced Cappuccino as prep w/ 2% milk	1 serv (8 oz)	180	3	5
Starbucks				
Frappuccino	1 bottle (9.5 fl oz)	190	2	3
COFFEE SUBSTITUTES				
powder	1 tsp	9	tr	tr
powder as prep	6 oz	9	tr	tr
powder as prep w/ milk	6 oz	121	4	6
Kava				
Instant	1 tsp	2	0	0
Natural Touch				
Kaffree Roma	1 tsp (2 g)	10	0	0
Roma Cappuccino	3 tbsp (0.4 oz)	50	3	3
Pero				
Instant Grain Beverage	1 tsp (1.5 g)	5	0	0
Postum				
Instant Coffee Flavor as prep	1 serv (8 oz)	10	0	0
Instant as prep	1 serv (8 oz)	10	0	0
COFFEE WHITENERS				
(see also MILK SUBSTITUTES)				
liquid nondairy frzn	1 tbsp (0.5 oz)	20	tr	2
powder nondairy	1 tsp	11	1	tr
Coffee-Mate				
Liquid	1 tbsp (0.5 fl oz)	16	tr	1
Powder	1 tsp (2 g)	10	1	1
Cremora				
Whitener	1 tsp	12	—	1
Hood				
Non Dairy	1 tbsp (0.5 oz)	20	0	2

FOOD	PORTION	CALS.	SAT. FAT	FAT
International Delight				
Amaretto	1 tbsp (0.6 fl oz)	45	0	2
Cinnamon Hazelnut	1 tbsp (0.6 fl oz)	45	0	2
Irish Creme	1 tbsp (0.6 fl oz)	45	0	2
No Fat Amaretto	1 tbsp (0.5 fl oz)	30	0	0
No Fat French Vanilla Royale	1 tbsp (0.5 fl oz)	30	0	0
No Fat Hawaiian Macadamia	1 tbsp (0.5 fl oz)	30	0	0
No Fat Irish Creme	1 tbsp (0.5 fl oz)	30	0	0
Suisse Chocolate Mocha	1 tbsp (0.6 fl oz)	45	0	2
Mocha Mix				
Fat-Free	1 tbsp (0.5 fl oz)	10	0	0
Lite	1 tbsp (0.5 fl oz)	10	0	tr
Lite	4 fl oz	80	2	7
Original	1 tbsp (0.5 fl oz)	20	0	2
Signature Flavors French Vanilla	1 tbsp (0.5 fl oz)	35	0	0
Signature Flavors Irish Creme	1 tbsp (0.5 fl oz)	35	0	0
Signature Flavors Kahlua	1 tbsp (0.5 fl oz)	35	0	0
Signature Flavors Mauna Loa Macadamia Nut	1 tbsp (0.5 fl oz)	35	0	0
N-Rich Creamer				
Whitener	1 tsp	10	—	tr
COLESLAW				
Fresh Express				
Cole Slaw	1½ cups (3 oz)	25	0	0
HOME RECIPE				
coleslaw w/ dressing	¾ cup	147	2	11
TAKE-OUT				
coleslaw w/ dressing	½ cup	42	tr	2
vinegar & oil coleslaw	3.5 oz	150	1	9
COLLARDS				
fresh cooked	½ cup	17	—	tr
frzn chopped cooked	½ cup	31	—	tr
Allen				
Canned	½ cup (4.1 oz)	30	0	1
Sunshine				
Canned	½ cup (4.1 oz)	30	0	1
COOKIES				
(see also BROWNIE, CAKE, DOUGHNUT, PIE)				
HOME RECIPE				
chocolate chip as prep w/ butter	1 (0.42 oz)	78	2	5
chocolate chip as prep w/ margarine	1 (0.56 oz)	78	1	5
oatmeal	1 (0.5 oz)	67	1	3

FOOD	PORTION	CALS.	SAT. FAT	FAT
oatmeal w/ raisins	1 (0.52 oz)	65	tr	2
peanut butter	1 (0.7 oz)	95	1	5
shortbread as prep w/ butter	1 (0.38 oz)	60	2	4
shortbread as prep w/ margarine	1 (0.38 oz)	60	1	4
sugar as prep w/ butter	1 (0.49 oz)	66	2	3
sugar as prep w/ margarine	1 (0.49 oz)	66	1	3
MIX				
chocolate chip	1 (0.56 oz)	79	1	4
oatmeal	1 (0.6 oz)	74	1	3
oatmeal raisin	1 (0.6 oz)	74	1	3
Betty Crocker				
Chocolate Peanut Butter	1 bar	200	3	9
Easy Layer Dessert Bar	1 bar	140	3	6
Hershey Bars	1 bar	150	2	6
Pouch Dessert Chocolate Chip	2	160	3	8
Pouch Dessert Double Chocolate Chunk	2	150	2	6
Pouch Dessert Oatmeal Chocolate Chip	2	160	2	7
Pouch Dessert Peanut Butter	2	160	2	8
Pouch Dessert Sugar	2	170	2	8
Sunkist Lemon	1 bar	140	1	5
GoldnBrown				
Fat Free	1 (1.1 oz)	120	0	0
READY-TO-EAT				
animal	11 crackers (1 oz)	126	1	4
animal crackers	1 box (2.4 oz)	299	4	9
animal crackers	1 (2.5 g)	11	tr	tr
australian anzac biscuit	1	98	1	3
butter	1 (5 g)	23	1	1
chocolate chip	1 (0.4 oz)	48	1	2
chocolate chip	1 box (1.9 oz)	233	5	12
chocolate chip low fat	1 (0.25 oz)	45	tr	2
chocolate chip low sugar low sodium	1 (0.24 oz)	31	1	1
chocolate chip soft-type	1 (0.5 oz)	69	1	4
chocolate w/ creme filling	1 (0.35 oz)	47	tr	2
chocolate w/ creme filling chocolate coated	1 (0.60 oz)	82	1	5
chocolate w/ creme filling sugar free low sodium	1 (0.35 oz)	46	1	2
chocolate w/ extra creme filling	1 (0.46 oz)	65	1	3
chocolate wafer	1 (0.2 oz)	26	tr	1
chocolate wafer cookie crumbs	½ cup (5.9 oz)	728	6	25

FOOD	PORTION	CALS.	SAT. FAT	FAT
fig bars	1 (0.56 oz)	56	tr	1
fortune	1 (0.28 oz)	30	tr	tr
fudge	1 (0.73 oz)	73	tr	1
gingersnaps	1 (0.24 oz)	29	tr	1
graham	1 squares (0.24 oz)	30	tr	1
graham chocolate covered	1 (0.49 oz)	68	2	3
graham honey	1 (0.24 oz)	30	tr	1
ladyfingers	1 (0.38 oz)	40	tr	1
macaroons	1 (0.8 oz)	97	3	3
marshmallow chocolate coated	1 (0.46 oz)	55	1	2
marshmallow pie chocolate coated	1 (1.4 oz)	165	2	7
meringue	1 (0.3 oz)	20	0	0
molasses	1 (0.5 oz)	65	tr	2
neapolitan tri-color cookie	1 (0.6 oz)	79	2	5
oatmeal	1 (0.52 oz)	71	1	4
oatmeal	1 (0.6 oz)	81	1	3
oatmeal soft-type	1 (0.5 oz)	61	tr	2
oatmeal raisin	1 (0.6 oz)	81	1	3
oatmeal raisin low sugar no sodium	1 (0.24 oz)	31	1	1
oatmeal raisin soft-type	1 (0.5 oz)	61	tr	2
peanut butter sandwich	1 (0.5 oz)	67	1	3
peanut butter sandwich sugar free low sodium	1 (0.35 oz)	54	1	3
peanut butter soft-type	1 (0.5 oz)	69	1	4
raisin soft-type	1 (0.5 oz)	60	1	2
shortbread	1 (0.28 oz)	40	tr	2
shortbread pecan	1 (0.49 oz)	79	1	5
sugar	1 (0.52 oz)	72	1	3
sugar low sugar sodium free	1 (0.24 oz)	30	tr	1
sugar wafers w/ creme filling	1 (0.12 oz)	18	tr	1
sugar wafers w/ creme filling sugar free sodium free	1 (0.14 oz)	20	tr	1
vanilla sandwich	1 (0.35 oz)	48	tr	2
vanilla wafers	1 (0.21 oz)	28	tr	1
zeppole	1 (0.8 oz)	78	2	6
Alternative Baking				
Vegan Chocolate Chip	1 serv (2.5 oz)	280	4	10
Vegan Expresso Chocolate Chip	1 serv (2 oz)	230	3	9
Vegan Lemon	1 serv (2.25 oz)	250	2	7
Vegan Oatmeal	1 serv (2.25 oz)	250	2	10
Vegan Peanut Butter	1 serv (2.25 oz)	270	2	10

FOOD	PORTION	CALS.	SAT. FAT	FAT
Alternative Baking (CONT.)				
Vegan Pumpkin	1 serv (2 oz)	200	2	6
Vegan Wheat Free Choco Cherry Chunk	1 serv (1.75 oz)	190	2	6
Vegan Wheat Free Hula Nut	1 serv (1.75 oz)	190	2	6
Vegan Wheat Free P-nut Fudge Fusion	1 serv (1.75 oz)	190	2	7
Vegan Wheat Free Snickerdoodle	1 serv (1.75 oz)	170	0	3
Amay's				
Chinese Style Almond	1 (0.5 oz)	80	2	4
Archway				
Almond Crescents	2 (0.8 oz)	100	1	4
Apple N'Raisin	1 (1.1 oz)	130	1	52
Apricot Filled	1 (1 oz)	110	1	4
Bells And Stars	3 (1 oz)	150	2	7
Blueberry Filled	1 (1 oz)	110	2	4
Carrot Cake	1 (1 oz)	120	1	5
Cherry Filled	1 (1 oz)	110	2	4
Cherry Nougat	3 (1 oz)	150	2	9
Chocolate Chip	1 (1 oz)	130	2	6
Chocolate Chip & Toffee	1 (1 oz)	140	2	7
Chocolate Chip Bag	3 (0.9 oz)	130	2	7
Chocolate Chip Drop	1 (1 oz)	140	3	10
Chocolate Chip Ice Box	1 (1 oz)	140	3	7
Chocolate Chip Mini	12 (1.1 oz)	150	2	7
Cinnamon Snaps	12 (1.1 oz)	150	1	7
Coconut Macaroon	1 (0.8 oz)	90	4	5
Cookie Jar Hermits	1 (1 oz)	110	1	3
Dark Chocolate	1 (1 oz)	110	1	4
Dutch Chocolate	1 (1 oz)	120	1	4
Fig Bars Low Fat	2 (1.1 oz)	100	0	1
Frosty Lemon	1 (1 oz)	120	1	5
Frosty Orange	1 (1 oz)	120	1	4
Fruit And Honey Bar	1 (1 oz)	110	1	4
Fruit Bar No Fat	1 (1 oz)	90	0	0
Fruit Cake	1 (1.1 oz)	140	2	7
Fudge Nut Bar	1 (1 oz)	110	1	5
Fun Chip Mini	12 (1.1 oz)	140	1	6
Gingersnaps	5 (1.1 oz)	130	1	5
Granola No Fat	1 (0.5 oz)	50	0	0
Holiday Pak	3 (1.1 oz)	150	2	8
Iced Gingerbread	3 (1.1 oz)	140	1	5
Iced Molasses	1 (1 oz)	110	1	5

FOOD	PORTION	CALS.	SAT. FAT	FAT
Archway (CONT.)				
Iced Oatmeal	1 (1 oz)	120	1	5
Lemon Snaps	12 (1.1 oz)	150	1	7
New Orleans Cake	1 (1 oz)	110	1	4
Nutty Nougat	3 (1.1 oz)	160	2	10
Oatmeal	1 (0.9 oz)	110	1	3
Oatmeal Apple Filled	1 (1 oz)	110	1	3
Oatmeal Date Filled	1 (1 oz)	110	1	4
Oatmeal Mini	12 (1.1 oz)	150	2	8
Oatmeal Pecan	1 (1 oz)	120	1	5
Oatmeal Raisin	1 (1 oz)	110	1	4
Oatmeal Raisin Bran	1 (1 oz)	110	1	4
Old Fashioned Molasses	1 (1 oz)	120	1	3
Old Fashioned Windmill	1 (0.7 oz)	100	1	4
Party Treats	3 (1.1 oz)	140	2	7
Peanut Butter	1 (1 oz)	140	—	7
Peanut Butter & Chip	3 (0.9 oz)	130	2	7
Peanut Butter N' Chips	1 (1 oz)	140	2	7
Peanut Butter Nougat	3 (1.1 oz)	160	2	9
Pecan Crunch	6 (1.1 oz)	150	2	8
Pecan Ice Box	1 (1 oz)	140	2	7
Pecan Malted Nougat	3 (1.1 oz)	160	2	10
Pfeffernusse	2 (1.3 oz)	140	0	1
Pineapple Filled	1 (0.9 oz)	100	1	4
Raisin Oatmeal	1 (1 oz)	130	1	5
Raisin Oatmeal Bag	3 (1 oz)	130	1	6
Raspberry Filled	1 (1 oz)	110	1	4
Rocky Road	1 (1 oz)	130	2	6
Ruth's Golden Oatmeal	1 (1 oz)	120	1	5
Select Assortment	3 (0.9 oz)	130	2	6
Soft Molasses Drop	1 (1 oz)	110	1	4
Soft Sugar	1 (1 oz)	110	1	4
Strawberry Filled	1 (1 oz)	110	1	4
Sugar	1 (1 oz)	120	1	4
Vanilla Wafer	5 (1.1 oz)	130	1	4
Wedding Cakes	3 (1.1 oz)	160	2	8
Bahlsen				
Afrika	8 (1.1 oz)	170	6	10
Butter Leaves	7 (1 oz)	140	4	7
Choco Leibniz	2 (1 oz)	140	4	7
Choco Star Dark Chocolate	3 (1.1 oz)	170	6	12
Choco Star Milk Chocolate	3 (1.1 oz)	180	6	12
Chocolate Hearts	4 (1 oz)	160	6	9
Delice	6 (1 oz)	140	2	6

FOOD	PORTION	CALS.	SAT. FAT	FAT
Bahlsen (CONT.)				
Deloba	4 (0.9 oz)	130	2	5
Hit Chocolate Vanilla Filled	2 (1 oz)	140	6	8
Hit Vanilla Chocolate Filled	2 (1 oz)	140	5	7
Leibniz	6 (1 oz)	130	2	4
Nuss Dessert	3 (1.1 oz)	180	5	11
Probiers	6 (1.1 oz)	150	3	6
Twingo	6 (1.1 oz)	170	9	11
Waffeletten	4 (1 oz)	160	6	9
Waffelin	5 (1 oz)	160	9	10
Baker's Harvest				
Animal	12 (0.9 oz)	130	1	3
Chocolate Graham	2 (0.9 oz)	130	1	3
Cinnamon Grahams	2 (0.9 oz)	130	1	5
Cinnamon Grahams Low Fat	2 (0.9 oz)	110	0	2
Fig Bars	2 (1.2 oz)	120	0	3
Graham	2 (0.9 oz)	120	1	4
Graham Low Fat	2 (0.9 oz)	110	0	2
Iced Oatmeal	1 (0.6 oz)	70	1	3
Pecan Shortbread	1 (0.5 oz)	80	1	5
Vanilla Wafers	7 (1.1 oz)	150	1	6
Bakery Wagon				
Cobbler Mixed Fruit Fat Free	1	70	0	0
Cobbler Raspberry Fat Free	1	70	0	0
Ginger Snaps	5	160	2	7
Honey Fruit Bars	1	100	1	3
Iced Molasses Mini	3	130	1	3
Oatmeal Raspberry Filled	1	100	1	3
Oatmeal Soft	1	100	1	4
Oatmeal Walnut Raisin	1	100	1	4
Vanilla Wafers Cholesterol Free	6	130	2	6
Barbara's				
Animal Cookies Vanilla	8 (1 oz)	130	3	5
Chocolate Chip	1 (0.6 oz)	80	2	4
Double Dutch Chocolate	1 (0.6 oz)	80	2	4
Fat Free Homestyle Chewy Chocolate	2 (0.9 oz)	80	0	0
Fat Free Homestyle Chocolate Mint	2 (0.9 oz)	80	0	0
Fat Free Homestyle Nutt'n Crispies	2 (0.9 oz)	80	0	0
Fat Free Homestyle Oatmeal Raisin	2 (0.9 oz)	80	0	0
Fat Free Mini Carmel Apple	6 (1 oz)	110	0	0

FOOD	PORTION	CALS.	SAT. FAT	FAT
Barbara's (CONT.)				
Fat Free Mini Cocoa Mocha	6 (1 oz)	100	0	0
Fat Free Mini Double Chocolate	6 (1 oz)	100	0	0
Fat Free Mini Oatmeal Raisin	6 (1 oz)	110	0	0
Fig Bars Fat Free	1 (0.7 oz)	60	0	0
Fig Bars Fat Free Raspberry	1 (0.7 oz)	60	0	0
Fig Bars Fat Free Whole Wheat	1 (0.7 oz)	60	0	0
Fig Bars Fat Free Whole Wheat Apple Cinnamon	1 (0.7 oz)	60	0	0
Fig Bars Low Fat	1 (0.7 oz)	60	0	1
Fig Bars Low Fat Blueberry	1 (0.7 oz)	60	0	1
Old Fashioned Oatmeal	1 (0.6 oz)	70	1	3
Snackimals Chocolate Chip	8 (1 oz)	120	0	5
Snackimals Oatmeal Wheat Free	8 (1 oz)	120	0	5
Snackimals Vanilla	8 (1 oz)	120	0	5
Traditional Shortbread	1 (0.6 oz)	80	3	4
Barnum's				
Animal Crackers	12 (1.1 oz)	140	1	4
Animal Crackers Chocolate	10 (1 oz)	130	1	4
Beigel's				
Black & White	1 (1 oz)	100	1	3
Biscos				
Sugar Wafers	8 (1 oz)	140	2	6
Waffle Cremes	4 (1.2 oz)	180	2	9
Breaktime				
Chocolate Chip	1 (0.3 oz)	37	tr	2
Coconut	1 (0.3 oz)	35	tr	1
Ginger	1 (0.3 oz)	34	tr	1
Oatmeal	1 (0.3 oz)	35	tr	1
Sprinkles	1 (0.3 oz)	36	tr	2
Brent & Sam's				
Chocolate Chip Pecan	2 (0.5 oz)	80	1	5
Chocolate Chip Raspberry	2 (0.5 oz)	70	1	4
Chocolate Chips	2 (0.5 oz)	70	1	4
Oatmeal Raisin Pecan	2 (0.5 oz)	70	1	7
Toffee Pecan	2 (0.5 oz)	80	1	5
White Chocolate Macadamia	2 (0.5 oz)	80	2	5
Bud's Best				
Caco Creme	7 (1 oz)	140	2	6
Chocolate Chip	6 (1 oz)	140	2	6
French Vanilla	7 (1 oz)	150	2	6
Oatmeal	6 (1 oz)	130	2	5

FOOD	PORTION	CALS.	SAT. FAT	FAT
Cadbury				
Fingers	3	85	3	4
Cafe				
Cinnamony Twists Chocolate Chip	1 (0.5 oz)	40	0	2
Sugar Free California Almond	4 (1 oz)	110	1	4
Twists Cinnamony	1 (0.3 oz)	40	0	2
Carr's				
Ginger Lemon Cremes	2 (1 oz)	140	4	7
Carriage Trade				
Finnish Ginger Snaps	3	60	—	7
Chips Ahoy!				
Bit Size Chocolate Chip	14 (1.1 oz)	170	3	7
Chewy Chocolate Chip	3 (1.3 oz)	170	3	8
Chunky Chocolate Chip	1 (0.5 oz)	80	3	4
Real Chocolate Chip	3 (1.1 oz)	160	3	8
Reduced Fat	3 (1.1 oz)	150	2	6
Sprinkled Real Chocolate Chip	3 (1.3 oz)	170	3	8
Striped Chocolate Chip	1 (0.5 oz)	80	2	4
Chortles				
Cookies	½ pkg. (1 oz)	125	1	3
Cookie Lover's				
Blue Ribbon Brownies	1 (0.8 oz)	90	1	3
Classic Shortbread	1 (0.8 oz)	110	2	7
Dutch Chocolate Chip	1 (0.8 oz)	90	1	4
Fancy Peanut Butter	1 (0.8 oz)	100	1	6
Fancy Peanut Butter	1 (0.8 oz)	100	1	6
Grahams Cinnamon Honey	2 (1 oz)	110	0	1
Grahams Honey	2 (1 oz)	100	0	2
Old-Time Raisin	1 (0.8 oz)	90	1	3
Dare				
Blueberry Cheesecake	1 (0.6 oz)	90	1	5
Butter Shortbread	1 (0.5 oz)	63	2	4
Butter Creme	1 (0.6 oz)	85	1	4
Carrot Cake	1 (0.6 oz)	92	1	5
Chocolate Chip	1 (0.5 oz)	77	1	4
Chocolate Fudge	1 (0.7 oz)	97	3	5
Cinnamon Danish	1 (0.4 oz)	47	tr	2
Coconut Creme	1 (0.7 oz)	99	3	5
French Creme	1 (0.5 oz)	80	3	5
Harvest From The Rain Forest	1 (0.5 oz)	70	1	4
Key Lime Creme	1 (0.6 oz)	86	1	4
Lemon Creme	1 (0.7 oz)	95	1	5
Maple Leaf Creme	1 (0.6 oz)	83	1	4

FOOD	PORTION	CALS.	SAT. FAT	FAT
Dare (CONT.)				
Maple Walnut Fudge	1 (0.7 oz)	99	3	5
Milk Chocolate Fudge	1 (0.7 oz)	99	3	5
Oatmeal Raisin	1 (0.4 oz)	59	1	3
Social Tea	1 (0.2 oz)	26	tr	1
Sun Maid Raisin Oatmeal	1 (0.5 oz)	52	1	3
De Beukelaer				
Pirouline	8 (1 oz)	130	3	4
Delacre				
Cookie Assortment	4 (1.1 oz)	130	6	<5
Dunkaroos				
Chocolate Chip w/ Chocolate Frosting	1 pkg (1 oz)	120	1	5
Cinnamon Graham w/ Vanilla Frosting	1 pkg (1 oz)	130	1	5
Cookies'n Creme	1 pkg (1 oz)	120	2	5
Dutch Mill				
Chocolate Chip	3 (1.1 oz)	160	3	10
Coconut Macaroons	3 (1 oz)	120	6	7
Oatmeal Raisin	3 (1 oz)	130	2	6
Ensemble				
Oatmeal	1 (1 oz)	120	1	4
Oatmeal Raisin	1 (1 oz)	120	1	4
Entenmann's				
Chocolate Chip	3 (0.9 oz)	140	—	7
Estee				
Chocolate Chip	4	150	2	7
Coconut	4	140	2	6
Fig Bars	2	100	0	1
Fudge	4	150	2	7
Lemon Thins	4	140	1	6
Oatmeal Raisin	4	130	1	5
Sandwich Chocolate	3	160	2	6
Sandwich Original	3	160	2	6
Sandwich Peanut Butter	3	160	1	7
Sandwich Vanilla	3	160	1	5
Shortbread	4	130	1	4
Sugar Free Chocolate Chip	3	110	1	4
Sugar Free Chocolate Walnut	3	110	0	4
Sugar Free Coconut	3	110	1	4
Sugar Free Grahams Chocolate	2	110	0	2
Sugar Free Grahams Cinnamon	2	90	0	2

FOOD	PORTION	CALS.	SAT. FAT	FAT
Estee (CONT.)				
Sugar Free Grahams Old Fashion	2	90	0	2
Sugar Free Lemon	3	110	0	3
Sugar Free Wafer Banana Split	5	155	2	9
Sugar Free Wafer Chocolate	5	150	2	9
Sugar Free Wafer Chocolate Peanut Butter Caramel	5	150	2	8
Sugar Free Wafer Lemon Creme	5	150	2	8
Sugar Free Wafer Peanut Butter Creme	5	150	2	8
Sugar Free Wafer Vanilla	5	150	2	8
Sugar Free Wafer Vanilla Strawberry	5	150	2	8
Vanilla Thins	4	140	1	6
Famous Amos				
Butter Shortie	1 (0.5 oz)	80	2	5
Chocolate Chip	4 (1 oz)	140	2	7
Chocolate Chip & Pecan	4 (1 oz)	140	2	8
Chocolate Chip Toffee	4 (1 oz)	130	3	6
Chocolate Creme Sandwich	3 (1.2 oz)	140	2	6
Chunky Chocolate Chip	1 (0.5 oz)	70	2	4
Fat Free Fig Bar	2 (1 oz)	90	0	0
Fat Free Strawberry Fruit Bar	2 (1 oz)	90	0	0
Fig Bar	2 (1.1 oz)	120	1	3
Oatmeal Chocolate Chip Walnut	4 (1 oz)	140	2	7
Oatmeal Raisin	4 (1 oz)	130	1	6
Oatmeal Macaroon Creme Sandwich	3 (1.2 oz)	160	2	7
Peanut Butter Chocolate Chunk	1 (0.5 oz)	80	2	5
Peanut Butter Creme Sandwich	3 (1.2 oz)	160	2	8
Pecan Shortie	1 (0.5 oz)	80	1	5
Vanilla Creme Sandwich	3 (1.2 oz)	160	2	7
Freihofer's				
Chocolate Chip	2 (0.9 oz)	120	3	6
Frookie				
Animal Frackers	14 (1 oz)	130	0	5
Chocolate Chip Wheat & Gluten Free	3 (1.1 oz)	140	2	5

FOOD	PORTION	CALS.	SAT. FAT	FAT
Frookie (CONT.)				
Double Chocolate Wheat & Gluten Free	3 (1.1 oz)	130	1	4
Dream Creams Strawberry	4 (1 oz)	140	2	8
Dream Creams Vanilla	4 (1 oz)	140	2	8
Funky Monkeys Chocolate	16 (1 oz)	120	1	4
Funky Monkeys Vanilla	16 (1 oz)	120	1	4
Graham Cinnamon	2 (1 oz)	100	0	3
Graham Honey	2 (1 oz)	110	0	3
Lemon Wafers	8 (1 oz)	110	0	0
Old Fashioned Ginger Snaps	8 (1 oz)	120	0	2
Organic Chocolate Chip	3 (1.1 oz)	150	2	7
Organic Double Chocolate Chip	3 (1.1 oz)	140	2	6
Organic Iced Lemon	3 (1.3 oz)	165	1	6
Organic Oatmeal Raisin	3 (1.1 oz)	140	1	5
Peanut Butter Chunk Wheat & Gluten Free	3 (1.1 oz)	140	1	5
Sandwich Chocolate	2 (0.7 oz)	100	0	4
Sandwich Lemon	2 (0.7 oz)	100	0	4
Sandwich Peanut Butter	2 (0.7 oz)	100	0	4
Sandwich Vanilla	2 (0.7 oz)	100	0	4
Shortbread	5 (1 oz)	130	3	5
Vanilla Wafers	8 (1 oz)	110	0	0
Girl Scout				
Apple Cinnamon Reduced Fat	3 (1 oz)	120	1	5
Do-si-dos	3 (1.2 oz)	170	1	8
Lemon Drops	3 (1.2 oz)	160	2	8
Samoas	2 (1 oz)	160	6	9
Striped Chocolate Chip	3 (1.2 oz)	180	4	10
Tagalongs	2 (0.9 oz)	150	4	10
Thin Mints	4 (1 oz)	140	2	8
Trefoils	5 (1.1 oz)	160	1	8
Golden Grahams Treats				
Chocolate Chunk	1 bar (0.8 oz)	90	1	3
Honey Graham	1 bar (0.8 oz)	90	0	2
King Size Chocolate Chunk	1 bar (1.6 oz)	190	1	5
King Size Honey Graham	1 bar (1.6 oz)	180	1	4
Grandma's				
Chocolate Chip	1 (1.4 oz)	190	3	9
Fudge Chocolate Chip	1 (1.4 oz)	170	3	7
Fudge Sandwich	3	180	2	5
Fudge Vanilla Sandwich	3	120	1	4
Mini Fudge	9	150	2	7

FOOD	PORTION	CALS.	SAT. FAT	FAT
Grandma's (CONT.)				
Mini Peanut Butter	9	150	2	7
Mini Vanilla	9	150	2	7
Oatmeal Raisin	1 (1.4 oz)	160	2	6
Old Time Molasses	1 (1.4 oz)	160	2	4
Peanut Butter	1 (1.4 oz)	190	2	9
Peanut Butter Chocolate Chip	1 (1.4 oz)	190	3	9
Peanut Butter Sandwich	5	210	3	10
Rich N'Chewy	1 pkg	270	4	12
Vanilla Sandwich	3	180	2	5
Vanilla Sandwich	5	210	3	10
Handi-Snack				
Cookie Jammers Cookies & Fruit Spread	1 pkg (1.3 oz)	130	0	3
Health Valley				
Apple Spice	3	100	0	0
Apricot Delight	3	100	0	0
Biscotti Amaretto	2	120	—	3
Biscotti Chocolate	2	120	—	3
Biscotti Fruit & Nut	2	120	—	3
Cheesecake Bars Blueberry	1 bar	160	—	2
Cheesecake Bars Raspberry	1 bar	160	—	2
Cheesecake Bars Strawberry	1 bar	160	—	2
Chips Double Chocolate	3	100	0	0
Chips Old Fashioned	3	100	0	0
Chips Original	3	100	0	0
Chocolate Fudge Center	2	70	0	0
Chocolate Sandwich Bar Bavarian Creme	1 bar	150	0	0
Chocolate Sandwich Bars Caramel Creme	1 bar	150	0	0
Chocolate Sandwich Bars Vanilla Creme	1 bar	150	0	0
Date Delight Date Delight	3	100	0	0
Graham Amaranth	8	100	0	0
Graham Oat Bran	8	100	0	0
Graham Original Amaranth	6	120	—	3
Hawaiian Fruit	3	100	0	0
Jumbo Apple Raisin	1	80	0	0
Jumbo Raisin Raisin	1	80	0	0
Jumbo Raspberry	1	80	0	0
Marshmallow Bars Chocolate Chip	1	90	0	0

FOOD	PORTION	CALS.	SAT. FAT	FAT
Health Valley (CONT.)				
Marshmallow Bars Old Fashioned	1	90	0	0
Marshmallow Bars Tropical Fruit	1	90	0	0
Oat Bran Fruit Bars Raisin Cinnamon	1 bar	160	—	1
Raisin Oatmeal	3	100	0	0
Raspberry Fruit Center	1	70	0	0
Tarts Baked Apple Cinnamon	1	150	0	0
Tarts California Strawberry	1	150	0	0
Tarts Chocolate Fudge	1	150	0	0
Tarts Cranberry Apple	1	150	0	0
Tarts Mountain Blueberry	1	150	0	0
Tarts Red Raspberry	1	150	0	0
Tarts Sweet Red Cherry	1	150	0	0
Heyday				
Caramel & Peanut	1 (0.8 oz)	110	1	5
Fudge	1 (0.8 oz)	110	1	5
Honey Maid				
Cinnamon Grahams	10 (1.1 oz)	140	1	3
Honey Grahams	8 (1 oz)	120	1	3
Joseph's				
Almond Sugar Free	2 (0.9 oz)	100	1	5
Chocolate Chip Sugar Free	2 (0.9 oz)	100	1	5
Chocolate Walnut Sugar Free	2 (0.9 oz)	100	1	6
Coconut Sugar Free	2 (0.9 oz)	105	1	5
Lemon Sugar Free	2 (0.9 oz)	95	1	4
Oatmeal Raisin Sugar Free	2 (0.9 oz)	100	1	5
Peanut Butter Sugar Free	2 (0.9 oz)	95	1	5
Pecan Shortbread Sugar Free	2 (0.9 oz)	100	1	5
Keebler				
All American Lemon Coolers	5 (1 oz)	140	2	6
Animal Crackers	1 pkg (2 oz)	250	2	9
Animal Crackers Frosted	1 pkg (2 oz)	290	9	14
Butter	5 (1.1 oz)	150	2	6
Chips Deluxe	1 (0.5 oz)	80	2	5
Chips Deluxe Chocolate Lovers	1 (0.6 oz)	90	3	5
Chips Deluxe Rainbow	1 (0.6 oz)	80	2	4
Chips Deluxe Soft 'n Chewy	1 (0.6 oz)	80	1	4
Chips Deluxe w/ Peanut Butter Cups	1 (0.6 oz)	90	2	5
Chips Deluxe w/ Coconut	1 (0.5 oz)	80	2	5

FOOD	PORTION	CALS.	SAT. FAT	FAT
Keebler (CONT.)				
Classic Collection Chocolate Fudge Sandwich	1 (0.6 oz)	80	1	5
Classic Collection French Vanllia Creme Sandwich	1 (0.6 oz)	80	1	4
Cookie Stix Butter	5 (1.2 oz)	160	3	6
Cookie Stix Chocolate Chip	4 (0.9 oz)	130	2	5
Cookie Stix Rainbow	5 (1.2 oz)	150	2	6
Danish Wedding	4 (1 oz)	120	2	5
Deluxe Grahams Fudge Covered	3 (1 oz)	140	5	7
Droxies	3 (1.1 oz)	140	1	6
E.L. Fudge Butter Sandwich w/ Fudge Creme	2 (0.9 oz)	120	1	6
E.L. Fudge Chocolate Sandwich w/ Peanut Butter Creme	2 (0.9 oz)	120	1	6
E.L. Fudge Fudge w/ Fudge Creme	2 (0.9 oz)	120	1	6
Fudge Sticks Creme Wafers	3 (1 oz)	150	5	8
Fudge Sticks Peanut Butter Creme Wafers	3 (1 oz)	150	4	8
Fudge Stripes	3 (1.1 oz)	160	5	8
Fudge Stripes 25% Reduced Fat	3 (1 oz)	140	3	5
Ginger Snaps	5 (1.1 oz)	150	1	6
Golden Fruit Cranberry	1 (0.7 oz)	80	0	2
Golden Fruit Raisin	1 (0.7 oz)	80	1	2
Golden Vanilla Wafers	8 (1.1 oz)	150	2	7
Graham Cinnamon Crisp	8 (1 oz)	140	1	5
Graham Cinnamon Crisp Low Fat	8 (1 oz)	110	1	2
Graham Honey	8 (1.1 oz)	150	2	6
Graham Honey Low Fat	8 (1.1 oz)	120	1	2
Graham Original	8 (1 oz)	130	1	3
Grahams Chocolate	8 (1.1 oz)	130	1	4
Grasshoppers	4 (1 oz)	150	5	7
Iced Animal	6 (1.1 oz)	150	1	5
Iced Animal Chocolate Chip	7 (1.1 oz)	130	1	5
Iced Animal w/ Sprinkles	6 (1.1 oz)	150	1	5
Krisp Kreem	5 (1 oz)	140	2	7
Oatmeal Country Style	2 (0.8 oz)	120	1	5
S'Mores	3 (1.2 oz)	160	5	8
Sandies	1 (0.5 oz)	80	2	5
Sandies w/ Almonds	1 (0.5 oz)	80	1	5

FOOD	PORTION	CALS.	SAT. FAT	FAT
Keebler (CONT.)				
Sandies w/ Pecans	1 (0.5 oz)	80	1	5
Sandies w/ Pecans 25% Reduced Fat	1 (0.5 oz)	80	1	3
Snack Size Chips Deluxe	1 pkg (2 oz)	300	5	16
Snack Size Mini Fudge Stripes	1 pkg (2 oz)	280	9	14
Snack Size Rainbow Chips Deluxe	1 pkg (2 oz)	290	4	16
Snack Size Sandies w/ Pecans	1 pkg (2 oz)	300	4	17
Snackin' Grahams Cinnamon Crisp	21 (1 oz)	130	1	3
Snackin' Grahams Honey	23 (1 oz)	130	1	4
Soft Batch Chocolate Chip	1 (0.6 oz)	80	1	4
Soft Batch Homestyle Chocolate Chunk	1 (0.9 oz)	130	3	7
Soft Batch Homestyle Chocolate Chunk	1 (0.9 oz)	130	3	7
Soft Batch Homestyle Double Chocolate	1 (0.9 oz)	130	2	7
Soft Batch Homestyle Oatmeal Raisin	1 (0.9 oz)	130	1	5
Soft Batch Oatmeal Raisin	1 (0.6 oz)	70	1	3
Sugar Wafers Peanut Butter	4 (1.1 oz)	170	2	9
Sugar Wafers Vanilla	3 (0.9 oz)	130	2	6
Vanilla Wafer 30% Reduced Fat	8 (1.1 oz)	130	1	4
Vienna Fingers	2 (1 oz)	140	2	6
Vienna Fingers Lemon	2 (1 oz)	140	2	6
Knott's Berry Farm				
Fruit Filled All Flavors	4 (1 oz)	120	1	5
LU				
Le Bastogne	2 (0.8 oz)	120	3	5
Le Chocolatiers	3 (1 oz)	150	7	8
Le Dore	4 (1 oz)	140	3	6
Le Fondant	4 (1.1 oz)	170	9	10
Le Palmier	4 (1.2 oz)	180	5	10
Le Petit Beurre	4 (1.2 oz)	150	3	4
Le Petit Ecolier Dark Chocolate	2 (0.9 oz)	130	4	6
Le Petit Ecolier Hazelnut Milk Chocolate	2 (0.9 oz)	130	3	7
Le Petit Ecolier Milk Chocolate	2 (0.9 oz)	130	4	6

FOOD	PORTION	CALS.	SAT. FAT	FAT
LU (CONT.)				
Le Pim's Orange	2 (0.9 oz)	90	1	3
Le Pim's Raspberry	2 (0.9 oz)	90	1	3
Le Raisin Dore	4 (1.2 oz)	160	5	7
Le Truffe Coconut	4 (1.2 oz)	190	11	12
Le Truffe Praline Chocolate	4 (1.2 oz)	170	7	9
Les Varietes	3 (0.9 oz)	140	5	7
Lance				
Apple Bar Fat Free	1 (1.75 oz)	160	0	0
Apple Oatmeal Bar	1 (1.8 oz)	190	2	6
Big Town Banana	1 pkg (2 oz)	250	3	10
Big Town Chocolate	1 pkg (2 oz)	250	3	8
Big Town Vanilla	1 pkg (2 oz)	250	3	11
Choc-O-Lunch	1 pkg (1.5 oz)	200	2	8
Choc-O-Mint	1 pkg (1¼ oz)	190	4	9
Coated Graham	1 pkg (1.3 oz)	190	2	8
Fig Bar	1 (1.75 oz)	180	1	4
Fudge Chocolate Chip	1 (2 oz)	130	2	5
Gourmet Chocolate Chip	1 (2 oz)	130	3	6
Lem-O-Lunch	1 pkg (3.4 oz)	240	3	11
Lemon Nekot	1 pkg (1.5 oz)	210	2	10
Nut-O-Lunch	1 pkg (3.3 oz)	240	3	11
Oatmeal	1 (2 oz)	130	1	6
Oatmeal Creme	1 (2 oz)	240	3	10
Peanut Butter	1 (2 oz)	140	2	8
Van-O-Lunch	1 pkg (1.5 oz)	210	2	8
Linden's				
Lemon	1 (1 oz)	120	1	5
Little Debbie				
Apple Flips	1 (1.2 oz)	150	2	5
Caramel Bars Bars	1 (1.2 oz)	160	2	8
Cherry Cordials	1 (1.3 oz)	170	2	8
Coconut Rounds	1 (1.2 oz)	150	3	7
Cookie Wreaths	1 (0.6 oz)	100	1	5
Easter Puffs	1 (1.2 oz)	140	2	6
Fig Bars	1 (1.5 oz)	150	1	4
Fudge Delights	1 (1.1 oz)	110	0	2
Fudge Rounds	1 (1.2 oz)	140	2	6
German Chocolate Ring	1 (1 oz)	140	4	8
Ginger	1 (0.7 oz)	90	1	3
Jelly Creme Pies	1 (1.2 oz)	160	2	7
Marshmallow Crispy Bar	1 (1.3 oz)	140	1	4
Marshmallow Supremes	1 (1.1 oz)	130	1	5
Marshmallow Pie Banana	1 pkg (1.5 oz)	180	2	6

FOOD	PORTION	CALS.	SAT. FAT	FAT
Little Debbie (CONT.)				
Marshmallow Pie Chocolate	1 (1.4 oz)	160	3	6
Nutty Bar	1 (2 oz)	310	3	18
Oatmeal Raisin	1 (1.3 oz)	160	2	7
Oatmeal Creme Pie	1 (1.3 oz)	170	2	7
Oatmeal Delights	1 (1.1 oz)	110	0	2
Oatmeal Lights	1 (1.3 oz)	130	1	3
Peanut Butter Bars	1 (1.9 oz)	270	3	15
Peanut Butter & Jelly Oatmeal Pie	1 (1.1 oz)	130	1	5
Peanut Clusters	1 (1.4 oz)	190	2	11
Pumpkin Delights	1 (1.2 oz)	150	2	5
Raisin Creme Pie	1 (1.2 oz)	140	1	5
Star Crunch	1 (1.1 oz)	140	2	6
Sugar Free Chocolate Chip	3 (1.1 oz)	140	3	7
Sugar Free Oatmeal	6 (1.1 oz)	120	1	4
Yo-Yo's	1 (1.2 oz)	130	2	6
Lorna Doone				
Cookies	4 (1 oz)	140	1	7
Manischewitz				
Macaroons Chocolate	2 (0.9 oz)	90	4	4
MoonPie				
Chocolate	1 (2.75 oz)	330	6	10
Mini Banana	1 (1.2 oz)	152	3	5
Mini Chocolate	1 (1.2 oz)	152	3	5
Mini Vanilla	1 (1.2 oz)	152	3	5
Mother's				
Almond Shortbread	3	180	4	11
Checkerboard Wafers	8	150	5	8
Chocolate Chip	2	160	3	8
Chocolate Chip Angel	3	180	4	9
Chocolate Chip Parade	4	130	2	5
Circus Animals	6	140	5	6
Classic Assortments	2	140	4	7
Cocadas	5	150	3	7
Cookie Parade	4	140	3	7
Dinosaur Grrrahams	2	130	1	3
Double Fudge	2	180	5	9
English Tea	2	180	4	7
Flaky Flix Fudge	2	140	5	7
Flaky Flix Vanilla	2	140	5	8
Gaucho Peanut Butter	2	190	3	10
Iced Oatmeal	2	130	2	4
Iced Raisin	2	180	7	8

FOOD	PORTION	CALS.	SAT. FAT	FAT
Mother's (CONT.)				
MLB Double Header Duplex	3	170	4	8
Macaroon	2	150	4	8
Marias	3	170	2	6
Oatmeal	2	110	2	5
Oatmeal Chocolate Chip	2	120	2	5
Oatmeal Raisin	5	150	2	7
Oatmeal Walnut Chocolate Chip	2	130	2	6
Rainbow Wafers	8	150	5	8
Striped Shortbread	3	170	5	8
Sugar	2	140	2	6
Taffy	2	180	2	8
Triplet Assortment	2	140	3	7
Vanilla Wafers	6	150	2	6
Wallops Boysenberry	1	80	1	2
Wallops Honey Crust Fig	1	80	5	2
Wallops Honey Graham Fig	1	80	1	2
Wallops Mixed Berry	1	80	1	2
Wallops Peach Apricot	1	80	1	2
Wallops Raspberry	1	80	1	2
Wallops Strawberry	1	80	1	2
Walnut Fudge	2	130	3	7
Zoo Pals	14	140	2	5
Mrs. Alison's				
Coconut Bar	2 (1 oz)	130	1	6
Creme Wafers	5 (1.1 oz)	170	2	10
Fudge Fingers	3 (1 oz)	160	6	10
Ginger Snaps	4 (1 oz)	130	1	3
Jelly Tops	5 (1 oz)	140	2	7
Lemon Creme	3 (1 oz)	130	2	5
Macaroons	2 (1 oz)	140	3	7
Pecan	2 (1 oz)	140	2	7
Shortbread	5 (1 oz)	120	1	5
Murray's				
Sugar Free Double Fudge	3 (1.2 oz)	140	3	6
Sugar Free Ginger Snap	6 (1 oz)	110	2	4
Sugar Free Peanut Butter	6 (1 oz)	130	2	7
Sugar Free Vanilla Sandwich Creme	3 (1 oz)	120	2	5
Sugar Free Vanilla Wafers	9 (1.1 oz)	120	1	4
Mystic Mint				
Cookies	1 (0.5 oz)	90	1	4
Nabisco				
Brown Edge Wafers	5 (1 oz)	140	2	6

FOOD	PORTION	CALS.	SAT. FAT	FAT
Nabisco (CONT.)				
Bugs Bunny Chocolate Graham	13 (1.1 oz)	140	1	5
Bugs Bunny Cinnamon Graham	13 (1.1 oz)	140	1	5
Bugs Bunny Graham	13 (1.1 oz)	140	1	7
Cameo	2 (1 oz)	130	1	5
Chocolate Grahams	3 (1.1 oz)	160	5	8
Chocolate Chip Snaps	7 (1.1 oz)	150	2	5
Chocolate Snaps	7 (1.1 oz)	140	2	5
Cookie Break	3 (1.1 oz)	160	2	6
Danish Imported	5 (1.1 oz)	170	2	8
Family Favorites Fudge Covered Grahams	3 (1 oz)	140	2	7
Family Favorites Fudge Striped Shortbread	3 (1.1 oz)	160	2	8
Family Favorites Oatmeal	1 (0.5 oz)	80	1	3
Family Favorites Vanilla Sandwich	3 (1.2 oz)	170	2	8
Famous Chocolate Wafers	5 (1.1 oz)	140	2	4
Ginger Snaps Old Fashioned	4 (1 oz)	120	1	3
Grahams	8 (1 oz)	120	1	3
Mallomars	2 (0.9 oz)	120	3	5
Marshmallow Puffs	1 (0.75 oz)	90	1	4
Marshmallow Twirls	1 (1 oz)	130	2	6
Nilla Wafers	8 (1.1 oz)	140	1	5
Pecan Passion	1 (0.5 oz)	90	1	5
Pinwheels	1 (1 oz)	130	3	5
National				
Arrowroot	1 (5 g)	20	0	1
Newman's Own				
Fig Newman's Organic	2 (1.3 oz)	120	0	0
Newtons				
Apple Fat Free	2 (1 oz)	100	0	0
Cranberry Fat Free	2 (1 oz)	100	0	0
Fig	2 (1.1 oz)	110	1	3
Fig Fat Free	1 (1 oz)	100	0	0
Raspberry Fat Free	2 (1 oz)	100	0	0
Strawberry Fat Free	2 (1 oz)	100	0	0
NutraBalance				
Fibre Oatmeal Raisin	1 (0.7 oz)	80	1	4
Protein Fortified	1 (2 oz)	260	5	14
ReNeph Spice	1 (2 oz)	210	0	7
Nutter Butter				
Bites Peanut Butter Sandwich	10 (1.1 oz)	150	2	7

FOOD	PORTION	CALS.	SAT. FAT	FAT
Nutter Butter (CONT.)				
Peanut Butter Sandwich	2 (1 oz)	130	1	6
Peanut Creme Patties	5 (1.1 oz)	160	2	9
Old Brussels				
Ginger Crisps	2 (0.9 oz)	140	1	4
Oreo				
Cookies	3 (1.2 oz)	160	2	7
Double Stuf	2 (1 oz)	140	1	7
Fudge Covered	1 (0.75 oz)	110	2	6
Halloween Treats	2 (1 oz)	140	2	7
Reduced Fat	3 (1.2 oz)	140	1	5
White Fudge Covered	1 (0.75 oz)	110	2	6
Otis Spunkmeyer				
Butter Sugar	1 med (1.3 oz)	160	3	8
Butter Sugar	1 (2 oz)	250	5	12
Carnival	1 med (1.3 oz)	170	3	7
Chocolate Chip	1 med (1.3 oz)	170	4	8
Chocolate Chip	1 bite size (0.75 oz)	100	2	5
Chocolate Chip	1 (2 oz)	250	6	11
Chocolate Chip Pecan	1 med (1.3 oz)	170	4	9
Chocolate Chip Walnut	1 bite size (0.75 oz)	100	3	5
Chocolate Chip Walnut	1 med (1.3 oz)	180	4	9
Chocolate Chip Walnut	1 (2 oz)	270	6	14
Double Chocolate Chip	1 bite size (0.75 oz)	100	3	5
Double Chocolate Chip	1 med (1.3 oz)	180	5	9
Oatmeal Raisin	1 med (1.3 oz)	160	5	7
Oatmeal Raisin	1 bite size (0.75 oz)	90	3	4
Otis Express Chocolate Chunk	1 (2 oz)	280	6	13
Otis Express Double Chocolate Chip	1 (2 oz)	270	7	14
Otis Express Oatmeal Raisin	1 (2 oz)	240	7	10
Otis Express Peanut Butter	1 (2 oz)	270	6	15
Peanut Butter	1 med (1.3 oz)	180	4	10
Pinnacle Checkpoint Chocolate Almond Coconut	1 (2.4 oz)	320	10	18
Pinnacle Mach One Mocha Chocolate Chunk	1 (2.4 oz)	300	6	13
Pinnacle Passport Peanut Butter Chocolate Chunk	1 (2.4 oz)	300	5	13
Pinnacle Ripcord Rocky Road	1 (2.4 oz)	310	6	15
Pinnacle Takeoff Triple Chocolate	1 (2.4 oz)	300	6	14
Pinnacle Transatlantic Turtle	1 (2.4 oz)	310	6	16

FOOD	PORTION	CALS.	SAT. FAT	FAT
Otis Spunkmeyer (CONT.)				
Travel Lite Low Fat Apple Cinnamon	1 (1.3 oz)	130	0	2
Travel Lite Low Fat Chocolate Chip	1 (1.3 oz)	130	1	2
Travel Lite Low Fat Ginger Spice	1 (1.3 oz)	130	0	2
Travel Lite Low Fat Oatmeal Rum Raisin	1 (1.3 oz)	130	0	2
White Chocolate Macadamia Nut	1 med (1.3 oz)	180	4	10
White Chocolate Macadamia Nut	1 (2 oz)	280	7	15
Pally				
Butter	4 (0.88 oz)	100	2	3
Pamela's				
Pecan Shortbread Rice Flour	1 (0.8 oz)	130	4	8
Peek Freans				
Petit Beret Creme Caramel	2 (0.8 oz)	110	4	5
Petit Beret Fudge Truffle	2 (0.8 oz)	110	4	5
Traditional Oatmeal	1 (0.7 oz)	90	1	3
Pepperidge Farm				
Biscotti Almond	1 (0.7 oz)	90	1	4
Biscotti Chocolate Hazelnut	1 (0.7 oz)	90	1	5
Biscotti Cranberry Pistachio	1 (0.7 oz)	90	1	3
Bordeaux	4	130	3	5
Brussels	3	150	3	7
Chessman	3	120	3	8
Chocolate Chip	3	140	3	7
Chocolate Chunk Soft Baked	1	130	3	6
Chocolate Chunk Soft Baked Milk Chocolate Macademia	1	130	3	7
Chocolate Chunk Soft Baked Reduced Fat	1	110	2	5
Chocolate Chunk Soft Baked White Chocolate Pecan	1	120	2	5
Fruitful Apricot-Raspberry Cut	3	140	2	6
Fruitful Strawberry Cut	3	140	2	5
Geneva	3	160	4	9
Lemon Nut Crunch	3	170	2	9
Lido	1	90	2	5
Milano	3	180	4	10
Milano Endless Chocolate	3	180	5	10

FOOD	PORTION	CALS.	SAT. FAT	FAT
Pepperidge Farm (CONT.)				
Milano Milk Chocolate	3	170	4	9
Mint Milano	2	130	4	7
Nantucket	1 (0.9 oz)	130	3	7
Nantucket Chocolate Chunk	1	140	3	7
Oatmeal Raisin	1	100	1	3
Orange Milano	2	130	3	7
Pirouettes Traditional	5 (1.2 oz)	170	3	9
Shortbread	2	140	—	7
Sugar	3	140	2	6
Ralston				
Animal	12 (0.9 oz)	130	1	3
Chocolate Graham	2 (0.9 oz)	130	1	3
Cinnamon Grahams	2 (0.9 oz)	130	1	5
Cinnamon Grahams Low Fat	2 (0.9 oz)	110	0	2
Fig Bars	2 (1.2 oz)	120	0	3
Vanilla Wafers	7 (1.1 oz)	150	1	6
Ritz				
Chocolate Covered	3 (1 oz)	150	5	9
Royal				
Apple Bars	1 (1.1 oz)	100	0	2
Apple Cake	1 (1.1 oz)	110	1	3
Brownie Rounds	1 (1.1 oz)	130	2	6
Chocolate Chip	1 (1.1 oz)	140	2	6
Devilfood	1 (1 oz)	110	1	5
Oatmeal	1 (1.1 oz)	130	1	6
Raisin	1 (1 oz)	110	1	5
Strawberry Bars	1 (1.1 oz)	100	0	2
Santa Fe Farms				
Chocolate Chocolate Chip Fat Free	2 (1 oz)	60	0	0
Chocolate Mint Fat Free	2 (1 oz)	60	0	0
Ginger Fat Free	2 (1 oz)	70	0	0
Sargento				
MooTown Snackers Honey Graham Sticks & Vanilla Creme w/ Sprinkles	1 pkg (1 oz)	140	1	7
MooTown Snackers Vanilla Sticks & Chocolate Fudge Creme	1 pkg (1 oz)	130	2	6
Scotto's				
Biscotti Fat Free French Vanilla	4 (1 oz)	80	0	0

FOOD	PORTION	CALS.	SAT. FAT	FAT
Season				
Hamantashen Poppy	1 (1 oz)	150	4	7
Hamantasken Apricot	1 (1 oz)	150	4	7
Simple Pleasures				
Almond	1 (0.3 oz)	37	tr	2
Cinnamon Snaps	1 (0.2 oz)	31	tr	1
Digestive	1 (0.3 oz)	46	tr	2
Encore Tea Cookie	1 (0.2 oz)	29	tr	1
Lemon Social Tea	1 (0.2 oz)	29	tr	1
Oatmeal	1 (0.5 oz)	74	1	3
Spice Snaps	1 (0.3 oz)	34	tr	1
Sugar	1 (0.4 oz)	45	1	2
SnackWell's				
Fat Free Double Fudge	1 (0.5 oz)	50	0	0
Golden Devil's Food	1 (0.5 oz)	50	0	1
Reduced Fat Chocolate Chip	13 (1 oz)	130	2	4
Reduced Fat Chocolate Sandwich	2 (0.8 oz)	100	0	2
Reduced Fat Oatmeal Raisin	2 (1 oz)	110	0	3
Reduced Fat Vanilla Sandwich	2 (0.9 oz)	110	1	3
Social Tea				
Cookies	6 (1 oz)	120	1	4
Stella D'Oro				
Almond Toast Mandel	1	60	—	1
Angel Bars	1	80	—	5
Angel Wings	1	70	—	5
Angelica Goodies	1	110	—	4
Anginetti	1	30	—	1
Anisette Sponge	1	50	—	1
Anisette Toast	1	50	—	1
Anisette Toast Jumbo	1	110	—	1
Apple Pastry Low Sodium	1	80	—	3
Biscottini Cashews	1	110	—	6
Breakfast Treats	1	100	—	4
Castelets Chocolate	1	60	—	3
Chinese Dessert Cookies	1	170	—	9
Como Delight	1	150	—	7
Deep Night Fudge	1	65	—	4
Dutch Apple Bars	1	110	—	3
Egg Biscuits Low Sodium	3	120	—	3
Egg Biscuits Sugared	1	80	—	1
Egg Jumbo	1	50	—	1
Fruit Delight Apple Cinnamon Fat Free	1	70	0	0

FOOD	PORTION	CALS.	SAT. FAT	FAT
Stella D'Oro (CONT.)				
Fruit Delight Peach Apricot Fat Free	1	70	0	0
Fruit Delight Raspberry Fat Free	1	70	0	0
Fruit Slices	1	60	—	2
Fruit Slices Fat Free	1	50	0	0
Golden Bars	1	110	—	4
Holiday Rings & Stars	1	47	—	1
Holiday Trinkets	1	40	—	2
Hostess Assortment	1	40	—	2
Indulgente Cashew Biscottini	1 (1.1 oz)	150	2	8
Kichel Low Sodium	21	150	—	9
Lady Stella Assortment	1	40	—	2
Margherite Chocolate	1	70	—	3
Margherite Vanilla	1	70	—	3
Peach Apricot Pastry Sodium Free	1	80	—	3
Pfeffernusse Spice Drops	1	40	—	1
Prune Pastry Dietetic	1	90	—	3
Roman Egg Biscuits	1	140	—	5
Royal Nuggets	1	2	—	tr
Sesame Regina	1	50	—	2
Swiss Fudge	1	70	—	3
Sunshine				
All American Butter	5 (1.1 oz)	140	2	6
All American Lemon Coolers	5 (1 oz)	140	2	6
All American Mini Chip-A-Roos	5 (1.1 oz)	160	3	8
Animal Crackers	14 (1.1 oz)	140	1	4
Ginger Snaps	7 (1 oz)	130	1	5
Golden Fruit Cranberry	1 (0.7 oz)	80	0	2
Golden Fruit Raisin	1 (0.7 oz)	80	1	2
Hydrox	3 (1.1 oz)	150	2	7
Hydrox Reduced Fat	3 (1.1 oz)	140	2	5
Oatmeal Country Style	2 (0.8 oz)	120	1	5
Sugar Wafers Peanut Butter Creme	4 (1.1 oz)	170	2	9
Sugar Wafers Vanilla Creme	3 (0.9 oz)	130	2	6
Vanilla Wafers	7 (1.1 oz)	150	2	7
Vienna Fingers	2 (1 oz)	140	2	6
Vienna Fingers Lemon	2 (1 oz)	140	2	6
Vienna Fingers Reduced Fat	2 (1 oz)	130	1	5
Sweet Rewards				
Fat Free Blueberry w/ Drizzle	1 bar (1.3 oz)	120	0	0

FOOD	PORTION	CALS.	SAT. FAT	FAT
Sweet Rewards (CONT.)				
Fat Free Double Fudge Supreme	1 bar (1.3 oz)	100	0	0
Fat Free Raspberry	1 bar (1.3 oz)	120	0	0
Fat Free Strawberry w/ Drizzle	1 bar (1.3 oz)	120	0	0
Low Fat Chocolate Chip	1 bar (1.1 oz)	110	1	2
Tastykake				
Chocolate Chip	1 (1.4 oz)	180	2	7
Chocolate Chip Bar	1 (2 oz)	270	4	12
Chocolate Fudge Iced	1 (1.4 oz)	170	2	7
Fudge Bar	1 (2 oz)	250	2	10
Lemon Bar	1 (2 oz)	260	1	10
Oatmeal Raisin Bar	1 (2 oz)	260	3	10
Oatmeal Raisin Boxed	3 (0.4 oz)	130	2	6
Oatmeal Raisin Iced	1 (1.4 oz)	170	2	6
Strawberry Bar	1 (2 oz)	260	1	10
Sugar Boxed	3 (0.4 oz)	120	2	6
Teddy Grahams				
Chocolate	24 (1 oz)	140	1	5
Cinnamon	24 (1 oz)	140	1	4
Honey	24 (1 oz)	140	1	4
The Source				
Barry's Raspberry Palmiers	1 (0.7 oz)	80	0	3
Tree Of Life				
Creme Supremes	2 (0.9 oz)	120	0	5
Creme Supremes Mint	2 (0.9 oz)	120	0	5
Fat Free Classic Carrot Cake	1 (0.8 oz)	60	0	0
Fat Free Devil's Food Chocolate	1 (0.8 oz)	70	0	0
Fat Free Golden Oatmeal Raisin	1 (0.8 oz)	70	0	0
Fat Free Harvest Fruit & Nut	1 (0.8 oz)	70	0	0
Fat Free Toasted Almond Butter	1 (0.8 oz)	70	0	0
Fruit Bars Apple Spice	2 (1.3 oz)	120	1	3
Fruit Bars Fat Free Fig	1 (0.8 oz)	70	0	0
Fruit Bars Fat Free Peach Apricot	1 (0.8 oz)	70	0	0
Fruit Bars Fat Free Wildberry	1 (0.8 oz)	70	0	0
Fruit Bars Fig	2 (1.3 oz)	120	1	3
Fruit Bars Peach Apricot	2 (1.3 oz)	120	1	3
Honey-Sweet Colossal Carrot Cake	1 (0.8 oz)	110	0	5
Honey-Sweet Lemon Burst	1 (0.8 oz)	110	0	5

FOOD	PORTION	CALS.	SAT. FAT	FAT
Tree Of Life (CONT.)				
Honey-Sweet Oh-So-Oatmeal	1 (0.8 oz)	110	0	5
Honey-Sweet Pecans-A-Plenty	1 (0.8 oz)	125	1	7
Monster Fat Free Carrot Cake	¼ cookie (0.9 oz)	60	0	0
Monster Fat Free Devil's Food Chocolate	¼ cookie (0.9 oz)	80	0	0
Monster Fat Free Gingerbread	¼ cookie (0.9 oz)	80	0	0
Monster Fat Free Maple Pecan	¼ cookie (0.9 oz)	90	0	0
Royal Vanilla	2 (0.9 oz)	120	0	5
Small World Animal Grahams	7 (1 oz)	120	0	3
Small World Chocolate Chip	7 (1 oz)	120	1	4
Soft-Bake Chocolate Chip	1 (0.8 oz)	125	2	7
Soft-Bake Double Fudge	1 (0.8 oz)	110	0	5
Soft-Bake Maui Macaroon	1 (0.8 oz)	135	6	10
Soft-Bake Oatmeal	1 (0.8 oz)	115	0	5
Soft-Bake Peanut Butter	1 (0.8 oz)	125	1	7
Wheat-Free American Oatmeal	1 (0.8 oz)	90	0	5
Wheat-Free California Carob	1 (0.8 oz)	105	0	5
Wheat-Free Georgia Peanut Butter	1 (0.8 oz)	95	1	6
Wheat-Free Mountain Maple Walnut	1 (0.8 oz)	100	0	6
Voortman				
Almonette	2 (1 oz)	150	2	8
Chocolate Chip	1 (0.7 oz)	100	2	5
Chocolate Wafers Sugar Free	3 (1 oz)	160	3	11
Coconut Delight	1 (0.6 oz)	90	3	5
Peanut Delight	1 (0.9 oz)	130	2	7
Strawberry Wafers Sugar Free	3 (1 oz)	160	3	11
Sugar	1 (0.6 oz)	80	1	4
Turnovers Blueberry	1 (0.9 oz)	100	1	3
Turnovers Cherry	1 (0.9 oz)	100	1	3
Turnovers Strawberry	1 (0.9 oz)	100	1	3
Vanilla Wafers Sugar Free	3 (1 oz)	160	3	11
Windmill	1 (0.7 oz)	90	1	4
Walkers				
Shortbread Triangles	2 (0.7 oz)	100	4	6
Weight Watchers				
Apple Raisin Bar	1 (0.75 oz)	70	1	2
Chocolate Chip	2 (1.06 oz)	140	2	5
Chocolate Sandwich	2 (1.06)	140	1	4
Fruit Filled Fig	1 (0.7 oz)	70	0	0
Fruit Filled Raspberry	1 (0.7 oz)	70	0	0

FOOD	PORTION	CALS.	SAT. FAT	FAT
Weight Watchers (CONT.)				
Oatmeal Raisin	2 (1.06 oz)	120	0	2
Vanilla Sandwich	2 (1.06 oz)	140	1	3
White Eagle Bakery				
Chruscik	2 (1 oz)	140	3	8
Wortz				
Animal	9 (1.1 oz)	140	1	5
Chocolate Graham	2 (0.9 oz)	130	1	3
Cinnamon Grahams	2 (0.9 oz)	130	1	5
REFRIGERATED				
chocolate chip	1 (0.42 oz)	59	1	3
chocolate chip unbaked	1 oz	126	2	6
oatmeal	1 (0.4 oz)	56	1	3
oatmeal raisin	1 (0.4 oz)	56	1	3
peanut butter	1 (0.4 oz)	60	1	3
peanut butter dough	1 oz	130	2	7
sugar	1 (0.42 oz)	58	1	3
sugar dough	1 oz	124	2	6
Pillsbury				
Bunny	2	130	2	7
Chocolate Chip	1 (1 oz)	130	3	6
Chocolate Chip Reduced Fat	1 (1 oz)	110	2	3
Chocolate Chip w/ Walnuts	1 (1 oz)	140	2	7
Chocolate Chunk	1 (1 oz)	130	2	6
Christmas Tree	2	130	2	7
Double Chocolate	1 (1 oz)	130	2	6
Flag	2	130	2	7
Frosty	2	130	2	7
M&M's	1 (1 oz)	130	2	6
Oatmeal Chocolate Chip	1 (1 oz)	120	2	6
One Step Pan Chocolate Chip	⅙ pan (1 oz)	130	2	6
One Step Pan M&M's	⅙ pan (1 oz)	130	2	6
Peanut Butter	1 (1 oz)	120	2	6
Pumpkin	2	130	2	7
Reeses	1 (1 oz)	130	3	6
Shamrock	2	130	2	7
Sugar	2	130	2	3
Sugar Holiday Red & Green	2	130	2	6
Valentine	2	130	2	7
White Chocolate Chunk	1 (1 oz)	130	2	6
TAKE-OUT				
biscotti with nuts chocolate dipped	1 (1.3 oz)	117	3	6
black & white	1 lg (3 oz)	302	5	9

FOOD	PORTION	CALS.	SAT. FAT	FAT
CORIANDER				
leaf dried	1 tsp	2	—	tr
leaf fresh	¼ cup	1	—	tr
seed	1 tsp	5	tr	tr
CORN				
(see also BRAN, CEREAL, CORNMEAL)				
CANNED				
cream style	½ cup	93	tr	1
w/ red & green peppers	½ cup	86	tr	1
white	½ cup	66	tr	1
Del Monte				
Cream Style Golden	½ cup (4.4 oz)	90	0	1
Cream Style Golden 50% Less Salt	½ cup (4.4 oz)	90	0	1
Cream Style Golden No Salt Added	½ cup (4.4 oz)	90	0	1
Cream Style Supersweet Golden	½ cup (4.4 oz)	60	0	1
Cream Style White	½ cup (4.4 oz)	100	0	0
Whole Kernel Golden	½ cup (4.4 oz)	90	0	0
Whole Kernel Golden Supersweet 50% Less Salt	½ cup (4.4 oz)	60	0	1
Whole Kernel Golden Supersweet No Salt Added	½ cup (4.4 oz)	60	0	1
Whole Kernel Golden Supersweet No Sugar	½ cup (4.4 oz)	60	0	0
Whole Kernel Golden Supersweet Vacuum Packed	½ cup (3.7 oz)	70	0	1
Whole Kernel Golden Supersweet Vacuum Packed No Salt Added	½ cup (3.7 oz)	70	0	1
Whole Kernel White Sweet	½ cup (4.4 oz)	80	0	0
Green Giant				
Cream Style	½ cup (4.5 oz)	100	0	1
Mexicorn	⅓ cup (2.7 oz)	60	0	0
Niblets	⅓ cup (2.7 oz)	70	0	0
Niblets 50% Less Sodium	⅓ cup (2.7 oz)	60	0	0
Niblets Extra Sweet	⅓ cup (2.6 oz)	50	0	1
Niblets No Added Sugar or Salt	⅓ cup (2.7 oz)	60	0	0
White Shoepeg	⅓ cup	80	0	0
Whole Sweet	½ cup (4.3 oz)	80	0	1
Whole Sweet 50% Less Sodium	½ cup (4.2 oz)	80	0	1

FOOD	PORTION	CALS.	SAT. FAT	FAT
Owatonna				
Cream Style	½ cup	100	—	1
Whole Kernel In Brine	½ cup	90	—	1
Whole Kernel Vacuum Pack	½ cup	100	—	1
Seneca				
Cream Style	½ cup	80	0	0
Whole Kernel	½ cup	90	0	0
Whole Kernel Natural Pack	½ cup	80	0	1
DRIED				
Goya				
Giant White	⅓ cup (1.6 oz)	160	1	2
FRESH				
on-the-cob w/ butter cooked	1 ear	155	2	3
white cooked	½ cup	89	tr	1
white raw	½ cup	66	tr	1
yellow cooked	1 ear (2.7 oz)	83	tr	1
yellow cooked	½ cup	89	tr	1
yellow raw	1 ear (3 oz)	77	tr	1
yellow raw	½ cup	66	tr	1
FROZEN				
cooked	½ cup	67	tr	tr
on-the-cob cooked	1 ear (2.2 oz)	59	tr	tr
Birds Eye				
Baby Corn Blend	⅔ cup (2.9 oz)	60	0	1
Baby Gold & White	⅔ cup (3.3 oz)	80	tr	1
In Butter Sauce	½ cup (4.6 oz)	110	2	3
Fresh Like				
Cob Corn	1 ear (3 in)	96	—	1
Cob Corn	1 ear (5 in)	96	—	1
Cut	3.5 oz	85	—	1
Green Giant				
Butter Sauce Niblets	⅔ cup (4.3 oz)	130	2	3
Butter Sauce Shoepeg White	¾ cup (4 oz)	120	2	3
Cream Corn	½ cup (4.1 oz)	110	0	1
Extra Sweet Niblets	⅔ cup (3.1 oz)	70	0	1
Harvest Fresh Niblets	⅔ cup (3.4 oz)	80	0	1
Harvest Fresh Shoepeg White	½ cup (2.6 oz)	70	0	1
Niblets	⅔ cup (2.9 oz)	80	0	1
On The Cob Extra Sweet	1 ear (4.4 oz)	120	0	2
On The Cob Nibblers	1 ear (2.1 oz)	70	0	1
On The Cob Niblets	1 ear (5 oz)	160	0	2
Select Extra Sweet White	⅔ cup (2.9 oz)	50	0	1
Select Shoepeg White	¾ cup (3.2 oz)	100	0	1

FOOD	PORTION	CALS.	SAT. FAT	FAT
Hanover				
White Shoepeg	½ cup	80	—	0
White Sweet	½ cup	80	—	0
Yellow Sweet	½ cup	80	—	0
Mrs. Paul's				
Fritters	2	240	—	9
Ore Ida				
Cob Corn	1 ear (6.1 oz)	180	0	3
Cob Corn Mini-Gold	1 ear (3.1 oz)	90	0	1
Stouffer's				
Souffle	½ cup (6 oz)	170	2	7
Tree Of Life				
Corn	⅔ cup (3.2 oz)	80	0	1

CORN CHIPS
(see CHIPS)

CORNISH HENS
(see CHICKEN)

CORNMEAL
(see also POLENTA)

FOOD	PORTION	CALS.	SAT. FAT	FAT
corn grits cooked	1 cup	146	tr	tr
corn grits uncooked	1 cup	579	tr	2
white	1 cup (4.8 oz)	505	tr	2
whole grain	1 cup (4.3 oz)	442	1	4
yellow	1 cup (4.8 oz)	505	tr	2
yellow self-rising	1 cup (4.3 oz)	407	1	4
Albers				
White	3 tbsp	110	0	0
Yellow	3 tbsp	110	0	0
Arrowhead				
Yellow	¼ cup (1.2 oz)	120	0	1
MIX				
Arrowhead				
Corn Bread	¼ cup (1.2 oz)	120	0	1
Hodgson Mill				
Yellow	¼ cup (1 oz)	100	0	1
Yellow Self Rising	¼ cup (1 oz)	90	0	1
Kentucky Kernal				
White Corn Meal Mix	¼ cup (1 oz)	100	0	1
Miracle Maize				
Complete as prep	1 piece (1.5 oz)	193	—	3
Country Style as prep	1 piece 2 in x 2 in (1.8 oz)	230	—	5
Sweet as prep	1 piece 2 in x 2 in (1.8 oz)	236	—	5

FOOD	PORTION	CALS.	SAT. FAT	FAT
Stone-Buhr				
Yellow Corn Meal	¼ cup (1 oz)	100	0	0
TAKE-OUT				
hush puppies	1 (0.75 oz)	74	tr	3
CORNSALAD				
raw	1 cup	12	—	tr
CORNSTARCH				
cornstarch	1 cup (4.5 oz)	488	tr	tr
Armour				
Cream Cornstarch	1 tbsp (0.4 oz)	40	0	0
Hodgson Mill				
Cornstarch	2 tsp (0.4 oz)	35	0	0
COTTAGE CHEESE				
creamed	4 oz	117	3	5
creamed	1 cup (7.4 oz)	217	6	9
creamed w/ fruit	4 oz	140	2	4
dry curd	1 cup (5.1 oz)	123	tr	1
dry curd	4 oz	96	tr	tr
lowfat 1%	1 cup (7.9 oz)	164	1	2
lowfat 1%	4 oz	82	1	1
lowfat 2%	1 cup (7.9 oz)	203	3	4
lowfat 2%	4 oz	101	1	2
Axelrod				
Nonfat	½ cup (4.4 oz)	90	0	0
Breakstone's				
2% Fat Large Curd	½ cup (4.2 oz)	90	2	3
4% Fat Large Curd	½ cup (4.2 oz)	120	3	5
4% Fat Small Curd	½ cup (4.2 oz)	120	3	5
Cottage Doubles Peach	1 pkg (5.5 oz)	140	2	3
Dry Curd	¼ cup (1.9 oz)	45	0	0
Free	½ cup (4.4 oz)	80	0	0
Snack 2% Fat Small Curd	1 pkg (4 oz)	90	2	2
Snack 4% Fat Small Curd	1 pkg (4 oz)	110	3	5
Snack Free	1 pkg (4 oz)	70	0	0
Cabot				
Cottage Cheese	4 oz	120	3	5
Light	4 oz	90	1	1
Friendship				
California Style	½ cup (4 oz)	115	3	5
Lowfat No Salt Added	½ cup (4 oz)	90	1	1
Lowfat Pineapple	½ cup (4 oz)	120	1	1
Lowfat 1%	½ cup (4 oz)	90	1	1
Nonfat	½ cup (4 oz)	80	0	0

FOOD	PORTION	CALS.	SAT. FAT	FAT
Friendship (CONT.)				
Nonfat Plus Peach	½ cup (4 oz)	110	0	0
Pot Style	½ cup (4 oz)	90	2	3
With Pineapple	½ cup (4 oz)	140	3	4
Hood				
1% Fat	½ cup (4 oz)	90	1	2
1% Fat Chive & Onion	½ cup (4 oz)	90	1	2
1% Fat No Salt Added	½ cup (4 oz)	90	1	2
1% Fat Pepper & Herb	½ cup (4 oz)	90	1	2
1% Fat Pineapple Cherry	½ cup (4 oz)	110	1	1
4% Fat	½ cup (4 oz)	120	3	4
4% Fat Chive	½ cup (4 oz)	130	3	4
4% Fat Pineapple	½ cup (4 oz)	130	3	4
Nonfat	½ cup (4 oz)	80	0	0
Nonfat Pineapple	½ cup (4 oz)	110	0	0
Knudsen				
1.5% Fat Small Curd Pineapple	½ cup (4.6 oz)	120	1	2
2% Fat Small Curd	½ cup (4.2 oz)	100	2	3
4% Fat Large Curd	½ cup (4.5 oz)	130	4	5
4% Fat Small Curd	½ cup (4.3 oz)	120	4	5
Free	½ cup (4.2 oz)	80	0	0
On The Go! 1.5% Fat Peach	1 pkg (4 oz)	110	1	2
On The Go! 1.5% Fat Pineapple	1 pkg (4 oz)	110	1	2
On The Go! 1.5% Fat Strawberry	1 pkg (4 oz)	110	1	2
On The Go! 1.5% Fat Tropical Fruit	1 pkg (4 oz)	110	2	2
On The Go! 2% Fat	1 pkg (4 oz)	90	2	2
On The Go! Free	1 pkg (4 oz)	70	0	0
Lactaid				
1%	4 oz	72	1	1
Light N'Lively				
1% Fat	½ cup (4 oz)	80	1	1
1% Fat Garden Salad	½ cup (4.2 oz)	80	1	2
1% Fat Peach & Pineapple	½ cup (4.3 oz)	110	1	1
Fat Free	½ cup (4.4 oz)	80	0	0
Lite Line				
Lowfat 1½%	½ cup	90	—	2
Viva				
Nonfat	½ cup	70	0	0

COTTONSEED

kernels roasted	1 tbsp	51	1	4

FOOD	PORTION	CALS.	SAT. FAT	FAT
COUGH DROPS				
Halls				
Cough Drops	1 (3.8 g)	15	0	0
Plus	1 (4.7 g)	18	0	0
With Vitamin C	1 (3.8 g)	14	0	0
Lifesavers				
Menthol	2 (0.5 oz)	60	0	0
COUSCOUS				
cooked	1 cup (5.5 oz)	176	tr	tr
dry	1 cup (6.1 oz)	650	tr	1
Casbah				
Almond Chicken Vegetarian	1 pkg (1.5 oz)	160	0	2
Asparagus Au Gratin Organic	1 pkg (1.5 oz)	150	0	2
Cheddar Broccoli	1 pkg (1.3 oz)	130	1	2
Hearty Harvest Zestful Organic as prep	1 pkg (10 fl oz)	180	—	1
Moroccan Stew	1 pkg (2 oz)	180	0	1
Pilaf as prep	1 cup	200	0	tr
Tomato Parmesan	1 pkg (1.8 oz)	170	0	2
Kitchen Del Sol				
Aegean Citrus as prep	½ cup (1.1 oz)	110	tr	3
Moroccan Ginger as prep	½ cup (1.1 oz)	120	tr	3
Spicy Vegetable as prep	½ cup (1.1 oz)	120	tr	3
Tomato & Olive	½ cup (1 oz)	120	1	4
Tomato & Olive	½ cup (1.1 oz)	120	1	4
Melting Pot				
Calypso Cranberry	1 cup	200	0	0
Lentil Curry	1 cup	170	0	0
Lucky Seven	1 cup	190	0	1
Mango Salsa	1 cup	190	0	0
Roasted Garlic	1 cup	170	0	0
Sesame Ginger	1 cup	180	0	1
Sun-Dried Tomatoes	1 cup	190	0	1
Wild Mushroom	1 cup	190	0	0
Near East				
As Prep	1¼ cup	260	2	6
COWPEAS				
catjang dried cooked	1 cup	200	tr	1
common canned	1 cup	184	tr	1
frozen cooked	½ cup	112	tr	tr
leafy tips chopped cooked	1 cup	12	tr	tr
leafy tips raw chopped	1 cup	10	tr	tr

FOOD	PORTION	CALS.	SAT. FAT	FAT
CRAB				
CANNED				
blue	1 cup	133	tr	2
blue	3 oz	84	tr	1
FRESH				
alaska king cooked	3 oz	82	tr	1
alaska king cooked	1 leg (4.7 oz)	129	tr	2
alaska king raw	3 oz	71	—	1
alaska king raw	1 leg (6 oz)	144	—	1
blue cooked	3 oz	87	tr	2
blue cooked	1 cup	138	tr	2
blue raw	1 crab (7 oz)	18	tr	tr
blue raw	3 oz	74	tr	1
dungeness raw	1 crab (5.7 oz)	140	tr	2
dungeness raw	3 oz	73	tr	1
queen steamed	3 oz	98	tr	1
FROZEN				
Mrs. Paul's				
Deviled Crab	1 cake	180	—	9
Deviled Crab Miniatures	3½ oz	240	—	12
TAKE-OUT				
baked	1 (3.8 oz)	160	tr	2
cake	1 (2 oz)	160	2	10
mousse	¼ cup	364	—	20
soft-shell fried	1 (4.4 oz)	334	4	18
CRACKER CRUMBS				
cracker meal	1 cup (4 oz)	440	tr	2
graham cracker crumbs	½ cup (4.4 oz)	540	3	13
Baker's Harvest				
Graham	⅓ cup (1 oz)	130	1	4
Honey Maid				
Graham Cracker	0.5 oz	70	0	2
Kellogg's				
Corn Flake Crumbs	2 tbsp (0.4 oz)	40	0	0
Nabisco				
Nilla Cookie Crumbs	2 tbsp (0.5 oz)	70	1	3
Oreo				
Cookie Crumbs	2 tbsp (0.5 oz)	80	1	3
Premium				
Fat Free Cracker Crumbs	¼ cup (1 oz)	100	0	0
Ritz				
Cracker Crumbs	⅓ cup (1 oz)	140	1	7
CRACKERS				
(see also CRACKER CRUMBS)				

FOOD	PORTION	CALS.	SAT. FAT	FAT
cheese	1 (1 in sq) (1 g)	5	tr	tr
cheese	14 (½ oz)	71	1	4
cheese low sodium	14 (½ oz)	71	1	4
cheese low sodium	1 (1 in sq) (1 g)	5	tr	tr
cheese w/ peanut butter filling	1 (0.24 oz)	34	tr	2
crispbread rye	1 (0.35 oz)	37	tr	tr
melba toast plain	1 (5 g)	19	tr	tr
melba toast pumpernickel	1 (5 g)	19	tr	tr
melba toast rye	1 (5 g)	19	tr	tr
melba toast wheat	1 (5 g)	19	tr	tr
milk	1 (0.42 oz)	55	tr	2
oyster cracker	1 (1 g)	4	tr	tr
peanut butter sandwich	1 (7 g)	34	tr	2
rusk toast	1 (0.35 oz)	41	tr	1
rye w/ cheese filling	1 (0.24 oz)	34	tr	2
rye wafers plain	1 (0.9 oz)	84	tr	tr
rye wafers seasoned	1 (0.8 oz)	84	tr	2
saltines	1 (3 g)	13	tr	tr
saltines fat free low sodium	6 (1 oz)	118	tr	tr
saltines fat free low sodium	3 (0.5 oz)	59	tr	tr
saltines low salt	1 (3 g)	13	tr	tr
snack cracker	1 (3 g)	15	tr	1
snack cracker low salt	1 (3 g)	15	tr	1
snack cracker w/ cheese filling	1 (7 g)	33	tr	2
soup cracker	1 (1 g)	4	tr	tr
wheat w/ cheese filling	1 (0.24 oz)	35	tr	2
wheat w/ peanut butter filling	1 (0.24 oz)	35	tr	2
wheat thins	1 (2 g)	9	tr	tr
wheat thins	7 (0.5 oz)	67	1	3
wheat thins low salt	7 (0.5 oz)	67	1	3
whole wheat	1 (4 g)	18	tr	1
whole wheat low salt	1 (4 g)	18	tr	1
Adrienne's				
Gourmet Flatbread Caraway & Rye	2	20	—	tr
Gourmet Flatbread Classic Island	2	20	—	tr
Gourmet Flatbread Slightly Onion	2	20	—	tr
Gourmet Flatbread Ten Grain	2	20	0	tr
Ak-mak				
100% Whole Wheat	5 (1 oz)	116	tr	2
Armenian Cracker Bread	1 sheet (1 oz)	100	1	2

FOOD	PORTION	CALS.	SAT. FAT	FAT
Ak-mak (CONT.)				
Armenian Cracker Bread Whole Wheat	1 sheet (1 oz)	116	tr	2
Round Cracker Bread No Seeds	1 (1 oz)	100	1	1
Round Cracker Bread Seeded	1 (1 oz)	100	1	2
Round Cracker Bread Whole Wheat	1 (1 oz)	116	tr	2
Baker's Harvest				
Cheese	23 (1 oz)	150	2	6
Cheese Reduced Fat	29 (1 oz)	130	1	4
Oyster	35 (0.5 oz)	70	0	2
Saltines Unsalted	5 (0.5 oz)	70	—	2
Saltines Deluxe	5 (0.5 oz)	60	—	2
Snackers	9 (1.1 oz)	160	2	8
Snackers Reduced Fat	10 (1.1 oz)	140	1	4
Snackers Unsalted	9 (1.1 oz)	160	2	8
Wheat Snacks	16 (1 oz)	140	1	6
Wheat Snacks Reduced Fat	16 (1.1 oz)	140	1	4
Woven Wheats	7 (1.1 oz)	140	1	5
Woven Wheats Reduced Fat	8 (1.1 oz)	130	1	3
Barbara's				
Cheese Bites	26 (1 oz)	120	0	2
French Onion	3	60	0	1
Rite Lite Rounds	5 (0.5 oz)	55	0	tr
Roasted Garlic & Herb	3	60	0	1
Sundried Tomato & Basil	3	60	0	1
Toasted Sesame	3	60	0	2
Wheatines All Flavors	1 lg sq (0.5 oz)	50	0	2
Better Cheddars				
Crackers	22 (1 oz)	70	2	8
Low Sodium	22 (1 oz)	150	2	7
Reduced Fat	24 (1 oz)	140	2	6
Burns & Ricker				
Bagel Crisps Garlic	5 (1 oz)	100	0	0
Cheetos				
Bacon Cheddar	1 pkg	190	3	9
Cheddar Cheese	1 pkg	210	3	11
Golden Toast	1 pkg	240	4	14
Cheez It				
Big	13 (1 oz)	150	2	8
Big Reduced Fat	15 (1 oz)	140	1	5
Heads & Tails	37 (1 oz)	140	2	6
Hot & Spicy	26 (1 oz)	150	2	8

FOOD	PORTION	CALS.	SAT. FAT	FAT
Cheez It (CONT.)				
Low Sodium	27 (1 oz)	160	2	8
Nacho	28 (1 oz)	150	2	7
Original	27 (1 oz)	160	2	8
Party Mix	½ cup (1 oz)	140	1	5
Party Mix Nacho	½ cup (1 oz)	130	1	5
Party Mix Reduced Fat	½ cup (1 oz)	130	1	3
Peanut Butter	1 pkg (1.3 oz)	190	2	10
Reduced Fat	29 (1 oz)	140	1	5
Snack Mix	½ cup (1 oz)	130	1	5
Snack Mix Big Crunch	¾ cup (1 oz)	110	1	6
White Cheddar	26 (1 oz)	150	2	7
Crown Pilot				
Crackers	1 (0.5 oz)	70	0	2
Dare				
Breton	1 (5 g)	21	tr	1
Breton 50% Less Salt	1 (5 g)	21	tr	1
Breton Garden Vegetable	1 (5 g)	20	1	1
Breton Light	1 (5 g)	20	tr	1
Breton Sesame	1 (5 g)	22	1	1
Breton Minis	20 (0.6 oz)	89	2	4
Breton Minis Cheddar Cheese	20 (0.6 oz)	87	3	4
Breton Minis Garden Vegetable	20 (0.6 oz)	87	3	4
Cabaret	1 (5 g)	23	tr	1
Vinta	1 (6 g)	30	1	1
Vivant Italian Bruschetta	1 (5 g)	22	1	1
Devonsheer				
Melba Rounds Garlic	½ oz	56	—	1
Melba Rounds Honey Bran	½ oz	52	—	1
Melba Rounds Onion	½ oz	51	—	1
Melba Rounds Plain	½ oz	53	—	1
Melba Rounds Plain Unsalted	½ oz	52	—	1
Melba Rounds Rye	½ oz	53	—	1
Melba Rounds Sesame	½ oz	57	—	2
Doritos				
Jalapeno Cheese	1 pkg	230	4	14
Nacho Cheddar	1 pkg	240	3	14
Eden				
Brown Rice	5 (1 oz)	120	0	2
Escort				
Crackers	3 (0.5 oz)	70	tr	4

FOOD	PORTION	CALS.	SAT. FAT	FAT
Estee				
Sugar Free Cracked Pepper	18	120	0	2
Sugar Free Golden	10	130	0	2
Sugar Free Wheat	17	100	0	2
Frito Lay				
Cheddar Snacks	1 pkg	200	3	10
Frookie				
Cheddar	17 (1 oz)	140	1	4
Cracked Pepper	8 (0.7 oz)	70	0	0
Garden Vegetable	13 (1 oz)	130	0	4
Garlic & Herb	8 (0.7 oz)	70	0	0
Pizza	17 (1 oz)	130	0	3
Snack & Party	10 (1 oz)	140	0	5
Water Crackers	8 (0.7 oz)	70	0	0
Wheat & Onion	12 (1 oz)	120	0	4
Wheat & Rye	13 (1 oz)	120	0	4
Goya				
Butter Crackers	1	40	—	1
Crackers	1	30	—	0
Hain				
Cheese	1 oz	130	—	6
Onion	1 oz	130	—	6
Onion No Salt Added	1 oz	130	—	6
Rich	1 oz	130	—	5
Rich No Salt Added	1 oz	130	—	5
Rye	1 oz	120	—	4
Rye No Salt Added	1 oz	120	—	4
Sesame	1 oz	140	—	7
Sesame No Salt Added	1 oz	140	—	7
Sour Cream & Chive	1 oz	130	—	6
Sour Cream & Chive No Salt Added	1 oz	130	—	6
Sourdough	½ oz	65	—	3
Sourdough Low Salt	1 oz	130	—	5
Vegetable	1 oz	130	—	5
Vegetable No Salt Added	1 oz	130	—	5
Harvest Crisps				
5 Grain	13 (1.1 oz)	130	1	4
Oat	13 (1.1 oz)	140	1	5
Health Valley				
Healthy Pizza Garlic & Herb	6	50	0	0
Healthy Pizza Italiano	6	50	0	0
Healthy Pizza Zesty Cheese	6	50	0	0
Low Fat Mild Jalapeno	6	60	—	2

FOOD	PORTION	CALS.	SAT. FAT	FAT
Health Valley (CONT.)				
Low Fat Mild Ranch	6	60	—	2
Low Fat Roasted Garlic	6	60	—	2
Original Oat Bran	6	120	—	3
Original Rice Bran	6	110	—	3
Whole Wheat	5	50	0	0
Whole Wheat Cheese	5	50	0	0
Whole Wheat Herb	5	50	0	0
Whole Wheat No Salt Vegetable	5	50	0	0
Whole Wheat Onion	5	50	0	0
Whole Wheat Vegetable	5	50	0	0
Healthy Choice				
Bread Crisps Garlic Herb	11 (1 oz)	110	0	2
J.J. Flats				
Breadflats Caraway	1	52	—	1
Breadflats Caraway And Salt	1	51	—	1
Breadflats Cinnamon	1	53	—	1
Breadflats Flavorall	1	52	—	1
Breadflats Garlic	1	52	—	1
Breadflats Oat Bran	1	49	—	1
Breadflats Onion	1	53	—	1
Breadflats Plain	1	53	—	1
Breadflats Poppy	1	53	—	1
Breadflats Sesame	1	55	—	2
Kavli				
Crackers	1 piece	40	—	tr
Keebler				
Club 33% Reduced Fat	5 (0.6 oz)	70	0	2
Club 50% Reduced Sodium	4 (0.5 oz)	70	1	3
Club Orignal	4 (0.5 oz)	70	1	3
Elfin	23 (1 oz)	130	0	2
Export Soda	3 (0.5 oz)	60	0	2
Munch'ems Cheddar	39 (1 oz)	140	1	5
Munch'ems Cheddar	30 (1 oz)	130	1	4
Munch'ems Chili Cheese	28 (1.1 oz)	130	2	4
Munch'ems Mexquite BBQ	40 (1 oz)	140	1	5
Munch'ems Ranch	40 (1 oz)	140	2	5
Munch'ems Ranch	33 (1 oz)	130	1	4
Munch'ems Salsa	28 (1.1 oz)	130	1	4
Munch'ems Seasoned Original	30 (1 oz)	130	1	5
Munch'ems Sour Cream & Onion	39 (1 oz)	140	2	5

FOOD	PORTION	CALS.	SAT. FAT	FAT
Keebler (CONT.)				
Munch'ems Sour Cream & Onion 55% Reduced Fat	33 (1 oz)	130	1	4
Paks Cheese & Peanut Butter	1 pkg	190	2	9
Paks Club & Cheddar	1 pkg	190	3	11
Paks Toast & Peanut Butter	1 pkg	190	2	9
Paks Wheat & Cheddar	1 pkg (1.3 oz)	180	3	10
Toasteds Buttercrisp	5 (0.5 oz)	80	1	4
Toasteds Buttercrisp	9 (1 oz)	140	2	7
Toasteds Medley	9 (1 oz)	140	2	6
Toasteds Onion	9 (1 oz)	140	1	6
Toasteds Sesame	5 (0.5 oz)	80	1	4
Toasteds Sesame	9 (1 oz)	140	1	6
Toasteds Sesame Reduced Fat	10 (1 oz)	120	1	3
Toasteds Wheat	5 (0.5 oz)	80	1	3
Toasteds Wheat	9 (1 oz)	140	2	6
Toasteds Wheat Reduced Fat	5 (0.5 oz)	60	0	2
Toasteds Wheat Reduced Fat	10 (1 oz)	120	1	3
Town House	5 (0.6 oz)	80	1	5
Town House	5 (0.5 oz)	80	1	5
Town House 50% Reduced Sodium	5 (0.6 oz)	80	1	5
Town House 50% Reduced Sodium	5 (0.5 oz)	80	1	5
Town House 50% Reduced Fat	5 (0.5 oz)	70	1	2
Town House Reduced Fat	6 (0.6 oz)	70	1	2
Town House Wheat	5 (0.6 oz)	80	1	4
Wheatables Honey Wheat	12 (1 oz)	140	2	6
Wheatables Original	12 (1 oz)	140	2	6
Wheatables Seven Grain	12 (1 oz)	140	2	6
Zesta Saltine 50% Reduced Sodium	5 (0.5 oz)	60	1	2
Zesta Saltine Fat Free	5 (0.5 oz)	50	0	0
Zesta Saltine Original	5 (0.5 oz)	60	1	2
Zesta Saltine Unsalted Top	5 (0.5 oz)	70	1	2
Zesta Soup & Oyster	42 (0.5 oz)	80	1	3
Lance				
Bonnie	6 (1⅛ oz)	160	3	7

FOOD	PORTION	CALS.	SAT. FAT	FAT
Lance (CONT.)				
Captain Wafers w/ Cream Cheese & Chives	1 pkg (1.3 oz)	190	2	9
Cheese-On-Wheat	1 pkg (1.3 oz)	190	2	10
Cranberry Bar Fat Free	1 (1.75 oz)	160	0	0
Lanchee	1 pkg (1.25 oz)	190	2	11
Malt	1 pkg (1.25 oz)	190	2	10
Nekot	1 pkg (1.5 oz)	210	2	10
Nip-Chee	1 pkg (1.3 oz)	190	2	10
Peanut Butter Wheat	1 pkg (1.3 oz)	190	2	11
Rye-Chee	1 pkg (1.4 oz)	210	3	11
Saltines Slug Pack	4 crackers	50	0	1
Sour Dough w/ Cheddar & Sour Cream	1 pkg (1.6 oz)	240	4	15
Toastchee	1 pkg (1.4 oz)	200	2	12
Toasty	1 pkg (1.25 oz)	190	2	11
Wheat Italian	¾ cup (1.4 oz)	200	2	11
Wheat Pizza	¾ cup (1.4 oz)	200	2	10
Lavash				
Bread Crisp Original	2 (0.5 oz)	60	tr	1
Bread Crisp Sesame	2 (0.5 oz)	60	tr	1
Little Debbie				
Cheese Crackers With Peanut Butter	1 (0.9 oz)	140	2	8
Cheese On Cheese Crackers	1 (0.9 oz)	140	2	8
Cream Cheese & Chive	1 (0.9 oz)	140	2	7
Toasty Crackers With Peanut Butter	1 (0.9 oz)	140	2	7
Wheat Crackers With Cheddar Cheese	1 (0.9 oz)	140	2	8
Nabisco				
Bacon Flavored	15 (1.1 oz)	160	2	8
Chicken In A Biskit	14 (1 oz)	160	2	9
Garden Crisps	15 (1 oz)	130	1	4
Oat Thins	18 (1 oz)	140	1	1
Royal Lunch	1 (0.4 oz)	50	0	2
Swiss	15 (1 oz)	140	2	7
Tid-Bit Cheese	32 (1 oz)	150	2	8
Vegetable Thins	14 (1.1 oz)	160	2	9
Wheat Thins Original	16 (1 oz)	140	1	6
Wheat Thins Reduced Fat	18 (1 oz)	120	1	4
Zings!	1 pkg (1.8 oz)	240	2	11

FOOD	PORTION	CALS.	SAT. FAT	FAT
NABS				
Cheese Peanut Butter Sandwich	6 (1.4 oz)	190	2	10
Peanut Butter Toast Sandwich	6 (1.4 oz)	190	2	10
Nips				
Cheese	29 (1 oz)	150	2	6
No-No				
Flatbreads Tortilla Corn Low Fat Sugar Free Everything	3 (1 oz)	95	0	1
Old London				
Melba Toast Pumpernickel	½ oz	54	—	1
Melba Toast Rye	½ oz	52	—	1
Melba Toast Sesame	½ oz	55	—	2
Melba Toast Sesame Unsalted	½ oz	55	—	2
Melba Toast Wheat	½ oz	51	—	1
Melba Toast White	½ oz	51	—	1
Melba Toast White Unsalted	½ oz	51	—	1
Melba Toast Whole Grain	½ oz	52	—	1
Melba Toast Whole Grain Unsalted	½ oz	53	—	1
Rounds Bacon	½ oz	53	—	1
Rounds Garlic	½ oz	56	—	1
Rounds Onion	½ oz	52	—	1
Rounds Rye	½ oz	52	—	1
Rounds Sesame	½ oz	56	—	2
Rounds White	½ oz	48	—	1
Rounds Whole Grain	½ oz	54	—	1
Oysterettes				
Crackers	19 (0.5 oz)	60	1	3
Partners				
Walla Walla Sweet Onion Perservative Free	0.5 oz	65	2	3
Pepperidge Farm				
Butter Thins	4 (0.5 oz)	70	1	3
English Water Biscuits	4 (0.5 oz)	70	0	2
Goldfish Cheddar	55	140	2	6
Goldfish Cheddar 30% Less Sodium	60 (1.1 oz)	150	2	6
Goldfish Cheese Trio	58	140	2	6
Goldfish Original	55	140	2	6
Goldfish Parmesan Cheese	60	140	2	5
Goldfish Pizza Flavored	55 (1 oz)	140	2	6
Goldfish Pretzel	43 (1 oz)	120	1	3
Goldfish Toasted Wheat	41	150	1	7

FOOD	PORTION	CALS.	SAT. FAT	FAT
Pepperidge Farm (CONT.)				
Hearty Wheat	3 (0.6 oz)	80	0	4
Sesame	3 (0.5 oz)	70	0	3
Snack Mix Fat Free Goldfish	⅔ cup (0.9 oz)	90	0	0
Peter Pan				
Cheese Peanut Butter	1 pkg	210	3	10
Toast Peanut Butter	1 pkg	210	3	11
Planters				
Cheese Peanut Butter Sandwiches	1 pkg (1.4 oz)	190	2	10
Toast Peanut Butter Sandwiches	1 pkg (1.4 oz)	190	2	10
Premium				
Saltine Bits	34 (1 oz)	150	1	7
Saltine Fat Free	5 (0.5 oz)	50	0	0
Saltine Low Sodium	5 (0.5 oz)	60	0	1
Saltine Multigrain	5 (0.5 oz)	60	0	2
Saltine Original	5 (0.5 oz)	60	0	2
Saltine Unsalted Tops	5 (0.5 oz)	60	0	2
Soup & Oyster	23 (0.5 oz)	60	0	2
Ralston				
Cheese	23 (1 oz)	150	2	6
Cheese Reduced Fat	29 (1 oz)	130	1	4
Oyster	35 (0.5 oz)	70	0	2
Rich & Crisp	1 (0.5 oz)	70	1	3
Saltines Fat Free	5 (0.5 oz)	60	0	0
Saltines Deluxe	5 (0.5 oz)	60	—	2
Snackers	9 (1.1 oz)	160	2	8
Snackers Reduced Fat	10 (1.1 oz)	140	1	4
Snackers Unsalted	9 (1.1 oz)	160	2	8
Wheat Snacks	16 (1 oz)	140	1	6
Wheat Snacks Reduced Fat	16 (1.1 oz)	140	1	4
Woven Wheats	7 (1.1 oz)	140	1	5
Woven Wheats Reduced Fat	8 (1.1 oz)	130	1	3
Ritz				
Bits	48 (1 oz)	160	2	9
Bits Sandwiches With Peanut Butter	13 (1 oz)	150	2	8
Bits Sanwiches With Real Cheese	14 (1.1 oz)	160	3	10
Crackers	5 (0.5 oz)	80	1	4
Low Sodium	5 (0.5 oz)	80	1	4

FOOD	PORTION	CALS.	SAT. FAT	FAT
Ritz (CONT.)				
Sandwiches With Real Cheese	1 pkg (1.4 oz)	210	3	12
Savory Thins				
Toasted Onion & Garlic	15 (1 oz)	110	0	1
Sesmark				
Brown Rice	15 (1 oz)	120	0	2
Cheese Thins	15 (1 oz)	130	0	3
Rice Thins Original	15 (1 oz)	130	0	3
Rice Thins Teriyaki Flavored	13 (1 oz)	130	0	3
Savory Thins Original	15 (1 oz)	125	0	2
Sesame Thins Cheddar	9 (1 oz)	150	1	8
Sesame Thins Garlic	9 (1 oz)	150	1	8
Sesame Thins Original	9 (1 oz)	150	1	8
Sesame Thins Unsalted	11 (1 oz)	150	1	8
SnackWell's				
Cracked Pepper	7 (0.5 oz)	60	0	0
Fat Free Wheat	5 (0.5 oz)	60	0	0
Reduced Fat Cheese	38 (1 oz)	130	1	2
Reduced Fat Classic Golden	6 (0.5 oz)	60	0	1
Salsa Cheddar	32 (1 oz)	120	0	2
Snorkles				
Cheddar	56 (1 oz)	140	2	5
Sociables				
Crackers	7 (0.5 oz)	80	1	4
Sunshine				
Hi Ho	4 (0.5 oz)	70	1	4
Hi Ho Reduced Fat	5 (0.5 oz)	70	1	3
Krispy	5 (0.5 oz)	60	0	2
Krispy Fat Free	5 (0.5 oz)	50	0	0
Krispy Mild Cheddar	5 (0.5 oz)	60	1	2
Krispy Soup & Oyster	17 (0.5 oz)	60	0	2
Krispy Unsalted Tops	5 (0.5 oz)	60	0	2
Krispy Whole Wheat	5 (0.5 oz)	60	0	2
Tree Of Life				
Bite Size Fat Free Corn & Salsa	12	60	0	0
Bite Size Fat Free Cracked Pepper	12	55	0	0
Bite Size Fat Free Garden Vegetable	12	55	0	0
Bite Size Fat Free Garlic & Herb	12	55	0	0

FOOD	PORTION	CALS.	SAT. FAT	FAT
Tree Of Life (CONT.)				
Bite Size Fat Free Soya Nut	12	60	0	0
Bite Size Fat Free Toasted Onion	12	60	0	0
Bite Size Fat Free Whole Wheat	12	60	0	0
Fat Free Oyster	40 (0.5 oz)	60	0	0
Saltine Cracked Pepper Fat Free	4 (0.5 oz)	60	0	0
Saltine Fat Free	4 (0.5 oz)	50	0	0
Triscuit				
Crackers	7 (1.1 oz)	140	1	5
Deli-Style Rye	7 (1.1 oz)	140	1	5
Garden Herb	6 (1 oz)	130	1	5
Low Sodium	7 (1.1 oz)	150	1	6
Reduced Fat	8 (1.1 oz)	130	1	3
Wheat 'n Bran	7 (1.1 oz)	140	1	5
Tuscany				
Pita Crisps	1 oz	90	—	1
Pita Crisps Sesame	1 oz	96	—	2
Toast	1 oz	95	—	2
Toast Pepato	1 oz	93	—	2
Toast Pesto	1 oz	96	—	2
Toast Tomato	1 oz	95	—	2
Twigs				
Sesame & Cheese Sticks	15 (1 oz)	150	2	7
Uneeda Biscuit				
Unsalted Tops	2 (0.5 oz)	60	0	2
Venus				
Fat Free Cracked Pepper	11 (0.5 oz)	60	0	0
Fat Free Garden Vegetable	5 (0.5 oz)	60	0	0
Fat Free Garlic & Herb	11 (0.5 oz)	60	0	0
Fat Free Multi-Grain	5 (0.5 oz)	60	0	0
Fat Free Spicy Chili	10 (0.5 oz)	60	0	0
Fat Free Toasted Onion	5 (0.5 oz)	60	0	0
Fat Free Toasted Wheat	5 (0.5 oz)	60	0	0
Fat Free Tomato & Basil	10 (0.5 oz)	60	0	0
Fat Free Zesty Italian	10 (0.5 oz)	60	0	0
Garden Vegetable	6 (1 oz)	150	2	8
Honey Wheat	1 oz	140	0	5
Low Fat Cracker Bread	5 (0.5 oz)	60	0	2
Low Fat Water Crackers	4 (0.5 oz)	60	0	1
Sesame & Flaxseed	1 oz	130	0	3
Soup Original	0.5 oz	60	0	2
Toasted Wheat	6 (1 oz)	150	2	7

FOOD	PORTION	CALS.	SAT. FAT	FAT
Venus (CONT.)				
Wine Cheese Caviar Original	0.5 oz	60	0	2
Wine Cheese Caviar Pepper & Poppy	0.5 oz	60	0	2
Wasa				
Crisp	3 (0.5 oz)	50	—	0
Crisp'N Light Sourdough Rye	3 (0.6 oz)	60	0	0
Crisp'N Light Wheat	2 (0.5 oz)	50	0	0
Crispbread Cinnamon Toast	1 (0.6 oz)	60	0	1
Crispbread Fiber Rye	1 (0.4 oz)	30	0	1
Crispbread Gluten & Wheat Free Corn	1 (0.4 oz)	40	0	1
Crispbread Hearty Rye	1 (0.5 oz)	45	0	0
Crispbread Light Rye	1 (0.3 oz)	25	0	0
Crispbread Multi Grain	1 (0.5 oz)	45	0	0
Crispbread Organic Rye	1 (0.3 oz)	25	0	0
Crispbread Sodium Free Rye	1 (0.3 oz)	30	0	0
Crispbread Sourdough Rye	1 (0.4 oz)	35	0	0
Crispbread Toasted Wheat	1 (0.5 oz)	50	0	2
Crispbread Whole Wheat	1 (0.5 oz)	50	0	1
Waverly				
Crackers	5 (0.5 oz)	70	1	4
Wheat Thins				
Low Salt	16 (1 oz)	140	1	6
Multi-Grain	17 (1 oz)	130	1	4
Wheatworth				
Stone Ground	5 (0.5 oz)	80	1	4
Wortz				
Cheese	23 (1 oz)	150	2	6
Oyster	35 (0.5 oz)	70	0	2
Rich & Crisp	1 (0.5 oz)	70	1	3
Saltines Fat Free	5 (0.5 oz)	60	0	0
Saltines Deluxe	5 (0.5 oz)	60	—	2
Wheat Snacks	16 (1 oz)	140	1	6
Wheat Snacks Reduced Fat	16 (1.1 oz)	140	1	4
Woven Wheats	7 (1.1 oz)	140	1	5
Zwieback				
Crackers	1 (8 g)	35	1	1
CRANBERRIES				
CANNED				
cranberry sauce sweetened	½ cup	209	—	tr

FOOD	PORTION	CALS.	SAT. FAT	FAT
Ocean Spray				
Cran*Fruit Cranberry Orange	¼ cup	120	0	0
Cranberry Sauce Jellied	¼ cup	110	0	0
Whole Berry Sauce	¼ cup	110	0	0
DRIED				
Craisins	⅓ cup (1.4 oz)	130	0	0
FRESH				
chopped	1 cup	54	—	tr
Ocean Spray				
Fresh	2 oz	25	—	0

CRANBERRY BEANS

canned	1 cup	216	tr	1
dried cooked	1 cup	240	tr	1
Bean Cuisine				
Dried	½ cup	115	—	1

CRANBERRY JUICE

cocktail	1 cup	147	—	tr
cranberry juice cocktail	6 oz	108	—	tr
cranberry juice cocktail low calorie	6 oz	33	0	0
cranberry juice cocktail frzn	12 oz can	821	0	0
cranberry juice cocktail frzn as prep	6 oz	102	0	0
After The Fall				
Cape Cod Cranberry	1 bottle (10 oz)	130	0	0
Cranberry Ginger Ale	1 can (12 oz)	140	0	0
Apple & Eve				
Juice	6 fl oz	100	0	0
Crystal Light				
Cranberry Breeze Drink	1 serv (8 oz)	5	0	0
Cranberry Breeze Drink Mix as prep	1 serv (8 oz)	5	0	0
Everfresh				
Cranberry Cocktail	1 can (8 oz)	140	0	0
Nantucket Nectars				
Cocktail	8 oz	140	0	0
Ocean Spray				
Cocktail	8 oz	140	0	0
Cocktail Reduced Calorie	8 oz	50	0	0
Lightstyle Cranberry Juice Cocktail	8 oz	40	0	0
Seneca				
Cocktail frzn as prep	8 fl oz	140	0	0

FOOD	PORTION	CALS.	SAT. FAT	FAT
Snapple				
Cranberry Royal	10 fl oz	150	0	0
Tree Of Life				
Concentrate	8 tsp (1.4 oz)	110	0	0
Tropicana				
Twister Ruby Red	1 bottle (10 oz)	160	0	0
Veryfine				
Cocktail	1 bottle (10 oz)	180	0	0
Wellfleet Farms				
Cranberry	8 oz	130	0	0

CRAYFISH

(see also LOBSTER)

cooked	3 oz	97	tr	1
raw	3 oz	76	tr	1
raw	8	24	tr	tr

CREAM

(see also SOUR CREAM, SOUR CREAM SUBSTITUTES, WHIPPED TOPPINGS)

LIQUID

half & half	1 tbsp (0.5 oz)	20	1	2
half & half	1 cup (8.5 oz)	315	17	28
heavy whipping	1 tbsp (0.5 oz)	52	3	6
light coffee	1 cup (8.4 oz)	496	29	46
light coffee	1 tbsp (0.5 oz)	29	2	3
light whipping	1 tbsp (0.5 oz)	44	3	5
Farmland				
Half & Half	2 tbsp	40	2	3
Light Cream	2 tbsp	30	2	3
Hood				
Half & Half	2 tbsp (1 oz)	40	2	4
Heavy	1 tbsp (0.5 oz)	50	4	5
Light	1 tbsp (0.5 oz)	30	2	3
Whipping Cream	1 tbsp (0.5 oz)	45	3	5
Organic Valley				
Half & Half	2 tbsp (1 oz)	40	2	3
Parmalat				
Half & Half	2 tbsp (1 oz)	40	2	3

WHIPPED

heavy whipping	1 cup (4.1 oz)	411	27	44
light whipping	1 cup (4.2 oz)	345	23	37

CREAM CHEESE

cream cheese	1 oz	99	6	10
cream cheese	1 pkg (3 oz)	297	19	30

FOOD	PORTION	CALS.	SAT. FAT	FAT
Alpine Lace				
Fat Free Garden Vegetable	2 tbsp (1 oz)	30	tr	tr
Fat Free Garlic & Herbs	2 tbsp (1 oz)	30	tr	tr
Boar's Head				
Cream Cheese	2 tbsp (1 oz)	100	7	10
Breakstone's				
Temp-Tee Whipped	2 tbsp (0.8 oz)	80	5	8
Fleur De Lait				
Bermuda Onion & Chives	2 tbsp (0.9 oz)	90	5	8
Cinnamon Raisin	2 tbsp (0.9 oz)	90	5	8
Date Nut Rum	2 tbsp (0.9 oz)	90	5	8
Fresh Cut Garden Vegetable	2 tbsp (0.9 oz)	80	5	8
Garden Vegetable	2 tbsp (0.9 oz)	80	5	8
Garlic & Spice	2 tbsp (0.9 oz)	90	6	9
Herb & Spice	2 tbsp (0.9 oz)	90	6	9
Irish Creme	2 tbsp (0.9 oz)	100	5	9
Lemon	2 tbsp (0.9 oz)	90	4	7
Lox	2 tbsp (0.9 oz)	90	5	8
Mandarin Orange	2 tbsp (0.9 oz)	90	5	7
Peach	2 tbsp (0.9 oz)	90	5	7
Pineapple	2 tbsp (0.9 oz)	90	5	8
Plain	2 tbsp (1 oz)	100	6	10
Strawberry	2 tbsp (0.9 oz)	90	5	8
Toasted Onion	2 tbsp (0.9 oz)	90	6	9
Wildberry	2 tbsp (0.9 oz)	90	5	7
Fresh Cut				
Bac'n & Horseradish	2 tbsp (0.9 oz)	90	5	9
Bermuda Onion & Chives	2 tbsp (0.9 oz)	90	5	8
Date Nut & Rum	2 tbsp (0.9 oz)	90	5	8
Garlic & Spice	2 tbsp (0.9 oz)	90	6	9
Herb & Spice	2 tbsp (0.9 oz)	90	6	9
Lox	2 tbsp (0.9 oz)	90	5	8
Peaches & Cream	2 tbsp (0.9 oz)	90	5	7
Strawberry	2 tbsp (0.9 oz)	90	5	8
Friendship				
NY Style Reduced Fat	2 tbsp (1 oz)	50	2	3
Galaxy				
Slices	1 slice (1 oz)	50	2	3
Healthy Choice				
Herbs & Garlic	2 tbsp (1 oz)	25	0	0
Plain	2 tbsp (1 oz)	25	0	0
Strawberry	2 tbsp (1 oz)	30	0	0

FOOD	PORTION	CALS.	SAT. FAT	FAT
Heluva Good Cheese				
Cream Cheese	1 tbsp (1 oz)	100	6	10
Organic Valley				
Cream Cheese	1 oz	100	6	9
Philadelphia				
Free	1 oz	30	0	0
Regular	1 oz	100	6	10
Soft	2 tbsp (1 oz)	100	7	10
Soft Apple Cinnamon	2 tbsp (1.1 oz)	100	5	8
Soft Cheesecake	2 tbsp (1 oz)	110	6	9
Soft Chives & Onions	2 tbsp (1.1 oz)	110	7	10
Soft Garden Vegetable	2 tbsp (1.1 oz)	110	7	11
Soft Honey Nut	2 tbsp (1.1 oz)	110	6	10
Soft Pineapple	2 tbsp (1.1 oz)	100	6	9
Soft Salmon	3 tbsp (1.1 oz)	100	6	9
Soft Strawberry	2 tbsp (1.1 oz)	100	6	9
Soft Free	2 tbsp (1.2 oz)	30	0	0
Soft Free Garden Vegetable	2 tbsp (1.2 oz)	30	0	0
Soft Free Strawberries	2 tbsp (1.2 oz)	45	0	0
Soft Light	2 tbsp (1.1 oz)	70	4	5
Soft Light Jalapeno	2 tbsp (1.1 oz)	60	3	5
Soft Light Raspberry	2 tbsp (1.1 oz)	70	3	5
Soft Light Roasted Garlic	2 tbsp (1.1 oz)	70	3	5
Whipped	2 tbsp (0.7 oz)	70	5	7
Whipped Chives	2 tbsp (0.7 oz)	70	4	6
Whipped Smoked Salmon	2 tbsp (0.7 oz)	70	4	6
With Chives	1 oz	90	6	9
Ultra Delight				
Cheddar Cream Cheese	2 tbsp (0.9 oz)	60	3	4
Chive	2 tbsp (0.9 oz)	60	3	4
Garlic	2 tbsp (0.9 oz)	60	3	4
Mixed Berry	2 tbsp (0.9 oz)	70	3	4
Nacho	2 tbsp (0.9 oz)	60	3	4
Salsa	2 tbsp (0.9 oz)	60	3	4
Shrimp	2 tbsp (0.9 oz)	60	3	4
Strawberry	2 tbsp (0.9 oz)	60	3	4
Vegetable	2 tbsp (0.9 oz)	50	3	4

CREAM CHEESE SUBSTITUTES

FOOD	PORTION	CALS.	SAT. FAT	FAT
Tofutti				
Better Than Cream Cheese French Onion	1 oz	80	2	8
Better Than Cream Cheese Herb & Chive	1 oz	80	2	8

FOOD	PORTION	CALS.	SAT. FAT	FAT
Tofutti (CONT.)				
Better Than Cream Cheese Plain	1 oz	80	2	8
CREAM OF TARTAR				
cream of tartar	1 tsp	8	0	0
CREPES				
basic crepe unfilled	1	75	—	2
Frieda's				
Ready-To-Use	2 (0.8 oz)	50	0	1
CRESS				
(*see also* WATERCRESS)				
garden cooked	½ cup	16	tr	tr
garden raw	½ cup	8	tr	tr
CROAKER				
atlantic breaded & fried	3 oz	188	3	11
atlantic raw	3 oz	89	1	3
CROISSANT				
apple	1 (2 oz)	145	3	5
cheese	1 (2 oz)	236	5	12
plain	1 (2 oz)	232	7	12
plain	1 mini (1 oz)	115	3	6
Rudy's Farm				
Ham & Swiss Sandwich	1 (3.4 oz)	310	5	18
TAKE-OUT				
w/ egg & cheese	1 (4.5 oz)	368	14	25
w/ egg cheese & bacon	1 (4.5 oz)	413	15	28
w/ egg cheese & ham	1 (5.3 oz)	474	17	34
w/ egg cheese & sausage	1 (5.6 oz)	523	18	38
CROUTONS				
plain	1 cup (1 oz)	122	tr	2
seasoned	1 cup (1.4 oz)	186	2	7
Arnold				
Crispy Cheddar Romano	½ oz	64	—	3
Crispy Cheese Garlic	½ oz	60	tr	2
Crispy Fine Herbs	½ oz	50	0	1
Crispy Italian	½ oz	60	tr	3
Crispy Onion & Garlic	½	60	tr	2
Crispy Seasoned	½ oz	60	tr	3
Pepperidge Farm				
Garlic	6 (0.2 oz)	30	0	1
Homestyle	6 (0.2 oz)	30	0	1
Sourdough	6 (0.2 oz)	35	1	2

FOOD	PORTION	CALS.	SAT. FAT	FAT
Up Country Naturals				
Organic Whole Wheat Garlic & Herb	¼ cup (0.3 oz)	35	0	2
CUCUMBER				
FRESH				
raw	1 (11 oz)	38	tr	tr
raw sliced	½ cup (1.8 oz)	7	tr	tr
JARRED				
Rosoff's				
Salad	3 slices (1 oz)	12	0	0
Schorr's				
Cucumber Garden Salad	3 slices (1 oz)	12	0	0
TAKE-OUT				
cucumber salad	3.5 oz	50	tr	tr
kirnchee	½ cup (1.8 oz)	36	tr	2
tzatziki	½ cup (3.4 oz)	72	1	6
CUMIN				
seed	1 tsp	8	—	tr
CURRANTS				
black fresh	½ cup	36	tr	tr
zante dried	½ cup	204	tr	tr
CUSK				
fillet baked	3 oz	106	—	1
CUSTARD				
HOME RECIPE				
baked	1 recipe 4 serv (19.8 oz)	549	13	26
flan	1 recipe 10 serv (53.7 oz)	2206	30	63
MIX				
as prep w/ 2% milk	½ cup (4.7 oz)	148	2	4
as prep w/ 2% milk	1 recipe 4 serv (18.7 oz)	595	8	15
as prep w/ whole milk	½ cup (4.7 oz)	163	3	5
as prep w/ whole milk	1 recipe 4 serv (18.7 oz)	652	12	22
flan as prep w/ 2% milk	½ cup (4.7 oz)	135	1	2
flan as prep w/ 2% milk	1 recipe 4 serv (18.7 oz)	542	6	9
flan as prep w/ whole milk	½ cup (4.7 oz)	150	3	4
flan as prep w/ whole milk	1 recipe 4 serv (18.7 oz)	600	10	16

FOOD	PORTION	CALS.	SAT. FAT	FAT
Jell-O				
Americana Custard Dessert as prep w/ 2% milk	½ cup (5 oz)	140	2	3
Flan as prep w/ 2% milk	½ cup (5.1 oz)	140	2	3
Royal				
Custard	mix for 1 serv	60	—	0
Flan Caramel Custard	mix for 1 serv	60	—	0
READY-TO-EAT				
Kozy Shack				
Flan	1 pkg (4 oz)	150	2	4
TAKE-OUT				
baked	½ cup (5 oz)	148	3	7
flan	½ cup (5.4 oz)	220	3	6
zabaione	½ cup (57.2 g)	135	2	5

CUTTLEFISH

FOOD	PORTION	CALS.	SAT. FAT	FAT
steamed	3 oz	134	tr	1

DANDELION GREENS

FOOD	PORTION	CALS.	SAT. FAT	FAT
fresh cooked	½ cup	17	—	tr
raw chopped	½ cup	13	—	tr

DANISH PASTRY
FROZEN

FOOD	PORTION	CALS.	SAT. FAT	FAT
Morton				
Honey Buns	1 (2.28 oz)	250	3	10
Honey Buns Mini	1 (1.23 oz)	160	2	8
READY-TO-EAT				
plain ring	1 (12 oz)	1305	22	71
Dolly Madison				
Danish Rollers	3 (2.8 oz)	290	2	10
Tastykake				
Cheese	1 (3 oz)	290	3	14
Lemon	1 (3 oz)	290	3	14
Raspberry	1 (3 oz)	290	3	14
TAKE-OUT				
almond	1 (4¼ in) (2.3 oz)	280	4	16
apple	1 (4¼ in) (2.5 oz)	264	3	13
cheese	1 (3.2 oz)	353	5	25
cheese	1 (4¼ in) (2.5 oz)	266	5	16
cinnamon	1 (3.1 oz)	349	3	17
cinnamon	1 (4¼ in) (2.3 oz)	262	4	15
cinnimon nut	1 (4¼ in) (2.3 oz)	280	4	16
fruit	1 (3.3 oz)	335	3	16
lemon	1 (4¼ in) (2.5 oz)	264	3	13
raisin	1 (4¼ in) (2.5 oz)	264	3	13

FOOD	PORTION	CALS.	SAT. FAT	FAT
raisin nut	1 (4¼ in) (2.3 oz)	280	4	16
raspberry	1 (4¼ in) (2.5 oz)	264	3	13
strawberry	1 (4¼ in) (2.5 oz)	264	3	13
DATES				
DRIED				
chopped	1 cup	489	—	1
deglet noor	10	240	—	0
whole	10	228	—	tr
Bordo				
Diced	2 oz	203	—	1
Dole				
Chopped	½ cup	230	0	0
Pitted	½ cup	280	0	0
Dromedary				
Chopped	¼ cup	130	0	0
Pitted	5	100	0	0
Sonoma				
Dried	5-6 (1.4 oz)	110	0	0
DEER				
(*see* VENISON)				
DELI MEATS/COLD CUTS				
(*see also* CHICKEN, HAM, MEAT SUBSTITUTES, TURKEY)				
barbecue loaf pork & beef	1 oz	49	1	3
beerwurst beef	1 slice (2¾ in x ⅟₁₆ in)	20	1	2
beerwurst beef	1 slice (4 in x ⅛ in)	75	3	7
beerwurst pork	1 slice (4 in x ⅛ in)	55	1	4
beerwurst pork	1 slice (2¾ in x ⅟₁₆ in)	14	tr	1
berliner pork & beef	1 oz	65	2	4
blood sausage	1 oz	95	3	9
bologna beef	1 oz	88	3	8
bologna beef & pork	1 oz	89	3	8
bologna pork	1 oz	70	2	6
braunschweiger pork	1 oz	102	3	9
braunschweiger pork	1 slice (2½ in x ¼ in)	65	2	6
corned beef loaf	1 oz	43	1	2
dried beef	5 slices (21 g)	35	—	tr
dried beef	1 oz	47	—	1
dutch brand loaf pork & beef	1 oz	68	2	5
headcheese pork	1 oz	60	1	5
honey loaf pork & beef	1 oz	36	tr	1
honey roll sausage beef	1 oz	42	1	2
lebanon bologna beef	1 oz	60	2	4
liver cheese pork	1 oz	86	3	7

FOOD	PORTION	CALS.	SAT. FAT	FAT
liverwurst pork	1 oz	92	3	8
luncheon meat beef	1 oz	87	3	7
luncheon meat pork & beef	1 oz	100	3	9
luncheon sausage pork & beef	1 oz	74	2	6
mortadella beef & pork	1 oz	88	3	7
mother's loaf pork	1 oz	80	2	6
new england sausage pork & beef	1 oz	46	1	2
olive loaf pork	1 oz	67	2	5
peppered loaf pork & beef	1 oz	42	1	2
pepperoni pork & beef	1 slice (0.2 oz)	27	1	2
pepperoni pork & beef	1 (9 oz)	1248	40	110
picnic loaf pork & beef	1 oz	66	2	5
salami cooked beef & pork	1 oz	71	2	6
salami hard pork	1 slice (⅓ oz)	41	1	4
salami hard pork	1 pkg (4 oz)	460	13	38
salami hard pork & beef	1 pkg (4 oz)	472	14	39
salami hard pork & beef	1 slice (⅓ oz)	42	1	3
sandwich spread pork & beef	1 tbsp	35	1	3
sandwich spread pork & beef	1 oz	67	2	5
summer sausage thuringer cervelat	1 oz	98	3	8
Boar's Head				
Bologna Beef	2 oz	150	4	13
Bologna Garlic	2 oz	150	5	13
Bologna Lowered Sodium	2 oz	150	5	13
Bologna Pork & Beef	2 oz	150	5	13
Braunschweiger Lite	2 oz	120	4	8
Head Cheese	2 oz	90	3	5
Liverwurst Strassburger	2 oz	170	6	15
Olive Loaf	2 oz	130	5	12
Pastrami	2 oz	90	2	4
Prosciutto	1 oz	60	1	3
Red Pastrami	2 oz	90	2	4
Salami Beef	2 oz	120	4	9
Salami Cooked	2 oz	130	5	11
Salami Genoa	2 oz	180	5	14
Salami Hard	1 oz	110	4	9
Spiced Ham	2 oz	120	5	10
Carl Buddig				
Beef	1 pkg (2.5 oz)	100	2	5
Corned Beef	1 pkg (2.5 oz)	100	2	5
Pastrami	1 pkg (2.5 oz)	100	2	5
Hansel n'Gretel				
Healthy Deli Bologna Beef & Pork	1 oz	41	—	2

FOOD	PORTION	CALS.	SAT. FAT	FAT
Hansel n'Gretel (CONT.)				
Healthy Deli Cooked Corn Beef	1 oz	35	—	1
Healthy Deli Italian Roast Beef	1 oz	31	—	1
Healthy Deli Pastrami Round	1 oz	34	—	1
Healthy Deli Regular Roast Beef	1 oz	30	—	tr
Healthy Deli St Paddy's Corned Beef	1 oz	24	—	tr
Healthy Choice				
Bologna	1 slice (1 oz)	30	0	1
Bologna Beef	1 slice (1 oz)	35	0	1
Deli-Thin Bologna	4 slices (1.8 oz)	60	1	2
Well-Pack Bologna	1 slice (1 oz)	30	0	1
Hebrew National				
Bologna Beef	2 oz	180	—	16
Bologna Beef Reduced Fat	2 oz	130	—	12
Bologna Lean Chub	2 oz	90	—	6
Bologna Midget	2 oz	180	—	16
Deli Pastrami	2 oz	80	—	3
Deli Express Corned Beef	2 oz	80	—	3
Deli Express Tongue Sliced	2 oz	120	—	9
Salami Beef	2 oz	170	—	14
Salami Beef Reduced Fat	2 oz	110	—	8
Salami Sean Chub	2 oz	90	—	6
Salami Midget	2 oz	170	—	14
Hillshire				
Bologna Large	1 oz	90	—	8
Bologna Ring	1 oz	90	—	8
Brunschweiger	1 oz	95	—	8
Deli Select Corned Beef	1 slice	10	—	tr
Deli Select Light Bologna	1 slice	12	—	1
Deli Select Oven Roasted Cured Beef	1 slice	10	—	tr
Deli Select Pastrami	1 slice	10	—	tr
Deli Select Roast Beef	1 slice	10	—	tr
Deli Select Smoked Beef	1 slice	10	—	tr
Flavor Pack 90-99% Fat Free Light Bologna	1 slice (0.73 oz)	30	—	2
Flavor Pack 90-99% Fat Free Pastrami	1 slice (0.6 oz)	18	—	tr

FOOD	PORTION	CALS.	SAT. FAT	FAT
Hillshire (CONT.)				
Lunch 'N Munch Bologna/ American/Snickers	1 pkg (4.25 oz)	490	—	34
Lunch 'N Munch Bologna/ American/Snickers/Hi-C	1 pkg (4.25 oz + 6 fl oz)	590	—	34
Lunch 'N Munch Bologna/American	1 pkg (4.5 oz)	480	—	37
Lunch 'N Munch Cotto Salami/ Monterey Jack	1 pkg (4.5 oz)	440	—	32
Lunch 'N Munch Pepperoni/ American	1 pkg (4.5 oz)	570	—	46
Pepperoni	1 oz	110	—	10
Salami Hard	1 oz	100	—	9
Salami Hard	1 oz	90	—	7
Summer Sausage	2 oz	180	—	16
Summer Sausage Beef	2 oz	190	—	17
Summer Sausage Light	2 oz	150	—	12
Summer Sausage w/Cheddar Cheese	2 oz	200	—	18
Hormel				
Liverwurst Spread	4 tbsp (2 oz)	130	4	10
Pepperoni Chunk	1 oz	140	6	13
Pepperoni Sliced	15 slices (1 oz)	140	6	13
Pepperoni Twin	1 oz	140	5	13
Pillow Pack Genoa Salami	2 oz	160	7	18
Pillow Pack Pepperoni	16 slices (1 oz)	140	6	13
Jordan's				
Healthy Trim 95% Fat Free Macaroni & Cheese Loaf	2 slices (1.6 oz)	50	1	2
Healthy Trim 95% Fat Free Olive Loaf	2 slices (1.6 oz)	50	1	2
Healthy Trim 95% Fat Free Pickle & Pepper Loaf	2 slices (1.6 oz)	50	1	2
Healthy Trim 97% Fat Free Corned Beef	2 slices (1.6 oz)	45	1	2
Healthy Trim Low Fat Cooked Salami	3 slices (2 oz)	70	1	3
Healthy Trim Low Fat German Brand Bologna	3 slices (2 oz)	70	1	3
Oscar Mayer				
Bologna	1 slice (1 oz)	90	3	8
Bologna Beef	1 slice (1 oz)	90	4	8
Bologna Garlic	1 slice (1.4 oz)	110	5	12

FOOD	PORTION	CALS.	SAT. FAT	FAT
Oscar Mayer (CONT.)				
Bologna Wisconsin Made Ring	2 oz	180	6	16
Braunschweiger Spread	2 oz	190	6	17
Brunschweiger	1 slice (1 oz)	100	3	9
Free Bologna	1 slice (1 oz)	20	0	0
Head Cheese	1 slice (1 oz)	50	2	4
Light Bologna	1 slice (1 oz)	60	2	4
Light Bologna Beef	1 slice (1 oz)	60	2	4
Liver Cheese	1 slice (1.3 oz)	120	4	10
Lunchables Bologna/American	1 pkg (4.5 oz)	450	15	34
Lunchables Deluxe Turkey/Ham	1 pkg (5.1 oz)	360	10	19
Lunchables Dessert Jello/ Honey Turkey/Cheddar	1 pkg (5.7 oz)	320	9	16
Lunchables Fun Pack Bologna/Wild Cherry	1 pkg (11.2 oz)	530	14	29
Lunchables Fun Pack Ham/Fruit Punch	1 pkg (11.2 oz)	450	10	20
Lunchables Ham/Swiss	1 pkg (4.5 oz)	320	8	17
Lunchables Pepperoni/ American	1 pkg (4.5 oz)	480	17	36
Lunchables Salami/American	1 pkg (4.5 oz)	430	15	32
Luncheon Loaf Spiced	1 slice (1 oz)	70	2	5
New England Brand Sausage	2 slices (1.6 oz)	60	1	3
Old Fashioned Loaf	1 slice (1 oz)	70	2	5
Olive Loaf	1 slice (1 oz)	70	2	6
Pepperoni	15 slices (1 oz)	140	5	13
Pickle And Pimiento Loaf	1 slice (1 oz)	80	2	6
Salami Cotto	1 slice (1 oz)	70	2	5
Salami Cotto Beef	1 slice (1 oz)	60	2	5
Salami For Beer	1 slices (1.6 oz)	110	3	9
Salami Genoa	3 slices (1 oz)	100	3	9
Salami Hard	3 slices (1 oz)	100	3	9
Salami Machaich Brand Beef	2 slices (1.6 oz)	120	5	10
Sandwich Spread	2 oz	130	4	10
Summer Sausage	2 slices (1.6 oz)	140	5	13
Summer Sausage Beef	2 slices (1.6 oz)	140	5	12
Russer				
Bologna	2 oz	180	7	15
Bologna Jalapeno Pepper	2 oz	170	6	14

FOOD	PORTION	CALS.	SAT. FAT	FAT
Russer (CONT.)				
Bologna Wunderbar German Brand	2 oz	190	6	16
Bologna Beef	2 oz	180	7	15
Bologna Garlic	2 oz	180	6	16
Bologna Italian Brand Sweet Red Pepper	2 oz	180	6	15
Braunschweiger	2 oz	170	6	14
Cooked Salami	2 oz	120	3	8
Dutch Brand	2 oz	130	3	8
Hot Cooked Salami	2 oz	110	3	7
Italian Brand Loaf	2 oz	130	3	8
Jalapeno Loaf With Monterey Jack Cheese	2 oz	160	5	13
Kielbasa Loaf	2 oz	120	3	8
Light Bologna	2 oz	120	4	8
Light Bologna Beef	2 oz	120	4	8
Light Braunschweiger	2 oz	120	3	8
Light Old Fashioned Loaf	2 oz	90	3	4
Light P&P Loaf	2 oz	100	3	6
Light Salami Cooked	2 oz	90	3	5
Olive Loaf	2 oz	160	5	13
P&P Loaf	2 oz	160	5	13
Pepper Loaf	2 oz	90	2	3
Polish Loaf	2 oz	140	4	10
Sara Lee				
Pastrami Beef	2 oz	100	3	6
Peppered Beef	2 oz	70	1	2
Shofar				
Salami Beef	2 oz	160	6	15
Spam				
Less Salt	2 oz	170	6	16
Lite	2 oz	110	3	8
Original	2 oz	170	6	16
Smoked	2 oz	170	6	16
Underwood				
Liverwurst	2.08 oz	180	—	15
TAKE-OUT				
corned beef	2 oz	70	1	2
corned beef brisket	2 oz	90	2	5

DIETING AIDS
(see NUTRITION SUPPLEMENTS)

DILL

FOOD	PORTION	CALS.	SAT. FAT	FAT
seed	1 tsp	6	tr	tr

FOOD	PORTION	CALS.	SAT. FAT	FAT
sprigs fresh	5	0	tr	tr
sprigs fresh	1 cup	4	tr	tr
weed dry	1 tsp	3	—	tr
Watkins				
Liquid Spice	1 tbsp (0.5 oz)	120	2	14

DINNER

(see also ASIAN FOOD, PASTA DISHES, POT PIES, SPANISH FOOD)

FROZEN

FOOD	PORTION	CALS.	SAT. FAT	FAT
Amy's Organic				
Whole Meals Country Dinner	1 pkg (11 oz)	380	4	12
Armour				
Classics Chicken Parmigiana	1 meal (10.75 oz)	360	6	18
Classics Chicken & Noodles	1 meal (11 oz)	280	5	9
Classics Chicken Mesquite	1 meal (9.5 oz)	280	4	13
Classics Chicken w/ Wine & Mushroom	1 meal (10 oz)	260	5	11
Classics Glazed Chicken	1 meal (10.75 oz)	280	4	14
Classics Meatloaf	1 meal (11.25 oz)	300	5	10
Classics Salisbury Steak	1 meal (11.25 oz)	330	8	18
Classics Turkey and Dressing	1 meal (11.25 oz)	270	4	7
Classics Veal Parmigiana	1 meal (11.25 oz)	400	11	22
Classics Lite Beef Pepper	1 meal (11 oz)	210	2	4
Classics Lite Chicken Burgundy	1 meal (10 oz)	210	2	5
Classics Lite Salisbury Steak	1 meal (11.5 oz)	260	4	7
Classics Lite Shrimp Creole	1 meal (10 oz)	220	0	1
Banquet				
BBQ Style Chicken	1 meal (9 oz)	320	2	12
Beef	1 meal (9 oz)	240	3	7
Chicken Parmigiana	1 pkg (9.5 oz)	290	4	15
Chicken & Dumplings	1 meal (10 oz)	260	3	8
Chicken Fried Steak	1 pkg (10 oz)	400	6	20
Chicken Nuggets	1 pkg (6.75 oz)	410	5	21
Extra Helping All White Chicken	1 meal (18 oz)	820	9	41
Extra Helping Chicken Parmigiana	1 meal (19 oz)	650	8	33

FOOD	PORTION	CALS.	SAT. FAT	FAT
Banquet (CONT.)				
Extra Helping Chicken Fried Steak	1 meal (18.5 oz)	800	14	44
Extra Helping Fried Chicken	1 meal (18 oz)	790	9	39
Extra Helping Meatloaf	1 meal (19 oz)	650	16	38
Extra Helping Mexican Style	1 meal (22 oz)	820	14	34
Extra Helping Salisbury Steak	1 meal (19 oz)	740	19	46
Extra Helping Southern Fried Chicken	1 meal (17.5 oz)	750	9	37
Extra Helping Turkey Dinner	1 meal (18.8 oz)	560	5	20
Family Entree Beef Stew	1 serv (8.13 oz)	160	2	4
Family Entree Chicken Parmigiana	1 serv (4.67 oz)	240	5	13
Family Entree Chicken & Dumplings	1 serv (7.47 oz)	290	5	14
Family Entree Gravy & Sliced Turkey	1 serv (4.8 oz)	100	2	5
Family Entree Gravy w/ Charbroiled Beef	1 serv (4.67 oz)	180	6	13
Family Entree Onion Gravy w/Beef	1 serv (4.67 oz)	180	6	14
Family Entree Salisbury Steak	1 serv (4.67 oz)	200	6	14
Family Entree Veal Parmigiana	1 serv (4.67 oz)	230	4	14
Family Entrees Dumplings & Chicken	7 oz	280	—	14
Family Entrees Gravy & Sliced Beef	1 serv (5.6 oz)	100	2	3
Family Entrees Gravy & Sliced Turkey	6 oz	120	—	6
Fried Chicken	1 meal (9 oz)	470	9	27
Gravy w/ Beef Patty	1 pkg (9.5 oz)	300	8	20
Hot Sandwich Toppers Chicken Ala King	1 pkg (4.5 oz)	100	2	4
Hot Sandwich Toppers Creamed Chipped Beef	1 pkg (4 oz)	100	2	3
Hot Sandwich Toppers Gravy & Sliced Beef	1 pkg (4 oz)	70	1	2
Hot Sandwich Toppers Gravy & Sliced Turkey	1 pkg (5 oz)	90	2	4

FOOD	PORTION	CALS.	SAT. FAT	FAT
Banquet (CONT.)				
Hot Sandwich Toppers Salisbury Steak	1 pkg (5 oz)	220	7	16
Hot Sandwich Toppers Sloppy Joe	1 meal (4 oz)	140	3	7
Meatloaf	1 meal (9.5 oz)	280	7	17
Mexican Style Combo Meal	1 pkg (11 oz)	380	5	11
Mexican Style Meal	1 pkg (11 oz)	340	5	13
Oriental Style Chicken	1 pkg (9 oz)	260	3	9
Salisbury Steak	1 meal (9.5 oz)	310	7	16
Southern Fried Chicken Meal	1 pkg (8.75 oz)	260	8	30
Turkey	1 meal (9.25 oz)	270	3	10
Veal Parmagiana	1 pkg (9 oz)	530	5	14
Western Style Meal	1 meal (9.5 oz)	210	9	20
White Meat Chicken Meal	1 pkg (8.75 oz)	470	11	28
Birds Eye				
Easy Recipe Meal Starter Cacciatore as prep	1 serv	280	2	8
Easy Recipe Meal Starter Orange Glaze Chicken as prep	1 serv	280	2	8
Easy Recipe Meal Starter Southwestern	1 serv	280	2	8
Easy Recipe Meal Starter Sweet & Sour as prep	1 serv	280	2	8
Budget Gourmet				
Beef Cantonese	1 meal (9.1 oz)	270	—	9
Beef Stroganoff	1 meal (8.75 oz)	260	5	10
Chicken And Egg Noodles	1 meal (10 oz)	440	—	26
Chicken Au Gratin	1 meal (9.1 oz)	230	5	8
Chicken Breast Parmigiana	1 pkg (11 oz)	270	3	9
Chicken Marsala	1 meal (9 oz)	260	—	8
Chicken With Fettucini	1 meal (10 oz)	400	—	21
Chinese Style Vegetables & Chicken	1 meal (10 oz)	280	1	7
French Recipe Chicken	1 meal (10 oz)	220	4	9
Glazed Turkey	1 meal (9 oz)	260	2	5
Ham & Asparagus Au Gratin	1 meal (8.7 oz)	300	7	14
Herbed Chicken Breast With Fettucini	1 pkg (11 oz)	240	2	6
Italian Style Vegetables & Chicken	1 meal (10.25 oz)	310	2	8
Mandarin Chicken	1 meal (10 oz)	240	1	5
Mesquite Chicken Breast	1 pkg (11 oz)	250	1	6

FOOD	PORTION	CALS.	SAT. FAT	FAT
Budget Gourmet (CONT.)				
Orange Glazed Chicken	1 meal (9 oz)	270	1	3
Oriental Beef	1 meal (10 oz)	290	3	8
Oriental Chicken With Vegetables	1 meal (9 oz)	280	1	6
Pepper Steak With Rice	1 meal (10 oz)	300	—	8
Pot Roast Beef	1 meal (10.5 oz)	230	3	7
Roast Chicken With Homestyle Gravy	1 meal (11 oz)	280	2	8
Roast Sirloin Supreme	1 meal (9 oz)	320	—	15
Sirloin Salisbury Steak	1 meal (11 oz)	280	4	9
Sirloin Salisbury Steak	1 meal (9 oz)	220	3	8
Sirloin Cheddar Melt	1 meal (9.4 oz)	380	—	21
Sirloin Of Beef In Herb Sauce	1 meal (9.5 oz)	250	3	9
Sirloin Of Beef In Wine Sauce	1 pkg (11 oz)	280	2	8
Sirloin Tips And Country Vegetables	1 meal (10 oz)	290	—	17
Special Recipe Sirloin Of Beef	1 meal (11 oz)	250	3	9
Stuffed Turkey Breast	1 pkg (11 oz)	250	2	6
Swedish Meatballs With Noodles	1 meal (10 oz)	590	—	38
Sweet And Sour Chicken	1 meal (10 oz)	340	—	5
Teriyaki Beef	1 pkg (10.75 oz)	260	2	7
Teriyaki Chicken Breast	1 meal (11 oz)	300	1	8
Green Giant				
Create A Meal Broccoli Stir Fry as prep	1⅓ cups (9.9 oz)	290	3	13
Create A Meal Cheese & Herb Primavera as prep	1¼ cups (10 oz)	330	4	11
Create A Meal Garlic Herb as prep	1¼ cups (10 oz)	340	6	14
Create A Meal Hearty Vegetable Stew as prep	1¼ cups (10 oz)	280	2	9
Create A Meal Lemon Herb as prep	1½ cups (10 oz)	360	4	11
Create A Meal Mushroom & Wine as prep	1¼ cups (10 oz)	390	6	16
Create A Meal Vegetable Almond Stir Fry as prep	1⅓ cups (10 oz)	320	2	11
Healthy Choice				
Beef & Peppers Cantonese	1 meal (11.5 oz)	270	3	5
Beef Pepper Steak Oriental	1 meal (9.5 oz)	250	2	4

FOOD	PORTION	CALS.	SAT. FAT	FAT
Healthy Choice (CONT.)				
Beef Tips Francais	1 meal (9.5 oz)	280	2	5
Beef Tips With Sauce	1 meal (11 oz)	290	3	6
Chicken Cantonese	1 meal (11.25)	210	0	1
Chicken Parmigiana	1 meal (11.5 oz)	300	1	2
Chicken & Vegetables Marsala	1 meal (11.5 oz)	220	0	1
Chicken Bangkok	1 meal (9.5 oz)	270	1	4
Chicken Dijon	1 meal (11 oz)	280	1	4
Chicken Imperial	1 meal (9 oz)	230	1	4
Chicken Picante	1 meal (11.25 oz)	220	2	2
Chicken Teriyaki	1 meal (12.25 oz)	270	1	2
Classics Beef Broccoli Beijing	1 meal (12 oz)	330	1	3
Classics Cacciatore Chicken	1 meal (12.5 oz)	260	1	3
Classics Chicken Fransesca	1 meal (12.5 oz)	360	2	5
Classics Country Inn Roast Turkey	1 meal (10 oz)	250	1	4
Classics Ginger Chicken Hunan	1 meal (12.6 oz)	350	1	3
Classics Mesquite Beef Barbecue	1 meal (11 oz)	310	2	4
Classics Salisbury Steak	1 meal (11 oz)	260	3	6
Classics Sesame Chicken Shanghai	1 meal (12 oz)	310	1	5
Classics Shrimp & Vegetables Maria	1 meal (12.5 oz)	260	1	2
Country Glazed Chicken	1 meal (8.5 oz)	200	1	2
Country Herb Chicken	1 meal (11.5 oz)	270	2	4
Country Roast Turkey With Mushroom	1 meal (8.5 oz)	220	1	4
Country Turkey & Pasta	1 meal (12.6 oz)	300	2	4
Homestyle Turkey With Vegetables	1 meal (9.5 oz)	260	1	2
Honey Mustard Chicken	1 meal (9.5 oz)	260	0	2
Lemon Pepper Fish	1 meal (10.7 oz)	290	1	5
Mandarin Chicken	1 meal (10 oz)	280	0	3
Mesquite Chicken Barbecue	1 meal (10.5 oz)	320	1	2
Shrimp Marinara	1 meal (10.5 oz)	220	0	1
Smoky Chicken Barbecue	1 meal (12.75 oz)	380	2	5
Southwestern Glazed Chicken	1 meal (12.5 oz)	300	1	3

FOOD	PORTION	CALS.	SAT. FAT	FAT
Healthy Choice (CONT.)				
Sweet & Sour Chicken	1 meal (11.5 oz)	310	1	5
Traditional Breast Of Turkey	1 meal (10.5 oz)	280	1	3
Traditional Meat Loaf	1 meal (12 oz)	320	4	8
Traditional Beef Tips	1 meal (11.25 oz)	260	2	5
Tradtional Salisbury Steak	1 meal (11.5 oz)	320	3	6
Yankee Pot Roast	1 meal (11 oz)	280	2	5
Kid Cuisine				
Chicken Sandwiche	1 pkg (9.43 oz)	480	4	15
Chicken Nuggets	1 pkg (9.1 oz)	440	5	16
Fish Sticks	1 pkg (8.25 oz)	370	3	12
Fried Chicken	1 pkg (10.1 oz)	440	5	19
Hot Dogs w/ Buns	6.7 oz	450	—	19
Macaroni & Beef	1 pkg (9.6 oz)	370	4	9
Le Menu				
Beef Sirloin Tips	11½ oz	400	—	18
Beef Stroganoff	10 oz	430	—	24
Chicken Parmigiana	11¾ oz	410	—	20
Chicken A La King	10¼ oz	330	—	13
Chicken Cordon Bleu	11 oz	460	—	20
Chicken In Wine Sauce	10 oz	280	—	7
Chopped Sirloin Beef	12¼ oz	430	—	24
Entree LightStyle Chicken A La King	8¼ oz	240	—	5
Entree LightStyle Chicken Dijon	8 oz	240	—	7
Entree LightStyle Empress Chicken	8¼ oz	210	—	5
Entree LightStyle Glazed Turkey	8¼ oz	260	—	6
Entree LightStyle Herb Roast Chicken	7¾ oz	260	—	6
Entree LightStyle Swedish Meatballs	8 oz	260	—	8
Entree LightStyle Traditional Turkey	8 oz	200	—	5
Ham Steak	10 oz	300	—	11
LightStyle Glazed Chicken Breast	10 oz	230	—	3
LightStyle Herb Roasted Chicken	10 oz	240	—	7
LightStyle Salisbury Steak	10 oz	280	—	9
LightStyle Sliced Turkey	10 oz	210	—	5

FOOD	PORTION	CALS.	SAT. FAT	FAT
Le Menu (CONT.)				
LightStyle Sweet & Sour Chicken	10 oz	250	—	7
LightStyle Turkey Divan	10 oz	260	—	7
LightStyle Veal Marsala	10 oz	230	—	3
Pepper Steak	11.5 oz	370	—	13
Salisbury Steak	10.5 oz	370	—	20
Sliced Breast Of Turkey w/ Mushroom Gravy	10.5 oz	300	—	7
Sweet & Sour Chicken	11.5 oz	400	—	18
Veal Parmigiana	11.5 oz	390	—	17
Yankee Pot Roast	10 oz	330	—	13
Lean Cuisine				
American Favorite Baked Chicken	1 pkg (8.6 oz)	230	2	4
American Favorite Baked Fish	1 pkg (9 oz)	270	2	6
American Favorite Beef Pot Roast	1 pkg (9 oz)	210	2	6
American Favorite Beef Tips Barbecue	1 pkg (8.75 oz)	290	2	6
American Favorite Chicken Medallions w/ Creamy Cheese	1 pkg (9.37 oz)	260	3	8
American Favorite Country Vegetables & Beef	1 pkg (9 oz)	210	1	4
American Favorite Honey Roasted Chicken	1 pkg (8.5 oz)	290	2	6
American Favorite Meatloaf & Whipped Potatoes	1 pkg (9.4 oz)	250	3	6
American Favorite Oven Roasted Beef	1 pkg (9.25 oz)	260	3	8
American Favorite Roasted Turkey Breast	1 pkg (9.75 oz)	270	1	3
American Favorite Salisbury Steak	1 pkg (9.5 oz)	280	4	8
American Favorite Scalloped Potatoes w/ Turkey Ham	1 pkg (10 oz)	250	3	6
Cafe Classics Chicken Carbonara	1 pkg (9 oz)	280	2	8
Cafe Classics Chicken Mediterranean	1 pkg (10.5 oz)	270	1	4
Cafe Classics Chicken Breast In Wine Sauce	1 pkg (8.1 oz)	210	2	6

FOOD	PORTION	CALS.	SAT. FAT	FAT
Lean Cuisine (CONT.)				
Cafe Classics Chicken Parmesan	1 meal (10.9 oz)	220	2	5
Cafe Classics Chicken Piccata	1 pkg (9 oz)	270	2	6
Cafe Classics Chicken w/ Basil Cream Sauce	1 pkg (8.5 oz)	270	2	7
Cafe Classics Glazed Turkey	1 pkg (9 oz)	240	1	5
Cafe Classics Grilled Chicken Salsa	1 pkg (8.9 oz)	270	3	7
Cafe Classics Herb Roasted Chicken	1 pkg (8 oz)	210	1	5
Cafe Classics Honey Mustard Chicken	1 pkg (8 oz)	250	2	5
Cafe Classics Mesquite Beef w/ Rice	1 pkg (9 oz)	290	2	6
Cafe Classics Sirlion Beef Peppercorn	1 pkg (8.75 oz)	220	2	7
Chicken & Vegetables	1 pkg (10.5 oz)	250	1	6
Chicken A L'Orange	1 pkg (9 oz)	250	1	2
Chicken In Peanut Sauce	1 pkg (9 oz)	290	1	6
Fiesta Chicken w/ Rice & Vegetables	1 pkg (8.5 oz)	250	1	5
Glazed Chicken w/ Vegetable Rice	1 pkg (8.5 oz)	240	1	6
Homestyle Turkey	1 pkg (9.4 oz)	230	1	5
Mandarin Chicken	1 pkg (9 oz)	250	1	4
Oriental Beef	1 pkg (9.25 oz)	220	2	5
Stuffed Cabbage w/ Whipped Potatoes	1 pkg (9.5 oz)	170	2	5
Swedish Meatballs w/ Pasta	1 pkg (9.1 oz)	280	3	7
Life Choice				
Garden Potato Casserole	1 meal (13.4 oz)	160	0	1
Lightlife				
Vegetarian Request French Country Stew	1 pkg (12 oz)	340	0	3
Vegetarian Request Meatloaf Dinner	1 pkg (12 oz)	300	1	5
Vegetarian Request Moroccan Lentil Stew	1 pkg (12 oz)	400	0	2
Vegetarian Request Thai Tofu	1 pkg (12 oz)	400	2	10

FOOD	PORTION	CALS.	SAT. FAT	FAT
Lightlife (CONT.)				
Vegetarian Request Tuscan White Bean Stew	1 pkg (12 oz)	340	0	3
Luigino's				
Chicken A La King With Noodles	1 pkg (8 oz)	240	3	7
Noodles With Chicken Peas & Carrots	1 cup (6.3 oz)	260	3	10
Noodles With Chicken Peas & Carrots	1 pkg (8 oz)	300	3	11
Sweet & Sour Chicken With Rice	1 pkg (8 oz)	300	3	6
Morton				
Breaded Chicken Pattie	1 meal (6.75 oz)	280	3	15
Chicken Nugget	1 meal (7 oz)	320	4	17
Fried Chicken	1 meal (9 oz)	420	8	25
Meatloaf	1 meal (9 oz)	250	4	13
Mexican	1 meal (10 oz)	260	3	7
Salisbury Steak	1 meal (9 oz)	210	4	9
Turkey	1 meal (9 oz)	230	3	8
Veal Parmagiana	1 meal (8.75 oz)	280	4	13
Western	1 meal (9 oz)	290	7	16
Patio				
Chili	1 cup (8 oz)	260	1	13
Ranchera	1 pkg (13 oz)	410	6	15
Stouffer's				
Baked Chicken Breast w/ Mashed Potatoes	1 serv (12.2 oz)	330	5	14
Beef Stroganoff	1 pkg (9.75 oz)	390	7	20
Chicken A La King	1 pkg (9.5 oz)	350	4	13
Creamed Chicken	1 pkg (6.5 oz)	260	10	19
Creamed Chipped Beef	½ cup (5.5 oz)	160	3	11
Creamy Chicken & Broccoli	1 pkg (8.9 oz)	320	5	15
Escalloped Chicken & Noodles	1 pkg (10 oz)	430	5	27
Fish w/ Macaroni & Cheese	1 serv (9.5 oz)	460	6	20
Glazed Chicken w/ Rice	1 serv (11.8 oz)	290	1	6
Green Pepper Steak	1 pkg (10.5 oz)	330	3	9
Homestyle Baked Chicken & Gravy & Whipped Potatoes	1 pkg (8.9 oz)	270	3	12
Homestyle Beef Pot Roast & Browned Potatoes	1 pkg (8.9 oz)	250	3	8
Homestyle Fish Filet w/ Macaroni & Cheese	1 pkg (9 oz)	430	5	21

FOOD	PORTION	CALS.	SAT. FAT	FAT
Stouffer's (CONT.)				
Homestyle Fried Chicken & Whipped Potatoes	1 pkg (7.5 oz)	310	4	12
Homestyle Meatloaf & Whipped Potatoes	1 pkg (9.9 oz)	330	6	16
Homestyle Roast Turkey w/ Gravy Stuffing & Whipped Potatoes	1 pkg (9.6 oz)	320	4	13
Homestyle Salisbury Steak & Gravy & Macaroni & Cheese	1 pkg (9.6 oz)	350	7	16
Meatloaf	1 serv (5.5 oz)	210	4	12
Meatloaf w/ Whipped Potatoes	1 serv (11.5 oz)	380	7	18
Stuffed Pepper	1 pkg (10 oz)	200	2	5
Swedish Meatballs	1 pkg (10.25 oz)	480	9	24
Swanson				
Beans & Franks	10.5 oz	440	—	19
Beef	11.25 oz	310	—	6
Beef In Barbecue Sauce	11 oz	460	—	17
Chicken Duet Gourmet Nuggets Pizza Style	3 oz	210	—	12
Chopped Sirloin Beef	10.75 oz	340	—	16
Fish 'n' Chips	10 oz	500	—	21
Fried Chicken Dark Meat	9.75 oz	560	—	28
Fried Chicken White Meat	10.25 oz	550	—	25
Homestyle Chicken Cacciatore	10.95 oz	260	—	8
Homestyle Chicken Nibbles	4.25 oz	340	—	20
Homestyle Fish & Fries	6.5 oz	340	—	16
Homestyle Fried Chicken	7 oz	390	—	21
Homestyle Salisbury Steak	10 oz	320	—	16
Homestyle Scalloped Potatoes & Ham	9 oz	300	—	13
Homestyle Seafood Creole With Rice	9 oz	240	—	6
Homestyle Sirloin Tips In Burgundy Sauce	7 oz	160	—	5
Homestyle Turkey With Dressing & Potatoes	9 oz	290	—	11
Homestyle Veal Parmigiana	10 oz	330	—	13
Hungry-Man Boneless Chicken	17.75 oz	700	—	28
Hungry-Man Chopped Beef Steak	16.75 oz	640	—	37

FOOD	PORTION	CALS.	SAT. FAT	FAT
Swanson (CONT.)				
Hungry-Man Fried Chicken Dark Meat	14.25 oz	860	—	45
Hungry-Man Fried Chicken White Meat	14.25 oz	870	—	46
Hungry-Man Salisbury Steak	16.5 oz	680	—	41
Hungry-Man Sliced Beef	15.25 oz	450	—	12
Hungry-Man Turkey	17 oz	550	—	18
Hungry-Man Veal Parmigiana	18.25 oz	590	—	26
Loin Of Pork	10.75 oz	280	—	12
Macaroni & Beef	12 oz	370	—	15
Meatloaf	10.75 oz	360	—	15
Noodles & Chicken	10.5 oz	280	—	8
Salisbury Steak	10.75 oz	400	—	17
Swedish Meatballs	8.5 oz	360	—	20
Swiss Steak	10 oz	350	—	11
Turkey	8.75 oz	270	—	11
Turkey	11.5 oz	350	—	11
Veal Parmigiana	12.25 oz	430	—	20
Western Style	11.5 oz	430	—	19
Tamarind Tree				
Alu Chole	1 pkg (9.2 oz)	350	1	6
Channa Dal Masala	1 pkg (9.2 oz)	340	1	5
Dal Makhini	1 pkg (9.2 oz)	330	2	6
Dhingri Mutter	1 pkg (9.2 oz)	290	1	5
Navratan Korma	1 pkg (9.2 oz)	430	4	15
Palak Paneer	1 pkg (9.2 oz)	380	6	15
Saag Chole	1 pkg (9.2 oz)	370	2	10
Vegetable Jalfrazi	1 pkg (9.2 oz)	310	1	6
Tyson				
BBQ Chicken Potato & Vegetable Medley	1 pkg (14.7 oz)	560	5	21
Blackened Chicken Spanish Rice & Corn	1 pkg (8.8 oz)	260	1	5
Chicken Primavera	1 pkg (11.3 oz)	350	3	6
Chicken Diev Rice Pilaf & Broccoli Carrots	1 pkg (9.1 oz)	440	11	25
Chicken Divan Candied Carrots & Pasta	1 pkg (9.8 oz)	370	4	15
Chicken Francais Sliced Potatoes & Green Beans	1 pkg (8.8 oz)	260	3	10

FOOD	PORTION	CALS.	SAT. FAT	FAT
Tyson (CONT.)				
Chicken Marsala Carrots & Red Potatoes	1 pkg (8.8 oz)	180	2	5
Chicken Mesquite Corn & Pea Medley & Au Gratin Potatoes	1 pkg (8.8 oz)	320	3	8
Chicken Picatta	1 pkg (8.8 oz)	190	2	6
Chicken w/ Broccoli & Cheese Carrots & Pasta	1 pkg (8.8 oz)	270	5	12
Chicken w/ Mushroom Sauce Rice Pilaf & Candied Carrots	1 pkg (8.8 oz)	220	2	6
Chicken w/ Tabasco BBQ Sauce	1 pkg (8.8 oz)	260	2	7
Fried Chicken & Gravy w/ Mashed Potatoes & Corn	1 pkg (10.8 oz)	360	3	15
Grilled Chicken Corn O'Brien & Ranch Beans	1 pkg (8.8 oz)	230	1	4
Grilled Italian Chicken Pasta & Vegetable Medley	1 pkg (8.8 oz)	190	2	4
Honey Dijon Chicken Pasta & Pea Medley	1 pkg (11.3 oz)	340	2	7
Roasted Chicken w/ Garlic Sauce Pasta & Vegetable Medley	1 pkg (8.8 oz)	210	2	7
Ultra Slim-Fast				
Beef Pepper Steak	12 oz	270	—	4
Chicken Fettucini	12 oz	380	—	12
Chicken & Vegetable	12 oz	290	—	3
Country Style Vegetable & Beef Tips	12 oz	230	—	5
Mesquite Chicken	12 oz	360	—	1
Roasted Chicken In Mushroom Sauce	12 oz	280	—	6
Shrimp Creole	12 oz	240	—	4
Shrimp Marinara	12 oz	290	—	3
Sweet & Sour Chicken	12 oz	330	—	2
Turkey Medallions In Herb Sauce	12 oz	280	—	6
Weight Watchers				
Smart One Grilled Salisbury Steak	1 pkg (8.5 oz)	250	4	9
Smart Ones Chicken Mirabella	1 pkg (9.2 oz)	180	1	2

FOOD	PORTION	CALS.	SAT. FAT	FAT
Weight Watchers (CONT.)				
Smart Ones Fiesta Chicken	1 pkg (8.5 oz)	210	1	2
Smart Ones Honey Mustard Chicken	1 pkg (8.5 oz)	200	1	2
Smart Ones Lemon Herb Chicken Piccata	1 pkg (8.5 oz)	190	1	2
Smart Ones Pepper Steak	1 pkg (10 oz)	240	2	5
Smart Ones Risotto w/ Cheese & Mushrooms	1 pkg (10 oz)	290	3	7
Smart Ones Roast Turkey Medallions & Mushrooms	1 pkg (8.5 oz)	180	1	2
Smart Ones Shrimp Marinara	1 pkg (9 oz)	180	1	2
Smart Ones Stuffed Turkey Breast	1 pkg (10 oz)	260	2	7
Smart Ones Swedish Meatballs	1 pkg (9 oz)	300	4	10
READY-TO-EAT				
Tyson				
Beef Stir Fry	1 pkg (14 oz)	430	2	5
Chicken Stir Fry Kit	2¾ cups (14 oz)	430	1	5
SHELF-STABLE				
My Own Meal				
Beef Stew	1 pkg (10 oz)	260	3	11
Chicken Mediterranean	1 pkg (10 oz)	270	2	9
Chicken Noodles	1 pkg (10 oz)	270	2	8
Chicken & Black Beans	1 pkg (10 oz)	240	1	5
Old World Stew	1 pkg (10 oz)	310	4	12
DIP				
Breakstone's				
Bacon & Onion	2 tbsp (1.1 oz)	60	3	5
Chesapeake Clam	2 tbsp (1.1 oz)	50	3	4
Free Creamy Salsa	2 tbsp (1.1 oz)	20	0	0
Free French Onion	2 tbsp (1.1 oz)	25	0	0
Free Ranch	2 tbsp (1.1 oz)	25	0	0
French Onion	2 tbsp (1.1 oz)	50	3	5
Toasted Onion	2 tbsp (1.1 oz)	50	3	5
Cheez Whiz				
Medium Cheese & Salsa	2 tbsp (1.2 oz)	100	5	8
Mild Cheese & Salsa	2 tbsp (1.2 oz)	100	5	8
Chi-Chi's				
Fiesta Bean	2 tbsp (0.9 oz)	35	1	2
Fiesta Cheese	2 tbsp (0.9 oz)	40	1	3

FOOD	PORTION	CALS.	SAT. FAT	FAT
Frito-Lay's				
French Onion	2 tbsp (1.1 oz)	60	3	5
Jalapeno & Cheddar Cheese	2 tbsp (1.2 oz)	50	1	4
Fritos				
Bean	2 tbsp (1.2 oz)	40	1	1
Chili Cheese	1.2 oz	45	1	3
Hot Bean	2 tbsp (1.2 oz)	40	0	1
Guiltless Gourmet				
Black Bean Mild	2 tbsp (1 oz)	30	0	0
Black Bean Spicy	2 tbsp (1 oz)	30	0	0
Hain				
Hot Bean	4 tbsp	70	—	1
Mexican Bean	4 tbsp	60	—	1
Onion Bean	4 tbsp	70	—	1
Taco Dip & Sauce	4 tbsp	25	—	1
Heluva Good Cheese				
Bacon Horseradish	2 tbsp (1.1 oz)	60	3	5
Clam	2 tbsp (1.1 oz)	50	3	5
French Onion	2 tbsp (1.1 oz)	50	3	5
Homestyle Onion	2 tbsp (1.1 oz)	60	3	5
Light French Onion	2 tbsp (1.1 oz)	35	1	2
Light Jalapeno Cheddar	2 tbsp (1.1 oz)	40	2	2
Ranch	2 tbsp (1.1 oz)	60	3	5
Knudsen				
Free Creamy Salsa	2 tbsp (1.1 oz)	20	0	0
Free French Onion	2 tbsp (1.1 oz)	25	0	0
Free Ranch	2 tbsp (1.1 oz)	25	0	0
Kraft				
Avocado	2 tbsp (1.1 oz)	60	3	4
Bacon & Horseradish	2 tbsp (1.1 oz)	60	3	5
Clam	2 tbsp (1.1 oz)	60	3	4
Free French Onion	2 tbsp (1.1 oz)	25	0	0
Free Ranch	2 tbsp (1.1 oz)	25	0	0
Free Salsa	2 tbsp (1.1 oz)	20	0	0
French Onion	2 tbsp (1.1 oz)	60	3	4
Green Onion	2 tbsp (1.1 oz)	60	3	4
Jalapeno Cheese	2 tbsp (1.1 oz)	60	3	4
Premium Sour Cream	2 tbsp (1.1 oz)	50	3	4
Premium Sour Cream Bacon & Horseradish	2 tbsp (1.1 oz)	60	3	5
Premium Sour Cream Bacon & Onion	2 tbsp (1.1 oz)	60	3	5
Premium Sour Cream Creamy Onion	2 tbsp (1.1 oz)	45	3	4

FOOD	PORTION	CALS.	SAT. FAT	FAT
Kraft (CONT.)				
Premium Sour Cream French Onion	2 tbsp (1.1 oz)	45	3	4
Premium Sour Cream Ranch	2 tbsp (1.1 oz)	50	3	4
Ranch	2 tbsp (1.1 oz)	60	3	5
Louise's				
Fat Free Honey Mustard	1 oz	40	0	0
Fat Free Sour Cream & Onion	1 oz	25	0	0
Fat Free White Cheese Peppercorn	1 oz	25	0	0
Marzetti				
Blue Cheese Veggie	2 tbsp	200	4	21
Lemon Dill Veggie	2 tbsp	140	3	14
Light Ranch Veggie	2 tbsp	60	2	7
Ranch Veggie	2 tbsp	140	3	14
Sour Cream & Onion	2 tbsp	130	3	14
Southwestern Veggie	2 tbsp	130	3	14
Spinach Veggie	2 tbsp	130	3	13
Old El Paso				
Black Bean	2 tbsp (1 oz)	20	0	0
Cheese 'n Salsa Medium	2 tbsp (1 oz)	40	1	3
Cheese 'n Salsa Mild	2 tbsp (1 oz)	40	1	3
Chunky Salsa Medium	2 tbsp (1 oz)	15	0	0
Chunky Salsa Mild	2 tbsp (1 oz)	15	0	0
Jalapeno	2 tbsp (1 oz)	30	0	1
Ruffles				
French Onion	2 tbsp	70	1	5
Ranch	2 tbsp (1.2 oz)	70	1	6
Snyder's of Hanover				
Mustard Pretzel	2 tbsp (1.2 oz)	90	2	4
Taco Bell				
Fat Free Black Bean	2 tbsp (1.2 oz)	30	0	0
Salsa Con Queso Medium	2 tbsp (1.2 oz)	45	1	3
Salsa Con Queso Mild	2 tbsp (1.2 oz)	45	1	3
Tyson				
Bleu Cheese For Dipping Wings	2 tbsp (1.4 oz)	140	3	14
Utz				
Fat Free Sour Cream & Onion	2 tbsp (1 oz)	30	0	0
Jalapeno & Cheddar	2 tbsp (1 oz)	30	1	3
Low Fat Desert Garden	2 tbsp (1.1 oz)	40	0	2
Low Fat Salsa Con Queso	2 tbsp (1 oz)	40	0	2
Mild Cheddar	2 tbsp (1 oz)	45	2	3
Sour Cream & Onion	2 tbsp (1 oz)	60	3	5

FOOD	PORTION	CALS.	SAT. FAT	FAT
Wise				
Jalapeno Bean	2 tbsp	25	0	0
Taco	2 tbsp	12	0	0
DOCK				
fresh cooked	3.5 oz	20	—	1
raw chopped	½ cup	15	—	tr
DOLPHINFISH				
fresh baked	3 oz	93	tr	1
fresh fillet baked	5.6 oz	174	tr	1
DOUGHNUTS				
(see also DUNKIN' DONUTS, KRISPY KREME, WINCHELL'S)				
cake type unsugared	1 (1.6 oz)	198	2	11
chocolate glazed	1 (1.5 oz)	175	3	8
chocolate sugared	1 (1.5 oz)	175	3	8
chocolate coated	1 (1.5 oz)	204	4	13
creme filled	1 (3 oz)	307	6	21
french cruller glazed	1 (1.4 oz)	169	2	8
frosted	1 (1.5 oz)	204	4	13
honey bun	1 (2.1 oz)	242	3	14
jelly	1 (3 oz)	289	4	16
old fashioned	1 (1.6 oz)	198	2	11
sugared	1 (1.6 oz)	192	3	10
wheat glazed	1 (1.6 oz)	162	1	9
wheat sugared	1 (1.6 oz)	162	1	9
yeast glazed	1 (2.1 oz)	242	3	14
Dolly Madison				
Chocolate Frosted	1 (1.1 oz)	140	5	8
Donut Gems Chocolate	4 (2 oz)	260	9	15
Donut Gems Crunch	3 (2 oz)	220	4	10
Donut Gems Powdered	4 (2 oz)	230	5	11
English Cruller	1 (2 oz)	250	6	14
Glazed Whirl	1 (1.6 oz)	210	5	11
Glazed Yeast	1 (1.5 oz)	190	5	9
Old Fashioned	1 (2.1 oz)	280	8	16
Plain	1 (1.2 oz)	140	3	7
Powdered	1 (1 oz)	120	3	6
Dutch Mill				
Cider	1 (2.1 oz)	240	2	10
Cinnamon	1 (1.8 oz)	210	5	11
Donut Holes Double-Dipped Chocolate	3 (1.4 oz)	220	6	16
Donut Holes Shootin' Stars	3 (1.4 oz)	190	3	10
Double-Dipped Chocolate	1 (2.1 oz)	280	7	17

FOOD	PORTION	CALS.	SAT. FAT	FAT
Dutch Mill (CONT.)				
Glazed	1 (2.1 oz)	250	3	12
Glazed Chocolate	1 (2.4 oz)	270	3	11
Plain	1 (1.8 oz)	210	5	12
Sugared	1 (1.8 oz)	220	5	11
Entenmann's				
Crumb Topped	1 (2.1 oz)	260	—	12
Devil's Food Crumb	1 (2.1 oz)	250	—	12
Rich Frosted	1 (2 oz)	280	—	18
Freihofer's				
Assorted	1 (2 oz)	270	4	17
Hostess				
Blueberry	1 (1.7 oz)	210	6	13
Donettes Crumb	3 (1.5 oz)	170	3	8
Donettes Frosted	3 (1.5 oz)	200	7	12
Donettes Powdered	3 (1.5 oz)	180	3	9
Frosted	1 (1.4 oz)	180	7	11
O's Raspberry Filled	1 (2.2 oz)	230	4	10
Old Fashioned Glazed	1 (2.1 oz)	260	6	13
Plain	1 (1.1 oz)	140	3	7
Powdered	1 (1.3 oz)	150	4	8
Little Debbie				
Donut Sticks	1 (1.6 oz)	210	3	12
Mini Powdered	1 pkg (2.5 oz)	290	4	14
Tastykake				
Mini Plain Glaze	1 pkg (2.5 oz)	260	2	11
Mini Powdered Sugar	1 pkg (2.5 oz)	260	2	12
Mini Rich Frosted	1 pkg (3 oz)	370	10	22

DRESSING
(see STUFFING/DRESSING)

DRINK MIXERS
(see *also* SODA, WATER)

FOOD	PORTION	CALS.	SAT. FAT	FAT
whiskey sour mix	2 oz	55	0	0
whiskey sour mix as prep	3.6 oz	169	0	0
Bacardi				
Margarita Mix w/ rum	8 fl oz	160	0	0
Margarita Mix w/o liquor	8 fl oz	100	0	0
Pina Colada	8 fl oz	140	0	0
Rum Runner	8 fl oz	140	0	0
Strawberry Daiquiri w/o liquor	8 fl oz	140	0	0
Canada Dry				
Collins Mixer	8 fl oz	120	0	0
Sour Mixer	8 fl oz	90	0	0

FOOD	PORTION	CALS.	SAT. FAT	FAT
Daily's				
Bloody Mary Original	1 serv (6 oz)	50	0	0
Margarita Daiquiri Strawberry	1 serv (4 oz)	180	0	0
Margarita Green Demon	1 serv (3 oz)	80	0	0
Pina Colada	1 serv (3 oz)	160	1	2
Schweppes				
Collins Mixer	8 fl oz	100	0	0
Tabasco				
Bloody Mary Mix	1 serv (8.4 oz)	56	tr	tr
Bloody Mary Mix Extra Spicy	1 serv (8.4 oz)	58	tr	tr
DRUM				
freshwater fillet baked	5.4 oz	236	2	10
freshwater baked	3 oz	130	1	5
DUCK				
w/ skin roasted	1 cup (4.9 oz)	472	14	40
w/ skin w/ bone leg roasted	3 oz	184	3	10
w/ skin w/o bone breast roasted	3 oz	172	2	9
w/o skin roasted	1 cup (4.9 oz)	281	6	16
w/o skin w/ bone leg braised	1 cup (6.1 oz)	310	2	10
w/o skin w/o bone breast broiled	1 cup (6.1 oz)	244	1	4
wild w/ skin raw	½ duck (9.5 oz)	571	14	41
wild w/o skin breast raw	½ breast (2.9 oz)	102	1	4
DUMPLING				
Pepperidge Farm				
Apple	1 (3 oz)	230	3	11
Peach	1 (3 oz)	320	3	11
EEL				
fresh cooked	1 fillet (5.6 oz)	375	5	24
fresh cooked	3 oz	200	3	13
raw	3 oz	156	2	10
smoked	3.5 oz	330	7	28
EGG				
(see also EGG DISHES, EGG SUBSTITUTES)				
CHICKEN				
frozen	1 cup	363	8	24
frozen	1	75	2	5
hard cooked	1	77	2	5
hard cooked chopped	1 cup	210	4	14
poached	1	74	2	5

FOOD	PORTION	CALS.	SAT. FAT	FAT
raw	1	75	2	5
white only	1 cup	121	0	0
white only	1	17	0	0
EggsPlus				
Fresh	1 (1.8 oz)	70	2	5
Organic Valley				
Brown Extra Large	1 (2.2 oz)	90	5	6
Brown Large	1 (2 oz)	80	4	6
Brown Medium	1 (1.8 oz)	70	3	5
OTHER POULTRY				
duck preserved hard core	1 (1.8 oz)	80	2	6
duck preserved soft core	1 (1.8 oz)	80	2	6
duck raw	1 (2.5 oz)	130	3	10
duck salted	1 (1.9 oz)	100	3	7
goose raw	1 (5 oz)	267	5	19
quail raw	1 (9 g)	14	tr	1
turkey raw	1 (2.7 oz)	135	3	9

EGG DISHES
FROZEN
Downyflake

FOOD	PORTION	CALS.	SAT. FAT	FAT
Scrambled Eggs With Ham & Hash Browns	1 pkg (6.25 oz)	360	—	26
Scrambled Eggs With Ham & Pecan Twirl	1 pkg (6.25 oz)	470	—	28
Scrambled Eggs With Hash Browns & Sausage	1 pkg (6.25 oz)	420	—	34
Scrambled Eggs With Sausage & Pecan Twirl	1 pkg (6.25 oz)	510	—	33
Quaker				
Scrambled Eggs & Sausage With Hash Browns	1 pkg (5.7 oz)	290	—	20
Scrambled Eggs & Sausage With Pancakes	1 pkg (5.2 oz)	270	—	14
Scrambled Eggs Cheddar Cheese & Fried Potatoes	1 pkg (5.9 oz)	250	—	13
Weight Watchers				
Handy Ham & Cheese Omelet	1 (4 oz)	220	3	5

TAKE-OUT

FOOD	PORTION	CALS.	SAT. FAT	FAT
omelette plain	1 serv (3.5 oz)	172	4	13
scrambled plain	2 (3.3 oz)	199	6	15
scrambled w/ whole milk & margarine	1 serv	365	8	27
sunny side up	1	91	2	7

FOOD	PORTION	CALS.	SAT. FAT	FAT
EGG ROLLS				
(see also ASIAN FOOD)				
egg roll wrapper fresh	1	83	tr	tr
Chun King				
Chicken	8 (4.4 oz)	270	2	9
Pork & Shrimp	8 (4.4 oz)	290	3	11
Shrimp	8 (4.4 oz)	260	2	8
Empire				
Large	1 (3 oz)	190	1	6
Miniature	6 (4.8 oz)	280	2	8
Lean Cuisine				
Vegetable	1 pkg (9 oz)	340	2	6
Lo-An				
White Meat Chicken	1 (2.7 oz)	140	1	4r
Luigino's				
Chicken	1 pkg (6 oz)	360	7	13
Pork & Shrimp	1 pkg (6 oz)	340	3	9
Shrimp	1 pkg (6 oz)	350	3	11
Sweet & Sour Chicken	1 pkg (6 oz)	400	3	12
Sweet & Sour Pork	1 pkg (6 oz)	360	3	10
Szechwan Vegetable	1 pkg (6 oz)	350	4	12
Worthington				
Vegetarian Egg Rolls	1 (3 oz)	180	2	8
TAKE-OUT				
lobster	1 (4.8 oz)	270	2	7
meat & shrimp	1 (4.8 oz)	320	3	12
pork & shrimp	1 (5 oz)	300	4	10
shrimp	1 (3 oz)	170	1	5
spicy pork	1 (3 oz)	200	2	9
vegetable	1 (3 oz)	170	1	4
EGG SUBSTITUTES				
frozen	¼ cup	96	1	7
frozen	1 cup	384	5	27
liquid	1 cup (8.8 oz)	211	2	8
liquid	1½ oz	40	tr	2
powder	0.35 oz	44	tr	1
powder	0.7 oz	88	1	3
Egg Beaters				
Eggs Substitute	¼ cup	25	0	0
Omelette Cheese	½ cup	110	2	5
Omelette Vegetable	½ cup	50	0	0
Healthy Choice				
Cholesterol Free	¼ cup (2 oz)	25	0	0

FOOD	PORTION	CALS.	SAT. FAT	FAT
Morningstar Farms				
Better'n Eggs	¼ cup (2 oz)	20	0	0
Breakfast Sandwich Bagel Scramblers Pattie Cheese	1 (5.9 oz)	320	1	5
Breakfast Sandwich English Muffin Scramblers Pattie	1 (5.1 oz)	240	1	3
Breakfast Sandwich English Muffin Scramblers Pattie Cheese	1 (6 oz)	280	1	3
Scramblers	¼ cup (2 oz)	35	0	0
Second Nature				
No Cholesterol	2 fl oz	60	tr	2
No Fat	2 fl oz	40	0	0
No Fat With Garden Vegetables	2.5 fl oz	40	0	0
Simply Eggs				
Egg Substitute	1.75 fl oz	35	tr	1
EGGNOG				
eggnog	1 cup	342	11	19
eggnog	1 qt	1368	45	76
eggnog flavor mix as prep w/ milk	9 oz	260	5	8
Hood				
Fat Free	4 fl oz	100	0	0
Golden	4 fl oz	180	5	8
Light	4 fl oz	120	1	2
Select	4 fl oz	210	8	12
EGGPLANT				
CANNED				
Progresso				
Appetizer	2 tbsp (1 oz)	30	0	2
FRESH				
cubed cooked	½ cup	13	tr	tr
raw cut up	½ cup (1.4 oz)	11	tr	tr
slices cooked	4 (7 oz)	38	0	0
whole peeled raw	1 (1 lb)	117	tr	1
FROZEN				
Mrs. Paul's				
Parmigiana	5 oz	240	—	16
TAKE-OUT				
baba ghannouj	¼ cup	55	—	4
caponata	2 tbsp (1 oz)	30	—	2
indian eggplant runi	1 serv	180	4	14

FOOD	PORTION	CALS.	SAT. FAT	FAT
ELDERBERRIES				
fresh	1 cup	105	—	1
ELK				
roasted	3 oz	124	1	2
ENDIVE				
raw chopped	½ cup	4	tr	tr
ENERGY BARS				
(see CEREAL BARS, NUTRITION SUPPLEMENTS)				
ENGLISH MUFFIN				
FROZEN				
Weight Watchers				
Sandwich	1 (4 oz)	210	3	5
READY-TO-EAT				
apple cinnamon	1	138	tr	2
granola	1	155	tr	1
mixed grain	1	155	tr	1
plain	1	134	tr	1
plain toasted	1	133	tr	1
raisin cinnamon	1	138	tr	2
sourdough	1	134	tr	1
wheat	1	127	tr	1
whole wheat	1	134	tr	1
Arnold				
Extra Crisp	1	130	0	1
Sourdough	1	130	0	1
Milton's				
Multi-Grain	1 (2 oz)	150	0	1
Roman Meal				
English Muffin	1 (2.2 oz)	135	tr	1
Thomas'				
Honey Wheat	1	128	—	1
Oat Bran	1	116	—	1
Raisin Cinnamon	1	151	—	1
Regular	1	130	—	1
Sandwich Size	1 (92 g)	210	1	2
Sour Dough	1	131	—	1
Wonder				
Cinnamon Raisin	1 (2.1 oz)	140	1	2
Original	1 (2 oz)	130	0	1
Sourdough	1 (2 oz)	130	0	1
REFRIGERATED				
Roman Meal				
English Muffin	½ muffin (1.1 oz)	66	tr	tr
Honey Nut Oat Bran	½ muffin (1.1 oz)	81	tr	1

FOOD	PORTION	CALS.	SAT. FAT	FAT
TAKE-OUT				
w/ butter	1 (2.2 oz)	189	2	6
w/ cheese & sausage	1 (4 oz)	393	10	24
w/ egg cheese & canadian bacon	1 (4.8 oz)	289	5	13
w/ egg cheese & sausage	1 (5.8 oz)	487	12	31
EPAZOTE				
fresh	1 tbsp (1 g)	tr	—	0
fresh sprig	1 (2 g)	1	—	tr
EPPAW				
raw	½ cup	75	—	1
FALAFEL				
Casbah				
as prep	5	130	0	3
Near East				
As Prep	2½ patties	230	2	15
TAKE-OUT				
falafel	1 (1.2 oz)	57	tr	3
FAST FOODS				
(see INDIVIDUAL NAMES IN PART TWO)				
FAT				
(see also BUTTER, BUTTER BLENDS, BUTTER SUBSTITUTES, MARGARINE, OIL)				
beef cooked	1 oz	193	8	20
beef suet	1 oz	242	15	27
beef tallow	1 tbsp (13 g)	115	6	13
chicken	1 cup	1846	61	205
chicken	1 tbsp	115	4	13
cocoa butter	1 tbsp	120	8	14
duck	1 tbsp (13 g)	115	4	13
goose	1 tbsp	115	4	13
goose	3.5 oz	900	6	100
lamb new zealand raw	1 oz	182	10	19
lard	1 cup (205 g)	1849	80	205
lard	1 tbsp (13 g)	115	5	13
nutmeg butter	1 tbsp	120	12	14
pork backfat	1 oz	230	9	25
pork cooked	1 oz	178	7	18
salt pork	1 oz	212	8	23
shortening	1 tbsp	113	3	13
shortening	1 cup	1812	41	205
turkey	1 tbsp	115	4	13
ucuhuba butter	1 tbsp	120	12	14

FOOD	PORTION	CALS.	SAT. FAT	FAT
Crisco				
Butter Flavor	1 tbsp	110	3	12
Shortening	1 tbsp	110	3	12
Shortening	1 tbsp (0.4 oz)	110	3	12
Sticks	1 tbsp (0.4 oz)	110	3	12
Sticks Butter Flavor	1 tbsp (0.4 oz)	110	3	12
Empire				
Chicken Fat Rendered	1 tbsp (0.5 oz)	120	4	13
Wesson				
Shortening	1 tbsp	100	3	12
FAT SUBSTITUTES				
Soy Is Us				
Fat Not! Organic	3 tbsp	66	tr	1
FAVA BEANS				
Progresso				
Fava Beans	½ cup (4.6 oz)	110	0	1
FEIJOA				
fresh	1 (1.75 oz)	25	—	tr
puree	1 cup	119	—	2
FENNEL				
fresh bulb	1 (8.2 oz)	72	—	tr
fresh sliced	1 cup	27	—	tr
leaves	3.5 oz	24	—	tr
seed	1 tsp	7	tr	tr
FENUGREEK				
seed	1 tsp	12	—	tr
FIBER				
Delta				
Natural Fiber	½ cup (1 oz)	20	—	tr
FIDDLEHEAD FERNS				
fresh	3.5 oz	34	—	tr
FIGS				
CANNED				
in heavy syrup	3	75	tr	tr
in light syrup	3	58	tr	tr
water pack	3	42	—	tr
DRIED				
California	½ cup (3.5 oz)	200	—	1
cooked	½ cup	140	tr	1
whole	10	477	tr	2

FOOD	PORTION	CALS.	SAT. FAT	FAT
Sonoma				
White Misson	3-4 (1.4 oz)	110	0	0
FRESH				
fig	1 med	50	tr	tr
FIREWEED				
leaves chopped	1 cup (0.8 oz)	24	—	1
FISH				
(see also INDIVIDUAL NAMES, FISH SUBSTITUTES, SUSHI)				
CANNED				
Holmes				
Finest Kippered Snacks drained	1 can (3.2 oz)	135	1	8
Port Clyde				
Fish Steaks In Louisiana Hot Sauce	1 can (3.75 oz)	150	2	9
Fish Steaks In Mustard Sauce	1 can (3.75 oz)	140	1	7
Fish Steaks In Soybean Oil With Hot Chilies drained	1 can (3.3 oz)	155	2	8
Fish Steaks In Soybean Oil drained	1 can (3.3 oz)	220	4	17
FROZEN				
breaded fillet	1 (2 oz)	155	2	7
sticks	1 stick (1 oz)	76	1	3
Cajun Cookin'				
Seafood Gumbo	17 oz	330	—	7
Gorton's				
Crispy Batter Dipped Fillets	2	290	8	19
Crispy Batter Sticks	4	260	6	18
Crunch Fillets	2	230	3	13
Crunchy Sticks	4	210	4	13
Grilled Fillets Cajun Blackened	1 piece (3.8 oz)	120	1	6
Light Recipe Lightly Breaded Fish Fillets	1 fillet	180	3	8
Light Recipe Tempura Fillets	1 fillet	200	4	14
Microwave Crispy Batter Large Cut Fillets	1	320	—	21
Microwave Entree Fillets In Herb Butter	1 pkg	190	5	8
Microwave Fillets	2	340	12	26
Microwave Larger Cut Fillets	1	320	10	22

FOOD	PORTION	CALS.	SAT. FAT	FAT
Gorton's (CONT.)				
Microwave Larger Cut Ranch Fillet	1	330	—	21
Microwave Sticks	6	340	7	22
Potato Crisp Fillets	2	300	6	20
Potato Crisp Sticks	4	260	5	16
Value Pack Portions	1 portion	180	—	11
Value Pack Sticks	4	190	—	9
Kineret				
Fish Sticks	5 pieces (4 oz)	280	3	14
Mrs. Paul's				
Buttered Fillet Microwave	1 fillet	80	—	4
Entree Light Seafood Dijon	8.75 oz	200	2	5
Entree Light Seafood Florentine	8 oz	220	—	8
Entree Light Seafood Mornay	9 oz	230	4	10
Fillet Sandwich Microwave	1	280	—	15
Fillets Microwave	1 fillet	280	—	19
Fish Cakes	2	190	—	7
Fish Fillets Batter Dipped	2 fillets	330	—	17
Fish Fillets Crispy Crunchy	2 fillets	220	—	9
Fish Fillets Crunchy Batter	2 fillets	280	—	14
Fish Sticks 40 Crunchy	4 (2.75 oz)	200	—	10
Fish Sticks Crispy Crunchy	4 sticks	190	—	8
Fish Sticks Microwave	5	290	—	20
In Butter Sauce Light Fillet	1 fillets	140	—	6
Portions Battered Fish	2 portions	300	—	19
Portions Crispy Crunchy Breaded Fish	2 portions	230	—	15
Seafood Platter Combination	9 oz	600	—	33
Sticks Battered Fish	4 sticks	210	—	12
Sticks Crispy Crunchy Breaded Fish	4 sticks	140	—	6
Van De Kamp's				
Battered Fish Fillets	1 (2.6 oz)	180	2	11
Battered Fish Nuggets	8 (4 oz)	280	3	18
Battered Fish Portions	2 pieces (5 oz)	350	4	22
Battered Fish Sticks	6 (4 oz)	260	3	16
Breaded Fillets	2 (3.5 oz)	280	3	19
Breaded Fish Portions	3 pieces (4.5 oz)	330	3	21
Breaded Fish Sticks	6 (4 oz)	290	3	17
Breaded Mini Fish Sticks	13 (3.3 oz)	250	2	14
Crisp & Healthy Breaded Fillets	2 (3.5 oz)	150	1	3

FOOD	PORTION	CALS.	SAT. FAT	FAT
Van De Kamp's (CONT.)				
Crisp & Healthy Fish Sticks	6 (4 oz)	180	1	3
Fish 'n Fries	1 pkg (6.6 oz)	380	3	18
TAKE-OUT				
fish cake	1 (4.7 oz)	166	2	7
jamaican brown fish stew	1 serv	426	5	22
mousse	1 serv (3.5 oz)	185	—	14
stew	1 cup (7.9 oz)	157	2	4
FISH SUBSTITUTES				
Loma Linda				
Ocean Platter not prep	⅓ cup (0.9 oz)	90	0	1
Worthington				
Fillets	2 (3 oz)	180	2	10
Tuno	½ cup (1.9 oz)	80	1	6
FLAXSEED				
Arrowhead				
Flaxseed	3 tbsp (1 oz)	140	1	10
Stone-Buhr				
Flaxseed	1 tsp (1 oz)	150	1	10
FLOUNDER				
FRESH				
cooked	3 oz	99	tr	1
cooked	1 fillet (4.5 oz)	148	tr	2
FROZEN				
Gorton's				
Fishmarket Fresh	5 oz	110	—	1
Microwave Entree Stuffed	1 pkg	350	7	18
Mrs. Paul's				
Crunchy Batter Fillets	2 fillets	220	—	9
Light Fillets	1 fillet	240	—	10
Van De Kamp's				
Lightly Breaded Fillets	1 (4 oz)	230	2	11
Natural Fillets	1 (4 oz)	110	0	2
TAKE-OUT				
battered & fried	3.2 oz	211	3	11
breaded & fried	3.2 oz	211	3	11
FLOUR				
buckwheat whole groat	1 cup (4.2 oz)	402	1	4
corn masa	1 cup (4 oz)	416	1	4
cottonseed lowfat	1 oz	94	tr	tr
potato	1 cup (6.3 oz)	628	tr	1
rice brown	1 cup (5.5 oz)	574	tr	4

FOOD	PORTION	CALS.	SAT. FAT	FAT
rice white	1 cup (5.5 oz)	578	1	2
rye dark	1 cup (4.5 oz)	415	tr	3
rye light	1 cup (3.6 oz)	374	tr	1
rye medium	1 cup (3.6 oz)	361	tr	2
sesame lowfat	1 oz	95	tr	tr
triticale whole grain	1 cup (4.6 oz)	439	tr	2
white all-purpose	1 cup (4.4 oz)	455	tr	1
white bread	1 cup (4.8 oz)	495	tr	2
white cake unsifted	1 cup (4.8 oz)	496	tr	1
white self-rising	1 cup (4.4 oz)	443	tr	1
white unbleached	1 cup (4.4 oz)	455	tr	1
whole wheat	1 cup (4.2 oz)	407	tr	2
All Trump				
Flour	¼ cup (1 oz)	100	0	0
Arrowhead				
Kamut	¼ cup (1.2 oz)	110	0	1
Pastry	⅓ cup (1.1 oz)	100	0	1
Rye Whole Grain	¼ cup (1.6 oz)	160	0	1
Spelt	¼ cup (1.2 oz)	100	0	1
Teff	¼ cup (1.4 oz)	140	0	1
Unbleached White	⅓ cup (1.6 oz)	160	0	1
Whole Grain Wheat	¼ cup (1.6 oz)	160	0	1
Whole Wheat	¼ cup (1.2 oz)	130	0	1
Aunt Jemima				
Self-Rising	3 tbsp	90	0	0
Betty Crocker				
Softasilk Velvet Cake Flour	¼ cup (1 oz)	100	0	0
General Mills				
Wondra	¼ cup (1 oz)	100	0	0
Gold Medal				
All Purpose	¼ cup (1 oz)	100	0	0
Better For Bread	¼ cup (1 oz)	100	0	0
Better For Bread Wheat Blend	¼ cup (1 oz)	110	0	1
Self Rising	¼ cup (1 oz)	100	0	0
Supreme Hygluten	¼ cup (1 oz)	100	0	0
Unbleached	¼ cup (1 oz)	100	0	0
Hodgson Mill				
50/50 Flour	¼ cup (1 oz)	100	0	1
Best For Bread	¼ cup (1 oz)	100	0	0
Buckwheat	⅓ cup (1.6 oz)	160	0	1
Oat Bran Blend	¼ cup (1 oz)	110	0	1
Oat Bran Flour	¼ cup (1 oz)	110	1	2
Rye	¼ cup (1 oz)	90	0	1

FOOD	PORTION	CALS.	SAT. FAT	FAT
Hodgson Mill (CONT.)				
Seasoned Flour	¼ cup (1 oz)	90	0	0
White	¼ cup (1 oz)	100	0	0
Whole Wheat	¼ cup (1 oz)	100	0	1
King Arthur				
All Purpose Unbleached	¼ cup (1 oz)	100	0	0
La Pina				
Flour	¼ cup (1 oz)	100	0	0
Red Band				
All Purpose	¼ cup (1 oz)	100	0	0
Bread	¼ cup (1 oz)	100	0	0
Self-Rising	¼ cup (1 oz)	100	0	0
Robin Hood				
All Purpose	¼ cup (1 oz)	100	0	0
Self-Rising	¼ cup (1 oz)	100	0	0
Unbleached	¼ cup (1 oz)	100	0	0
Whole Wheat	¼ cup (1 oz)	90	0	1
Stone Ground Mills				
White Unbleached Organic	¼ cup (1.4 oz)	130	0	0
Whole Wheat 100% Stone Ground	3 tbsp (1 oz)	90	0	1

FRANKFURTER
(see HOT DOG)

FRENCH BEANS

dried cooked	1 cup	228	tr	1

FRENCH FRIES
(see POTATO)

FRENCH TOAST
FROZEN

french toast	1 slice (2 oz)	126	1	4
Aunt Jemima				
Cinnamon Swirl	2 pieces (4.1 oz)	240	2	6
Slices	2 pieces (4.1 oz)	240	2	6
Downyflake				
Extra Thick	1	150	—	9
French Toast	2 slices	270	—	12
Texas Style & Sausage	1 pkg (4.25 oz)	400	—	24
Quaker				
French Toast Sticks & Syrup	1 pkg (5.2 oz)	400	—	20
French Toast Wedges & Sausage	1 pkg (5.3 oz)	360	—	17

FOOD	PORTION	CALS.	SAT. FAT	FAT
HOME RECIPE				
as prep w/ 2% milk	1 slice	149	2	7
as prep w/ whole milk	1 slice	151	2	7
TAKE-OUT				
sticks	5 (4.9 oz)	513	5	29
w/ butter	2 slices (4.7 oz)	356	8	19
FROSTING				
(see CAKE ICING)				
FRUCTOSE				
Estee				
Fructose	1 tsp	15	0	0
Packet	1 pkg	10	0	0
FRUIT DRINKS				
(see also INDIVIDUAL NAMES, LEMONADE)				
FROZEN				
citrus juice drink as prep	1 cup	114	0	0
citrus juice drink not prep	1 can (12 fl oz)	684	tr	tr
fruit punch as prep w/water	1 cup	113	tr	tr
fruit punch not prep	1 can (12 fl oz)	678	tr	tr
limeade	1 can (6 oz)	408	tr	tr
limeade as prep w/ water	1 cup	102	tr	tr
Bright & Early				
Fruit Punch	8 fl oz	130	0	0
Five Alive				
Berry Citrus	8 fl oz	120	0	0
Citrus	8 fl oz	120	0	0
Tropical Citrus	8 fl oz	120	0	0
Minute Maid				
Berry Punch	8 fl oz	130	0	0
Citrus Punch	8 fl oz	120	0	0
Fruit Punch	8 fl oz	120	0	0
Limeade	8 fl oz	100	0	0
Pineapple Orange	8 fl oz	120	0	0
Tropical Punch	8 fl oz	120	0	0
Seneca				
Cranberry-Apple Juice Cocktail frzn as prep	8 fl oz	140	0	0
Raspberry-Cranberry Juice Cocktail frzn as prep	8 fl oz	140	0	0
MIX				
fruit punch as prep w/water	9 oz	97	0	0
Crystal Light				
Fruit Punch as prep	1 serv (8 oz)	5	0	0

FOOD	PORTION	CALS.	SAT. FAT	FAT
Crystal Light (CONT.)				
Lemon-Lime Drink as prep	1 serv (8 oz)	5	0	0
Passion Fruit Pineapple Drink as prep	1 serv (8 oz)	5	0	0
Pineapple Orange Drink as prep	1 serv (8 oz)	5	0	0
Strawberry Orange Banana as prep	1 serv (8 oz)	5	0	0
Strawberry Kiwi as prep	1 serv (8 oz)	5	0	0
Watermelon Strawberry as prep	1 serv (8 oz)	5	0	0
Kool-Aid				
Cherry as prep	1 serv (8 oz)	60	0	0
Grape Berry Splash Drink as prep	1 serv (8 oz)	70	0	0
Grape Berry Splash Drink as prep w/ sugar	1 serv (8 oz)	100	0	0
Kickin' Kiwi Lime Drink as prep	1 serv (8 oz)	60	0	0
Kickin' Kiwi Lime Drink as prep w/ sugar	1 serv (8 oz)	100	0	0
Lemon-Lime Drink as prep w/ sugar	1 serv (8 oz)	100	0	0
Man-O-Mango Berry Drink as prep w/ sugar	1 serv (8 oz)	100	0	0
Mon-O-Mango Berry Drink as prep	1 serv (8 oz)	60	0	0
Oh Yeah Orange Pineapple Drink as prep w/ sugar	1 serv (8 oz)	100	0	0
Oh Yeah Orange Pineapple Drink as prep	1 serv (8 oz)	60	0	0
Pina-Pineapple Drink as prep	1 serv (8 oz)	60	0	0
Pina-Pineapple Drink as prep w/ sugar	1 serv (8 oz)	100	0	0
Rainbow Punch	8 oz	98	0	0
Roarin' Raspberry Cranberry Drink as prep	1 serv (8 oz)	70	0	0
Roarin' Raspberry Cranberry Drink as prep w/ sugar	1 serv (8 oz)	100	0	0
Slammin' Strawberry Kiwi Drink as prep	1 serv (8 oz)	70	0	0
Slammin' Strawberry Kiwi Drink as prep w/ sugar	1 serv (8 oz)	100	0	0

FOOD	PORTION	CALS.	SAT. FAT	FAT
Kool-Aid (CONT.)				
Strawberry Raspberry Drink as prep	1 serv (8 oz)	60	0	0
Strawberry Raspberry Drink as prep w/ sugar	1 serv (8 oz)	100	0	0
Sugar Free Tropical Punch as prep	1 serv (8 oz)	5	0	0
Tropical Punch as prep	1 serv (8 oz)	60	0	0
Tropical Punch as prep w/ sugar	1 serv (8 oz)	100	0	0
Watermelon Cherry Drink as prep	1 serv (8 oz)	60	0	0
Watermelon Cherry Drink as prep w/ sugar	1 serv (8 oz)	100	0	0
Tang				
Orange Pineapple as prep	1 serv (8 oz)	100	0	0
READY-TO-DRINK				
cranberry apple drink	6 fl oz	123	—	0
cranberry apricot drink	6 fl oz	118	0	0
fruit punch	6 fl oz	87	0	tr
orange grapefruit juice	8 fl oz	107	tr	tr
orange & apricot	8 fl oz	128	tr	tr
pineapple & grapefruit	8 fl oz	117	tr	tr
pineapple & orange drink	8 fl oz	125	0	0
After The Fall				
Amaretto Almond	1 can (12 oz)	170	0	0
American Pie Cherry	1 can (12 oz)	190	0	0
Apple Apricot	1 cup (8 oz)	100	0	0
Apple Raspberry	1 bottle (10 oz)	110	0	0
Apple Strawberry	1 bottle (10 oz)	120	0	0
Banana Casablanca	1 bottle (10 oz)	120	0	0
Berrymeister	1 can (12 oz)	160	0	0
Cranberry Meets Raspberry	1 bottle (10 oz)	120	0	0
Georgia Peach Blend	1 bottle (10 oz)	130	0	0
Mango Montage	1 bottle (10 oz)	140	0	0
Maui Grove	1 bottle (10 oz)	120	0	0
Nantucket Ginger Ale	1 can (12 oz)	140	0	0
Orange Icicle Cream	1 can (12 oz)	170	0	0
Oregon Berry	1 bottle (10 oz)	130	0	0
Passion Of The Islands	1 bottle (10 oz)	125	0	0
Peach Vanilla	1 can (12 oz)	170	0	0
Strawberry Vanilla	1 can (12 oz)	160	0	0
Twist O' Strawberry	1 can (12 oz)	190	0	0
Vanilla Bean Cream	1 can (12 oz)	170	0	0

FOOD	PORTION	CALS.	SAT. FAT	FAT
Apple & Eve				
Apple Cranberry	6 fl oz	80	0	0
Apple Grape	6 fl oz	120	0	0
Cranberry Grape	6 fl oz	100	0	0
Fruit Punch	6 fl oz	78	0	0
Raspberry Cranberry	6 fl oz	90	0	0
BAMA				
Fruit Punch	8.45 fl oz	130	0	0
Boku				
White Grape Raspberry	16 fl oz	120	0	0
Capri Sun				
Fruit Punch	1 pkg (7 oz)	100	0	0
Maui Punch	1 pkg (7 oz)	100	0	0
Mountain Cooler	1 pkg (7 oz)	90	0	0
Pacific Cooler	1 pkg (7 oz)	100	0	0
Red Berry	1 pkg (7 oz)	100	0	0
Safari Punch	1 pkg (7 oz)	100	0	0
Strawberry Kiwi Drink	1 pkg (7 oz)	100	0	0
Surfer Cooler Drink	1 pkg (7 oz)	100	0	0
Citrus Squeeze				
California Punch	8 oz	130	0	0
Florida Punch	8 oz	120	0	0
Coco Lopez				
Mango Kiwi	8 fl oz	130	0	0
Crystal Geyser				
Juice Squeeze Citrus Grape	1 bottle (12 fl oz)	145	0	0
Juice Squeeze Orange & Passion Fruit	1 bottle (12 fl oz)	130	0	0
Juice Squeeze Passion Fruit & Mango	1 bottle (12 fl oz)	125	0	0
Juice Squeeze Wild Berry	1 bottle (12 fl oz)	130	0	0
Crystal Light				
Fruit Punch	1 serv (8 oz)	5	0	0
Kiwi Strawberry	1 serv (8 oz)	5	0	0
Orange Strawberry Banana Drink	1 serv (8 oz)	5	0	0
Dole				
Apple Berry Burst	8 fl oz	120	0	0
Cranberry Apple	8 fl oz	120	0	0
Fruit Fiesta	8 fl oz	140	0	0
Fruit Punch	1 carton (10 oz)	160	0	0
Mountain Cherry	8 fl oz	150	0	0
Orange Peach Mango	8 oz	120	0	0
Orange Strawberry Banana	8 oz	120	0	0

FOOD	PORTION	CALS.	SAT. FAT	FAT
Dole (CONT.)				
Orchard Peach	8 oz	140	0	0
Pineapple Orange	8 oz	120	0	0
Pineapple Orange Strawberry	8 oz	130	0	0
Tropical Fruit	8 oz	160	0	0
Everfresh				
Cranberry-Apple Drink	1 can (8 oz)	120	0	0
Grape-Strawberry	1 can (8 oz)	120	0	0
Kiwi-Strawberry	1 can (8 oz)	120	0	0
Mandarin Orange Mango Drink	1 can (8 oz)	120	0	0
Orange Banana Strawberry Drink	1 can (8 oz)	120	0	0
Tropical Fruit Punch	1 can (8 oz)	120	0	0
Wild Blackberry Lime Drink	1 can (8 oz)	120	0	0
Five Alive				
Citrus	6 fl oz	90	0	0
Citrus	1 bottle (16 fl oz)	120	0	0
Citrus	1 can (11.5 fl oz)	170	0	0
Citrus Chilled	8 fl oz	120	0	0
Fresh Samantha				
Banana Strawberry	1 cup (8 oz)	148	tr	1
Beta Yet	1 cup (8 oz)	98	0	1
Carrot Orange	1 cup (8 oz)	107	0	1
Colossal C	1 cup (8 oz)	116	0	0
Desperately Seeking C	1 cup (8 oz)	129	tr	1
Protein Blast	1 cup (8 oz)	156	tr	1
Spirulina Fruit Blend	1 cup (8 oz)	129	0	1
Strawberry Orange	1 cup (8 oz)	120	0	1
The Big Bang	1 cup (8 oz)	97	0	1
Fruitopia				
Fruit Integration	8 fl oz	110	0	0
Hi-C				
Boppin Berry Box	8.45 fl oz	140	0	0
Boppin' Berry	8 fl oz	130	0	0
Double Fruit Box	8.45 fl oz	130	0	0
Double Fruit Cooler	8 fl oz	130	0	0
Ecto Cooler	8 fl oz	130	0	0
Ecto Cooler	1 can (11.5 fl oz)	180	0	0
Ecto Cooler Box	8.45 fl oz	130	0	0
Fruit Punch	8 fl oz	130	0	0
Fruit Punch	1 can (11.5 fl oz)	190	0	0
Fruit Punch Box	8.45 fl oz	140	0	0
Fruity Bubble Gum	8 fl oz	120	0	0

FOOD	PORTION	CALS.	SAT. FAT	FAT
Hi-C (CONT.)				
Fruity Bubble Gum Box	8.45 fl oz	130	0	0
Hula Punch	8 fl oz	120	0	0
Hula Punch	1 can (11.5 fl oz)	170	0	0
Hula Punch Box	8.45 fl oz	120	0	0
Jammin' Apple Box	8.45 fl oz	130	0	0
Stompin' Banana Berry	8 fl oz	130	0	0
Stompin' Banana Berry Box	8.45 fl oz	130	0	0
Wild Berry	8 fl oz	120	0	0
Wild Berry Box	8.45 fl oz	130	0	0
Hood				
Natural Blenders Apple Cranberry Raspberry	1 cup (8 oz)	130	0	0
Natural Blenders Apple Grape Cherry	1 cup (8 oz)	130	0	0
Natural Blenders Apple Peach Pear	1 cup (8 oz)	120	0	0
Natural Blenders Apple Wild Blueberry Strawberry	1 cup (8 oz)	120	0	0
Natural Blenders Pineapple Orange Kiwi	1 cup (8 oz)	120	0	0
Juicy Juice				
Apple Grape	1 box (8.45 fl oz)	120	0	0
Berry	1 box (8.45 fl oz)	130	0	0
Berry	1 bottle (6 fl oz)	90	0	0
Punch	1 box (8.45 fl oz)	140	0	0
Punch	1 bottle (6 fl oz)	100	0	0
Tropical	1 bottle (6 fl oz)	110	0	0
Tropical	1 box (8.45 fl oz)	150	0	0
Kern's				
Apple Strawberry Nectar	6 fl oz	110	0	0
Apricot Pineapple Nectar	6 fl oz	110	0	0
Banana Pineapple Nectar	6 fl oz	110	0	0
Coconut Pineapple Nectar	6 fl oz	140	0	0
Orange Banana Nectar	6 fl oz	110	0	0
Strawberry Banana Nectar	6 fl oz	110	0	0
Tropical Nectar	6 fl oz	110	0	0
Kool-Aid				
Bursts Great Bluedini	1 (7 oz)	100	0	0
Bursts Kickin' Kiwi Lime	1 (7 oz)	100	0	0
Bursts Oh Yeah Orange Pineapple	1 (7 oz)	100	0	0
Bursts Slammin' Strawberry Kiwi	1 (7 oz)	100	0	0

FOOD	PORTION	CALS.	SAT. FAT	FAT
Kool-Aid (CONT.)				
Bursts Tropical Punch	1 (7 oz)	100	0	0
Splash Grape Berry Punch	1 serv (8 oz)	120	0	0
Splash Kiwi Strawberry Drink	1 serv (8 oz)	110	0	0
Splash Tropical Punch	1 serv (8 oz)	120	0	0
Libby				
Strawberry Banana Nectar	1 can (11.5 fl oz)	220	0	0
Mauna La'i				
Island Guava	8 oz	130	0	0
Paradise Passion	8 oz	130	0	0
Minute Maid				
Berry Punch Box	8.45 fl oz	130	0	0
Berry Punch Chilled	8 fl oz	130	0	0
Citrus Punch Chilled	8 fl oz	130	0	0
Fruit Punch Box	8.45 fl oz	120	0	0
Fruit Punch Chilled	8 fl oz	120	0	0
Juices To Go Citrus Punch	1 can (11.5 fl oz)	180	0	0
Juices To Go Citrus Punch	1 bottle (10 oz)	160	0	0
Juices To Go Concord Punch	1 can (11.5 fl oz)	180	0	0
Juices To Go Concord Punch	1 bottle (10 oz)	160	0	0
Juices To Go Concord Punch	1 bottle (16 fl oz)	130	0	0
Juices To Go Fruit Punch	1 can (11.5 fl oz)	180	0	0
Juices To Go Fruit Punch	1 bottle (10 oz)	160	0	0
Juices To Go Fruit Punch	1 bottle (16 fl oz)	120	0	0
Juices To Go Orange Blend	1 bottle (10 oz)	150	0	0
Juices To Go Orange Blend	1 can (11.5 fl oz)	170	0	0
Naturals Apple Cranberry	8 fl oz	170	0	0
Naturals Concord Medley	8 fl oz	130	0	0
Naturals Fruit Medley	8 fl oz	120	0	0
Naturals Orange Grape Medley	8 fl oz	120	0	0
Naturals Tropical Medley	8 fl oz	120	0	0
Tropical Punch Box	8.45 fl oz	130	0	0
Tropical Punch Chilled	8 fl oz	120	0	0
Mott's				
Apple Cranberry Blend	10 fl oz	180	0	0
Apple Cranberry From Concentrate as prep	8 fl oz	120	0	0
Apple Grape From Concentrate as prep	8 fl oz	120	0	0
Apple Raspberry Blend	10 fl oz	140	0	0

FOOD	PORTION	CALS.	SAT. FAT	FAT
Mott's (CONT.)				
Apple Raspberry From Concentrate	8.45 fl oz	120	0	0
Fruit Basket Apple Raspberry Juice Cocktail as prep	8 fl oz	130	0	0
Fruit Basket Tropical Blend Juice Cocktail as prep	8 fl oz	120	0	0
Fruit Punch From Concentrate	10 fl oz	170	0	0
Fruit Punch From Concentrate	8.45 fl oz	120	0	0
Grape Apple	10 fl oz	170	0	0
Pineapple Orange	10 fl oz	170	0	0
Nantucket Nectars				
Apple Raspberry	8 oz	140	0	0
California Melonberry	8 oz	110	0	0
Cranberry Apple	8 oz	140	0	0
Fruit Punch	8 oz	130	0	0
Kiwi Berry	8 oz	120	0	0
Orange Mango	8 oz	130	0	0
Pineapple Orange Banana	8 oz	140	0	0
Pineapple Orange Guava	8 oz	120	0	0
Watermelon Strawberry	8 oz	120	0	0
Ocean Spray				
Cran*Blueberry	8 oz	160	0	0
Cran*Cherry	8 oz	160	0	0
Cran*Currant	8 oz	140	0	0
Cran*Grape	8 oz	170	0	0
Cran*Mango	8 oz	130	0	0
Cran*Raspberry	8 oz	140	0	0
Cran*Raspberry Reduced Calorie	8 oz	50	0	0
Cran*Strawberry	8 oz	140	0	0
Cran*Tangerine	8 oz	130	0	0
Cranapple	8 oz	160	0	0
Cranapple Reduced Calorie	8 oz	50	0	0
Cranicot	8 oz	160	0	0
Crazy Kiwi Passion	8 oz	130	0	0
Fruit Punch	8 oz	130	0	0
Kiwi Strawberry	8 oz	120	0	0
Lightstyle Cran*Grape	8 oz	40	0	0
Lightstyle Cran*Mango	8 oz	40	0	0
Lightstyle Cran*Raspberry	8 oz	40	0	0
Mandarin Magic	8 oz	120	0	0

FOOD	PORTION	CALS.	SAT. FAT	FAT
Ocean Spray (CONT.)				
Ruby Red & Tangerine Grapefruit	8 oz	130	0	0
Ruby Red & Mango	8 oz	130	0	0
Odwalla				
Boyzenberry Mango	8 fl oz	140	0	0
C Monster	16 fl oz	300	0	0
Fruitshake Blackberry	8 fl oz	160	0	0
Guanaba Dabba Doo!	8 fl oz	130	0	0
Lotta Colada	8 fl oz	160	—	3
Mango Tango	8 fl oz	150	—	3
Mo Beta	16 fl oz	280	—	1
Raspberry Smoothie	8 fl oz	140	0	0
Strawberry Banana Smoothie	8 fl oz	100	0	0
Strawberry Go Man Go	8 fl oz	100	—	1
Super Protein	16 fl oz	400	—	6
Pek				
Mango Guava Ecstasy	1 bottle (20 fl oz)	110	0	0
Passionate Peach Grapefruit	8 fl oz	110	0	0
Shasta Plus				
Apple-Strawberry	1 can (11.5 oz)	160	0	0
Fruit Punch	1 can (11.5 oz)	160	0	0
Pineapple-Cherry	1 can (11.5 oz)	160	0	0
Sipps				
Fruit Punch	8.45 oz	130	—	0
Snapple				
Diet Cranberry Raspberry	8 fl oz	10	0	0
Diet Kiwi Strawberry	8 fl oz	13	0	0
Fruit Punch	8 fl oz	120	0	0
Kiwi Strawberry	8 fl oz	110	0	0
Vitamin Supreme	10 fl oz	150	0	0
Squeezit				
Berry B. Wild	1 bottle (7 oz)	110	0	0
Blue Raspberry	1 bottle (7 oz)	110	0	0
Cherry Cola	1 bottle (7 oz)	110	0	0
Chucklin' Cherry	1 bottle (7 oz)	110	0	0
Green Apple	1 bottle (7 oz)	110	0	0
Grumpy Grape	1 bottle (7 oz)	110	0	0
Lemon Lime	1 bottle (7 oz)	110	0	0
Rockin' Red Puncher	1 bottle (7 oz)	110	0	0
Smarty Arty Orange	1 bottle (7 oz)	110	0	0
Strawberry	1 bottle (7 oz)	110	0	0
Tropical Punch	1 bottle (7 oz)	110	0	0
Watermelon	1 bottle (7 oz)	110	0	0

FOOD	PORTION	CALS.	SAT. FAT	FAT
Sunny Delight				
Drink	6 fl oz	90	—	0
Tropicana				
Berry Punch	8 fl oz	130	0	0
Citrus Punch	8 fl oz	140	0	0
Fruit Punch	8 oz	130	0	0
Fruit Punch	1 container (10 fl oz)	160	0	0
Orange Pineapple	8 fl oz	110	0	0
Tangerine Orange Juice	8 fl oz	110	0	0
Tropics Orange Strawberry Banana	8 fl oz	110	0	0
Tropics Orange Kiwi Passion	8 fl oz	100	0	0
Tropics Orange Peach Mango	8 fl oz	110	0	0
Tropics Orange Pineapple	8 fl oz	110	0	0
Twister Apple Raspberry Blackberry	1 bottle (10 fl oz)	160	—	1
Twister Citrus Punch	1 bottle (10 oz)	180	0	0
Twister Cranberry Punch	1 bottle (10 oz)	170	0	0
Twister Fruit Punch	1 bottle (10 oz)	170	0	0
Twister Light Orange Strawberry Banana	1 bottle (10 oz)	45	0	0
Twister Orange Cranberry	1 bottle (10 fl oz)	160	0	0
Twister Orange Strawberry Banana	1 bottle (10 oz)	160	0	0
Twister Ruby Red Tangerine	1 bottle (10 oz)	160	0	0
Twister Strawberry Kiwi	1 bottle (10 oz)	160	0	0
V8				
Splash Berry Blend	8 oz	110	0	0
Veryfine				
Apple Cherryberry	8 fl oz	130	0	0
Apple Cranberry	1 bottle (10 oz)	190	0	0
Apple Quenchers Black Cherry White Grape	8 fl oz	120	0	0
Apple Quenchers Cranberry Tangerine	8 fl oz	120	0	0
Apple Quenchers Peach Kiwi	8 fl oz	130	0	0
Apple Quenchers Peach Plum	8 fl oz	130	0	0
Apple Quenchers Pear Passionfruit	8 fl oz	120	0	0
Apple Quenchers Raspberry Cherry	8 fl oz	120	0	0
Apple Quenchers Raspberry Lime	8 fl oz	120	0	0
Apple Quenchers Strawberry Banana	8 fl oz	120	0	0

FOOD	PORTION	CALS.	SAT. FAT	FAT
Veryfine (CONT.)				
Chillers Artic Mango Tangerine	8 fl oz	110	0	0
Chillers Freezing Fruit Punch	8 fl oz	130	0	0
Chillers Lemon Lime Blizzard	8 fl oz	120	0	0
Chillers Shivering Strawberry Melon	1 can (11.5 oz)	160	0	0
Chillers Tropical Freeze	8 fl oz	120	0	0
Cranberry Raspberry	8 fl oz	160	0	0
Fruit Punch	1 bottle (10 oz)	170	0	0
Juice-Ups Berry	8 fl oz	140	0	0
Juice-Ups Fruit Punch	8 fl oz	140	0	0
Juice-Ups Orange Punch	8 fl oz	140	0	0
Orange Strawberry	8 fl oz	120	0	0
Papaya Punch	1 bottle (10 oz)	160	0	0
Pineapple Orange	1 bottle (10 oz)	160	0	0
Strawberry Banana	1 can (11.5 oz)	160	0	0
Strawberry Banana Punch	1 can (11.5 oz)	190	0	0
Wellfleet Farms				
Cranberry & Georgia Peach	8 oz	140	0	0
Cranberry & Granny Smith Apple	8 oz	130	0	0
Cranberry & Key Lime	8 oz	140	0	0

FRUIT MIXED

(see also INDIVIDUAL NAMES)

CANNED

FOOD	PORTION	CALS.	SAT. FAT	FAT
fruit cocktail in heavy syrup	½ cup	93	tr	tr
fruit cocktail juice pack	½ cup	56	tr	tr
fruit cocktail water pack	½ cup	40	tr	tr
fruit salad in heavy sirup	½ cup	94	tr	tr
fruit salad in light syrup	½ cup	73	tr	tr
fruit salad juice pack	½ cup	62	tr	tr
fruit salad water pack	½ cup	37	tr	tr
mixed fruit in heavy syrup	½ cup	92	tr	tr
tropical fruit salad in heavy sirup	½ cup	110	—	tr
Del Monte				
Fruit Cocktail Fruit Naturals	½ cup (4.4 oz)	60	0	0
Fruit Cocktail In Heavy Syrup	½ cup (4.5 oz)	100	0	0
Fruit Cocktail Lite	½ cup (4.4 oz)	60	0	0
Lite Mixed Fruits Chunky	½ cup (4.4 oz)	60	0	0
Mixed Fruits Chunky Fruit Naturals	½ cup (4.4 oz)	60	0	0
Mixed Fruits Chunky In Heavy Syrup	½ cup (4.5 oz)	100	0	0

FOOD	PORTION	CALS.	SAT. FAT	FAT
Del Monte (CONT.)				
Orchard Select California Mixed	½ cup (4.4 oz)	80	0	0
Snack Cups Mixed Fruit Fruit Naturals	1 serv (4.5 oz)	60	0	0
Snack Cups Mixed Fruit Fruit Naturals EZ-Open Lid	1 serv (4.5 oz)	60	0	0
Snack Cups Mixed Fruit In Heavy Syrup	1 serv (4.5 oz)	100	0	0
Snack Cups Mixed Fruit In Heavy Syrup EZ-Open Lid	1 serv (4.2 oz)	90	0	0
Snack Cups Mixed Fruit Lite	1 serv (4.5 oz)	60	0	0
Snack Cups Mixed Fruit Lite EZ-Open Lid	1 serv (4.5 oz)	60	0	0
Dole				
Tropical Fruit Salad	½ cup	70	—	0
Hunt's				
Fruit Cocktail	½ cup (4.5 oz)	90	0	0
Libby				
Chunky Mixed Lite	½ cup (4.3 oz)	60	0	0
Fruit Cocktail Lite	½ cup (4.3 oz)	60	0	0
Mott's				
Fruitsations Mixed Berry	1 pkg (4 oz)	90	0	0
Ocean Spray				
Cran*Fruit Cranberry Raspberry	¼ cup	120	0	0
Cran*Fruit Cranberry Strawberry	¼ cup	120	0	0
DRIED				
mixed	11 oz pkg	712	tr	1
Del Monte				
Mixed	⅓ cup (1.4 oz)	110	0	0
Paradise				
Old English Fruit & Peel Mix	1 tbsp (0.8 oz)	70	0	0
Planters				
Fruit'n Nut Mix	1 oz	140	2	9
Sonoma				
Diced	⅓ cup (1.4 oz)	120	0	0
Mixed Fruit	5–8 pieces (1.4 oz)	120	0	0
FROZEN				
mixed fruit sweetened	1 cup	245	tr	tr
Big Valley				
Burst O' Berries	⅔ cup (4.9 oz)	70	0	0
California Tropics	⅔ cup (4.9 oz)	60	0	0

FOOD	PORTION	CALS.	SAT. FAT	FAT
Big Valley (CONT.)				
Cup A Fruit	1 pkg (4 oz)	50	0	0
Mixed	4.9 oz	60	0	0
Birds Eye				
Mixed Fruit	½ cup (4.4 oz)	90	0	0

FRUIT SNACKS

FOOD	PORTION	CALS.	SAT. FAT	FAT
fruit leather	1 bar (0.8 oz)	81	1	1
fruit leather pieces	1 pkg (0.9 oz)	92	tr	2
fruit leather pieces	1 oz	97	tr	2
fruit leather rolls	1 lg (0.7 oz)	73	tr	1
fruit leather rolls	1 sm (0.5 oz)	49	tr	tr
Betty Crocker				
Fruit By The Foot All Flavors	1 roll (0.9 oz)	80	1	2
Fruit Gushers All Flavors	1 pkg (0.9 oz)	90	0	1
Fruit Roll-Ups All Flavors	1 (0.5 oz)	50	0	1
Fruit String Thing All Flavors	1 pkg (0.7 oz)	80	0	1
Brock				
Beauty & The Beast	1 pkg (0.9 oz)	90	0	0
Cinderella	1 pkg (0.9 oz)	90	0	0
Dinosaurs	1 pkg (0.9 oz)	90	0	0
Ninja Trolls	1 pkg (0.9 oz)	90	0	0
Sharks	1 pkg (0.9 oz)	90	0	0
Del Monte				
Sierra Trail Mix	¼ cup (1.2 oz)	150	3	8
Sierra Trail Mix	1 pkg (1 oz)	120	2	6
Sierra Trail Mix	1 pkg (0.9 oz)	110	2	6
Favorite Brands				
Cherry Fruit Snack	1 pkg (0.9 oz)	80	0	0
Creepy Crawler Fruit Snacks	1 pkg (0.9 oz)	80	0	0
Dinosaur Fruit Snack	1 pkg (0.9 oz)	80	0	0
Grape Fruit Snack	1 pkg (0.9 oz)	80	0	0
Space Alien Fruit Snack	1 pkg (0.9 oz)	80	0	0
Sports Fruit Snacks	1 pkg (0.9 oz)	80	0	0
Strawberry Fruit Snack	1 pkg (0.9 oz)	80	0	0
Teenage Mutant Ninja Turtle Fruit Snacks	1 pkg (0.9 oz)	80	0	0
The Mega Roll Strawberry	1 pkg (1 oz)	110	2	3
The Roll Cherry	1 pkg (0.75 oz)	80	1	2
The Roll Strawberry	1 pkg (0.75 oz)	80	1	2
Troll Fruit Snacks	1 pkg (0.9 oz)	80	0	0
Zoo Animal Fruit Snacks	1 pkg (0.9 oz)	80	0	0
General Mills				
Fruit Snacks All Flavors	1 pkg (0.9 oz)	80	0	0

FOOD	PORTION	CALS.	SAT. FAT	FAT
Health Valley				
Bakes Apple	1 bar	70	0	0
Bakes Date	1 bar	70	0	0
Bakes Raisin	1 bar	70	0	0
Fruit Bars Apple	1	140	0	0
Fruit Bars Apricot	1	140	0	0
Fruit Bars Date	1	140	0	0
Fruit Bars Raisin	1	140	0	0
Seneca				
Apple Chips	12 chips (1 oz)	140	1	7
Sensible Foods				
Crackin' Fruit Cherry Berry	1 pkg (0.6 oz)	51	0	0
Crackin' Fruit Tropical Fruit	1 pkg (0.6 oz)	65	0	1
Sonoma				
Trail Mix	¼ cup (1.4 oz)	160	3	7
Sovex				
Fruit Bites Jungle Pals	1 pkg (0.9 oz)	90	—	1
Stretch Island				
Fruit Leather Berry Blackberry	2 pieces (1 oz)	90	0	0
Fruit Leather Chunky Cherry	2 pieces (1 oz)	90	0	0
Fruit Leather Great Grape	2 pieces (1 oz)	90	0	0
Fruit Leather Organic Apple	2 pieces (1 oz)	90	0	0
Fruit Leather Organic Grape	2 pieces (1 oz)	90	0	0
Fruit Leather Organic Raspberry	2 pieces (1 oz)	90	0	0
Fruit Leather Rare Raspberry	2 pieces (1 oz)	90	0	0
Fruit Leather Snappy Apple	2 pieces (1 oz)	90	0	0
Fruit Leather Tangy Apricot	2 pieces (1 oz)	90	0	0
Fruit Leather Truly Tropical	2 pieces (1 oz)	90	0	0
Sunbelt				
Fruit Jammers	1 pkg (1 oz)	100	1	1
Sunkist				
100% Fruit Roll All Flavors	1 (0.5 oz)	50	0	0
Weight Watchers				
Apple & Cinnamon	1 pkg (0.5 oz)	50	0	0
Apple Chips	1 pkg (0.75 oz)	70	0	0
Peach & Strawberry	1 pkg (0.5 oz)	50	0	0

GARBANZO

(see CHICKPEAS)

GARLIC

clove	1	4	tr	tr
powder	1 tsp	9	—	tr

FOOD	PORTION	CALS.	SAT. FAT	FAT
Watkins				
Garlic & Chive Seasoning	1 tbsp (7 g)	25	0	2
Garlic Lover's Herb Blend	¼ tsp (0.5 oz)	0	0	0
Liquid Spice	1 tbsp (0.5 oz)	120	2	14
GEFILTE FISH				
sweet	1 piece (1.5 oz)	35	tr	1
GELATIN				
MIX				
low calorie	½ cup	8	0	0
mix artifically sweetened as prep	½ cup (4.1 oz)	8	—	0
mix artifically sweetened as prep	1 pkg 4 serv (16.5 oz)	33	—	0
mix as prep	½ cup (4.7 oz)	80	0	0
mix as prep	1 pkg 4 serv (19 oz)	319	0	0
mix not prep	1 pkg (3 oz)	324	0	0
mix w/ fruit as prep	½ cup (3.7 oz)	73	—	tr
mix w/ fruit as prep	1 pkg 8 serv (19 oz)	588	—	2
powder unsweetened	1 pkg (7 g)	23	tr	0
powder unsweetened	1 oz	94	tr	0
Emes				
Kosher-Jel	½ cup (4 fl oz)	60	0	0
Kosher-Jel Plain	1 tbsp (7 g)	21	0	0
Jell-O				
1-2-3-Brand Strawberry as prep	⅔ cup (5.2 oz)	130	1	2
Apricot as prep	½ cup (5 oz)	80	0	0
Berry Black as prep	½ cup (5 oz)	80	0	0
Berry Blue as prep	½ cup (5 oz)	80	0	0
Black Cherry as prep	½ cup (5 oz)	80	0	0
Cherry as prep	½ cup (5 oz)	80	0	0
Cranberry Raspberry as prep	½ cup (5 oz)	80	0	0
Cranberry Strawberry as prep	½ cup (5 oz)	80	0	0
Cranberry as prep	½ cup (5 oz)	80	0	0
Grape as prep	½ cup (5 oz)	80	0	0
Lemon as prep	½ cup (5 oz)	80	0	0
Lime as prep	½ cup (5 oz)	80	0	0
Mango as prep	½ cup (5 oz)	80	0	0
Mixed Fruit as prep	½ cup (5 oz)	80	0	0
Orange as prep	½ cup (5 oz)	80	0	0
Peach as prep	½ cup (5 oz)	80	0	0
Peach Passion Fruit as prep	½ cup (5 oz)	80	0	0
Pineapple as prep	½ cup (5 oz)	80	0	0
Raspberry as prep	½ cup (5 oz)	80	0	0

FOOD	PORTION	CALS.	SAT. FAT	FAT
Jell-O (CONT.)				
Sparkling White Grape as prep	½ cup (5 oz)	80	0	0
Strawberry Banana as prep	½ cup (5 oz)	80	0	0
Strawberry Kiwi as prep	½ cup (5 oz)	80	0	0
Strawberry as prep	½ cup (5 oz)	80	0	0
Sugar Free Cherry as prep	½ cup (4.2 oz)	10	0	0
Sugar Free Cranberry as prep	½ cup (4.2 oz)	10	0	0
Sugar Free Lemon	½ cup (4.2 oz)	10	0	0
Sugar Free Lime as prep	½ cup (4.2 oz)	10	0	0
Sugar Free Mixed Fruit as prep	½ cup (4.2 oz)	10	0	0
Sugar Free Orange as prep	½ cup (4.2 oz)	10	0	0
Sugar Free Raspberry as prep	½ cup (4.2 oz)	10	0	0
Sugar Free Strawberry Banana as prep	½ cup (4.2 oz)	10	0	0
Sugar Free Strawberry as prep	½ cup (4.2 oz)	10	0	0
Sugar Free Strawberry Kiwi as prep	½ cup (4.2 oz)	10	0	0
Sugar Free Watermelon as prep	½ cup (4.2 oz)	10	0	0
Watermelon as prep	½ cup (5 oz)	80	0	0
Wild Strawberry as prep	½ cup (5 oz)	80	0	0
Kojel				
Diet	1 serv	10	—	tr
Royal				
Apple	½ cup	80	0	0
Blackberry	½ cup	80	0	0
Cherry	½ cup	80	0	0
Cherry Sugar Free	½ cup	8	0	0
Concord Grape	½ cup	80	0	0
Fruit Punch	½ cup	80	0	0
Lemon	½ cup	80	0	0
Lemon-Lime	½ cup	80	0	0
Lime	½ cup	80	0	0
Lime Sugar Free	½ cup	8	0	0
Mixed Berry	½ cup	80	0	0
Orange	½ cup	80	0	0
Orange Sugar Free	½ cup	10	0	0
Peach	½ cup	80	0	0
Pineapple	½ cup	80	0	0
Raspberry	½ cup	80	0	0

FOOD	PORTION	CALS.	SAT. FAT	FAT
Royal (CONT.)				
Raspberry Sugar Free	½ cup	8	0	0
Strawberry	½ cup	80	0	0
Strawberry Banana Sugar Free	½ cup	8	0	0
Strawberry Orange	½ cup	80	0	0
Strawberry Sugar Free	½ cup	8	0	0
Tropical Fruit	½ cup	80	0	0
READY-TO-EAT				
Del Monte				
Gel Snack Cups Blue Berry	1 serv (3.5 oz)	70	0	0
Gel Snack Cups Cherry	1 serv (3.5 oz)	70	0	0
Gel Snack Cups Orange	1 serv (3.5 oz)	70	0	0
Gel Snack Cups Strawberry	1 serv (3.5 oz)	70	0	0
Handi-Snacks				
Gels Blue Raspberry	1 serv (4 oz)	80	0	0
Gels Cherry	1 serv (4 oz)	80	0	0
Gels Orange	1 serv (3.5 oz)	80	0	0
Gels Strawberry	1 serv (3.5 oz)	80	0	0
Hunt's				
Snack Pack Juicy Gels Cherry	1 (4 oz)	100	0	0
Snack Pack Juicy Gels Lemon Lime	1 (4 oz)	100	0	0
Snack Pack Juicy Gels Mixed Fruit	1 (4 oz)	100	0	0
Snack Pack Juicy Gels Orange	1 (4 oz)	100	0	0
Snack Pack Juicy Gels Strawberry	1 (4 oz)	100	0	0
Jell-O				
Berry Black	1 serv (3.5 oz)	70	0	0
Berry Blue	1 serv (3.5 oz)	70	0	0
Cherry	1 serv (3.5 oz)	70	0	0
Orange	1 serv (3.5 oz)	70	0	0
Orange Strawberry Banana	1 serv (3.5 oz)	70	0	0
Raspberry	1 serv (3.5 oz)	70	0	0
Rhymin' Lymon	1 serv (3.5 oz)	70	0	0
Strawberry	1 serv (3.5 oz)	70	0	0
Strawberry Kiwi	1 serv (3.5 oz)	10	0	0
Sugar Free Orange	1 serv (3.2 oz)	10	0	0
Sugar Free Raspberry	1 serv (3.2 oz)	10	0	0
Sugar Free Strawberry	1 serv (3.2 oz)	10	0	0
Tropical Berry	1 serv (3.5 oz)	10	0	0
Tropical Fruit Punch	1 serv (3.5 oz)	70	0	0
Wild Watermelon	1 serv (3.5 oz)	70	0	0

FOOD	PORTION	CALS.	SAT. FAT	FAT
Kozy Shack				
Gel Treat Cherry	1 pkg (4 oz)	100	0	0
Gel Treat Lemon Lime	1 pkg (4 oz)	100	0	0
Gel Treat Orange	1 pkg (4 oz)	100	0	0
Gel Treat Strawberry	1 pkg (4 oz)	100	0	0
Gel Treat Sugar Free Orange	1 pkg (4 oz)	10	0	0
Gel Treat Sugar Free Strawberry	1 pkg (4 oz)	10	0	0
GIBLETS				
capon simmered	1 cup (5 oz)	238	3	8
chicken floured & fried	1 cup (5 oz)	402	6	19
chicken simmered	1 cup (5 oz)	228	2	7
turkey simmered	1 cup (5 oz)	243	2	7
GINGER				
ground	1 tsp (1.8 g)	6	tr	tr
root fresh	¼ cup	17	tr	tr
root fresh	5 slices	8	tr	tr
root fresh sliced	¼ cup	17	tr	tr
GINKGO NUTS				
canned	1 oz	32	tr	tr
dried	1 oz	99	tr	tr
raw	1 oz	52	tr	tr
GIZZARDS				
chicken simmered	1 cup (5 oz)	222	2	5
turkey simmered	1 cup (5 oz)	236	2	6
Shady Brook				
Turkey	4 oz	130	1	4
GOAT				
roasted	3 oz	122	1	3
GOOSE				
w/ skin roasted	½ goose (1.7 lbs)	2362	53	170
w/ skin roasted	6.6 oz	574	13	41
w/o skin roasted	5 oz	340	7	18
w/o skin roasted	½ goose (1.3 lbs)	1406	27	75
GOOSEBERRIES				
canned in light sirup	½ cup	93	tr	tr
fresh	1 cup	67	tr	1
GRANOLA				
(*see* CEREAL, CEREAL BARS)				

FOOD	PORTION	CALS.	SAT. FAT	FAT
GRAPE JUICE				
bottled	1 cup	155	tr	tr
frzn sweetened as prep	1 cup	128	tr	tr
frzn sweetened not prep	6 oz	386	tr	1
grape drink	6 oz	84	0	0
BAMA				
Juice	8.45 fl oz	120	0	0
Bright & Early				
Frozen	8 fl oz	140	0	0
Capri Sun				
Drink	1 pkg (7 oz)	100	0	0
Daily				
Drink	8 oz	110	0	0
Everfresh				
Juice	1 can (8 oz)	150	0	0
Hi-C				
Box	8.45 fl oz	130	0	0
Drink	8 fl oz	130	0	0
Drink	1 can (11.5 fl oz)	180	0	0
Juicy Juice				
Drink	1 bottle (6 fl oz)	90	0	0
Drink	1 box	130	0	0
Kool-Aid				
Bursts Grape Drink	1 (7 oz)	100	0	0
Drink as prep w/ sugar	1 serv (8 oz)	100	0	0
Drink Mix as prep	1 serv (8 oz)	60	0	0
Sugar Free Drink Mix as prep	1 serv (8 oz)	5	0	0
Minute Maid				
Chilled	8 fl oz	130	0	0
Grape Punch frzn	8 fl oz	130	0	0
Punch Chilled	8 fl oz	130	0	0
Mott's				
Drink	10 fl oz	170	0	0
Fruit Basket Cocktail as prep	8 fl oz	130	0	0
Nantucket Nectars				
100% Juice	8 oz	160	0	0
Grapeade	8 oz	130	0	0
Seneca				
Blush Grape Juice frzn as prep	8 fl oz	170	0	0
Fortified With Vitamin C frzn as prep	8 fl oz	170	0	0
Sweetened frzn as prep	8 fl oz	140	0	0

FOOD	PORTION	CALS.	SAT. FAT	FAT
Seneca (CONT.)				
White Grape Juice frzn as prep	8 fl oz	140	0	0
Shasta Plus				
Grape Drink	1 can (11.5 oz)	160	0	0
Sippin' Pak				
100% Pure	8.45 fl	130	0	0
Snapple				
Grapeade	8 fl oz	120	0	0
Veryfine				
100% Juice	1 bottle (10 oz)	200	0	0
Chillers Glacial Grape	1 can (11.5 oz)	160	0	0
Grape Drink	1 bottle (10 oz)	160	0	0
Juice-Ups	8 fl oz	130	0	0
GRAPE LEAVES				
canned	1 (4 g)	3	tr	tr
fresh raw	1 (3 g)	3	tr	tr
Cedar's				
Grape Leaves Stuffed With Rice	6 pieces (4.9 oz)	180	1	8
GRAPEFRUIT				
CANNED				
juice pack	½ cup	46	tr	tr
unsweetened	1 cup	93	tr	tr
water pack	½ cup	44	tr	tr
FRESH				
pink	½	37	tr	tr
pink sections	1 cup	69	tr	tr
red	½	37	tr	tr
red sections	1 cup	69	tr	tr
white	½	39	tr	tr
white sections	1 cup	76	tr	tr
Dole				
Grapefruit	½	50	—	0
Ocean Spray				
Fresh	2 oz	50	0	0
GRAPEFRUIT JUICE				
fresh	1 cup	96	tr	tr
frzn as prep	1 cup	102	tr	tr
frzn not prep	6 oz	302	tr	1
sweetened	1 cup	116	tr	tr
After The Fall				
Pink	1 bottle (10 oz)	100	0	0

FOOD	PORTION	CALS.	SAT. FAT	FAT
Apple & Eve				
Made In The Shade Ruby Red	8 fl oz	130	0	0
Crystal Geyser				
Juice Squeeze	1 bottle (12 fl oz)	150	0	0
Del Monte				
Juice	8 fl oz	100	0	0
Everfresh				
Juice	1 can (8 oz)	90	0	0
Ruby Red Cocktail	1 can (8 oz)	130	0	0
Fresh Samantha				
Juice	1 cup (8 oz)	101	0	0
Hood				
Select	1 cup (8 oz)	100	0	0
Minute Maid				
Frozen	8 fl oz	100	0	0
Juices To Go	1 can (11.5 fl oz)	140	0	0
Juices To Go	1 bottle (10 fl oz)	120	0	0
Juices To Go	1 bottle (16 fl oz)	100	0	0
Juices To Go Pink Cocktail	1 bottle (10 fl oz)	140	0	0
Juices To Go Pink Cocktail	1 bottle (16 fl oz)	110	0	0
Juices to Go Pink Cocktail	8 fl oz	160	0	0
Mott's				
From Concentrate as prep	8 fl oz	120	0	0
Nantucket Nectars				
100% Juice	8 oz	100	0	0
100% Ruby Red	8 oz	100	0	0
Ocean Spray				
100% Juice	8 oz	100	0	0
100% Juice Pink	8 oz	110	0	0
Ruby Red Drink	8 oz	130	0	0
Odwalla				
Juice	8 fl oz	90	0	0
Snapple				
Juice	10 fl oz	110	0	0
Pink Grapefruit Cocktail	8 fl oz	120	0	0
Tree Of Life				
Juice	8 fl oz	100	0	0
Tropicana				
Golden	8 oz	90	0	0
Ruby Red	8 oz	90	0	0
Season's Best	8 oz	90	0	0
Twister Pink	1 bottle (10 oz)	140	0	0
W/ Double Vitamin C	8 fl oz	110	0	0

FOOD	PORTION	CALS.	SAT. FAT	FAT
Veryfine				
100% Juice	1 bottle (10 oz)	110	0	0
Pink	1 bottle (10 oz)	150	0	0
Ruby Red	8 fl oz	120	0	0
GRAPES				
fresh	10	36	tr	tr
thompson seedless in heavy sirup	½ cup	94	tr	tr
thompson seedless water pack	½ cup	48	tr	tr
Dole				
Fresh	1½ cup	85	—	0
GRAVY				
(see also SAUCE)				
CANNED				
au jus	1 cup	38	tr	tr
beef	1 cup	124	3	6
chicken	1 cup	189	3	14
mushroom	1 cup	120	1	6
turkey	1 cup	122	1	5
Franco-American				
Au Jus	2 oz	10	—	0
Beef	2 oz	25	—	1
Chicken	2 oz	45	—	4
Chicken Giblet	2 oz	30	—	2
Cream	2 oz	35	—	2
Mushroom	2 oz	25	—	1
Pork	2 oz	40	—	3
Turkey	2 oz	30	—	2
Gravymaster				
Seasoning	¼ tsp	3	0	0
Rudy's Farm				
Sausage Gravy	¼ cup (2 oz)	50	1	1
MIX				
au jus as prep w/ water	1 cup	32	1	1
brown as prep w/ water	1 cup	75	1	2
chicken as prep	1 cup	83	1	2
mushroom as prep	1 cup	70	1	2
pork as prep	1 cup	76	1	2
turkey as prep	1 cup	87	1	2
Cajun King				
Oil-Less Roux And Gravy Mix	3.5 oz	394	—	4
Durkee				
Au Jus as prep	¼ cup	5	0	0
Brown as prep	¼ cup	10	0	1

FOOD	PORTION	CALS.	SAT. FAT	FAT
Durkee (CONT.)				
Brown Mushroom as prep	¼ cup	15	0	0
Brown Onion as prep	¼ cup	15	0	0
Chicken as prep	¼ cup	20	0	1
Country as prep	¼ cup	35	1	2
Homestyle as prep	¼ cup	15	0	1
Mushroom as prep	¼ cup	15	0	0
Onion as prep	¼ cup	10	0	0
Pork as prep	¼ cup	10	0	0
Sausage as prep	¼ cup	35	1	2
Swiss Steak as prep	¼ cup	15	0	0
Turkey as prep	¼ cup	20	0	0
French's				
Au Jus as prep	¼ cup	5	0	0
Brown as prep	¼ cup	10	0	1
Chicken as prep	¼ cup	25	0	1
Country as prep	¼ cup	35	1	2
Herb Brown as prep	¼ cup	15	0	1
Homestyle as prep	¼ cup	10	0	1
Mushroom as prep	¼ cup	10	0	1
Onion	¼ cup	15	0	1
Pork as prep	¼ cup	10	0	1
Turkey as prep	¼ cup	20	0	0
Hain				
Brown	¼ pkg	16	0	0
Loma Linda				
Gravy Quik Brown	1 tbsp (5 g)	20	0	0
Gravy Quik Chicken	1 tbsp (5 g)	20	0	0
Quik Gravy Country	1 tbsp (5 g)	25	0	1
Quik Gravy Mushroom	1 tbsp (5 g)	15	0	0
Quik Gravy Onion	1 tbsp (5 g)	20	0	0
Pillsbury				
Brown	¼ cup	15	0	0
Chicken	¼ cup	25	—	1
Home Style	¼ cup	15	0	0

GREAT NORTHERN BEANS
CANNED

FOOD	PORTION	CALS.	SAT. FAT	FAT
great northern	1 cup	300	tr	1
Allen				
Great Northern	½ cup (4.5 oz)	100	0	1
Green Giant				
Great Northern	½ cup (4.4 oz)	100	0	1
Hanover				
Great Northern	½ cup	110	—	0

FOOD	PORTION	CALS.	SAT. FAT	FAT
Trappey				
With Sausage	½ cup (4.5 oz)	100	1	1
DRIED				
cooked	1 cup	210	tr	1
Bean Cuisine				
Dried	½ cup	115	—	1
Hurst				
HamBeens w/ Ham	3 tbsp (1.2 oz)	120	0	1

GREEN BEANS
CANNED

FOOD	PORTION	CALS.	SAT. FAT	FAT
italian	½ cup	13	tr	tr
Allen				
Cut	½ cup (4.2 oz)	30	0	1
Cut No Added Salt	½ cup (4.2 oz)	15	0	0
French Style	½ cup (4.2 oz)	25	0	0
Italian	½ cup (4.2 oz)	35	0	1
Shell Outs	½ cup (4.5 oz)	30	0	0
Alma				
Cut	½ cup (4.2 oz)	30	0	1
Crest Top				
Cut	½ cup (4.2 oz)	30	0	1
Del Monte				
Cut	½ cup (4.3 oz)	20	0	0
Cut 50% Less Salt	½ cup (4.3 oz)	20	0	0
Cut Italian	½ cup (4.3 oz)	30	0	0
Cut No Salt Added	½ cup (4.3 oz)	20	0	0
French Style	½ cup (4.3 oz)	20	0	0
French Style 50% Less Salt	½ cup (4.3 oz)	20	0	0
French Style No Salt Added	½ cup (4.3 oz)	20	0	0
French Style Seasoned	½ cup (4.3 oz)	20	0	0
Whole	½ cup (4.3 oz)	20	0	0
GaBelle				
Cut	½ cup (4.2 oz)	30	0	1
Green Giant				
Cut	½ cup (4.2 oz)	20	0	0
Cut 50% Less Sodium	½ cup (4.2 oz)	20	0	0
French Style	½ cup (4.1 oz)	20	0	0
Kitchen Sliced	½ cup (4.2 oz)	20	0	0
Whole	½ cup (4.1 oz)	25	0	0
Hanover				
Cut	½ cup	20	—	0
Owatonna				
Cut	½ cup	20	—	0
French	½ cup	20	—	0

FOOD	PORTION	CALS.	SAT. FAT	FAT
Seneca				
Cut	½ cup	20	0	0
Cuts Natural Pack	½ cup	25	0	0
French	½ cup	20	0	0
French Natural Pack	½ cup	25	0	0
Whole	½ cup	20	0	0
Sunshine				
Cut	½ cup (4.2 oz)	30	0	1
Italian	½ cup (4.2 oz)	35	0	1
FRESH				
cooked	½ cup	22	tr	tr
raw	½ cup	17	tr	tr
FROZEN				
cooked	½ cup	18	tr	tr
Birds Eye				
French w/ Toasted Almonds	¾ cup (4.1 oz)	80	0	4
Fresh Like				
Cut	3.5 oz	29	—	tr
French	3.5 oz	29	—	tr
Italian	3.5 oz	35	—	tr
Whole	3.5 oz	29	—	tr
Green Giant				
Cut	¾ cup (2.8 oz)	25	0	0
Harvest Fresh & Almonds	⅔ cup (2.8 oz)	60	0	3
Harvest Fresh Cut	⅔ cup (2.9 oz)	25	0	0
Hanover				
Cut	½ cup	20	—	0
French Style Blue Lake	½ cup	25	—	0
Italian Cut	½ cup	35	—	0
Whole Blue Lake	½ cup	30	—	0
Southland				
Cut Beans	3 oz	25	—	0
French	3 oz	25	—	0
Stouffer's				
Green Bean Mushroom Casserole	1 serv (4 oz)	130	2	8
Tree Of Life				
Green Beans	⅔ cup (2.8 oz)	25	0	0
GREENS				
Allen				
Mixed	½ cup (4.2 oz)	30	0	1
Sunshine				
Mixed	½ cup (4.2 oz)	30	0	1

FOOD	PORTION	CALS.	SAT. FAT	FAT
GROUNDCHERRIES				
fresh	½ cup	37	—	tr
GROUPER				
cooked	3 oz	100	tr	1
cooked	1 fillet (7.1 oz)	238	1	3
raw	3 oz	78	tr	1
GUANABANA JUICE				
Libby				
Nectar	1 can (11.5 fl oz)	210	0	0
GUAVA				
fresh	1	45	tr	1
guava sauce	½ cup	43	tr	tr
GUAVA JUICE				
Kern's				
Nectar	6 fl oz	110	0	0
Libby				
Nectar	1 can (11.5 fl oz)	220	0	0
Nantucket Nectars				
Cocktail	8 oz	130	0	0
Snapple				
Guava Mania	8 fl oz	110	0	0
GUINEA HEN				
w/ skin raw	½ hen (12.1 oz)	545	—	22
w/o skin raw	½ hen (9.3 oz)	292	—	7
HADDOCK				
FRESH				
cooked	1 fillet (5.3 oz)	168	tr	1
cooked	3 oz	95	tr	1
raw	3 oz	74	tr	1
roe raw	3½ oz	130	—	2
FROZEN				
Gorton's				
Fishmarket Fresh	5 oz	110	—	1
Microwave Entree Haddock In Lemon Butter	1 pkg	360	10	21
Mrs. Paul's				
Crunchy Batter Fillets	2 fillets	190	—	5
Light Fillets	1 fillet	220	—	9
Van De Kamp's				
Battered Fillets	2 (4 oz)	260	3	16
Breaded Fillets	2 (3.5 oz)	280	3	17
Lightly Breaded Fillets	1 (4 oz)	220	2	10

FOOD	PORTION	CALS.	SAT. FAT	FAT
SMOKED				
smoked	3 oz	99	tr	1
smoked	1 oz	33	tr	tr
TAKE-OUT				
breaded & fried	1 piece (3.5 oz)	187	3	9
HALIBUT				
FRESH				
atlantic & pacific cooked	½ fillet (5.6 oz)	223	1	5
atlantic & pacific cooked	3 oz	119	tr	2
atlantic & pacific raw	3 oz	93	tr	2
greenland baked	3 oz	203	2	15
FROZEN				
Van De Kamp's				
Battered Fillets	3 (4 oz)	300	3	21
HALVA				
(see SESAME)				
HAM				
(see also HAM DISHES, PORK, TURKEY)				
boneless 11% fat roasted	3 oz	151	3	8
canned extra lean roasted	3 oz	116	1	4
canned extra lean roasted	1 cup	190	2	7
canned extra lean 4% fat	3 oz	116	1	4
center slice country style lean roasted	4 oz	220	3	9
chopped	1 oz	65	2	5
chopped canned	1 oz	68	2	5
ham & cheese loaf	1 oz	73	4	6
ham & cheese spread	1 oz	69	2	5
ham & cheese spread	1 tbsp	37	1	3
ham salad spread	1 tbsp	32	1	2
ham salad spread	1 oz	61	1	4
minced	1 oz	75	2	6
patty cooked	1 patty (2 oz)	203	7	18
steak boneless extra lean	1 (2 oz)	69	1	2
Alpine Lace				
Boneless Cooked	2 oz	60	1	2
Armour				
Chopped Ham canned	2 oz	130	4	11
Deviled Ham Spread	1 pkg (3 oz)	210	6	18
Lean Slices Brown Sugar	1 pkg (2.5 oz)	90	1	2
Star Canned	1 oz	34	—	1
Boar's Head				
Black Forest Smoked	2 oz	60	0	1
Cappy	2 oz	60	1	2

FOOD	PORTION	CALS.	SAT. FAT	FAT
Boar's Head (CONT.)				
Deluxe	2 oz	60	0	1
Deluxe Lowered Sodium	2 oz	50	0	1
Fresh Roasted Seasoned	2 oz	80	2	3
Maple Glazed Honey	2 oz	60	0	1
Pepper	2 oz	60	0	1
Sweet Slice Smoked	3 oz	110	2	5
Virgina	2 oz	60	0	1
Virginia Smoked	2 oz	60	0	1
Carl Buddig				
Ham Sliced w/ Natural Juices	1 pkg (2.5 oz)	120	3	7
Honey Ham Sliced w/ Natural Juice	1 pkg (2.5 oz)	120	3	7
Lean Slices Oven Roasted Honey Ham	1 pkg (2.5 oz)	90	1	2
Lean Slices Smoked	1 pkg (2.5 oz)	80	1	2
Hansel n'Gretel				
Baked Virginia	1 oz	34	—	1
Black Forest	1 oz	32	—	1
Cappy	1 oz	31	—	1
Cooked Fresh	1 oz	33	—	1
Deluxe	1 oz	31	—	1
Honey Valley	1 oz	31	—	1
Jalapeno	1 oz	25	—	1
Lessalt	1 oz	30	—	1
Light AM	1 oz	27	—	1
Travane	1 oz	31	—	1
Healthy Choice				
Baked Cooked	3 slices (2.2 oz)	70	1	2
Cooked	3 slices (2.2 oz)	70	1	2
Deli-Thin Baked Cooked With Natural Juices	6 slices (2 oz)	60	1	2
Deli-Thin Cooked	6 slices (2 oz)	60	1	2
Deli-Thin Honey With Natural Juices	6 slices (2 oz)	60	1	2
Deli-Thin Smoked With Natural Juices	6 slices (2 oz)	60	1	2
Fresh-Trak Cooked	1 slice (1 oz)	30	0	1
Fresh-Trak Honey	1 slice (1 oz)	30	0	1
Honey Boneless	3 oz	100	1	3
Smoked	3 slices (2.2 oz)	70	1	2
Variety Pack Regular	3 slice (2.2 oz)	70	1	2
Hillshire				
Brown Sugar	1 oz	40	—	2
Cooked Ham	1 oz	30	—	1

FOOD	PORTION	CALS.	SAT. FAT	FAT
Hillshire (CONT.)				
Deli Select Baked Ham	1 slice	10	—	tr
Deli Select Brown Sugar Baked	1 slice	10	—	tr
Deli Select Cajun Ham	1 slice	10	—	tr
Deli Select Honey Ham	1 slice	10	—	tr
Deli Select Lower Salt	1 slice	10	—	tr
Deli Select Smoked Ham	1 slice	10	—	tr
Flavor Pack 90-99% Fat Free Brown Sugar Baked	1 slice (0.6 oz)	20	—	tr
Flavor Pack 90-99% Fat Free Honey Ham	1 slice (0.6 oz)	20	—	tr
Flavor Pack 90-99% Fat Free Smoked	1 slice (0.6 oz)	20	—	tr
Genuine Baked	1 oz	35	—	1
Honey Ham	1 oz	40	—	2
Lower Salt	1 oz	30	—	1
Lunch 'N Munch Cooked Ham/Swiss	1 pkg (4.5 oz)	360	—	22
Lunch 'N Munch Cooked Ham/Swiss Oreo	1 pkg (4.125 oz)	370	—	21
Lunch 'N Munch Cooked Ham/Swiss Snickers/Hi-C	1 pkg (4.25 oz + 6 fl oz)	470	—	21
Lunch 'N Munch Honey Ham/ Cheddar/ Snickers/ Hi-C	1 pkg (4.25 oz + 6 fl oz)	500	—	23
Hormel				
Black Label Canned (refrigerated)	3 oz	100	2	5
Black Label Canned (self stable)	3 oz	110	2	5
Cure 81 Half Ham	3 oz	100	2	5
Curemaster	3 oz	80	1	3
Deviled Ham	4 tbsp (2 oz)	150	4	12
Ham & Cheese Patties	1 patty (2 oz)	190	6	17
Ham Patties	1 (2 oz)	180	6	17
Light & Lean 97 Sliced	1 slice (1 oz)	25	0	1
Primissimo Proscuitti	2 oz	120	3	7
Spiral Cure 81	3 oz	150	5	9
Jordan's				
Healthy Trim 97% Fat Free Cooked	1 slice (1 oz)	30	0	1
Healthy Trim 97% Fat Free EZ Serve	1 slice (1 oz)	30	1	1
Healthy Trim 97% Fat Free Virginia	1 slice (1 oz)	30	1	1

FOOD	PORTION	CALS.	SAT. FAT	FAT
Krakus				
Ham	1 oz	25	—	1
Louis Rich				
Carving Board Baked	2 slices (1.6 oz)	50	1	2
Carving Board Honey Glazed Thin	6 slices (2.1 oz)	70	1	2
Carving Board Honey Glazed Traditional	2 slices (1.6 oz)	50	1	2
Carving Board Smoked	1 slice (1.6 oz)	45	1	2
Dinner Slices Baked	1 slice (3.3 oz)	80	1	2
Mr. Turkey				
Deli Cuts Honey Cured	3 slices	35	—	1
Oscar Mayer				
Baked	3 slices (2.2 oz)	70	1	3
Boiled	3 slices (2.2 oz)	60	1	3
Chopped	1 slice (1 oz)	50	2	3
Dinner Slice	3 oz	80	1	3
Dinner Steaks	1 (2 oz)	60	1	2
Free Baked	3 slices (1.6 oz)	35	0	0
Free Honey	3 slices (1.6 oz)	35	0	0
Free Smoked	3 slices (1.6 oz)	35	0	0
Ham & Cheese Loaf	1 slice (1 oz)	70	3	5
Honey	3 slices (2.2 oz)	70	1	3
Lower Sodium	3 slices (2.2 oz)	70	1	3
Lunchables Cookies/Ham/Swiss	1 pkg (4.2 oz)	360	8	19
Lunchables Dessert Chocolate Pudding/Ham/American	1 pkg (6.2 oz)	390	9	20
Lunchables Ham/Cheddar	1 pkg (4.5 oz)	340	11	20
Smoked	3 slices (2.2 oz)	60	1	3
Russer				
Baked	2 oz	70	1	3
Canadian Brand Maple	2 oz	70	1	2
Chopped	2 oz	130	3	9
Cooked Ham	2 oz	60	1	2
Ham & Cheese Loaf	2 oz	120	2	8
Honey & Maple Cured	2 oz	70	1	3
Honey Cured	2 oz	60	1	3
Hot	2 oz	70	1	3
Light Cooked	2 oz	60	1	2
Light Smoked	2 oz	60	1	2
Smoked Virginia	2 oz	70	1	3
Spiced	2 oz	160	3	12

FOOD	PORTION	CALS.	SAT. FAT	FAT
Sara Lee				
Bavarian Brand Baked	2 oz	80	1	4
Bavarian Brand Baked Honey	2 oz	80	1	4
Golden Cure Smoked	2 oz	80	2	4
Honey Ham	2 oz	60	1	2
Honey Roasted	2 oz	90	2	5
Spam				
Spread	4 tbsp (2 oz)	140	4	12
Spreadables				
Ham Salad	¼ can	100	—	6
Underwood				
Deviled	2.08 oz	220	6	19
Deviled Light	2.08 oz	120	1	8
Deviled Smoked	2.08 oz	190	6	18
Wampler				
Black Forest	2 oz	60	—	2

HAM DISHES
FROZEN
Croissant Pocket

Stuffed Sandwich Ham & Cheddar	1 piece (4.5 oz)	360	7	17

Hot Pocket

Stuffed Sandwich Ham & Cheese	1 (4.5 ox)	340	7	15

HAMBURGER
(see also BEEF)

FOOD	PORTION	CALS.	SAT. FAT	FAT
Jimmy Dean				
Burger	1 (2 oz)	220	7	21
Flamed Broiled Cheeseburger	1 (6.3 oz)	540	14	34
Mini Cheeseburger	2 (3 oz)	270	9	14
Kid Cuisine				
Beef Patty Sandwich w/ Cheese	1 (8.5 oz)	410	5	15
Rudy's Farm				
Mild Burger	1 (3 oz)	360	12	35
White Castle				
Cheeseburger	2 (3.6 oz)	310	9	17
Hamburger	2 (3.2 oz)	270	6	14
TAKE-OUT				
double patty w/ bun	1 reg	544	10	28
double patty w/ cheese & bun	1 reg	457	13	28
double patty w/ cheese & double bun	1 reg	461	10	22

FOOD	PORTION	CALS.	SAT. FAT	FAT
double patty w/ cheese ketchup mayonnaise onion pickle tomato & bun	1 reg	416	8	21
double patty w/ ketchup mayonnaise onion pickle tomato & bun	1 reg	649	13	35
double patty w/ ketchup cheese mayonnaise mustard pickle tomato & bun	1 lg	706	18	44
double patty w/ ketchup mustard mayonnaise onion pickle tomato & bun	1 lg	540	11	27
double patty w/ ketchup mustard onion pickle & bun	1 reg	576	12	32
single patty w/ bacon ketchup cheese mustard onion pickle & bun	1 lg	609	16	37
single patty w/ bun	1 reg	275	4	12
single patty w/ bun	1 lg	400	8	23
single patty w/ cheese & bun	1 reg	320	6	15
single patty w/ cheese & bun	1 lg	608	15	33
single patty w/ ketchup cheese ham mayonnaise pickle tomato & bun	1 lg	745	21	48
single patty w/ ketchup mustard mayonnaise onion pickle tomato & bun	1 reg	279	4	13
triple patty w/ cheese & bun	1 lg	769	22	51
triple patty w/ ketchup mustard pickle & bun	1 lg	693	16	41

HAZELNUTS

dried blanched	1 oz	191	1	19
dried unblanched	1 oz	179	1	18
dry roasted unblanched	1 oz	188	1	19
Crumpy				
Chocolate Hazelnut Spread	1 tbsp (0.5 oz)	80	1	5

HEART

beef simmered	3 oz	148	1	5
chicken simmered	1 cup (5 oz)	268	3	11
lamb braised	3 oz	158	3	7
pork braised	1 cup	215	2	7
pork braised	1	191	2	7
turkey simmered	1 cup (5 oz)	257	3	9
veal braised	3 oz	158	2	6

FOOD	PORTION	CALS.	SAT. FAT	FAT
HEARTS OF PALM				
canned	1 (1.2 oz)	9	tr	tr
canned	1 cup (5.1 oz)	41	tr	1
HERBAL TEA				
(see TEA/HERBAL TEA)				
HERBS/SPICES				
(see also INDIVIDUAL NAMES)				
curry powder	1 tsp	6	—	tr
poultry seasoning	1 tsp	5	—	tr
pumpkin pie spice	1 tsp	6	—	tr
Ac'cent				
Flavor Enhancer	½ tsp	5	0	0
Herbal All Purpose Seasoning	½ tsp	0	0	0
Chi-Chi's				
Seasoning Mix	1 tsp (3 g)	10	0	0
Lawry's				
Seasoning Blend Sloppy Joe	1 pkg	126	—	tr
Mcllhenny				
Crab Boil	3 oz	378	5	17
Mrs. Dash				
Extra Spicy	⅛ tsp (0.02 oz)	2	—	0
Garlic & Herb	⅛ tsp (0.02 oz)	2	—	tr
Lemon & Herb	⅛ tsp (0.02 oz)	2	—	0
Low Pepper No Garlic	⅛ tsp (0.02 oz)	2	—	0
Original Blend	⅛ tsp (0.02 oz)	2	0	0
Table Blend	⅛ tsp (0.02 oz)	2	—	0
Watkins				
Apple Bake Seasoning	¼ tsp (0.5 g)	0	0	0
Barbecue Spice	¼ tsp (0.5 g)	0	0	0
Bean Soup Seasoning	¾ tsp (2 g)	5	0	0
Beef Jerky Seasoning	2 tsp (6 g)	15	0	0
Chicken Seasoning	½ tsp (1 g)	0	0	0
Cole Slaw Seasoning	½ tsp (1.5 g)	5	0	0
Egg Sensations	1 tsp (3 g)	10	0	0
Fajita Seasoning	½ tsp (3 g)	10	0	0
Grill Seasoning	¼ tsp (1 g)	0	0	0
Ground Beef Seasoning	⅛ tsp (0.5 g)	0	0	0
Italian Blend	1 tsp (3 g)	1	0	0
Meat Tenderizer	⅛ tsp (0.5 g)	0	0	0
Meatloaf Seasoning	½ tsp (5 g)	15	0	0
Mexican Blend	½ tbsp (4 g)	15	0	0
Omelet & Souffle Seasoning	¾ tsp (2 g)	5	0	0
Oriental Ginger Garlic Liquid Spice Blend	1 tbsp (0.5 oz)	120	2	14

FOOD	PORTION	CALS.	SAT. FAT	FAT
Watkins (CONT.)				
Potato Salad Seasoning	¼ tsp (1 g)	0	0	0
Pumpkin Pie Spice	¼ tsp (0.5 g)	0	0	0
Smokehouse Liquid Blend	1 tbsp (0.5 oz)	120	2	14
Soup & Vegetable Seasoning	¼ tsp (0.5 g)	0	0	0
Spanish Seasoning Blend	¼ tsp (0.5 oz)	0	0	0
HERRING				
atlantic cooked	1 fillet (5 oz)	290	4	17
atlantic cooked	3 oz	172	2	10
atlantic raw	3 oz	134	2	8
pacific baked	3 oz	213	4	15
roe canned	3.5 oz	118	—	3
roe raw	3.5 oz	130	—	2
smoked	3.5 oz	210	3	14
TAKE-OUT				
atlantic kippered	1 fillet (1.4 oz)	87	1	5
atlantic pickled	0.5 oz	39	tr	3
fried	1 serv (3.5 oz)	233	—	15
HICKORY NUTS				
dried	1 oz	187	2	18
HOMINY				
CANNED				
white	1 cup (5.6 oz)	482	tr	1
Allen				
Golden	½ cup (4.5 oz)	120	0	1
Mexican	½ cup (4.5 oz)	120	0	1
White	½ cup (4.5 oz)	100	0	1
Uncle William				
Golden	½ cup (4.5 oz)	120	0	1
Mexican	½ cup (4.5 oz)	120	0	1
White	½ cup (4.5 oz)	100	0	1
Van Camp's				
Golden	½ cup (4.3 oz)	80	0	1
White	½ cup (4.3 oz)	80	0	1
HONEY				
honey	1 cup (11.9 oz)	1031	0	0
honey	1 tbsp (0.7 oz)	64	0	0
Burleson's				
Clover	1 tbsp	60	0	0
Creamed	1 tbsp	60	0	0
Natural	1 tbsp	60	0	0
Pure	1 tbsp	60	0	0

FOOD	PORTION	CALS.	SAT. FAT	FAT
Burleson's (CONT.)				
Raw	1 tbsp	60	0	0
Rocky Mountain Clover	1 tbsp	60	0	0
Tree Of Life				
Alfalfa	1 tbsp (0.7 oz)	60	0	0
Avocado	1 tbsp (0.7 oz)	60	0	0
Buckwheat	1 tbsp (0.7 oz)	60	0	0
Clover	1 tbsp (0.7 oz)	60	0	0
Honeybear Wildflower	1 tbsp (0.7 oz)	60	0	0
Orange	1 tbsp (0.7 oz)	60	0	0
Tupelo	1 tbsp (0.7 oz)	60	0	0
Wildflower	1 tbsp (0.7 oz)	60	0	0
HONEYDEW				
FRESH				
cubed	1 cup	60	—	tr
wedge	1/10 melon	46	—	tr
Dole				
Honeydew	1/10 melon	50	—	0
FROZEN				
Big Valley				
Balls	3/4 cup (4.9 oz)	45	0	0
HORSE				
roasted	3 oz	149	2	5
HORSERADISH				
Boar's Head				
Horseradish	1 tsp (5 g)	5	0	0
Hebrew National				
White	1 tbsp	7	0	0
Heluva Good Cheese				
Horseradish	1 tsp (5 g)	0	0	0
Kraft				
Cream Style	1 tsp (5 g)	0	0	0
Horseradish Sauce	1 tsp (5 g)	20	0	2
Prepared	1 tsp (5 g)	0	0	0
Rosoff's				
Red	1 tbsp (0.5 oz)	8	0	0
White	1 tbsp (0.5 oz)	7	0	0
Schorr's				
Red	1 tbsp (0.5 oz)	8	0	0
White	1 tbsp (0.5 oz)	7	0	0

HOT CAKES
(see PANCAKES)

FOOD	PORTION	CALS.	SAT. FAT	FAT
HOT COCOA				
(see COCOA)				
HOT DOG				
(see also MEAT SUBSTITUTES, SAUSAGE, SAUSAGE SUBSTITUTES)				
beef & pork	1 (2 oz)	183	6	17
beef & pork	1 (1.5 oz)	144	5	13
chicken	1 (1.5 oz)	116	2	9
pork cheesefurter smokie	1 (1.5 oz)	141	5	12
turkey	1 (1.5 oz)	102	—	8
Applegate Farms				
Chicken Natural Uncured	1 (1.5 oz)	120	2	5
Natural Turkey	1 (1.5 oz)	120	2	5
Armour				
Star Jumbo Beef	1	190	—	18
Boar's Head				
Beef	1 (1.6 oz)	120	5	11
Beef Lite	1 (1.6 oz)	90	3	6
Pork & Beef	1 (2 oz)	150	5	14
Empire				
Chicken	1 (2 oz)	100	2	7
Turkey	1 (2 oz)	90	2	6
Healthy Choice				
Beef	1 (1.8 oz)	60	1	2
Bunsize	1 (2 oz)	70	1	2
Franks	1 (1.6 oz)	50	1	2
Jumbo	1 (2 oz)	70	1	2
Hebrew National				
Beef	1 (1.7 oz)	150	—	14
Cocktail Beef	6 (1.8 oz)	160	—	15
Dinner Beef	1 (4 oz)	350	—	34
Reduced Fat Beef	1 (1.7 oz)	120	—	10
Hillshire				
Franks Bun Size Beef	2 oz	180	—	16
Light & Mild Franks Jumbo	1 link	110	—	8
Light & Mild Wieners	1 link	90	—	7
Lit'l Franks Beef	2 oz	180	—	16
Lit'l Wieners	2 oz	180	—	16
Weiners Natural Casing	2 oz	180	—	17
Wieners Bun Size	2 oz	180	—	16
Hormel				
Fat Free	1 (1.8 oz)	45	0	0
Fat Free Beef	1 (1.8 oz)	45	0	0

FOOD	PORTION	CALS.	SAT. FAT	FAT
Jordan's				
Healthy Trim Low Fat	1 (1.8 oz)	70	1	3
Healthy Trim Low Fat Skinless	1 (1.8 oz)	70	1	3
Louis Rich				
Bun Length	1 (2 oz)	110	3	8
Cheese	1 (1.6 oz)	90	3	6
Franks	1 (1.6 oz)	80	2	6
Mr. Turkey				
Bun Size	1	130	—	11
Cheese	1	140	—	12
Hot Dog	1	110	—	9
Organic Valley				
All-Natural Beef	1 (1.6 oz)	90	3	6
Oscar Mayer				
Beef	1 (1.6 oz)	140	6	13
Big & Juicy Franks Deli Style	1 (2.7 oz)	230	10	22
Big & Juicy Franks Original	1 (2.7 oz)	240	9	22
Big & Juicy Franks Quarter Pound	1 (4 oz)	350	13	32
Big & Juicy Weiners Hot 'N Spicy	1 (2.7 oz)	220	8	20
Big & Juicy Weiners Smokie Links	1 (2.7 oz)	220	7	19
Big & Juicy Weiners Original	1 (2.7 oz)	240	9	22
Bun-Length Beef	1 (2 oz)	180	7	17
Cheese	1 (1.6 oz)	140	5	13
Free Beef	1 (1.8 oz)	40	0	0
Free Turkey & Beef	1 (1.8 oz)	35	0	0
Jumbo Beef	1 (2 oz)	180	7	17
Light Beef	1 (2 oz)	110	4	8
Wieners	1 (1.6 oz)	150	5	13
Wieners Bun-Length	1 (2 oz)	190	6	17
Wieners Jumbo	1 (2 oz)	180	6	17
Wieners Light	1 (2 oz)	110	4	8
Wieners Little	6 (2 oz)	180	6	17
Russer				
Lil'Salt Deli Franks	1 (2.67 oz)	160	4	11
Shofar				
Kosher Beef	1 (1.8 oz)	150	5	14
Kosher Beef Reduced Fat Reduced Sodium	1 (1.8 oz)	120	4	10
Wampler				
Chicken	1 (2 oz)	120	3	11

FOOD	PORTION	CALS.	SAT. FAT	FAT
TAKE-OUT				
corndog	1	460	5	19
w/ bun chili	1	297	5	13
w/ bun plain	1	242	5	15
HUMMUS				
hummus	1 cup	420	3	21
Athenos				
Roasted Red Pepper	2 tbsp (1.1 oz)	60	1	4
Casbah				
Mix as prep	¼ cup	120	0	5
Cedar's				
No Salt Added Hommus Tahini	2 tbsp (1 oz)	50	0	2
TAKE-OUT				
hummus	⅓ cup	140	1	7
HYACINTH BEANS				
dried cooked	1 cup	228	—	1
ICE CREAM AND FROZEN DESSERTS				
(see also ICES AND ICE POPS, PUDDING POPS, SHERBET, YOGURT FROZEN)				
chocolate	½ cup (4 fl oz)	143	4	7
dixie cup chocolate	1 (3.5 fl oz)	125	4	6
dixie cup strawberry	1 (3.5 fl oz)	112	—	5
dixie cup vanilla	1 (3.5 fl oz)	116	4	6
freeze dried ice cream chocolate strawberry & vanilla	1 pkg (0.75 oz)	158	2	5
french vanilla soft serve	½ gal	3014	108	180
french vanilla soft serve	½ cup (4 fl oz)	185	6	11
strawberry	½ cup (4 fl oz)	127	—	6
vanilla	½ cup (4 fl oz)	132	4	7
vanilla light	½ cup (2.3 oz)	92	2	3
vanilla rich	½ cup (2.6 oz)	178	7	12
vanilla soft serve	½ cup	111	1	2
vanilla 10% fat	½ gal	2153	71	115
vanilla 16% fat	½ gal	2805	118	190
vanilla light	1 cup	184	4	6
vanilla light	½ gal	1469	28	45
vanilla light soft serve	1 cup	223	3	5
vanilla light soft serve	½ gal	1787	23	37
3 Musketeers				
Single Chocolate	1 (2 fl oz)	160	6	10
Single Vanilla	1 (2 fl oz)	160	6	10
Snack Chocolate	1 (0.72 fl oz)	60	2	4
Snack Vanilla	1 (0.72 fl oz)	60	2	4

FOOD	PORTION	CALS.	SAT. FAT	FAT
Ben & Jerry's				
Bovinity Divinity	½ cup	290	13	18
Butter Pecan	½ cup	330	12	25
Cherry Garcia	½ cup	260	11	16
Chocolate Chip Cookie Dough	½ cup	300	10	16
Chocolate Fudge Brownie	½ cup	280	10	15
Chubby Hubby	½ cup	350	12	21
Chunky Monkey	½ cup	310	11	19
Coconut Almond Fudge Chip	½ cup	310	14	22
Coffee Heath Bar Crunch	½ cup	310	12	18
Dilbert's World Totally Nuts	½ cup	310	11	21
Low Fat Blackberry Cobbler	½ cup	180	2	3
Low Fat Coconut Cream Pie	½ cup	160	2	3
Low Fat Mocha Latte	½ cup	150	2	2
Low Fat S'mores	½ cup	190	1	2
Mint Chocolate Cookie	½ cup	280	11	17
New York Super Fudge Chunk	½ cup	320	12	21
No Fat Chocolate Comfort	½ cup	150	2	2
Orange & Cream	½ cup	230	10	14
Peanut Butter Cup	½ cup	380	13	25
Phish Food	½ cup	300	10	14
Phish Stick	1	330	12	20
Pistachio Pistachio	½ cup	240	10	15
Pop Cookie Dough	1	420	14	25
Pop Totally Nuts	1	370	14	29
Pop Vanilla	1	330	16	23
Pop Vanilla Heath Bar Crunch	1	330	14	22
S'mores Bar	1	350	11	18
Smooth White Russian	½ cup (3.8 oz)	240	10	16
Triple Caramel Chunk	½ cup	290	12	17
Vanilla World's Best	½ cup	250	11	16
Vanilla Caramel Fudge	½ cup	300	10	17
Vanilla Heath Bar Crunch	½ cup	310	11	19
Wavy Gravy	½ cup	340	10	20
Bon Bons				
Vanilla With Milk Chocolate Coating	8 pieces	330	13	23
Vanilla With Milk Chocolate Coating	5 pieces	200	8	14
Borden				
Buttered Pecan	½ cup	180	—	12
Chocolate Swirl	½ cup	130	—	6

FOOD	PORTION	CALS.	SAT. FAT	FAT
Borden (CONT.)				
Dutch Chocolate Olde Fashioned Recipe	½ cup	130	—	6
Fat Free Black Cherry	½ cup	90	tr	tr
Fat Free Chocolate	½ cup	100	tr	tr
Fat Free Peach	½ cup	90	tr	tr
Fat Free Strawberry	½ cup	90	tr	tr
Fat Free Vanilla	½ cup	90	tr	tr
Ice Milk Chocolate	½ cup	100	—	2
Ice Milk Strawberry	½ cup	90	—	2
Ice Milk Vanilla	½ cup	90	—	2
Strawberries 'N Cream Olde Fashioned Recipe	½ cup	130	—	5
Strawberry	½ cup	130	—	6
Sundae Cone	1	210	—	12
Vanilla Olde Fashioned Recipe	½ cup	130	—	7
Bounty				
Cherry/Dark	1 (0.84 fl oz)	70	3	5
Coconut/Dark	1 (0.84 fl oz)	70	3	5
Coconut/Milk	1 (0.84 fl oz)	70	3	5
Breyers				
Butter Pecan	½ cup (2.4 oz)	180	6	12
Caramel Praline Crunch	½ cup (2.6 oz)	180	5	9
Cherry Vanilla	½ cup (2.4 oz)	150	5	8
Chocolate	½ cup (2.4 oz)	160	6	9
Chocolate Chip	½ cup (2.4 oz)	170	7	10
Chocolate Chip Cookie Dough	½ cup (2.5 oz)	180	6	10
Chocolate Rainbow	½ cup (2.4 oz)	120	6	10
Coffee	½ cup (2.4 oz)	150	6	9
Cookies N Cream	½ cup (2.4 oz)	170	6	9
Creamsicle	½ cup (2.8 oz)	130	3	4
Double Chocolate Fudge	½ cup (2.6 oz)	150	6	9
Fat Free Caramel Praline	½ cup (2.5 oz)	120	0	0
Fat Free Chocolate	½ cup (2.4 oz)	90	0	0
Fat Free Mint Cookies N Cream	½ cup (2.4 oz)	100	0	0
Fat Free Strawberry	½ cup (2.4 oz)	90	0	0
Fat Free Take Two Vanilla Strawberry	½ cup (2.4 oz)	80	0	0
Fat Free Vanilla	½ cup (2.4 oz)	90	0	0
Fat Free Vanilla Chocolate Strawberry	½ cup (2.4 oz)	90	0	0

FOOD	PORTION	CALS.	SAT. FAT	FAT
Breyers (CONT.)				
Fat Free Vanilla Fudge Twirl	½ cup (2.5 oz)	100	0	0
French Vanilla	½ cup (2.4 oz)	160	6	10
Fruit Rainbow	½ cup (2.4 oz)	140	5	8
Hershey w/ Almonds	½ cup (2.7 oz)	190	5	8
Light Butter Pecan	½ cup (2.3 oz)	120	1	4
Light Caramel Praline Pecan	½ cup (3 oz)	180	3	5
Light French Chocolate	½ cup (2.4 oz)	150	3	5
Light Mint Chocolate Chip	½ cup (2.4 oz)	140	3	5
Light Vanilla	½ cup (2.4 oz)	130	3	5
Light Vanilla Chocolate Strawberry	½ cup (2.4 oz)	120	2	3
Light Low Fat Brown Marble Fudge	½ cup (2.6 oz)	130	1	2
Light Low Fat French Vanilla	½ cup (2.3 oz)	110	1	2
Light Low Fat Swiss Almond Fudge	½ cup (2.5 oz)	130	2	3
Low Fat Butter Pecan	½ cup (2.6 oz)	150	2	7
Low Fat Vanilla	½ cup (2.6 oz)	120	2	3
Low Fat Vanilla Chocolate Strawberry	½ cup (2.6 oz)	120	2	3
Mint Chocolate Chip	½ cup (2.4 oz)	170	7	10
No Sugar Added Fudge Twirl	½ cup (2.6 oz)	100	3	5
No Sugar Added Mint Chocolate Chip	½ cup (2.4 oz)	100	4	5
No Sugar Added Vanilla	½ cup (2.4 oz)	90	3	5
No Sugar Added Vanilla Chocolate Strawberry	½ cup (2.4 oz)	90	3	5
Peach	½ cup (2.4 oz)	130	4	6
Peanut Butter Cup	½ cup (2.7 oz)	210	6	12
Rocky Road	½ cup (2.5 oz)	180	5	9
Soft'N Creamy Vanilla	½ cup (2.3 oz)	150	5	7
Soft'N Creamy Vanilla Chocolate Strawberry	½ cup (2.3 oz)	150	5	7
Strawberry	½ cup (2.4 oz)	130	5	7
Take Two Vanilla Chocolate	½ cup (2.5 oz)	160	6	9
Take Two Vanilla Orange Sherbet	½ cup (2.7 oz)	130	3	5
Vanilla	½ cup (2.4 oz)	150	6	9
Vanilla Chocolate Strawberry	½ cup (2.4 oz)	150	5	8
Vanilla Fudge Twirl	½ cup (2.6 oz)	160	5	8
Viennetta Cappuccino	½ cup (2.4 oz)	190	7	11
Viennetta Chocolate	½ cup (2.4 oz)	190	8	12
Viennetta Vanilla	½ cup (2.4 oz)	190	7	11

FOOD	PORTION	CALS.	SAT. FAT	FAT
Butterfinger				
Bar	1 (2.5 oz)	170	7	12
Nuggets	8	340	13	24
California Joe				
Soft Serve Chocolate	½ cup (2.5 oz)	72	0	0
Soft Serve Vanilla	½ cup (2.5 oz)	70	0	0
Carnation				
Berry Swirl Bar Raspberry	1 bar	70	—	3
Berry Swirl Bar Strawberry	1 bar	70	—	3
Cheesecake Bar Original	1 bar	120	—	6
Cheesecake Bar Strawberry	1 bar	125	—	6
Chocolate Malted Bar	1 bar	70	—	3
Creamy Lites Bar Chocolate	1 bar	50	—	2
Creamy Lites Bar Strawberry	1 bar	50	—	2
Sundae Cup Strawberry	1 (3.3 oz)	200	5	8
Cool Creations				
Cookies & Cream Sandwich	1 (3.5 oz)	240	4	11
Mini Sandwich	1 (2.3 oz)	110	2	5
Dippin' Dots				
Dipping Dots Chocolate	⅝ cup (3 oz)	190	6	9
DoveBar				
Almond	1 (3.67 fl oz)	335	12	22
Bite Size Almond Praline	1 (0.75 fl oz)	80	3	5
Bite Size Cherry Royale	1 (0.75 fl oz)	70	3	5
Bite Size Classic Vanilla	1 (0.75 fl oz)	70	3	5
Bite Size French Vanilla	1 (0.75 fl oz)	70	3	5
Bite Size Mint Supreme	1 (0.75 fl oz)	80	3	5
Caramel Pecan	1 (3.67 fl oz)	350	12	35
Chocolate Milk Chocolate	1 (3.8 fl oz)	340	13	21
Coffee Cashew	1 (3.67 fl oz)	335	13	22
Crunchy Cookie	1 (3.8 fl oz)	340	13	21
Peanut	1 (3.8 fl oz)	380	13	25
Single Vanilla/Dark	1 (2 fl oz)	200	7	12
Vanilla Dark Chocolate	1 (3.8 fl oz)	340	13	22
Vanilla Milk Chocolate	1 (3.8 fl oz)	340	13	21
Drumstick				
Cone Chocolate	1 (4.6 oz)	340	10	19
Cone Chocolate Dipped	1 (4.6 oz)	340	10	17
Cone Vanilla	1 (4.6 oz)	350	11	20
Cone Vanilla Caramel	1 (4.6 oz)	360	12	20
Cone Vanilla Fudge	1 (4.6 oz)	370	11	21
Eagle Brand				
Vanilla	½ cup	150	—	9
Edy's				
American Dream Chocolate	3 oz	90	—	1

FOOD	PORTION	CALS.	SAT. FAT	FAT
Edy's (CONT.)				
American Dream Chocolate Chip	3 oz	100	—	1
American Dream Cookies'N'Cream	3 oz	100	—	1
American Dream Mocha Almond Fudge	3 oz	110	—	1
American Dream Rocky Road	3 oz	110	—	1
American Dream Strawberry	3 oz	70	—	tr
American Dream Toasted Almond	3 oz	110	—	1
American Dream Vanilla	3 oz	80	—	tr
American Dream Vanilla Chocolate Strawberry	3 oz	80	—	1
Light Almond Praline	4 oz	140	2-3	5
Light Banana-Politan	4 oz	110	2-3	4
Light Butter Pecan	4 oz	140	2-3	5
Light Cafe Au Lait	4 oz	110	2-3	4
Light Candy Bar	4 oz	140	2-3	5
Light Chocolate Chip	4 oz	120	2-3	4
Light Chocolate Fudge Mousse	4 oz	130	2-3	5
Light Cookies'N'Cream	4 oz	120	2-3	5
Light Dreamy Caramel Cream	4 oz	140	2-3	4
Light Malt Ball 'N' Fudge	4 oz	140	2-3	5
Light Marble Fudge	4 oz	120	2-3	4
Light Mocha Almond Fudge	4 oz	140	2-3	5
Light Peanut Butter & Chocolate	4 oz	130	2-3	5
Light Raspberry Truffle	4 oz	110	2-3	5
Light Rocky Road	4 oz	130	2-3	5
Light Strawberry	4 oz	110	2-3	4
Light Vanilla	4 oz	100	2-3	4
Vanilla Chocolate Strawberry	4 oz	110	2-3	4
Fi-Bar				
Banana Cream	1 bar	93	—	tr
Cocoa-Fudge 'N Cream	1 bar	93	—	tr
Raspberries 'N Cream	1 bar	93	—	tr
Wildberry Cream	1 bar	93	—	tr
Flintstones				
Cool Cream	1 (2.75 oz)	90	1	2
Push-Up	1 (2.75 oz)	100	1	2
Friendly's				
Black Raspberry	½ cup	150	5	7
Chocolate Almond Chip	½ cup	170	6	10

FOOD	PORTION	CALS.	SAT. FAT	FAT
Friendly's (CONT.)				
Forbidden Chocolate	½ cup	150	5	9
Fudge Nut Brownie	½ cup	200	7	11
Heath English Toffee	½ cup (2.7 oz)	190	6	10
Purely Pistachio	½ cup	160	6	10
Vanilla	½ cup	150	5	8
Vanilla Chocolate Strawberry	½ cup	150	5	8
Vienna Mocha Chunk	½ cup	180	7	11
Good Humor				
Banana Bob	1 (3 fl oz)	155	6	7
Bar Classic Toasted Almond	1 (3.1 fl oz)	170	4	9
Bar Classic Vanilla	1 (3.1 fl oz)	190	8	10
Bar Classic Almond	1 (3.1 fl oz)	210	8	12
Bar Sidewalk Sundae	1	280	17	20
Bubble O'Bill	1 (3.6 fl oz)	170	8	10
Bubble Play	1	110	1	1
Chip Burrrger	1 (4.7 oz)	320	9	15
Chip Sandwich	1 (4.7 fl oz)	320	9	15
Choco Taco	1 (4.4 fl oz)	320	11	17
Chocolate Eclair Classic	1 (3.1 fl oz)	170	3	9
Classic Candy Center Crunch Vanilla	1	280	17	21
Colonel Crunch Chocolate	1 (3.1 oz)	160	4	7
Colonel Crunch Strawberry	1 (3.1 oz)	170	6	8
Combo Cup	1 (6.2 fl oz)	200	7	10
Cone Olde Nut Sundae	1 (3.9 oz)	230	6	9
Cone Sidewalk Sundae	1 (4.2 oz)	270	11	14
Creamee Burrrger	1 (4.7 oz)	310	12	17
Crunch Classic Candy Center	1 (3.1 oz)	260	14	19
Dinosaur Bar	1	110	1	2
Far Frog	1 (3.6 fl oz)	150	7	8
Fun Box Ice Cream Sandwich	1 (3.1 oz)	160	3	5
King Cone	1 (5.7 fl oz)	300	11	14
King Cone Classic Vanilla	1 (4.8 oz)	300	6	10
King Cone Strawberry	1 (5.7 oz)	250	7	10
Light Chocolate Chocolate Chip	½ cup (2.4 oz)	130	3	4
Light Chocolate Chip	½ cup (2.4 oz)	130	3	4
Light Coffee	½ cup (2.4 oz)	110	2	3
Light Cookies N'Cream	½ cup (2.4 oz)	130	2	3
Light Heavenly Hash	½ cup (2.4 oz)	140	2	4
Light Praline Almond Crunch	½ cup (2.4 oz)	130	2	3
Light Toffee Bar Crunch	½ cup (2.4 oz)	130	3	4

FOOD	PORTION	CALS.	SAT. FAT	FAT
Good Humor (CONT.)				
Light Vanilla	½ cup (2.4 oz)	110	2	3
Light Vanilla Chocolate Strawberry	½ cup (2.4 oz)	110	2	3
Light Vanilla Fudge	½ cup (2.6 oz)	120	2	3
Magmun Almond	1 (4.2 fl oz)	270	7	12
Magnum Chocolate	1 (4.2 fl oz)	260	8	12
Number One Bar	1 (4.1 fl oz)	190	9	11
Popsicle Ice Cream Bar	1 (3.1 fl oz)	160	9	11
Popsicle Ice Cream Sandwich	1 (3.6 fl oz)	190	4	8
Sandwich Classic Chip Cookie	1 (4.1 fl oz)	300	8	13
Sandwich Giant Neapolitan	1 (5.2 fl oz)	260	7	10
Sandwich Giant Vanilla	1 (5.2 fl oz)	240	6	10
Sandwich Ice Cream	1	190	4	8
Sandwich Sidewalk Sundae	1 (3.1 oz)	160	3	5
Sandwich Sprinkle	1 (3.1 oz)	180	4	6
Strawberry Shortcake Bar Classic	1 (3.1 oz)	160	4	8
Sundae Twist Cup	1	160	2	3
Toffee Taco	1 (4.4 fl oz)	300	10	16
WWF Bar	1 (3.7 fl oz)	200	8	10
X-Men Bar	1 (3 fl oz)	150	3	6
Haagen-Dazs				
Baileys Original Irish Cream	½ cup (3.6 oz)	280	11	18
Brownies A La Mode	½ cup (3.7 oz)	280	11	18
Butter Pecan	½ cup (3.7 oz)	320	11	24
Cappuccino Commotion	½ cup (3.6 oz)	310	12	21
Caramel Cone Explosion	½ cup (3.6 oz)	310	12	20
Chocolate	½ cup (3.7 oz)	270	11	18
Chocolate Chocolate Chip	½ cup (3.7 oz)	300	12	20
Coffee	½ cup (3.7 oz)	270	11	18
Cookie Dough Dynamo	½ cup (3.6 oz)	300	12	19
Cookies & Cream	½ cup (3.6 oz)	270	11	17
DiSaronno Amaretto	½ cup (3.6 oz)	260	9	15
Macadamia Brittle	½ cup (3.7 oz)	300	11	20
Multi Pack Bars Caramel Cone Explosion	1 (3.1 oz)	330	13	22
Multi Pack Bars Chocolate & Dark Chocolate	1 (3.2 oz)	320	15	22
Multi Pack Bars Coffee & Almond Crunch	1 (3 oz)	290	12	21
Multi Pack Bars Iced Cappuccino Explosion	1 (2.9 oz)	290	12	21

FOOD	PORTION	CALS.	SAT. FAT	FAT
Haagen-Dazs (CONT.)				
Multi Pack Bars Triple Brownie Overload	1 (3 oz)	320	12	23
Multi Pack Bars Vanilla & Almonds	1 (3 oz)	300	12	22
Multi Pack Bars Vanilla & Dark Chocolate	1 (3.2 oz)	320	15	22
Multi Pack Bars Vanilla & Milk Chocolate	1 (3 oz)	280	12	20
Peanut Butter Burst	½ cup (3.6 oz)	330	11	22
Rum Raisin	½ cup (3.7 oz)	270	10	17
Single Pack Bars Caramel Cone Explosion	1 (3.3 oz)	350	14	23
Single Pack Bars Chocolate & Dark Chocolate	1 (3.9 oz)	400	18	27
Single Pack Bars Coffee & Almond Crunch	1 (3.7 oz)	360	15	26
Single Pack Bars Cookie Dough Dynamo	1 (3.5 oz)	380	14	25
Single Pack Bars Iced Cappuccino	1 (3.4 oz)	330	14	24
Single Pack Bars Triple Brownie Overload	1 (3.5 oz)	380	14	27
Single Pack Bars Vanilla & Almonds	1 (3.7 oz)	370	14	27
Single Pack Bars Vanilla & Dark Chocolate	1 (3.9 oz)	400	18	27
Single Pack Bars Vanilla & Milk Chocolate	1 (3.5 oz)	330	14	25
Strawberry	½ cup (3.7 oz)	250	10	16
Strawberry Cheesecake Craze	½ cup (3.7 oz)	290	10	18
Triple Brownie Overload	½ cup (3.5 oz)	300	11	20
Vanilla	½ cup (3.7 oz)	270	11	18
Vanilla Fudge	½ cup (3.7 oz)	280	11	18
Vanilla Swiss Almond	½ cup (3.7 oz)	310	11	21
Healthy Choice				
Black Forest	½ cup (2.5 oz)	120	1	2
Bordeaux Cherry Chocolate Chip	½ cup (2.5 oz)	110	2	2
Butter Pecan Crunch	½ cup (2.5 oz)	120	1	2
Cappuccino Chocolate Chunk	½ cup (2.5 oz)	120	1	2
Cookies 'N Cream	½ cup (2.5 oz)	120	2	2
Double Fudge Swirl	½ cup (2.5 oz)	120	2	2
Fudge Brownie	½ cup (2.5 oz)	120	1	2

FOOD	PORTION	CALS.	SAT. FAT	FAT
Healthy Choice (CONT.)				
Malt Caramel Cone	½ cup (2.5 oz)	120	1	2
Mint Chocolate Chip	½ cup (2.5 oz)	120	1	2
Peanut Butter Cookie Dough 'N Fudge	½ cup (2.5 oz)	120	1	2
Praline & Caramel	½ cup (2.5 oz)	130	1	2
Rocky Road	½ cup (2.5 oz)	140	1	2
Vanilla	½ cup	100	2	2
Heath				
Bar	1 (2.5 oz)	160	8	12
Nuggets	8	180	7	11
Heaven				
Sundae Bars Chocolate Fudge	1 bar	150	—	9
Sundae Bars Vanilla Fudge	1 bar	150	—	9
Vanilla Caramel Nut	1 bar	225	—	15
Vanilla Nut Fudge	1 bar	222	—	15
Hood				
Bar Orange Cream	1 bar (1.8 oz)	90	1	2
Bar Vanilla	1 bar (1.6 oz)	160	9	12
Caramel Butterscotch Blast	½ cup (2.3 oz)	160	5	8
Chocolate	½ cup (2.3 oz)	140	5	7
Chocolate Chip	½ cup (2.3 oz)	160	6	9
Chocolate Eclair	1 bar (1.6 oz)	150	3	10
Christmas Tree	½ cup (2.3 oz)	140	5	7
Coffee	½ cup (2.3 oz)	140	5	7
Cookie Dough Delight	½ cup (2.3 oz)	160	5	8
Cookies N Cream	½ cup (2.3 oz)	160	5	8
Cooler Cups	1 (2.1 oz)	80	1	1
Crispy Bar	1 (1.9 oz)	180	10	13
Egg Nog	½ cup (2.3 oz)	130	4	6
Fabulous Fudge & Peanut Butter Swirled Fudge Bars	1 bar (2.1 oz)	110	2	4
Fabulous Fudgies Assorted Bars	1 bar (2.1 oz)	100	2	3
Fat Free Chocolate Passion	½ cup (2.5 oz)	100	0	0
Fat Free Classic Harlequin	½ cup (2.5 oz)	100	0	0
Fat Free Double Brownie Sundae	½ cup (2.5 oz)	120	0	0
Fat Free Heavenly Hash	½ cup (2.5 oz)	120	0	0
Fat Free Mississippi Mud Pie	½ cup (2.5 oz)	130	0	0
Fat Free Praline Pecan Delight	½ cup (2.5 oz)	120	0	0
Fat Free Raspberry Blush	½ cup (2.5 oz)	120	0	0

FOOD	PORTION	CALS.	SAT. FAT	FAT
Hood (CONT.)				
Fat Free Super Strawberry Swirl	½ cup (2.5 oz)	100	0	0
Fat Free Vanilla Fudge Twist	½ cup (2.5 oz)	120	0	0
Fat Free Very Vanilla	½ cup (2.5 oz)	100	0	0
Fudge Bars	1 bar (2.7 oz)	100	0	1
Grasshopper Pie	½ cup (2.3 oz)	160	4	7
Heavenly Hash	½ cup (2.3 oz)	140	4	6
Hendrie's Cherry Chocolate Dips	1 bar (1.3 oz)	120	7	9
Hoodsie Cup Vanilla & Chocolate	1 (1.7 oz)	100	4	5
Light Almond Praline Delight	½ cup (2.4 oz)	110	3	5
Light Brownie Nut Sundae	½ cup (2.4 oz)	140	3	5
Light Caribbean Coffee Royale	½ cup (2.4 oz)	110	2	4
Light Chocolate Almond Chip Sundae	½ cup (2.4 oz)	140	3	5
Light Chocolate Chocolate Chip Cookie Dough	½ cup (2.4 oz)	140	3	5
Light Cookies N Cream	½ cup (2.4 oz)	130	3	4
Light Heath Toffee Chunk Swirl	½ cup (2.4 oz)	140	3	5
Light Heavenly Hash	½ cup (2.4 oz)	130	2	4
Light Maple Sugar Shack	⅓ cup (2.4 oz)	130	2	4
Light Massachusetts Mud Pie	½ cup (2.4 oz)	140	3	5
Light Raspberry Swirl	½ cup (2.4 oz)	120	2	3
Light Strawberry Supreme	½ cup (2.4 oz)	110	2	3
Light Triple Nut Cluster Sundae	½ cup (2.4 oz)	140	2	5
Light Vanilla	½ cup (2.4 oz)	110	3	4
Light Vanilla Chocolate Strawberry	½ cup (2.4 oz)	110	2	4
Low Fat No Sugar Added Caramel Swirl	½ cup (2.4 oz)	120	2	3
Low Fat No Sugar Added Chocolate Supreme	½ cup (2.4 oz)	120	2	3
Low Fat No Sugar Added Mocha Fudge	½ cup (2.4 oz)	110	2	3
Low Fat No Sugar Added Raspberry Swirl	½ cup (2.4 oz)	110	2	3
Low Fat No Sugar Added Vanilla	½ cup (2.4 oz)	100	2	3
Maple Walnut	½ cup (2.3 oz)	160	5	9

FOOD	PORTION	CALS.	SAT. FAT	FAT
Hood (CONT.)				
Rockets	1 (2 oz)	120	4	5
Sandwich Light	1 (2.2 oz)	160	2	4
Sandwich Vanilla	1 (2.2 oz)	180	4	7
Sports Bar	1 (2.9 oz)	250	13	17
Spumoni	½ cup (2.3 oz)	140	5	9
Strawberry	½ cup (2.3 oz)	130	5	7
Super Sortment Chocolate & Banana Fudge Bar	1 bar (2.1 oz)	100	2	3
Super Sortment Root Beer Float & Orange Cream Bar	1 bar (1.5 oz)	70	2	3
Vanilla	½ cup (2.3 oz)	140	5	7
Vanilla Chocolate Patchwork	½ cup (2.3 oz)	140	5	7
Vanilla Chocolate Strawberry	½ cup (2.3 oz)	140	5	7
Vanilla Fudge	½ cup (2.3 oz)	140	4	6
Klondike				
Almond Bar	1 (5.2 fl oz)	310	14	21
Caramel Crunch	1 (5.2 fl oz)	300	13	18
Chocolate Chocolate Bar	1 (5.2 fl oz)	280	14	20
Coffee Bar	1 (5.2 fl oz)	290	14	20
Dark Chocolate Bar	1 (5.2 fl oz)	290	14	20
Gold Bar	1 (5.2 fl oz)	340	12	23
Krispy Bar	1 (5.2 fl oz)	300	13	20
Krunch	1 (3.1 fl oz)	200	9	13
Lite Bar	1 (2.3 fl oz)	110	4	6
Lite Bar Caramel	1 (2.4 fl oz)	120	5	6
Movie Bites Chocolate	8 pieces (4.6 fl oz)	340	3	26
Movie Bites Vanilla	8 pieces (4.6 fl oz)	320	18	22
Original	1 (3.3 oz)	290	14	19
Original Bar	1 (5.2 fl oz)	290	14	20
Sandwich Chocolate	1 (5.2 fl oz)	270	6	10
Sandwich Lite	1 (2.9 fl oz)	100	2	2
Mars				
Almond Bar	1 (1.85 fl oz)	210	6	14
Meadow Gold				
Sundae Cone	1	210	—	12
Milky Way				
Single Chocolate/Milk	1 (2 fl oz)	210	7	11
Snack Chocolate/Milk	1 (0.72 fl oz)	70	3	4
Snack Vanilla/Dark	1 (0.72 fl oz)	70	3	4
Mocha Mix				
Berry Berry Berry	½ cup	140	2	6
Dutch Chocolate	½ cup (2.3 oz)	140	2	8
Mocha Almond Fudge	½ cup (2.3 oz)	150	2	8

FOOD	PORTION	CALS.	SAT. FAT	FAT
Mocha Mix (CONT.)				
Neapolitan	½ cup (2.3 oz)	140	2	7
Strawberry Swirl	½ cup (2.3 oz)	140	2	6
Vanilla	½ cup (2.3 oz)	140	2	7
Nestle Crunch				
Chocolate	1 bar (3 oz)	200	9	14
Cones	1 (4.6 oz)	300	10	16
Crunch King	1 (4 oz)	270	14	19
Nuggets	8 pieces	140	5	9
Reduced Fat	1 (2.5 oz)	130	5	7
Vanilla	1 bar (3 oz)	200	9	14
NutraShake				
High Calorie High Protein All Flavors	1 serv (4 oz)	200	—	10
Perry's				
No Fat No Sugar Added Caramel	½ cup (2.8 oz)	90	0	0
No Fat No Sugar Added Chocolate	½ cup (2.6 oz)	80	0	0
No Fat No Sugar Added Peach	½ cup (2.9 oz)	90	0	0
No Fat No Sugar Added Strawberry	½ cup (2.8 oz)	90	0	0
No Fat No Sugar Added Vanilla	½ cup (2.6 oz)	80	0	0
Rice Dream				
Bar Chocolate	1	270	—	16
Bar Chocolate Nutty	1	330	—	23
Bar Strawberry	1	260	—	15
Bar Vanilla	1	275	—	16
Bar Vanilla Nutty	1	330	—	23
Cappuccino	½ cup	130	—	5
Carob	½ cup	130	—	5
Carob Almond	½ cup	140	—	6
Carob Chip	½ cup	140	—	6
Carob Chip Mint	½ cup	140	—	6
Cocoa Marble Fudge	½ cup	140	—	6
Dream Pie Chocolate	1	380	—	19
Dream Pie Mint	1	380	—	19
Dream Pie Mocha	1	380	—	19
Dream Pie Vanilla	1	380	—	19
Lemon	½ cup	130	—	5
Peanut Butter Fudge	½ cup	160	—	7
Strawberry	½ cup	130	—	5
Vanilla	½ cup	130	—	5
Vanilla Fudge	½ cup	140	—	6

FOOD	PORTION	CALS.	SAT. FAT	FAT
Rice Dream (CONT.)				
Vanilla Swiss Almond	½ cup	140	—	6
Wildberry	½ cup	130	—	5
Sealtest				
American Glory	½ cup (2.4 oz)	130	4	6
Butter Pecan	½ cup (2.4 oz)	160	5	9
Candy Cane Crunch	½ cup (2.4 oz)	150	4	6
Chocolate	½ cup (2.4 oz)	140	4	7
Chocolate Butter Pecan	½ cup (2.4 oz)	150	5	8
Chocolate Chip	½ cup (2.4 oz)	150	5	8
Coconut Chocolate	½ cup (2.4 oz)	160	6	8
Coffee	½ cup (2.4 oz)	140	4	7
Cupid's Scoops	½ cup (2.5 oz)	140	4	6
Dessert Bar Free Chocolate Fudge	1	90	0	0
Dessert Bar Free Vanilla Strawberry Swirl	1	80	0	0
Dessert Bar Free Vanilla Fudge	1	80	0	0
Free Black Cherry	½ cup	100	0	0
Free Chocolate	½ cup	100	0	0
Free Peach	½ cup	100	0	0
Free Strawberry	½ cup	100	0	0
Free Vanilla	½ cup	100	0	0
Free Vanilla Fudge Royale	½ cup	100	0	0
Free Vanilla Strawberry Royale	½ cup	100	0	0
French Vanilla	½ cup (2.4 oz)	140	5	8
Fudge Royale	½ cup (2.5 oz)	150	4	7
Heavenly Hash	½ cup (2.4 oz)	150	4	7
Maple Walnut	½ cup (2.4 oz)	160	5	9
Strawberry	½ cup (2.4 oz)	130	4	6
Triple Chocolate Passion	½ cup (2.5 oz)	160	5	7
Vanilla	½ cup (2.4 oz)	140	5	7
Vanilla Chocolate Strawberry	½ cup (2.4 oz)	140	4	6
Vanilla With Orange Sherbet	½ cup (2.7 oz)	130	3	4
Snickers				
Single	1 (2 fl oz)	220	6	13
Snack	1 (1 fl oz)	110	3	7
Starbucks				
Biscotti Bliss	½ cup	240	7	12
Caffe Almond Fudge	½ cup	260	7	13
Caffe Almond Roast	1 bar	280	9	18
Dark Roast Expresso Swirl	½ cup	220	6	10

FOOD	PORTION	CALS.	SAT. FAT	FAT
Starbucks (CONT.)				
Frappuccino	1 bar (2.8 oz)	110	1	2
Italian Roast Coffee	½ cup	230	7	12
Javachip	½ cup	250	8	13
Low Fat Latte	½ cup	170	2	3
Low Fat Mocha Mambo	½ cup	170	2	3
Vanilla Mochachip	½ cup	270	10	16
Tofu Ice Creme				
Carob	4 fl oz	190	—	8
Vanilla	4 fl oz	190	—	8
Tofutti				
Cuties Chocolate	1 (1.4 oz)	130	1	5
Cuties Vanilla	1 (1.4 oz)	121	1	5
Frutti Vanilla Apple Orchard	4 fl oz	100	0	0
Turkey Hill				
Black Cherry	½ cup (2.3 oz)	140	5	7
Butter Pecan	½ cup (2.3 oz)	170	5	11
Choco Mint Chip	½ cup (2.3 oz)	160	6	10
Cookies 'N Cream	½ cup (2.3 oz)	160	5	9
Lite Butter Pecan	½ cup (2.3 oz)	130	3	6
Lite Choco Mint Chip	½ cup (2.3 oz)	140	4	5
Lite Cookies 'N Cream	½ cup (2.3 oz)	130	3	5
Lite Vanilla & Chocolate	½ cup (2.3 oz)	110	2	3
Lite Vanilla Bean	½ cup (2.3 oz)	110	2	3
Neapolitan	½ cup (2.3 oz)	150	5	8
Rocky Road	½ cup (2.3 oz)	170	4	8
Tin Roof Sundae	½ cup (2.3 oz)	160	5	9
Vanilla	½ cup (2.3 oz)	140	5	8
Vanilla & Chocolate	½ cup (2.3 oz)	150	5	8
Vanilla Bean	½ cup (2.3 oz)	140	5	8
Ultra Slim-Fast				
Bar Fudge	1	90	—	tr
Bar Vanilla Cookie Crunch	1	90	—	4
Chocolate	4 oz	100	—	tr
Chocolate Fudge	4 oz	120	—	tr
Peach	4 oz	100	—	tr
Pralines & Caramel	4 oz	120	—	tr
Sandwich Vanilla	1	140	—	2
Sandwich Vanilla Chocolate	1	140	—	2
Sandwich Vanilla Oatmeal	1	150	—	3
Vanilla	4 oz	90	—	tr
Vanilla Fudge Cookie	4 oz	110	—	tr
Weight Watchers				
Chocolate Chip Cookie Dough Sundae	1 (2.64 oz)	190	2	5

FOOD	PORTION	CALS.	SAT. FAT	FAT
Weight Watchers (CONT.)				
Chocolate Mousse	1 bar	40	1	1
Chocolate Treat	1 bar	100	0	1
English Toffee Crunch	1 bar	110	3	6
Orange Vanilla Treat	1 bar	40	0	1
Vanilla Sandwich	1 bar	150	1	3
TAKE-OUT				
cone vanilla light soft serve	1 (4.6 oz)	164	4	6
gelato chocolate hazelnut	½ cup (5.3 oz)	370	4	29
gelato vanilla	½ cup (3 oz)	211	8	15
sundae caramel	1 (5.4 oz)	303	5	9
sundae hot fudge	1 (5.4 oz)	284	5	9
sundae strawberry	1 (5.4 oz)	269	4	8

ICE CREAM CONES AND CUPS

sugar cone	1	40	tr	tr
wafer cone	1	17	tr	tr
Comet				
Cups	1 (5 g)	20	—	0
Sugar Cones	1 (12 g)	50	—	0
Waffle Cone	1 (17 g)	70	0	1
Dutch Mill				
Chocolate Covered Wafer Cups	1 (0.5 oz)	80	2	5
Frookie				
Chocolate Crunch	1 (0.4 oz)	50	0	1
Honey Crunch	1 (0.4 oz)	45	0	1
Keebler				
Fudge Dipped Cup	1 (0.3 oz)	35	1	2
Sugar Cone	1 (0.4 oz)	50	0	1
Vanilla Cup	1 (0.2 oz)	15	0	0
Waffle Bowl	1 (0.4 oz)	50	0	1
Waffle Cone	1 (0.4 oz)	50	0	1
Oreo				
Chocolate Cones	1 (13 g)	50	0	1
Teddy Grahams				
Cinnamon Cones	1 (0.5 oz)	60	0	1

ICE CREAM TOPPINGS

(see also SYRUP)

butterscotch	2 tbsp (1.4 oz)	103	tr	tr
caramel	2 tbsp (1.4 oz)	103	tr	tr
marshmallow cream	1 oz	88	—	tr
marshmallow cream	1 jar (7 oz)	615	—	tr
pineapple	2 tbsp (1.5 oz)	106	—	0
strawberry	2 tbsp (1.5 oz)	107	—	tr

FOOD	PORTION	CALS.	SAT. FAT	FAT
strawberry	1 cup (11.5 oz)	863	—	1
walnuts in syrup	2 tbsp (1.4 oz)	167	1	9
Ben & Jerry's				
Hot Fudge	(1.3 oz)	140	3	7
Crumpy				
Chocolate Hazelnut Spread	1 tbsp (0.5 oz)	80	1	5
Hershey				
Chocolate Shop Double Chocolate	1 tbsp (0.7 oz)	50	0	0
Chocolate Shoppe Apple Pie A La Mode	1 tbsp (1.3 oz)	100	0	0
Chocolate Shoppe Butterscotch Caramel	1 tbsp (0.7 oz)	70	1	1
Chocolate Shoppe Caramel	2 tbsp (1.3 oz)	100	0	0
Chocolate Shoppe Chocolate Mini	1 tbsp (0.7 oz)	50	0	0
Chocolate Shoppe Double Chocolate	1 tbsp (0.6 oz)	60	1	1
Chocolate Shoppe Hot Fudge	1 tbsp (0.7 oz)	70	1	3
Chocolate Shoppe Hot Fudge Fat Free	2 tbsp (1.4 oz)	100	0	0
Chocolate Shoppe Sprinkles Milk Chocolate	1 tbsp (0.5 oz)	70	2	3
Chocolate Shoppe Sprinkles Reeses	1 tbsp (0.5 oz)	70	2	4
Chocolate Shoppe Sprinkles York	1 tbsp (0.6 oz)	80	3	4
Kraft				
Butterscotch	2 tbsp (1.4 oz)	130	1	2
Caramel	2 tbsp (1.4 oz)	120	0	0
Chocolate	2 tbsp (1.4 oz)	110	0	0
Hot Fudge	2 tbsp (1.4 oz)	140	2	5
Pineapple	2 tbsp (1.4 oz)	110	0	0
Strawberry	2 tbsp (1.4 oz)	110	0	0
Marzetti				
Caramel Apple	2 tbsp	60	2	7
Caramel Apple Reduced Fat	2 tbsp	30	2	3
Peanut Butter Caramel	2 tbsp	60	1	6
Planters				
Nut	2 tbsp (0.5 oz)	100	1	9

ICED TEA
(see also TEA/HERBAL TEA)

FOOD	PORTION	CALS.	SAT. FAT	FAT
MIX				
instant artifically sweetened lemon flavored as prep w/ water	8 oz	5	0	0
instant sweetened lemon flavor as prep w/ water	9 oz	87	tr	tr
instant unsweetened lemon flavor as prep w/ water	8 oz	4	0	0
Bigelow				
Nice Over Ice	5 fl oz	1	—	tr
Celestial Seasonings				
Iced Delight	8 fl oz	4	—	tr
Crystal Light				
Decaffeinated as prep	1 serv (8 oz)	5	0	0
Iced Tea as prep	1 serv (8 oz)	5	0	0
Peach Tea as prep	1 serv (8 oz)	5	0	0
Raspberry Tea as prep	1 serv (8 oz)	5	0	0
Lipton				
100% Tea Decaffeinated as prep	1 serv	0	0	0
100% Tea Unsweetened as prep	1 serv	0	0	0
100% Tea as prep	1 serv	0	0	0
Calorie Free as prep	1 serv	0	0	0
Decaffeinated Ice Tea Brew as prep	1 serv (8 oz)	0	0	0
Decaffeinated Lemon as prep	1 serv	90	0	0
Diet Decaffeinated Lemon as prep	1 serv	5	0	0
Diet Lemon as prep	1 serv	5	0	0
Diet Peach as prep	1 serv	5	0	0
Diet Raspberry as prep	1 serv	5	0	0
Diet Tea & Lemondage as prep	1 serv	10	0	0
Herbal Iced Collection	1 tea bag	0	0	0
Ice Tea Brew as prep	1 serv (8 oz)	0	0	0
Lemon as prep	1 serv	90	0	0
Lemon as prep	1 pkg (0.5 oz)	50	0	0
Natrual Brew Tropical as prep	1 serv	90	0	0
Natural Brew 100% Tea Decaffeinated as prep	1 serv	0	0	0
Natural Brew 100% Tea as prep	1 serv	0	0	0
Natural Brew Diet Lemon as prep	1 serv	5	0	0

FOOD	PORTION	CALS.	SAT. FAT	FAT
Lipton (CONT.)				
Natural Brew Diet Peach as prep	1 serv	5	0	0
Natural Brew Diet Tropical as prep	1 serv	5	0	0
Natural Brew Unsweetened Lemon as prep	1 serv	0	0	0
Peach as prep	1 serv	90	0	0
Rasberry as prep	1 serv	90	0	0
Tea & Lemonade as prep	1 serv	90	0	0
Nestea				
Peach as prep	8 oz	88	—	tr
Raspberry as prep	8 oz	88	—	tr
READY-TO-DRINK				
Arizona				
Lemon	1 bottle (16 oz)	180	0	0
Raspberry	8 fl oz	95	0	0
Clearly Canadian				
Clearly Tea Original	8 fl oz	80	—	0
Clearly Tea Tangy Lemon	8 fl oz	80	—	0
Crystal Light				
Lemon	1 serv (8 oz)	5	0	0
Peach Tea	1 serv (8 oz)	5	0	0
Raspberry Tea	1 serv (8 oz)	5	0	0
Lipton				
Carribean Cooler	1 can (12 oz)	130	0	0
Diet Lemon	8 oz	0	0	0
Diet Lemon	1 bottle (16 oz)	10	0	0
Green Tea & Passion Fruit	1 bottle (16 oz)	160	0	0
Lemon	8 oz	80	0	0
Lemon	1 can (12 oz)	120	0	0
Lemon	1 bottle (16 oz)	180	0	0
Natural Lemon	1 box (8 oz)	100	0	0
Peach	8 oz	80	0	0
Peach	1 bottle (16 oz)	220	0	0
Raspberry	8 oz	80	0	0
Raspberry	1 bottle (16 oz)	220	0	0
Raspberry Blast	1 can (12 oz)	130	0	0
Southern Style Extra Sweet No Lemon	1 bottle (16 oz)	240	0	0
Southern Style Lemon	1 bottle (16 oz)	200	0	0
Southern Style Sweetened No Lemon	1 bottle (16 oz)	200	0	0
Sweet	8 oz	80	0	0
Sweetened No Lemon	1 bottle (16 oz)	140	0	0

FOOD	PORTION	CALS.	SAT. FAT	FAT
Lipton (CONT.)				
Sweetened Lemon	8 oz	80	0	0
Tangerine Twist	1 can (12 oz)	120	0	0
Tea & Lemonade	1 bottle (16 oz)	220	0	0
Unsweetened No Lemon	1 bottle (16 oz)	0	0	0
Mad River				
Red Tea w/ Guarana	8 oz	90	0	0
Nantucket Nectars				
Diet	8 oz	5	0	0
Diet Green Tea	8 oz	5	0	0
Half & Half	8 oz	90	0	0
Iced Tea	8 oz	80	0	0
Matt Fee	8 oz	80	0	0
Raspberry	8 oz	90	0	0
Savannah	8 oz	80	0	0
Nestea				
With Sugar & Lemon	1 bottle (16 fl oz)	176	0	0
With Sugar & Lemon	1 can (11.5 fl oz)	127	0	0
Royal Mistic				
Diet	12 fl oz	8	0	0
Lemon	12 fl oz	144	0	0
Orange	12 fl oz	144	0	0
Wild Berry	12 fl oz	144	0	0
Schweppes				
Ice Tea	8 fl oz	90	0	0
Snapple				
Cranberry Raspberry	8 fl oz	120	0	0
Diet	8 fl oz	0	0	0
Diet Peach	8 fl oz	0	0	0
Diet Raspberry	8 fl oz	0	0	0
Lemon	8 fl oz	100	0	0
Mango	8 fl oz	110	0	0
Mint	8 fl oz	120	0	0
Old Fashioned	8 fl oz	80	0	0
Orange	8 fl oz	110	0	0
Peach	8 fl oz	100	0	0
Raspberry	8 fl oz	100	0	0
Strawberry	8 fl oz	100	0	0
Turkey Hill				
Diet Decaffeinated	1 cup (8 oz)	0	0	0
Raspberry Cooler	1 cup (8 oz)	110	0	0
Regular	1 cup (8 oz)	90	0	0

ICES AND ICE POPS
(see *also* ICE CREAM AND FROZEN DESSERTS, PUDDING POPS, SHERBET, YOGURT FROZEN)

FOOD	PORTION	CALS.	SAT. FAT	FAT
fruit & juice bar	1 (3 fl oz)	75	—	tr
gelatin pop	1 (1.5 oz)	31	0	0
ice coconut pineapple	½ cup (4 fl oz)	109	—	3
ice fruit w/ Equal	1 bar (1.7 oz)	12	0	0
ice lime	½ cup (4 fl oz)	75	0	0
ice pop	1 (2 fl oz)	42	0	0
Ben & Jerry's				
Sorbet Doonesberry	½ cup	140	0	0
Sorbet Lemon Swirl	½ cup	120	0	0
Sorbet Purple Passion Fruit	½ cup	140	0	0
Cool Creations				
10 Pack	1 pop (2 oz)	60	0	0
Lion King Cone	1 (4 oz)	280	9	14
Mickey Mouse Bar	1 (4 oz)	170	4	11
Mickey Mouse Bar	1 (2.5 oz)	110	3	7
Surprise Pops	1 (2 oz)	60	0	0
Fi-Bar				
Juice Bar Lemoney-Lime	1 bar	63	—	tr
Juice Bar Strawberry Nectar	1 bar	63	—	tr
Juice Bar Tropical Delight	1 bar	63	—	tr
Flintstones				
Rock Pops	1 (3.5 oz)	80	0	0
Frozfruit				
Banana Cream	1 bar (4 oz)	150	5	7
Cantaloupe	1 bar (4 oz)	60	0	0
Cappuccino Cream	1 bar (3 oz)	140	4	6
Cherry	1 bar (4 oz)	70	0	0
Coconut Cream	1 bar (4 oz)	170	8	11
Kiwi Strawberry	1 bar (4 oz)	90	0	0
Lemon	1 bar (4 oz)	90	0	0
Lemon Iced Tea	1 bar (4 oz)	80	0	0
Lime	1 bar (4 oz)	90	0	0
Orange	1 bar (4 oz)	90	0	0
Pina Colada Cream	1 bar (4 oz)	170	6	8
Pineapple	1 bar (4 oz)	80	0	0
Raspberry	1 bar (4 oz)	80	0	0
Strawberry	1 (4 oz)	80	0	0
Strawberry Banana Cream	1 bar (4 oz)	140	3	6
Strawberry Cream	1 bar (4 oz)	130	3	5
Tropical	1 bar (4 oz)	90	0	0
Watermelon	1 bar (4 oz)	50	0	0
Good Humor				
Big Stick Cherry Pineapple	1 (3.6 fl oz)	50	0	0
Big Stick Popsicle	1 (3.6 fl oz)	50	0	0

FOOD	PORTION	CALS.	SAT. FAT	FAT
Good Humor (cont.)				
Calippo Cherry	1 (3.8 fl oz)	100	0	0
Calippo Grape Lemon	1 (3.9 fl oz)	90	0	0
Calippo Orange	1 (3.9 fl oz)	90	0	0
Citrus Bites	1 (1.8 fl oz)	35	0	0
Creamsicle Orange	1 (2.8 fl oz)	110	2	3
Creamsicle Orange	1 (1.8 fl oz)	70	1	2
Creamsicle Orange Raspberry	1 (2.6 fl oz)	100	2	3
Creamsicle Sugar Free	1 (1.8 fl oz)	25	0	0
Flinstones Push-Up Yabba Dabba Doo Orange	1 (2.75 fl oz)	90	—	1
Fudgsicle Bar	1 (2.8 fl oz)	90	1	1
Fudgsicle Pop	1 (1.8 fl oz)	60	1	1
Fudgsicle Sugar Free	1 (1.8 fl oz)	40	1	1
Fun Box Fudge Bar	1 (2.3 fl oz)	80	1	1
Fun Box Pops	1 (2 fl oz)	35	0	0
Fun Box Twin Box Cherry	1 (2.6 fl oz)	50	0	0
Fun Box Twin Pop Banana	1 (2.6 fl oz)	50	0	0
Fun Box Twin Pop Blue Raspberry	1 (2.6 fl oz)	50	0	0
Fun Box Twin Pop Cherry Lemon	1 (2.6 fl oz)	50	0	0
Fun Box Twin Pop Orange Cherry Grape	1 (2.6 oz)	50	0	0
Fun Box Twin Pop Root Beer	1 (2.6 fl oz)	50	0	0
Garfield Bar	1 (3.9 fl oz)	90	0	0
Great White	1 (3.1 fl oz)	70	—	1
Hyperstripe	1 (2.8 fl oz)	80	0	0
Ice Stripe Cherry Orange	1 (1.5 fl oz)	35	0	0
Jumbo Jet Star	1 (4.7 fl oz)	80	0	0
Laser Blazer	1 (2.6 oz)	70	0	0
Popsicle All Natural	1 (1.8 fl oz)	45	0	0
Popsicle Orange Cherry Grape	1 (1.8 fl oz)	45	0	0
Popsicle Rainbow Pops	1 (1.8 fl oz)	45	0	0
Popsicle Rootbeer Banana Lime	1 (1.8 fl oz)	45	0	0
Popsicle Strawberry Raspberry Wildberry	1 (1.8 fl oz)	45	0	0
Popsicle Supersicle Traffic Signal	1	80	0	0
Popsicle Twin Pop Cherry	1 (2.6 fl oz)	70	0	0
Popsicle Twin Pop Orange Cherry Grape Lime	1 (2.6 fl oz)	70	0	0

FOOD	PORTION	CALS.	SAT. FAT	FAT
Good Humor (CONT.)				
Snow Cone	1	60	—	0
Snowfruit Coconut Bar	1 (3.75 fl oz)	150	3	4
Snowfruit Orange Bar	1	140	0	0
Snowfruit Strawberry Bar	1	120	0	0
Snowfruit Tropical Fruit Bar	1	110	0	0
Sugar Free Pop Orange Cherry Grape	1 (1.8 fl oz)	15	0	0
Super Mario Bar	1	120	1	1
Supersicle Cherry Banana	1 (4.7 fl oz)	80	0	0
Supersicle Cherry Cola	1 (4.7 fl oz)	80	0	0
Supersicle Double Fudge	1 (4.7 fl oz)	150	1	2
Supersicle Firecracker	1 (4.7 fl oz)	90	0	0
Supersicle Firecracker Jr.	1	72	0	0
Supersicle Sour Tower	1	80	0	0
Swirl Bubble Gum	1 (2.7 fl oz)	55	0	0
Swirl Cherry Banana	1 (2.7 fl oz)	55	0	0
Torpedo Cherry	1 (1.8 fl oz)	35	0	0
Twister Blue Raspberry Cherry Cherry Cola Cherry	1 (1.8 fl oz)	45	0	0
Twister Cherry Lemon Orange Lemon	1 (1.8 fl oz)	45	0	0
Vampire's Deadly Secret	1 (2.8 fl oz)	100	0	0
Watermelon Bar	1 (3.6 fl oz)	80	0	0
Haagen-Dazs				
Sorbet Banana Strawberry	½ cup (4 oz)	140	0	0
Sorbet Chocolate	½ cup (4 oz)	130	—	0
Sorbet Manago	½ cup (4 oz)	120	—	0
Sorbet Orchard Peach	½ cup (4 oz)	140	0	0
Sorbet Raspberry	½ cup (4 oz)	120	—	0
Sorbet Strawberry	½ cup (4 oz)	130	—	0
Sorbet Zesty Lemon	½ cup (4 oz)	130	—	0
Sorbet & Cream Orange	½ cup (3.7 oz)	200	5	9
Sorbet & Cream Raspberry	½ cup (3.7 oz)	190	5	9
Sorbet Bar Chocolate	1 (2.7 oz)	80	—	0
Sorbet Bar Wild Berry	1 (2.7 oz)	90	—	0
Hood				
Hendrie's Sizzle'N Sour Stix	1 bar (2 oz)	80	0	tr
Hoodsie Pop	1 (3.3 oz)	60	0	0
Natural Blenders Pineappple	1 bar (1 oz)	60	0	0
Natural Blenders Raspberry	1 bar (1 oz)	60	0	0
Natural Blenders Strawberry	1 bar (1 oz)	60	0	0
Pop Banana	1 (3.3 oz)	60	0	0
Pop Blue Raspberry	1 (3.3 oz)	60	0	0

FOOD	PORTION	CALS.	SAT. FAT	FAT
Hood (CONT.)				
Pop Cherry	1 (3.3 oz)	60	0	0
Pop Grape	1 (3.3 oz)	60	0	0
Pop Orange	1 (3.3 oz)	60	0	0
Pop Root Beer	1 (3.3 oz)	60	0	0
Super Sortment Juice Bars	1 bar (1.9 oz)	40	0	0
Lifesavers				
Ice Pops	1	35	0	0
Ice Pops	1 (1.75 oz)	35	0	0
Mr. Freeze				
Assorted	2 bars (3 oz)	45	0	0
Tropical	2 bars (3 oz)	45	0	0
Natural Choice				
Organic Banana	½ cup (3.6 oz)	110	0	0
Organic Blueberry	½ cup (3.6 oz)	100	0	0
Organic Kiwi	½ cup (3.6 oz)	110	0	0
Organic Lemon	½ cup (3.6 oz)	110	0	0
Organic Mango	½ cup (3.6 oz)	110	0	0
Organic Strawberry	½ cup (3.6 oz)	110	0	0
Organic Strawberry Kiwi	½ cup (3.6 oz)	110	0	0
Sunkist				
Orange Juice Bar	1 (3.4 fl oz)	80	—	1
Wildberry	1 (3.4 fl oz)	120	—	1
Tofutti				
Frutti Apricot Mango	4 fl oz	100	0	0
Frutti Three Berry	4 fl oz	100	0	0

ICING

(see CAKE ICING)

INSTANT BREAKFAST

(see BREAKFAST DRINKS)

JALAPENO

(see PEPPERS)

JAM/JELLY/PRESERVES

all flavors jam	1 tbsp (0.7 oz)	48	0	0
all flavors jam	1 pkg (0.5 oz)	34	0	0
all flavors jelly	1 tbsp (0.7 oz)	52	0	0
all flavors jelly	1 pkg (0.5 oz)	38	0	0
all flavors preserve	1 pkg (0.5 oz)	34	0	0
all flavors preserve	1 tbsp (0.7 oz)	48	0	0
apple butter	1 tbsp (0.6 oz)	33	0	0
apple butter	1 cup (9.9 oz)	519	—	1
apple jelly	1 tbsp (0.7 oz)	52	0	0

FOOD	PORTION	CALS.	SAT. FAT	FAT
apple jelly	1 pkg (0.5 oz)	38	0	0
linganberry jam	0.5 oz	23	tr	tr
orange marmalade	1 pkg (0.5 oz)	34	0	0
orange marmalade	1 tbsp (0.7 oz)	49	0	0
strawberry jam	1 pkg (0.5 oz)	34	0	0
strawberry jam	1 tbsp (0.7 oz)	48	0	0
strawberry preserve	1 pkg (0.5 oz)	34	0	0
strawberry preserve	1 tbsp (0.7 oz)	48	0	0
BAMA				
Apple Butter	2 tsp	25	0	0
Apple Jelly	2 tsp	30	0	0
Grape Jelly	2 tsp	30	0	0
Peach Preserves	2 tsp	30	0	0
Red Plum Jam	2 tsp	30	0	0
Strawberry Preserves	2 tsp	30	0	0
Estee				
Fruit Spread Apple Spice	1 tbsp	16	0	0
Fruit Spread Apricot	1 tbsp	16	0	0
Fruit Spread Grape	1 tbsp	16	0	0
Fruit Spread Peach	1 tbsp	16	0	0
Fruit Spread Red Raspberry	1 tbsp	16	0	0
Fruit Spread Strawberry	1 tbsp	16	0	0
Harvest Moon				
Apricot Fruit Spread	1 tbsp (0.6 oz)	35	0	0
Blueberry Fruit Spread	1 tbsp (0.6 oz)	35	0	0
Cherry Fruit Spread	1 tbsp (0.6 oz)	35	0	0
Grape Fruit Spread	1 tbsp (0.6 oz)	35	0	0
Peach Fruit Spread	1 tbsp (0.6 oz)	35	0	0
Raspberry Fruit Spread	1 tbsp (0.6 oz)	35	0	0
Strawberry Fruit Spread	1 tbsp (0.6 oz)	35	0	0
Red Wing				
Apple Jelly	1 tbsp (0.7 oz)	50	0	0
Apple Blackberry Jelly	1 tbsp (0.7 oz)	50	0	0
Apple Cherry Jelly	1 tbsp (0.7 oz)	50	0	0
Apple Currant Jelly	1 tbsp (0.7 oz)	50	0	0
Apple Grape Jelly	1 tbsp (0.7 oz)	50	0	0
Apple Raspberry Jelly	1 tbsp (0.7 oz)	50	0	0
Apple Strawberry Jelly	1 tbsp (0.7 oz)	50	0	0
Black Raspberry Jelly	1 tbsp (0.7 oz)	50	0	0
Blackberry Jelly	1 tbsp (0.7 oz)	50	0	0
Cherry Jelly	1 tbsp (0.7 oz)	50	0	0
Concord Grape Jelly	1 tbsp (0.7 oz)	50	0	0
Crabapple Jelly	1 tbsp (0.7 oz)	50	0	0
Cranberry Jelly	1 tbsp (0.7 oz)	50	0	0
Cranberry Grape Jelly	1 tbsp (0.7 oz)	50	0	0

FOOD	PORTION	CALS.	SAT. FAT	FAT
Red Wing (CONT.)				
Currant Jelly	1 tbsp (0.7 oz)	50	0	0
Damson Plum Jelly	1 tbsp (0.7 oz)	50	0	0
Elderberry Jelly	1 tbsp (0.7 oz)	50	0	0
Grape Jelly	1 tbsp (0.7 oz)	50	0	0
Mint Jelly	1 tbsp (0.7 oz)	50	0	0
Mint Apple Jelly	1 tbsp (0.7 oz)	50	0	0
Mixed Fruit Jelly	1 tbsp (0.7 oz)	50	0	0
Red Plum Jelly	1 tbsp (0.7 oz)	50	0	0
Red Raspberry Jelly	1 tbsp (0.7 oz)	50	0	0
Strawberry Jelly	1 tbsp (0.7 oz)	50	0	0
Strawberry Apple Jelly	1 tbsp (0.7 oz)	50	0	0
Tabasco				
Spicy Pepper Jelly	1 tbsp (0.6 oz)	50	0	0
Tree Of Life				
Apricot Fruit Spread	1 tbsp (0.6 oz)	45	0	0
Blueberry Fruit Spread	1 tbsp (0.6 oz)	35	0	0
Cherry Fruit Spread	1 tbsp (0.6 oz)	40	0	0
Grape Fruit Spread	1 tbsp (0.6 oz)	35	0	0
Peach Fruit Spread	1 tbsp (0.6 oz)	45	0	0
Raspberry Fruit Spread	1 tbsp (0.6 oz)	30	0	0
Strawberry Fruit Spread	1 tbsp (0.6 oz)	35	0	0
Whistling Wings				
Blueberry Jam	1 oz	50	—	tr
Raspberry Jam	1 oz	60	—	tr
White House				
Apple Butter	1 tbsp (0.6 oz)	35	0	0
JAVA PLUM				
fresh	3	5	—	tr
fresh	1 cup	82	—	tr

JAPANESE FOOD
(see ASIAN FOOD, SUSHI)

JELLY
(see JAM/JELLY/PRESERVE)

JERUSALEM ARTICHOKE
(see ARTICHOKE)

FOOD	PORTION	CALS.	SAT. FAT	FAT
KALE				
FRESH				
chopped cooked	½ cup	21	tr	tr
raw chopped	½ cup	21	tr	tr
scotch chopped cooked	½ cup	18	tr	tr
Dole				
Chopped	½ cup	17	—	1

FOOD	PORTION	CALS.	SAT. FAT	FAT
FROZEN				
chopped cooked	½ cup	20	tr	tr
KETCHUP				
ketchup	1 tbsp	16	tr	tr
ketchup	1 pkg (0.2 oz)	6	tr	tr
Del Monte				
Ketchup	1 tbsp (0.5 oz)	15	0	0
Estee				
Ketchup	1 tbsp	15	0	0
Hain				
Natural	1 tbsp	16	0	0
Natural No Salt Added	1 tbsp	16	0	0
Healthy Choice				
Ketchup	1 tbsp (0.5 oz)	9	0	0
Heinz				
Hot	1 tbsp	14	0	0
Ketchup	1 tbsp (0.6 oz)	15	0	0
Lite	1 tbsp	8	0	0
Hunt's				
Ketchup	1 tbsp (0.6 oz)	16	0	tr
No Salt Added	1 tbsp (0.6 oz)	16	0	tr
McIlhenny				
Spicy	1 tbsp (0.6 oz)	20	0	0
Muir Glen				
Organic	1 tbsp (0.6 oz)	15	—	0
Red Wing				
Extra Fancy	1 tbsp (0.6 oz)	20	0	0
Tree Of Life				
Ketchup	1 tbsp (0.5 oz)	10	0	0
Salsa Ketchup	1 tbsp (0.5 oz)	10	0	0
KIDNEY				
beef simmered	3 oz	122	1	3
lamb braised	3 oz	117	1	3
pork cooked	1 cup	211	2	7
pork cooked	3 oz	128	1	4
veal braised	3 oz	139	1	5
KIDNEY BEANS				
CANNED				
kidney beans	1 cup	208	tr	1
red	1 cup	216	tr	1
B&M				
Red Baked Beans	½ cup (4.6 oz)	170	1	2

FOOD	PORTION	CALS.	SAT. FAT	FAT
Eden				
Organic	½ cup (4.6 oz)	100	0	0
Friend's				
Red Baked Beans	½ cup (4.6 oz)	160	0	1
Goya				
Spanish Style	7.5 oz	140	—	1
Green Giant				
Dark Red	½ cup (4.5 oz)	110	0	0
Light Red	½ cup (4.5 oz)	110	0	0
Hanover				
Dark Red	½ cup	110	—	0
Light Red In Sauce	½ cup	120	—	0
Hunt's				
Red	½ cup (4.5 oz)	94	0	1
Progresso				
Red	½ cup (4.6 oz)	110	0	1
Trappey				
Dark Red	½ cup (4.5 oz)	130	0	1
Light Red	½ cup (4.5 oz)	120	0	1
Light Red New Orleans Style With Bacon	½ cup (4.5 oz)	110	1	1
Light Red With Jalapeno	½ cup (4.5 oz)	110	0	1
With Chili Gravy	½ cup (4.5 oz)	110	0	1
Van Camp's				
Dark Red	½ cup (4.6 oz)	90	0	0
Light Red	½ cup (4.6 oz)	90	0	0
DRIED				
california red cooked	1 cup	219	tr	tr
cooked	1 cup	225	tr	1
red cooked	1 cup	225	tr	1
royal red cooked	1 cup	218	tr	tr
Arrowhead				
Red	¼ cup (1.6 oz)	160	0	1
KIWI JUICE				
After The Fall				
Kiwi Bear	1 cup (8 oz)	100	0	0
KIWIS				
fresh	1 med	46	—	tr
Dole				
Fresh	2	90	—	1
Sonoma				
Dried	7-8 pieces (1 oz)	90	0	1

FOOD	PORTION	CALS.	SAT. FAT	FAT

KNISH
Joshua's

| Coney Island Potato | 1 (4.6 oz) | 280 | 2 | 8 |

TAKE-OUT

cheese & blueberry	1 (7 oz)	378	—	13
cheese & cherry	1 (7 oz)	378	—	13
everything	1 (7 oz)	221	—	8
kashe	1 (7 oz)	270	—	8
potato	1 lg (7 oz)	332	3	12
potato	1 med (3.5 oz)	166	2	6
potato w/ broccoli & cheese	1 (7 oz)	312	—	15
potato w/ spinach & mushroom	1 (7 oz)	214	—	8

KOHLRABI

| raw sliced | ½ cup | 19 | tr | tr |
| sliced cooked | ½ cup | 24 | tr | tr |

KUMQUATS

| fresh | 1 | 12 | — | tr |

LAMB
(see also LAMB DISHES)

FRESH

cubed lean only braised	3 oz	190	3	7
cubed lean only broiled	3 oz	158	2	6
ground broiled	3 oz	240	7	17
leg lean & fat Choice roasted	3 oz	219	6	14
loin chop w/ bone lean & fat Choice broiled	1 chop (2.3 oz)	201	6	15
loin chop w/ bone lean only Choice broiled	1 chop (1.6 oz)	100	2	5
rib chop lean & fat Choice broiled	3 oz	307	11	25
rib chop lean only Choice broiled	3 oz	200	4	11
shank lean & fat Choice braised	3 oz	206	5	11
shank lean & fat Choice roasted	3 oz	191	4	11
shoulder chop w/ bone lean & fat Choice braised	1 chop (2.5 oz)	244	7	17
shoulder chop w/ bone lean only Choice braised	1 chop (1.9 oz)	152	3	8
sirloin lean & fat Choice roasted	3 oz	248	7	21

FOOD	PORTION	CALS.	SAT. FAT	FAT
FROZEN				
New Zealand lean & fat cooked	3 oz	259	9	19
New Zealand lean only cooked	3 oz	175	3	8
LAMBSQUARTERS				
chopped cooked	½ cup	29	tr	1
LECITHIN				
(see soy)				
LEEKS				
chopped cooked	¼ cup	8	tr	tr
cooked	1 (4.4 oz)	38	tr	tr
freeze dried	1 tbsp	1	0	0
raw	1 (4.4 oz)	76	tr	tr
raw chopped	¼ cup	16	tr	tr
LEMON				
fresh	1 med	22	tr	tr
peel	1 tbsp	0	tr	tr
wedge	1	5	tr	tr
Dole				
Fresh	1	18	—	0
LEMON EXTRACT				
Virginia Dare				
Extract	1 tsp	22	—	0
LEMON GRASS				
fresh	1 cup (2.4 oz)	66	tr	tr
fresh	1 tbsp (5 g)	5	tr	tr
LEMON JUICE				
bottled	1 tbsp	3	tr	tr
fresh	1 tbsp	4	—	0
frzn	1 tbsp	3	tr	tr
After The Fall				
Spicy Lemon	1 can (12 oz)	150	0	0
Realemon				
Juice	1 tsp (5 ml)	0	0	0
LEMONADE				
FROZEN				
as prep w/ water	1 cup	100	tr	tr
not prep	1 can (6 oz)	397	tr	tr
Bright & Early				
Lemonade	8 fl oz	120	0	0

FOOD	PORTION	CALS.	SAT. FAT	FAT
Minute Maid				
Country Style	8 fl oz	120	0	0
Cranberry Lemonade	8 fl oz	80	0	0
Lemonade	8 fl oz	110	0	0
Pink	8 fl oz	120	0	0
Raspberry	8 fl oz	120	0	0
Seneca				
as prep	8 fl oz	110	0	0
MIX				
powder as prep w/ water	9 fl oz	113	tr	tr
powder w/ equal	1 pitcher (67 oz)	40	0	0
Country Time				
Lem'n Berry Sippers Cranberry Raspberry Lemonade as prep	1 serv (8 oz)	90	0	0
Lem'n Berry Sippers Raspberry Lemonade as prep	1 serv (8 oz)	90	0	0
Lem'n Berry Sippers Strawberry Lemonade as prep	1 serv (8 oz)	90	0	0
Lem'n Berry Sippers Wildberry Lemonade as prep	1 serv (8 oz)	90	0	0
Lem'n Berry Sippers Sugar Free Strawberry Lemonade as prep	1 serv (8 oz)	5	0	0
Lemonade as prep	1 serv (8 oz)	70	0	0
Pink as prep	1 serv (8 oz)	70	0	0
Sugar Free Pink as prep	1 serv (8 oz)	5	0	0
Sugar Free as prep	1 serv (8 oz)	5	0	0
Crystal Light				
Lemonade as prep	1 serv (8 oz)	5	0	0
Pink as prep	1 serv (8 oz)	5	0	0
Kool-Aid				
Lemonade as prep	1 serv (8 oz)	70	0	0
Mix as prep w/ sugar	1 serv (8 oz)	100	0	0
Pink as prep w/ sugar	1 serv (8 oz)	100	0	0
Soarin' Strawberry Lemonade as prep	1 serv (8 oz)	70	0	0
Soarin' Strawberry Lemonade as prep w/ sugar	1 serv (8 oz)	100	0	0
Sugar Free Soarin' Strawberry Lemonade as prep	1 serv (8 oz)	5	0	0
Sugar Free Mix as prep	1 serv (8 oz)	5	0	0
READY-TO-DRINK				
After The Fall				
Apple Raspberry	1 bottle (10 oz)	120	0	0

FOOD	PORTION	CALS.	SAT. FAT	FAT
Crystal Geyser				
Juice Squeeze Pink	1 bottle (12 fl oz)	140	0	0
Crystal Light				
Lemonade	1 serv (8 oz)	5	0	0
Pink	1 serv (8 oz)	5	0	0
Diet Rite				
Salt/Sodium Free	8 fl oz	2	0	0
Everfresh				
Lemonade	1 can (8 oz)	120	0	0
Ruby Red	1 can (8 oz)	110	0	0
Fruitopia				
Lemonade	8 fl oz	120	0	0
Minute Maid				
Chilled	8 fl oz	110	0	0
Cranberry Chilled	8 fl oz	120	0	0
Juices To Go	1 bottle (16 fl oz)	110	0	0
Juices To Go	1 can (11.5 fl oz)	160	0	0
Juices To Go Cranberry Lemonade	1 bottle (16 fl oz)	110	0	0
Juices To Go Raspberry Lemonade	1 bottle (16 fl oz)	120	0	0
Pink Chilled	8 fl oz	110	0	0
Raspberry Chilled	8 fl oz	120	0	0
Mott's				
Lemonade	10 fl oz	160	0	0
Nehi				
Lemonade	8 fl oz	130	0	0
Newman's Own				
Lemonade	1 bottle (10 oz)	140	0	0
Roadside Virginia	8 fl oz	110	0	0
Odwalla				
Honey	8 fl oz	70	0	0
Strawberry	8 fl oz	150	0	0
Royal Mistic				
Lemonade Limeade	16 fl oz	230	0	0
Tropical Pink	16 fl oz	230	0	0
Santa Cruz				
Organic	8 oz	100	0	0
Shasta Plus				
Lemonade	1 can (11.5 oz)	160	0	0
Snapple				
Diet Pink	8 fl oz	20	0	0
Lemonade	8 fl oz	110	0	0
Pink	8 fl oz	120	0	0
Strawberry	8 fl oz	110	0	0

FOOD	PORTION	CALS.	SAT. FAT	FAT
Turkey Hill				
Lemonade	8 fl oz	110	0	0
Veryfine				
Chillers	1 can (11.5 oz)	190	0	0
Chillers Cherry	8 fl oz	120	0	0
Chillers Peach	8 fl oz	120	0	0
Chillers Pink	1 can (11.5 oz)	180	0	0
Chillers Strawberry	1 can (11.5 oz)	170	0	0

LENTILS

FOOD	PORTION	CALS.	SAT. FAT	FAT
dried cooked	1 cup	231	tr	1
Casbah				
Pilaf as prep	1 cup	200	0	tr
Eden				
Organic w/ Sweet Onion & Bay Leaf	½ cup (4.6 oz)	90	0	0
Natural Touch				
Lentil Rice Loaf	1 in slice (3.2 oz)	170	3	9
TAKE-OUT				
indian sambar	1 serv	236	2	5
yemiser selatta ethiopian lentil salad	1 serv (3 oz)	115	1	7

LETTUCE
(see also SALAD)

FOOD	PORTION	CALS.	SAT. FAT	FAT
bibb	1 head (6 oz)	21	tr	tr
boston	2 leaves	2	tr	tr
boston	1 head (6 oz)	21	tr	tr
iceberg	1 leaf	3	tr	tr
iceberg	1 head (19 oz)	70	tr	1
looseleaf shredded	½ cup	5	tr	tr
romaine shredded	½ cup	4	tr	tr
Dole				
Butter	1 head	21	—	tr
Iceberg	1 cup (3 oz)	15	0	0
Romaine	1½ cups (3 oz)	15	0	0
Shredded	1½ cup (3 oz)	15	0	0
Western Express				
Heart's Of Romaine	6 leaves (3 oz)	20	0	1

LIMA BEANS
CANNED

FOOD	PORTION	CALS.	SAT. FAT	FAT
large	1 cup	191	tr	tr
lima beans	½ cup	93	tr	tr
Allen				
Green	½ cup (4.5 oz)	120	0	1

FOOD	PORTION	CALS.	SAT. FAT	FAT
Allen (CONT.)				
Green & White	½ cup (4.5 oz)	110	1	1
Del Monte				
Green	½ cup (4.4 oz)	80	0	0
Dennison's				
With Ham	7.5 oz	250	—	7
East Texas Fair				
Green	½ cup (4.5 oz)	120	0	1
Seneca				
Limas	½ cup	80	0	0
Trappey				
Baby Green With Bacon	½ cup (4.5 oz)	120	1	1
DRIED				
cooked	½ cup	104	tr	tr
Hurst				
HamBeens Baby Limas w/ Ham	1 serv	120	0	1
HamBeens Large Limas w/ Ham	1 serv	120	0	1
FROZEN				
cooked	½ cup	94	tr	tr
fordhook cooked	½ cup	85	tr	tr
Birds Eye				
Baby	½ cup (3.3 oz)	130	0	0
Fordhook	½ cup (3.3 oz)	100	0	0
Fresh Like				
Baby	3.5 oz	138	—	1
Green Giant				
Butter Sauce	⅔ cup (3.6 oz)	120	2	3
Harvest Fresh Baby	½ cup (2.7 oz)	80	0	0
Hanover				
Baby	½ cup	110	—	0
Fordhook	½ cup	100	—	0
LIME				
fresh	1	20	tr	tr
LIME JUICE				
bottled	1 tbsp	3	tr	tr
fresh	1 tbsp	4	tr	tr
After The Fall				
Caribbean Lime	1 can (12 oz)	170	0	0
Key West	1 cup (8 oz)	100	0	0
Odwalla				
Summertime Lime	8 fl oz	90	0	0

FOOD	PORTION	CALS.	SAT. FAT	FAT
Realime				
Juice	1 tsp (5 ml)	0	0	0
LING				
fresh baked	3 oz	95	—	1
LIQUOR/LIQUEUR				
(see also BEER AND ALE, CHAMPAGNE, DRINK MIXERS, MALT, WINE, WINE COOLERS)				
aquavit	3.5 oz	229	0	0
bloody mary	5 oz	116	tr	tr
bourbon & soda	4 oz	105	0	0
coffee liqueur	1.5 oz	174	tr	tr
coffee w/ cream liqueur	1.5 oz	154	5	7
cognac	3.5 oz	233	0	0
creme de menthe	1.5 oz	186	tr	tr
daiquiri	2 oz	111	0	0
gin	1.5 oz	110	0	0
gin & tonic	7.5 oz	171	0	0
gin ricky	4 oz	150	0	0
long island ice tea	1 serv (7.5 oz)	159	0	0
manhattan	2 oz	128	0	0
martini	2.5 oz	156	0	0
pina colada	4.5 oz	262	1	3
planter's punch	3.5 oz	175	0	0
rum	1.5 oz	97	0	0
screwdriver	7 oz	174	tr	tr
tequila sunrise	5.5 oz	189	tr	tr
tom collins	7.5 oz	121	0	0
vodka	1.5 oz	97	0	0
whiskey	1.5 oz	105	0	0
whiskey sour	3 oz	123	tr	tr
whiskey sour mix not prep	1 pkg (0.6 oz)	64	0	0
LIVER				
(see also PATE)				
beef braised	3 oz	137	2	4
beef pan-fried	3 oz	184	2	7
chicken stewed	1 cup (5 oz)	219	3	8
duck raw	1 (1.5 oz)	60	1	2
goose raw	1 (3.3 oz)	125	1	4
lamb braised	3 oz	187	3	7
lamb fried	3 oz	202	4	11
pork braised	3 oz	140	1	4
turkey simmered	1 cup (5 oz)	237	3	8
veal braised	3 oz	140	2	6
veal fried	3 oz	208	4	10

FOOD	PORTION	CALS.	SAT. FAT	FAT
Shady Brook				
Turkey	4 oz	160	2	5
LOBSTER				
(see also CRAYFISH)				
CANNED				
Progresso				
Rock Lobster Sauce	½ cup (4.3 oz)	100	1	7
FRESH				
northern cooked	1 cup	142	tr	1
northern cooked	3 oz	83	tr	1
northern raw	1 lobster (5.3 oz)	136	—	1
northern raw	3 oz	77	—	1
spiny steamed	3 oz	122	tr	2
spiny steamed	1 (5.7 oz)	233	tr	3
FROZEN				
Cajun Cookin'				
Crawfish Etouffee	12 oz	390	—	10
LOGANBERRIES				
frzn	1 cup	80	—	tr
LONGANS				
fresh	1	2	0	0
LOQUATS				
fresh	1	5	tr	tr
LOTUS				
root raw sliced	10 slices	45	tr	tr
root sliced cooked	10 slices	59	tr	tr
seeds dried	1 oz	94	tr	1
LOX				
(see SALMON)				
LUPINES				
dried cooked	1 cup	197	1	5
LYCHEES				
fresh	1	6	—	tr
MACADAMIA NUTS				
dried	1 oz	199	3	21
oil roasted	1 oz	204	3	22
MacFarms of Hawaii				
Chocolate Covered	¼ cup (1.3 oz)	210	6	16
Dry Roasted Salted	¼ cup (1.3 oz)	220	4	23
Kona Coffee Dark Chocolate Covered	¼ cup (1.3 oz)	210	6	16

FOOD	PORTION	CALS.	SAT. FAT	FAT
Mauna Loa				
Candy Glazed	1 oz	170	—	14
Chocolate Covered	1 oz	170	—	13
Honey Roasted	1 oz	200	—	17
Macadamia Nut Brittle	1 oz	150	—	8
Roasted & Salted	1 oz	210	—	21
MACARONI				
(see PASTA)				
MACE				
ground	1 tsp	8	tr	1
MACKEREL				
FRESH				
atlantic cooked	3 oz	223	4	15
atlantic raw	3 oz	174	3	12
jack baked	3 oz	171	2	9
king baked	3 oz	114	tr	2
pacific baked	3 oz	171	2	9
spanish cooked	1 fillet (5.1 oz)	230	3	9
spanish cooked	3 oz	134	2	5
spanish raw	3 oz	118	2	5
SMOKED				
atlantic	3.5 oz	296	5	24
MALANGA				
fresh	½ cup	137	—	tr
MALT				
nonalcoholic	12 fl oz	32	0	0
Bartles & Jaymes				
Malt Cooler Berry	12 fl oz	210	0	0
Malt Cooler Black Cherry	12 fl oz	190	0	0
Malt Cooler Light Berry	12 fl oz	140	0	0
Malt Cooler Mandarin Lemon	12 fl oz	210	0	0
Malt Cooler Margarita	12 fl oz	250	0	0
Malt Cooler Original	12 fl oz	180	0	0
Malt Cooler Peach	12 fl oz	200	0	0
Malt Cooler Pina Colada	12 fl oz	270	0	0
Malt Cooler Planter's Punch	12 fl oz	220	0	0
Malt Cooler Red Sangria	12 fl oz	190	0	0
Malt Cooler Strawberry	12 fl oz	200	0	0
Malt Cooler Strawberry Daiquiri	12 fl oz	220	0	0
Malt Cooler Tropical	12 fl oz	220	0	0

FOOD	PORTION	CALS.	SAT. FAT	FAT
MALTED MILK				
chocolate as prep w/ milk	1 cup	229	6	9
chocolate flavor powder	3 heaping tsp (¾ oz)	79	tr	1
natural flavor as prep w/ milk	1 cup	237	6	10
natural flavor powder	3 heaping tsp (¾ oz)	87	1	2
Carnation				
Chocolate	3 tbsp (0.7 oz)	90	1	1
Original	3 tbsp (0.7 oz)	90	1	2
MAMMY-APPLE				
fresh	1	431	—	4
MANGO				
fresh	1	135	tr	1
DRIED				
Rainforest Farms				
Slices	6 slices (1.3 oz)	140	0	1
Sonoma				
Pieces	8 pieces (2 oz)	180	0	1
MANGO JUICE				
After The Fall				
Hawaiian Mango	1 can (12 oz)	180	0	0
Mango Ginger	1 can (12 oz)	150	0	0
Fresh Samantha				
Mango Mama	1 cup (8 oz)	125	0	1
Kern's				
Nectar	6 fl oz	100	0	0
Libby				
Nectar	1 can (11.5 fl oz)	210	0	0
Ocean Spray				
Mango Mango	8 oz	130	0	0
Snapple				
Diet Mango Madness	8 fl oz	13	0	0
Mango Madness	8 fl oz	110	0	0
Tang				
Drink Mix as prep	1 serv (8 oz)	100	0	0
MARGARINE				
(see also BUTTER BLENDS, BUTTER SUBSTITUTES)				
squeeze soybean & cottonseed	1 tsp	34	1	4
stick corn	1 stick (4 oz)	815	15	91
stick corn	1 tsp	34	1	4
stick salted	1 stick (4 oz)	815	18	91
stick salted	1 tsp	39	1	4
stick unsalted	1 stick (4 oz)	809	17	91

FOOD	PORTION	CALS.	SAT. FAT	FAT
stick unsalted	1 tsp	34	1	4
tub corn	1 cup	1626	32	183
tub corn	1 tsp	34	1	4
tub diet	1 cup	800	18	90
tub diet	1 tsp	17	tr	2
tub safflower	1 cup	1626	21	183
tub safflower	1 tsp	34	tr	4
tub salted	1 cup	1626	31	183
tub salted	1 tsp	34	1	4
tub soybean salted	1 tsp	34	1	4
tub soybean salted	1 cup	1626	31	183
tub soybean unsalted	1 cup	1626	31	182
tub soybean unsalted	1 tsp	34	1	4
tub unsalted	1 tsp	34	1	4
tub unsalted	1 cup	1626	31	182
Blue Bonnet				
Stick	1 tbsp	100	2	11
Tub	1 tbsp	100	2	11
Whipped	1 tbsp	80	1	9
Fleischmann's				
Stick	1 tbsp	100	2	11
Stick Light Corn Oil	1 tbsp	80	1	8
Stick Sweet Unsalted	1 tbsp	100	2	11
Hain				
Stick Safflower	1 tbsp	100	2	11
Stick Safflower Unsalted	1 tbsp	100	2	11
Tub Safflower	1 tbsp	100	2	11
Hollywood				
Safflower	1 tbsp	100	2	11
Safflower Unsalted Sweet	1 tbsp	100	2	11
Soft Spread	1 tbsp	90	1	10
I Can't Believe Its Not Butter				
Tub	1 tbsp	90	—	10
Krona				
Stick	1 tbsp	100	—	11
Land O'Lakes				
Stick	1 tbsp (0.5 oz)	90	2	10
Stick With Sweet Cream	1 tbsp (0.5 oz)	90	2	10
Stick With Sweet Cream Unsalted	1 tbsp (0.5 oz)	90	2	10
Tub	1 tbsp (0.5 oz)	80	2	8
Tub With Sweet Cream	1 tbsp (0.5 oz)	80	2	8
Mother's				
Stick Unsalted	1 tbsp	100	—	11
Sticks	1 tbsp	100	—	11

FOOD	PORTION	CALS.	SAT. FAT	FAT
Hain				
Canola	1 tbsp	100	1	11
Canola	1 tbsp	60	0	5
Cold Processed	1 tbsp	110	2	12
Eggless No Salt Added	1 tbsp	110	2	12
Light Low Sodium	1 tbsp	60	1	6
Real No Salt Added	1 tbsp	110	2	12
Safflower	1 tbsp	110	1	12
Hollywood				
Canola	1 tbsp	100	3	11
Mayonnaise	1 tbsp	110	1	12
Safflower	1 tbsp	100	1	12
Kraft				
Fat Free	1 tbsp (0.6 oz)	10	0	0
Light	1 tbsp (0.5 oz)	50	1	5
Real	1 tbsp (0.5 oz)	100	2	11
McIlhenny				
Spicy	1 tbsp (0.5 oz)	108	3	12
Mother's				
Mayonnaise	1 tbsp	100	—	11
Red Wing				
"H" Style	1 tbsp (0.5 oz)	110	2	11
Smart Beat				
Canola Oil	1 tbsp	40	tr	4
Corn Beat	1 tbsp	40	tr	4
Fat Free	1 tbsp	10	0	0
Weight Watchers				
Fat Free	1 tbsp	10	0	0
Light	1 tbsp	25	0	2
Light Low Sodium	1 tbsp	25	0	2

MAYONNAISE TYPE SALAD DRESSING

(see also MAYONNAISE, RELISH)

home recipe	1 tbsp	25	1	2
home recipe	1 cup	400	7	24
mayonnaise type salad dressing	1 cup	916	12	78
mayonnaise type salad dressing	1 tbsp	57	1	5
reduced calorie w/o cholesterol	1 tbsp	68	1	7
reduced calorie w/o cholesterol	1 cup	1084	17	107
BAMA				
Dressing	1 tbsp	50	—	4
Miracle Whip				
Free	1 tbsp (0.5 oz)	15	0	0
Light	1 tbsp (0.5 oz)	35	0	3
Salad Dressing	1 tbsp (0.6 oz)	70	1	7

FOOD	PORTION	CALS.	SAT. FAT	FAT
Nayonaise				
Cholesterol Free	1 tbsp (0.5 oz)	35	tr	3
Fat Free	1 tbsp (0.5 oz)	11	tr	tr
Spin Blend				
Cholesterol Free	1 tbsp	40	1	4
Dressing	1 tbsp	60	1	5
Weight Watchers				
Fat Free Whipped Dressing	1 tbsp	15	0	0

MEAT STICKS

(see also BEEF DRIED)

FOOD	PORTION	CALS.	SAT. FAT	FAT
jerky beef	1 lg piece (0.7 oz)	67	1	3
jerky beef	1 oz	96	1	4
smoked	1 oz	156	6	14
smoked	1 (0.7 oz)	109	4	10
Big Ones				
BBQ	1 (1 oz)	130	5	12
Hot n'Spicy	1 (1 oz)	130	5	12
Original	1 (1 oz)	130	5	12
Teriyaki	1 (1 oz)	130	5	12
Jack Link's				
Kippered Beefsteak Teriyaki	1 oz	80	1	1
Lance				
Beef & Cheese	1 pkg (1.5 oz)	150	6	11
Beef Jerky	1 piece (0.25 oz)	30	1	2
Beef Snack	1 piece (0.63 oz)	100	4	8
Hot Sausage	1 piece (0.9 oz)	60	2	5
Lowrey's				
Smokehouse Tender Hickory Smoked	1 pkg (1 oz)	80	1	2
Smokehouse Tender Original	1 pkg (1 oz)	60	0	1
Smokehouse Tender Peppered	1 pkg (1 oz)	60	0	1
Pemmican				
Original Tender Kippered Beef Steak	1	110	3	5
Peppered Tender Kippered Beef Steak	1	110	3	5
Rustlers Roundup				
Beef Jerky	1 serv (5 g)	20	1	2
Flamin' Hot	1 serv (8 g)	40	2	3
Smoky Steak	1 serv (0.8 oz)	60	1	2
Spicy	1 serv (0.5 oz)	70	3	6
Slim Jim				
Spicy	1 (4½ in) (0.3 oz)	50	2	4
Spicy Big	1 (.44 oz)	70	3	6

FOOD	PORTION	CALS.	SAT. FAT	FAT
Slim Jim (CONT.)				
Spicy Giant	1 (0.97 oz)	150	6	14
Spicy Super	1 (0.64 oz)	100	4	9

MEAT SUBSTITUTES

(see also BACON SUBSTITUTES, CHICKEN SUBSTITUTES, SAUSAGE SUBSTITUTES, TURKEY SUBSTITUTES)

FOOD	PORTION	CALS.	SAT. FAT	FAT
simulated sausage	1 link (25 g)	64	1	5
simulated sausage	1 patty (38 g)	97	1	7
simulated meat product	1 oz	88	tr	1
Amy's Organic				
Veggie Burger California	1 (2.5 oz)	100	0	3
Veggie Burger Chicago	1 (2.5 oz)	100	1	4
Veggie Burger Texas	1 (2.5 oz)	130	0	3
Whole Meals Veggie Loaf	1 pkg (10 oz)	260	5	5
Boca Burgers				
Chef Max's Original	1 patty (2.5 oz)	110	1	2
Hint of Garlic	1 patty (2.5 oz)	110	1	2
Vegan Original	1 patty (2.5 oz)	84	0	0
Frieda's				
SoyTaco	1 oz	50	1	3
Soyrizo	4 tbsp (1.9 oz)	120	1	9
GardenVegan				
Fat-Free Patty	1 patty (2.5 oz)	140	0	0
Gardenburger				
Classic Greek	1 (2.5 oz)	120	2	3
Fire Roasted Vegetable	1 (2.5 oz)	120	2	3
Hamburger Style	1 (2.5 oz)	90	0	0
Hamburger Style w/ Cheese	1 (2.5 oz)	110	2	3
Savory Mushroom	1 (2.5 oz)	120	2	3
Green Giant				
Southwestern Style	1 patty (3.2 oz)	140	2	4
Harvest Burgers				
For Recipes	⅔ cup (2.1 oz)	90	0	0
Italian Style	1 patty (3.2 oz)	140	2	5
Original	1 (3 oz)	140	2	4
Harvest Direct				
TVP Beef Chunks	3.5 oz	280	tr	1
TVP Beef Chunks Flavored	3.5 oz	250	tr	1
TVP Beef Strips	3.5 oz	280	tr	1
TVP Ground Beef	3.5 oz	280	tr	1
TVP Ground Beef Flavored	3.5 oz	250	tr	1
Ken & Robert's				
Veggie Burger	1 (62 g)	110	0	2

FOOD	PORTION	CALS.	SAT. FAT	FAT
Knox Mountain Farm				
Wheat Balls Mix	1 serv (⅒ pkg)	110	—	1
Lightlife				
Barbecue Grilles	1 patty	120	2	4
Foney Baloney	3 slices (1.5 oz)	60	1	3
Gimme Lean Beef	2 oz	70	0	0
Lemon Grilles	1 patty	140	2	6
Light Burgers	3 oz	130	0	1
Savory Seitan Barbecue	4 oz	160	1	2
Savory Seitan Teriyaki	4 oz	160	1	2
Smart Deli Bologna	3 slices (1.5 oz)	50	0	0
Smart Deli Ham	3 slices (1.5 oz)	50	0	0
Smart Deli Jumbo's	1 link (2.7 oz)	80	0	0
Smart Deli Peppercorn	3 slices (1.5 oz)	45	0	0
Smart Deli Sticks Pepperoni	1 oz	45	0	0
Smart Deli Turkey	3 slices (1.5 oz)	40	0	0
Smart Dogs	1 (1.5 oz)	45	0	0
Smart Ground	2 oz	70	0	0
Tamari Grilles	1 patty	120	2	5
Tofu Pups	1 (1.5 oz)	60	1	3
Wonder Dogs	1 (1.5 oz)	55	0	1
Loma Linda				
Big Franks	1 (1.8 oz)	110	1	7
Big Franks Low Fat	1 (1.8 oz)	80	1	3
Corn Dogs	1 (2.5 oz)	200	2	9
Dinner Cuts	2 pieces (3.2 oz)	90	1	2
Nuteena	⅜ in slice (1.9 oz)	160	5	13
Patty Mix not prep	⅓ cup (0.9 oz)	90	0	1
Redi-Burger	⅝ in slice (3 oz)	120	1	3
Sandwich Spread	¼ cup (1.9 oz)	80	1	5
Savory Dinner Loaf Mix not prep	⅓ cup (0.9 oz)	90	0	2
Swiss Stake	1 piece (3.2 oz)	120	1	6
Tender Bits	6 pieces (3 oz)	110	1	5
Tender Rounds	6 pieces (2.8 oz)	120	1	5
Vege-Burger	¼ cup (1.9 oz)	70	1	2
Vita Burger Chunks not prep	¼ cup (0.7 oz)	70	0	1
Vita Burger Granules	3 tbsp (0.7 oz)	70	0	1
Midland Harvest				
Burger n' Loaf Chili w/o Beans	0.8 oz	90	1	3
Burger n' Loaf Herbs & Spice	3.2 oz	140	1	5
Burger n' Loaf Italian	3.2 oz	140	1	5
Burger n' Loaf Original	3.2 oz	140	1	5

FOOD	PORTION	CALS.	SAT. FAT	FAT
Midland Harvest (CONT.)				
Burger n' Loaf Sloppy Joe w/o Sauce	0.8 oz	80	1	2
Burger n' Loaf Taco	2.7 oz	90	tr	2
Morningstar Farms				
Better'n Burger	1 (2.7 oz)	70	0	0
Burger Style Recipe Crumbles	⅔ cup (1.9 oz)	90	0	3
Deli Franks	1 (1.6 oz)	110	1	7
Garden Grille	1 patty (2.5 oz)	120	1	3
Garden Veggie Patties	1 patty (2.4 oz)	100	1	3
Ground Meatless	½ cup (1.9 oz)	60	0	0
Prime Patties	1 (2.7 oz)	110	0	2
Quarter Prime	1 patty (3.4 oz)	140	0	2
Southwestern Veggie Burger Kit	¼ pkg (0.9 oz)	90	0	0
Spicy Black Bean Burger	1 (2.7 oz)	110	0	1
Natural Touch				
Dinner Entree	1 patty (3 oz)	220	3	15
Garden Veggie Pattie	1 (2.4 oz)	110	1	3
Loaf Mix not prep	4 tbsp (1 oz)	100	0	1
Okara Pattie	1 (2.2 oz)	110	1	5
Orignal Veggie Burger Kit not prep	¼ pkg (0.8 oz)	80	0	0
Southwestern Veggie Burger Kit not prep	¼ pkg (0.9 oz)	90	0	0
Spicy Black Bean Burger	1 (2.7 oz)	100	0	1
Stroganoff Mix not prep	4 tbsp (0.8 oz)	90	2	4
Taco Mix not prep	3 tbsp (0.6 oz)	90	0	1
Vegan Burger	1 (2.7 oz)	70	0	0
Vegan Burger Crumbles	½ cup (1.9 oz)	60	0	0
Vege Frank	1 (1.6 oz)	100	1	6
NewMenu				
VegiBurger	1 patty (3 oz)	110	0	1
VegiDogs	1 (1.5 oz)	45	0	0
Quorn				
Burger	1 patty (3 oz)	100	2	4
Sovex				
Better Than Burger?	½ cup (1.9 oz)	165	1	2
Soy Is Us				
Beef Not!	½ cup (1.75 oz)	140	1	2
Veggie Patch				
Burgeriffics	1 (2.5 oz)	110	—	3
Perfectly Franks	1 (1.7 oz)	70	—	2
Veggie Rounds	1 (2.5 oz)	120	—	3
Veggitinos Meatballs	5 (2.8 oz)	120	—	4

FOOD	PORTION	CALS.	SAT. FAT	FAT
White Wave				
Meatless Healthy Franks	1 (1.5 oz)	90	0	2
Meatless Jumbo Franks	1 (3 oz)	170	1	3
Meatless Sandwich Slices Beef	2 slices (1.6 oz)	90	0	0
Meatless Sandwich Slices Bologna	2 slices (1.6 oz)	120	2	8
Meatless Sandwich Slices Pastrami	2 slices (1.6 oz)	90	0	0
Meatless Healthy Franks	1 (1.5 oz)	90	0	2
Veggie Burger	1 patty (2.5 oz)	110	0	3
Worthington				
Beef Style Meatless	⅜ in slice (1.9 oz)	110	1	7
Bolono	3 slices (2 oz)	80	1	4
Choplets	2 slices (3.2 oz)	90	1	2
Corn Beef Meatless	4 slices (2 oz)	140	2	9
Country Stew	1 cup (8.4 oz)	210	2	9
Dinner Roast	¾ in slice (3 oz)	180	2	12
FriPats	1 patty (2.2 oz)	60	1	6
Granburger not prep	3 tbsp (0.6 oz)	60	0	1
Multigrain Cutlet	2 slices (3.2 oz)	100	1	2
Numete	⅜ in slice (1.9 oz)	130	3	10
Prime Stakes	1 piece (3.2 oz)	140	2	9
Prosage Patties	1 (1.3 oz)	100	1	3
Prosage Roll	⅝ in slice (1.9 oz)	140	2	10
Protose	⅜ in slice (1.9 oz)	130	1	7
Salami Meatless	3 slices (2 oz)	130	1	8
Savory Slices	3 slices (2.9 oz)	150	4	9
Smoked Beef Meatless	6 slices (2 oz)	120	1	6
Stakelets	1 piece (2.5 oz)	140	2	8
Veelets	1 patty (2.5 oz)	180	2	9
Vegetable Skallops	½ cup (3 oz)	90	1	2
Vegetable Steaks	2 pieces (2.5 oz)	80	1	2
Vegetarian Burger	¼ cup (1.9 oz)	60	0	2
Veja Links Low Fat	1 (1.1 oz)	40	0	2
Wham	2 slices (1.6 oz)	80	1	5
Zoglo's				
Crispy Vegetarian Cutlets	1 (3.5 oz)	200	2	10
Savory Vegetarian Kebabs	1 serv (2.8 oz)	135	1	5
Tender Vegetarian Burgers	1 (2.6 oz)	150	1	7
Vegetable Patties	1 (2.6 oz)	130	1	5
Vegetarian Franks	1 (2.6 oz)	125	1	5

MELON
(see also INDIVIDUAL NAMES)

FOOD	PORTION	CALS.	SAT. FAT	FAT
FROZEN				
melon balls	1 cup	55	—	tr
Big Valley				
Mixed	¾ cup (4.9 oz)	40	0	0
MELON JUICE				
Ocean Spray				
Mega Melon	8 oz	130	0	0
MEXICAN FOOD				
(see SALSA, SAUCE, SPANISH FOOD, TORTILLA)				
MILK				
(see also CHOCOLATE, COCOA, MILK DRINKS, MILKSHAKE)				
CANNED				
condensed sweetened	1 oz	123	2	3
condensed sweetened	1 cup	982	17	27
evaporated	½ cup	169	6	10
evaporated skim	½ cup	99	tr	tr
Carnation				
Evaporated	2 tbsp	40	2	3
Evaporated Lowfat	2 tbsp	25	—	1
Lite Evaporated Skimmed	½ cup (4 fl oz)	100	—	tr
Sweetened Condensed	2 tbsp	130	2	3
Eagle				
Sweetened Condensed	⅓ cup	320	—	9
Pet				
Evaporated	½ cup	170	—	10
Evaporated Filled	½ cup	150	1	8
Evaporated Light Skimmed	½ cup	100	—	tr
DRIED				
buttermilk	1 tbsp	25	tr	tr
nonfat instantized	1 pkg (3.2 oz)	244	tr	tr
Carnation				
Nonfat	⅓ cup dry	80	—	0
Saco				
Cultured Buttermilk	4 tbsp (0.8 oz)	80	0	tr
Sanalac				
As Prep	8 oz	80	—	tr
REFRIGERATED				
1%	1 cup	102	2	3
1%	1 qt	409	6	10
1% protein fortified	1 qt	477	7	12
1% protein fortified	1 cup	119	2	3
2%	1 cup	121	3	5

FOOD	PORTION	CALS.	SAT. FAT	FAT
2%	1 qt	485	12	19
buttermilk	1 cup	99	1	2
buttermilk	1 qt	396	5	9
goat	1 cup	168	7	10
goat	1 qt	672	26	40
human	1 cup	171	5	11
indian buffalo	1 cup	236	11	17
low sodium	1 cup	149	5	8
nonfat	1 cup	86	tr	tr
nonfat	1 qt	342	1	2
nonfat protein fortified	1 qt	400	2	2
nonfat protein fortified	1 cup	100	tr	1
sheep	1 cup	264	11	17
whole	1 cup	150	5	8
BodyWise				
Nonfat	8 fl oz	100	0	0
Borden				
Acidophilus 1%	8 fl oz	100	—	2
Buttermilk Lowfat Golden Churn	8 fl oz	120	—	4
Hi-Calcium	8 fl oz	150	—	8
Hi-Protein 2%	8 fl oz	140	—	5
Milk	8 fl oz	150	—	8
Skim	8 fl oz	90	—	1
Skim-line	8 fl oz	100	—	1
CalciMilk				
CalciMilk	8 fl oz	102	2	3
Cool Cow				
Low Fat	1 cup (8 oz)	110	1	3
Farmland				
1%	8 fl oz	100	2	3
2%	8 fl oz	130	3	5
Cholesterol Reduced	1 cup (8 oz)	150	—	8
Easylac 1%	8 fl oz	100	—	2
Easylac Nonfat	8 fl oz	90	—	0
Skim	8 fl oz	80	0	0
Skim Plus	1 cup (8 oz)	110	0	0
Friendship				
Buttermilk	8 fl oz	120	3	4
Hood				
1%	1 cup (8 oz)	110	2	3
Better Taste 2%	1 cup (8 oz)	130	3	5
Buttermilk	1 cup (8 oz)	90	0	0
Whole	1 cup (8 oz)	150	5	8

FOOD	PORTION	CALS.	SAT. FAT	FAT
Lactaid				
1%	8 fl oz	102	2	3
Nonfat	8 fl oz	86	tr	tr
Nuform				
1%	1 cup (8 oz)	120	2	3
Skim	1 cup (8 oz)	100	0	0
NutraBalance				
LactaCare	1 pkg (8 oz)	500	—	18
Organic Valley				
Low Fat	1 cup	100	2	3
Nonfat	1 cup	80	0	0
Reduced Fat	1 cup	130	3	5
Whole	1 cup	150	5	8
Silovet				
Skim	1 cup (8 oz)	90	0	0
Viva				
2%	8 fl oz	120	—	5
Skim	8 fl oz	100	—	1
SHELF-STABLE				
Parmalat				
1%	1 cup (8 oz)	110	2	3
2%	1 cup (8 oz)	130	3	5
Skim	1 cup (8 oz)	90	0	1
Whole	1 cup (8 oz)	160	5	8

MILK DRINKS

(see also BREAKFAST DRINKS, CHOCOLATE, COCOA, MILKSHAKES)

FOOD	PORTION	CALS.	SAT. FAT	FAT
chocolate milk	1 cup	208	5	8
chocolate milk	1 qt	833	21	34
chocolate milk 1%	1 cup	158	2	3
chocolate milk 1%	1 qt	630	6	10
chocolate milk 2%	1 cup	179	3	5
strawberry flavor mix as prep w/ whole milk	9 oz	234	5	8
Body Wise				
Chocolate Nonfat Milk	1 cup (8 fl oz)	180	0	0
Borden				
Chocolate Lowfat Dutch Brand	8 fl oz	180	—	5
Bosco				
Chocolate Milk	1 cup (8 fl oz)	230	—	8
Hood				
Chocolate Lowfat	1 cup (8 oz)	150	1	2
Horizon				
Organic 1% Chocolate Milk	1 cup (8 oz)	160	2	3

FOOD	PORTION	CALS.	SAT. FAT	FAT
Lactaid				
Chocolate Milk 1%	8 fl oz	158	2	3
Meadow Gold				
Chocolate Milk	8 fl oz	210	—	8
Organic Valley				
Chocolate Milk Reduced Fat	1 cup	180	3	5
Parmalat				
Chocolate 2%	1 box (8 oz)	180	3	5
Quik				
Banana Powder	2 tbsp (0.8 oz)	90	0	0
Cookies n Cream Powder	2 tbsp (0.8 oz)	100	1	1
Strawberry Powder	2 tbsp (0.8 oz)	90	0	0

MILK SUBSTITUTES
(see also COFFEE WHITENERS)

FOOD	PORTION	CALS.	SAT. FAT	FAT
imitation milk	1 cup	150	2	8
imitation milk	1 qt	600	7	33
Better Than Milk				
Carob	8 fl oz	130	—	5
Chocolate	8 fl oz	125	—	5
Light	8 fl oz	80	—	tr
Natural	8 fl oz	90	—	5
EdenBlend				
Original	8 fl oz	120	1	3
Edensoy				
Carob	8 fl oz	150	1	4
Extra Original	8 fl oz	130	1	5
Extra Original	8 oz	130	1	4
Extra Vanilla	8 oz	150	0	3
Original	8 oz	130	1	4
Vanilla	8 oz	150	0	3
Galaxy				
Veggi Milk Chocolate	1 cup (8 oz)	150	0	2
Veggie Milk Original	1 cup (8 oz)	110	0	3
Health Valley				
Soo Moo	1 cup	110	—	0
Rice Dream				
Carob Lite	8 fl oz	150	—	3
Chocolate	8 fl oz	190	—	3
Chocolate	8 fl oz	190	—	3
Lite Organic Original	8 fl oz	130	—	2
Lite Vanilla	8 fl oz	130	—	2
Vegelicious				
Milk	8 fl oz	100	—	2

FOOD	PORTION	CALS.	SAT. FAT	FAT
Vitamite				
Non-Dairy 2% Fat	1 cup (8 oz)	110	2	5
Non-Diary Nonfat	1 cup (8 oz)	90	0	0
Vitasoy				
Carob Supreme	8 fl oz	210	1	6
Cocoa Light	8 fl oz	130	0	2
Original Creamy	8 fl oz	160	1	7
Original Light	8 fl oz	90	0	2
Rich Cocoa	8 fl oz	210	1	6
Vanilla Light	8 fl oz	110	0	2
Vanilla Delite	8 fl oz	190	1	6
Westsoy				
Cocoa Lite	8 fl oz	140	tr	2
Plain Lite	8 fl oz	100	tr	2
Vanilla Lite	8 fl oz	110	tr	2

MILKFISH

baked	3 oz	162	—	7

MILKSHAKE

chocolate	10 oz	360	7	11
strawberry	10 oz	319	—	8
thick shake chocolate	10.6 oz	356	5	8
thick shake vanilla	11 oz	350	6	10
vanilla	10 oz	314	5	8
D'Frosta Shake				
Vanilla	1 serv (13.5 oz)	340	6	9
Freeze Flip				
Fruit Shake No Fat Lactose Free Black Raspberry	1 serv (6 oz)	150	0	0
Frostee				
Chocolate	8 fl oz	200	—	8
Strawberry	8 fl oz	180	—	7
Hood				
Shake Up Chocolate	1 cup (8 oz)	240	4	6
Shake Up Strawberry	1 cup (8 oz)	220	3	5
Shake Up Vanilla	1 cup (8 oz)	220	3	5
Milky Way				
Shake	1 (10 fl oz)	390	10	16
Parmalat				
Shake A Shake Chocolate	1 box (6 oz)	180	2	4
Shake A Shake Orange Vanilla	1 box (6 oz)	110	2	3
Shake A Shake Vanilla	1 box (6 oz)	170	2	3

MILLET

cooked	1 cup (6.1 oz)	207	tr	2

FOOD	PORTION	CALS.	SAT. FAT	FAT
MINERAL WATER				
(see WATER)				
MISO				
miso	½ cup	284	1	8
Eden				
Genmai Miso Organic	1 tbsp (0.5 oz)	25	0	1
Hacho Miso Organic	1 tbsp (0.5 oz)	35	0	2
Kome Miso Organic	1 tbsp (0.6 oz)	25	0	1
Mugi Miso Organic	1 tbsp (0.6 oz)	25	0	1
Shiro Miso Organic	1 tbsp (0.6 oz)	35	0	1
MOLASSES				
blackstrap	1 tbsp (0.7 oz)	47	0	0
blackstrap	1 cup (11.5 oz)	771	—	tr
molasses	1 tbsp (0.7 oz)	53	0	0
molasses	1 cup (11.5 oz)	873	—	1
Brer Rabbit				
Dark	2 tbsp	110	0	0
Light	2 tbsp	110	0	0
McIlhenny				
Molasses	1 tbsp (0.7 oz)	66	tr	tr
Tree Of Life				
Blackstrap	1 tbsp (0.5 oz)	45	0	0
MONKFISH				
baked	3 oz	82	—	2
MOOSE				
roasted	3 oz	114	tr	1
MOTH BEANS				
dried cooked	1 cup	207	tr	1
MOUSSE				
FROZEN				
Sara Lee				
Chocolate Mint Mousse	⅓ pkg (4.3 oz)	440	21	28
Weight Watchers				
Chocolate Mousse	1 (2.75 oz)	190	2	5
HOME RECIPE				
orange	½ cup	87	—	5
MIX				
Royal				
Chocolate Mousse No-Bake	⅛ pie	130	0	4
TAKE-OUT				
chocolate	½ cup (7.1 oz)	447	19	33

FOOD	PORTION	CALS.	SAT. FAT	FAT
MUFFIN				
FROZEN				
Pepperidge Farm				
Blueberry	1 (2 oz)	180	1	7
Bran w/ Raisins	1 (2 oz)	180	1	6
Corn	1 (2 oz)	190	1	7
Orange Cranberry	1 (2 oz)	180	1	6
Sara Lee				
Blueberry	1 (2.2 oz)	220	2	11
Corn	1 (2.2 oz)	260	3	14
Oat Bran	1	210	—	8
Weight Watchers				
Chocolate Chocolate Chip	1 (2.5 oz)	190	1	2
Fat Free Banana	1 (2.5 oz)	170	0	0
Fat Free Blueberry	1 (2.5 oz)	160	0	0
HOME RECIPE				
blueberry as prep w/ 2% milk	1 (2 oz)	163	1	6
blueberry as prep w/ whole milk	1 (2 oz)	165	1	6
corn as prep w/ 2% milk	1 (2 oz)	180	1	7
corn as prep w/ whole milk	1 (2 oz)	183	2	7
plain as prep w/ 2% milk	1 (2 oz)	169	1	7
plain as prep w/ whole milk	1 (2 oz)	172	1	7
wheat bran as prep w/ 2% milk	1 (2 oz)	161	1	7
wheat bran as prep w/ whole milk	1 (2 oz)	164	1	7
MIX				
blueberry	1 (1.75 oz)	149	1	4
corn	1 (1.75 oz)	160	1	5
wheat bran as prep	1 (1.75 oz)	138	1	5
Arrowhead				
Bran	⅓ cup (1.4 oz)	150	0	2
Oat Bran Wheat Free	⅓ cup (1.5 oz)	160	2	4
Betty Crocker				
Apple Cinnamon Low Fat Recipe	1	120	0	1
Banana Nut	1	150	1	5
Banana Nut No Cholesterol Recipe	1	140	1	4
Cinnamon Streusel	1	170	2	7
Fat Free Apple Cinnamon	1	120	0	0
Fat Free Blueberry	1	120	0	0
Fat Free Blueberry Low Fat Recipe	1	120	0	1
Lemon Poppyseed	1	190	2	7

FOOD	PORTION	CALS.	SAT. FAT	FAT
Betty Crocker (CONT.)				
Lemon Poppyseed No Cholesterol Recipe	1	190	1	7
Twice The Blueberry	1	140	1	4
Twice The Blueberry No Cholesterol Recipe	1	130	1	3
Dromedary				
Corn Muffin	1	120	—	4
Flako				
Corn	⅓ cup (1.4 oz)	160	1	4
Gold Medal				
Banana Nut	1	170	2	8
Caramel Nut	1	170	2	7
Corn	1	160	2	6
Hain				
Oat Bran Apple Cinnamon	1	140	—	3
Oat Bran Banana Nut	1	140	—	4
Oat Bran Raspberry Spice	1	140	—	3
Jiffy				
Apple Cinnamon as prep	1	190	3	7
Banana Nut as prep	1	180	4	7
Blueberry as prep	1	190	4	7
Bran With Dates as prep	1	170	3	6
Corn as prep	1	180	2	4
Honey Date as prep	1	170	2	5
Oatmeal as prep	1	180	2	7
Robin Hood				
Apple Cinnamon	1	170	2	8
Banana Nut	1	170	2	8
Blueberry	1	160	2	6
Caramel Nut	1	170	2	7
Sweet Rewards				
Fat Free Apple Cinnamon	1	120	0	0
Fat Free Wild Blueberry	1	120	0	0
Low Fat Recipe Apple Cinnamon	1	130	1	1
Low Fat Recipe Wild Blueberry	1	120	0	1
Wanda's				
Blue Corn	¼ cup mix per serv (1.2 oz)	130	0	1
READY-TO-EAT				
blueberry	1 (2 oz)	158	1	4
corn	1 (2 oz)	174	1	5
oat bran wheat free	1 (2 oz)	154	1	4

FOOD	PORTION	CALS.	SAT. FAT	FAT
toaster type blueberry	1	103	tr	3
toaster type corn	1	114	1	4
toaster type wheat bran w/ raisins	1 (1.3 oz)	106	1	3
Arnold				
Bran'nola	1 (2.3 oz)	160	0	1
Raisin	1 (2.3 oz)	160	0	1
Dolly Madison				
Blueberry	1 (1.75 oz)	170	1	7
Mega Banana Nut	1 (5.9 oz)	620	5	31
Mega Blueberry	1 (5.9 oz)	590	4	28
Mega Chocolate Chip	1 (5.9 oz)	620	5	29
Mega Cranberry Orange	1 (5.9 oz)	590	5	28
Mega Cream Cheese	1 (5.9 oz)	620	7	33
Dutch Mill				
Apple Oat Bran	1 (2 oz)	180	1	5
Banana Walnut	1 (2 oz)	220	2	6
Carrot	1 (2 oz)	190	2	7
Corn	1 (2 oz)	190	3	6
Cranberry Orange	1 (2 oz)	170	3	6
Raisin Bran	1 (2 oz)	230	3	5
Entenmann's				
Blueberry	1 (2 oz)	200	—	8
Freihofer's				
Corn Toasters	1 (1.3 oz)	130	1	6
Hostess				
Banana Bran Low Fat	1 (2.7 oz)	240	1	3
Blueberry Low Fat	1 (2.7 oz)	230	1	3
Hearty Banana Nut	1 (5.9 oz)	620	5	31
Hearty Blueberry	1 (5.9 oz)	590	4	28
Hearty Chocolate Chip	1 (5.9 oz)	620	2	29
Hearty Cranberry Orange	1 (5.9 oz)	590	5	28
Hearty Cream Cheese	1 (5.9 oz)	620	7	33
Mini Banana Walnut	3 (1.2 oz)	160	1	9
Mini Blueberry	3 (1.2 oz)	150	1	8
Mini Chocolate Chip	3 (1.2 oz)	160	3	9
Mini Cinnamon Apple	3 (1.2 oz)	160	2	9
Mini Cinnamon Bites	3 (1.1 oz)	130	1	6
Mini Rocky Road	3 (1.2 oz)	160	3	9
Muffin Loaf Apple Spice	1 (3.7 oz)	430	4	18
Muffin Loaf Banana Nut	1 (3.8 oz)	460	3	20
Muffin Loaf Blueberry	1 (3.8 oz)	440	3	19
Muffin Loaf Chocolate Chocolate Chip	1 (3.8 oz)	400	4	17

FOOD	PORTION	CALS.	SAT. FAT	FAT
Hostess (CONT.)				
Muffin Loaf Raspberry	1 (3.8 oz)	440	3	19
Oat Bran	1 (1.5 oz)	160	1	8
Otis Spunkmeyer				
Mayport Almond Poppy Seed	½ muffin (2 oz)	210	3	12
Mayport Apple Cinnamon	1 (2.25 oz)	240	2	13
Mayport Banana Nut	1 (2.25 oz)	270	3	14
Mayport Cheese Streusel	½ muffin (2 oz)	220	3	10
Mayport Chocolate Chocolate Chip	1 (2.25 oz)	260	3	13
Mayport Chocolate Chip	½ muffin (2 oz)	240	3	13
Mayport Cinnamon Spice	½ muffin (2 oz)	230	3	13
Mayport Corn	½ muffin (2 oz)	230	2	13
Mayport Harvest Bran	1 (2.25 oz)	240	2	10
Mayport Lemon	½ muffin (2 oz)	230	3	13
Mayport Orange	½ muffin (2 oz)	230	3	13
Mayport Pineapple	½ muffin (2 oz)	210	3	12
Mayport Wild Blueberry	1 (2.25 oz)	230	3	13
Mayport Low Fat Apple Cinnamon	1 (4 oz)	380	1	6
Mayport Low Fat Banana Nut	1 (4 oz)	350	1	6
Mayport Low Fat Chocolate Chocolate Chip	1 (4 oz)	370	2	6
Mayport Low Fat Wild Blueberry	1 (4 oz)	350	1	6
Weight Watchers				
Fat Free Apple Crisp	1 (2.5 oz)	160	0	0
Fat Free Cranberry Orange	1 (2.5 oz)	160	0	0
Fat Free Double Chocolate	1 (2.5 oz)	180	0	0
Fat Free Wild Blueberry	1 (2.5 oz)	160	0	0
Low Fat Apple Cinnamon	1 (2.5 oz)	170	0	3
Low Fat Blueberry	1 (2.5 oz)	180	0	3
Low Fat Carrot	1 (2.5 oz)	160	0	3
Low Fat Chocolate Chip	1 (2.5 oz)	180	1	3
Low Fat Cranberry Orange	1 (2.5 oz)	180	0	3
Low Fat Lemon Poppy	1 (2.5 oz)	190	0	3

MULBERRIES

fresh	1 cup	61	—	1

MULLET

striped cooked	3 oz	127	1	4
striped raw	3 oz	99	1	3

MUNG BEANS

DRIED

cooked	1 cup	213	tr	1

FOOD	PORTION	CALS.	SAT. FAT	FAT
MUNGO BEANS				
dried cooked	1 cup	190	tr	1
MUSHROOMS				
CANNED				
pieces	½ cup	19	tr	tr
straw	1 cup (6.4 oz)	58	tr	1
whole	1 (0.4 oz)	3	tr	tr
BinB				
Pieces & Stems	1 can (4.2 oz)	30	0	0
Sliced	1 can (4.2 oz)	30	0	0
Sliced With Garlic	1 can (4.2 oz)	35	0	1
Whole	1 can (4.2 oz)	30	0	0
Green Giant				
Pieces & Stems	½ cup (4.2 oz)	30	0	0
Sliced	½ cup (4.2 oz)	30	0	0
Whole	½ cup (4.2 oz)	30	0	0
Seneca				
Mushrooms	½ cup	25	0	0
DRIED				
cloud ear	1 (5 g)	13	—	tr
cloud ears	1 cup (1 oz)	80	—	tr
shiitake	4 (0.5 oz)	44	tr	tr
straw	1 piece (6 g)	2	0	tr
FRESH				
enoki raw	1 (4 in)	2	tr	tr
morel	3.5 oz	9	—	tr
oyster raw	1 sm (0.5 oz)	6	—	tr
oyster raw	1 lg (5.2 oz)	55	—	1
portabella sliced	1 serv (2 oz)	4	0	0
raw	1 (0.5 oz)	5	tr	tr
raw sliced	½ cup	9	tr	tr
shitake cooked	4 (2.5 oz)	40	tr	tr
sliced cooked	½ cup	21	tr	tr
whole cooked	1 (0.4 oz)	3	tr	tr
Mother Earth				
Organic	4 oz	35	—	1
FROZEN				
Empire				
Breaded	7 (2.8 oz)	90	0	1
Fresh Like				
Mushrooms	3.5 oz	28	—	tr
MUSKRAT				
roasted	3 oz	199	—	10

FOOD	PORTION	CALS.	SAT. FAT	FAT
MUSSELS				
blue raw	3 oz	73	tr	2
blue raw	1 cup	129	1	3
fresh blue cooked	3 oz	147	1	4
MUSTARD				
dry mustard seed yellow	1 tsp	15	tr	1
yellow ready-to-use	1 tsp	5	tr	tr
Blanchard & Blanchard				
Mustard	1 tsp (5 g)	0	0	0
Boar's Head				
Delicatessen Style	1 tsp (5 g)	0	0	0
Honey	1 tsp (5 g)	10	0	0
Grey Poupon				
Country Dijon	1 tsp	6	0	0
Dijon	1 tsp	6	0	0
Parisian	1 tsp	6	0	0
Gulden's				
Diablo	1 tsp	8	—	0
Mild	1 tsp	6	—	0
Spicy Brown	1 tsp	8	—	0
Hain				
Stone Ground	1 tbsp	14	—	1
Stone Ground No Salt Added	1 tbsp	14	—	1
Heinz				
Mild Yellow	1 tbsp	8	0	tr
Spicy Brown	1 tbsp	14	—	1
Kosciuszko				
Spicy Brown	1 tsp	5	—	tr
Kraft				
Horseradish Mustard	1 tsp (5 g)	0	0	0
Mustard	1 tsp (5 g)	0	0	0
McIlhenny				
Coarse Ground	1 tsp (0.2 oz)	4	tr	tr
Spicy	1 tsp (0.2 oz)	6	tr	tr
Plochman				
Dijon	1 tsp (5 g)	7	—	tr
Spoonable Salad	1 tsp (5 g)	4	—	tr
Squeeze Salad	1 tsp (5 g)	4	—	tr
Stone Ground	1 tsp (5 g)	6	—	tr
Russer				
Deli	1 tsp (5 g)	4	0	0
Tree Of Life				
Dijon	1 tsp (5 g)	0	0	0
Dijon Imported	1 tsp (5 g)	5	0	0

FOOD	PORTION	CALS.	SAT. FAT	FAT
Tree Of Life (CONT.)				
Low Sodium	1 tsp (5 g)	3	0	0
Stone Ground	1 tsp (5 g)	0	0	0
Yellow	1 tsp (5 g)	0	0	0
Watkins				
Country Mill	1 tsp (7 g)	15	0	1
Dusseldorf	1 tsp (7 g)	10	0	0
Horseradish	1 tsp (7 g)	10	0	0
Jalapeno	1 tsp (7 g)	10	0	0
Onion	1 tsp (7 g)	10	0	0
Parisienne	1 tsp (7 g)	10	0	0
MUSTARD GREENS				
fresh chopped cooked	½ cup	11	tr	tr
fresh raw chopped	½ cup	7	tr	tr
frozen chopped cooked	½ cup	14	tr	tr
Allen				
Mustard Greens	½ cup (4.1 oz)	30	0	1
Birds Eye				
Chopped	1 cup (3 oz)	30	0	0
Sunshine				
Mustard Greens	½ cup (4.1 oz)	30	0	1
NATTO				
natto	½ cup	187	1	10
NAVY BEANS				
CANNED				
navy	1 cup	296	tr	1
Allen				
Navy Beans	½ cup (4.5 oz)	110	0	1
Eden				
Organic	½ cup (4.3 oz)	100	0	1
Organic	½ cup (4.6 oz)	110	—	1
Hanover				
Navy	½ cup	100	—	0
Trappey				
With Bacon	½ cup (4.5 oz)	110	1	2
With Bacon & Jalapeno	½ cup (4.5 oz)	110	1	2
DRIED				
cooked	1 cup	259	tr	1
Hurst				
HamBeens w/ Ham	3 tbsp (1.2 oz)	120	0	1
NECTARINE				
fresh	1	67	—	1

FOOD	PORTION	CALS.	SAT. FAT	FAT
Dole				
Nectarine	1	70	—	1
NEUFCHATEL				
neufchatel	1 oz	74	4	7
neufchatel	1 pkg (3 oz)	221	13	20
Organic Valley				
Neufchatel	1 oz	70	4	6
Philadelphia				
Neufchatel	1 oz	70	4	6
WisPride				
Garden Vegetable Cup	2 tbsp (1.1 oz)	60	3	5
Garlic & Herb Cup	2 tbsp (1.1 oz)	60	3	5

NON-DAIRY CREAMERS
(see COFFEE WHITENERS)

NON-DAIRY WHIPPED TOPPINGS
(see WHIPPED TOPPINGS)

NOODLE DISHES
(see also NOODLES, PASTA DINNERS)

FOOD	PORTION	CALS.	SAT. FAT	FAT
CANNED				
Van Camp's				
Noodlee Weenee	1 can (8 oz)	230	2	8
FROZEN				
Luigino's				
Stroganoff	1 pkg (8 oz)	310	5	17
MIX				
Kraft				
Noodle Classics Cheddar Cheese as prep	1 cup (7.4 oz)	400	5	19
Noodle Classics Savory Chicken as prep	1 cup (8.5 oz)	340	3	13
Lipton				
Noodles & Sauce Alfredo Broccoli as prep	1 cup (2.2 oz)	340	6	14
Noodles & Sauce Alfredo as prep	1 cup (2.2 oz)	330	6	14
Noodles & Sauce Beef as prep	1 cup (2.1 oz)	280	2	10
Noodles & Sauce Butter as prep	1 cup (2.2 oz)	310	6	14
Noodles & Sauce Butter & Herb as prep	1 cup (2.2 oz)	300	5	13
Noodles & Sauce Chicken Broccoli as prep	1 cup (2.1 oz)	310	4	11

FOOD	PORTION	CALS.	SAT. FAT	FAT
Lipton (CONT.)				
Noodles & Sauce Chicken Tetrazzini as prep	1 cup (2 oz)	300	4	12
Noodles & Sauce Chicken as prep	1 cup (2.1 oz)	290	3	11
Noodles & Sauce Creamy Chicken as prep	1 cup (2.1 oz)	320	5	13
Noodles & Sauce Parmesan as prep	1 cup (2.1 oz)	330	6	15
Noodles & Sauce Sour Cream & Chives as prep	1 cup (2.2 oz)	310	6	14
Noodles & Sauce Stroganoff as prep	1 cup (2 oz)	300	4	11
Noodles By Leonardo				
Macaroni & Cheese as prep	1 cup (2.5 oz)	250	0	1
Ultra Slim-Fast				
Noodles & Alfredo Sauce	2.3 oz	240	—	4
Noodles & Beef	2.3 oz	230	—	3
Noodles & Cheese	2.3 oz	230	—	4
Noodles & Chicken Sauce	2.3 oz	220	—	3
Noodles & Tomato Herb Sauce	2.3 oz	220	—	3
SHELF-STABLE				
Hormel				
Microcup Meals Noodles & Chicken	1 cup (7.5 oz)	200	3	9
NOODLES				
cellophane	1 cup	492	tr	tr
chow mein	1 cup (1.6 oz)	237	2	14
egg	1 cup (38 g)	145	tr	2
egg cooked	1 cup (5.6 oz)	213	tr	2
japanese soba cooked	1 cup (4 oz)	113	tr	tr
japanese somen cooked	1 cup (6.2 oz)	231	tr	tr
rice cooked	1 cup (6.2 oz)	192	tr	tr
spinach/egg cooked	1 cup (5.6 oz)	211	1	3
Creamette				
Egg	2 oz	221	—	3
Egg	2 oz	220	—	3
Herb's				
Egg Fine	2 oz	220	0	2
Egg Medium	2 oz	220	0	2
Kluski Medium	2 oz	220	0	2
Kluski Wide	2 oz	220	0	2
Hodgson Mill				
Veggie Egg	2 oz	200	1	2

FOOD	PORTION	CALS.	SAT. FAT	FAT
Hodgson Mill (CONT.)				
Whole Wheat Egg	2 oz	190	1	2
Whole Wheat Spinach Egg	2 oz	190	1	2
Noodles By Leonardo				
Egg Fine	2 oz	210	1	2
Egg Medium	2 oz	210	1	2
Egg Wide	2 oz	210	1	2
San Giorgio				
Egg	2 oz	210	—	3
Shofar				
No Yolks	2 oz	210	0	0
NOPALES				
cooked	1 cup (5.2 oz)	23	—	tr
raw sliced	1 cup (3 oz)	14	—	tr
raw sliced	½ cup (1.5 oz)	7	—	tr
NUTMEG				
ground	1 tsp	12	1	1
Watkins				
Ground	¼ tsp (0.5 g)	0	0	0
NUTRITION SUPPLEMENTS				
(see also BREAKFAST BAR, BREAKFAST DRINKS, CEREAL BARS, SPORTS DRINKS)				
BeneFit				
Chocolate	1 serv	120	—	2
Nutrition Bar	1 (2 oz)	240	—	8
Vanilla	1 serv	120	—	2
Boost				
Chocolate	1 can (8 oz)	240	1	4
Vanilla	8 oz	240	1	4
Breakthru				
Organic Chocolate Fudge	1 bar (2.1 oz)	230	2	3
Organic Cinnamon Crunch	1 bar (2.1 oz)	220	1	3
Organic Honey Graham	1 bar (2.1 oz)	220	1	3
Organic Mocha Fudge	1 bar (2.1 oz)	230	2	3
California Joe				
All Natural Protein Drink Mix as prep	1 serv (8 oz)	165	2	4
Calorie Shed				
Shake Fat Free No Sugar Caramel Ripple	½ cup (4 fl oz)	70	0	0
Shake Fat Free No Sugar Chocolate	½ cup (4 fl oz)	70	0	0
Shake Fat Free No Sugar Marshmellow Nougat	½ cup (4 fl oz)	70	0	0

FOOD	PORTION	CALS.	SAT. FAT	FAT
Clif Bar				
Apple Cherry	1 bar (2.4 oz)	250	1	2
Apricot	1 bar (2.4 oz)	250	1	2
Carrot Cake	1 bar (2.4 oz)	240	1	4
Chocolate Expresso	1 bar (2.4 oz)	250	1	3
Chocolate Almond Fudge	1 bar (2.4 oz)	250	1	5
Chocolate Chip	1 bar (2.4 oz)	250	1	3
Chocolate Chip Peanut Crunch	1 bar (2.4 oz)	250	1	6
Cookie 'N Cream	1 bar (2.4 oz)	250	1	5
Crunchy Peanut Butter	1 bar (2.4 oz)	250	1	4
Real Berry	1 bar (2.4 oz)	250	1	2
Dynatrim				
Dutch Chocolate as prep w/ 1% milk	8 oz	220	—	4
Strawberry Royale as prep w/ 1% milk	8 oz	220	—	4
Vanilla as prep w/ 1% milk	8 oz	220	—	4
Ensure				
Honey Graham Crunch	1 bar (2.23 oz)	130	1	3
Essential				
Protein Powder	1 serv (0.6 oz)	70	0	tr
Fat Burner				
Diet Fruit Punch	8 fl oz	0	0	0
Fi-Bar				
Apple	1 (1 oz)	90	—	3
Cocoa Almond	1	130	—	4
Cocoa Peanut	1	130	—	4
Cranberry & Wild Berries	1 (1 oz)	100	—	3
Lemon	1 (1 oz)	90	—	3
Mandarin Orange	1 (1 oz)	99	—	4
Nuggets Almond Cappuccino Crunch	1 pkg	136	—	6
Nuggets Almond Butter Crunch	1 pkg	163	—	11
Nuggets Coconut Almond Crunch	1 pkg	136	—	6
Nuggets Peanut Butter Crunch	1 pkg	160	—	10
Raspberry	1 (1 oz)	100	—	3
Strawberry	1 (1 oz)	100	—	3
Treat Yourself Right Almond	1	152	—	6
Treat Yourself Right Peanutty Butter	1	152	—	5
Vanilla Almond	1	130	—	4
Vanilla Peanut	1	130	—	4
Gatorade				
GatorBar	1 (1.17 oz)	110	0	1

FOOD	PORTION	CALS.	SAT. FAT	FAT
Gatorade (CONT.)				
GatorLode	1 can (11.6 fl oz)	280	0	0
GatorPro	1 can (11 fl oz)	360	1	6
ReLode	1 pkt (0.75 oz)	80	0	0
GeniSoy				
Soy Protein Powder	1 scoop (0.6 oz)	60	0	0
Soy Protein Shake Chocolate	1 scoop (1.2 oz)	120	0	0
Soy Protein Shake Vanilla	1 scoop (1.2 oz)	130	0	0
Soy Protein Bar Chocolate	1 bar (2.2 oz)	210	0	0
Soy Protein Bar Chocolate Coated	1 bar (2.2 oz)	220	3	4
Healthy Pleasures				
Chocolate Irish Cream	1 bottle (10.5 oz)	260	1	2
Luna				
Chocolate Pecan Pie	1 bar (1.7 oz)	180	3	5
Lemonzest	1 bar (1.7 oz)	180	3	4
Nutz Over Chocolate	1 bar (1.7 oz)	180	3	5
Trail Mix	1 bar (1.7 oz)	180	0	3
Malsovit				
Mealwafers	2	152	—	8
Nancy Grey's				
Shake Hi-Protein Black Raspberry	1 cup (8 fl oz)	340	10	16
Shake Hi-Protein Chocolate	1 cup (8 fl oz)	340	10	15
Shake Hi-Protein Vanilla	1 cup (8 fl oz)	340	10	16
Nantucket Nectars				
Super Nectars Ginkgo Mango	8 oz	150	0	0
Super Nectars Green Angel	8 oz	140	0	0
Super Nectars Protein Smoothie	8 oz	170	—	1
Super Nectars Red Guarana Tea	8 oz	110	0	0
Super Nectars Vital C	8 oz	130	0	0
NiteBite				
Chocolate Fudge	1 bar (0.9 oz)	100	1	4
Peanut Butter	1 bar (0.9 oz)	100	1	4
NutraBalance				
EggPro	1 tbsp (7.5 g)	30	0	0
Frozen Pudding Chocolate	4 oz	225	—	8
NutraShake				
Citrus	1 pkg (4 oz)	200	0	0
Citrus Free	1 serv (4 oz)	200	0	0
Vanilla	1 serv (8 oz)	400	—	12
Vanilla No Added Sugar	1 serv (4 oz)	200	—	8

FOOD	PORTION	CALS.	SAT. FAT	FAT
Pounds Off				
All Flavors	1 bar (2.1 oz)	210	1	5
Dark Chocolate Ectasy	1 can (11 oz)	200	0	3
French Vanilla	1 can (11 oz)	220	1	3
PowerBar				
Apple Cinnamon	1 bar (2.3 oz)	230	1	3
Banana	1 bar (2.3 oz)	230	1	2
Chocolate	1 bar (2.3 oz)	230	1	2
Harvest Strawberry	1 bar (2.3 oz)	240	1	4
Malt-Nut	1 bar (2.3 oz)	230	1	3
Mocha	1 bar (2.3 oz)	230	1	3
Oatmeal Raisin	1 bar (2.3 oz)	230	1	3
Peanut Butter	1 bar (2.3 oz)	230	1	3
Power Gel Strawberry Banana	1 pkg	110	0	0
Wild Berry	1 bar (2.3 oz)	230	1	3
Resource				
Fructose Sweetened	1 pkg (8 oz)	250	—	11
Fruit Beverage	1 pkg (8 oz)	180	—	0
Liquid Food	1 pkg (8 oz)	250	—	9
Plus Liquid Food	1 pkg (8 oz)	355	—	13
Sego				
Lite Chocolate	10 fl oz	150	—	3
Lite Dutch Chocolate	10 fl oz	150	—	3
Lite French Vanilla	10 fl oz	150	—	4
Lite Strawberry	10 fl oz	150	—	4
Lite Vanilla	10 fl oz	150	—	4
Very Chocolate	10 fl oz	225	—	1
Very Chocolate Malt	10 fl oz	225	—	1
Very Strawberry	10 fl oz	225	—	5
Very Vanilla	10 fl oz	225	—	5
Slim-Fast				
Powder Chocolate as prep w/ skim milk	8 oz	190	—	1
Powder Chocolate Malt as prep w/ skim milk	8 oz	190	—	tr
Powder Strawberry as prep w/ skim milk	8 oz	190	—	1
Powder Vanilla as prep w/ skim milk	8 oz	190	—	1
Sobe				
Drive	8 oz	120	0	0
Jing Essentials	1 bottle (14 oz)	140	0	0
Karma	8 oz	120	0	0
Qi Essentials	1 bottle (14 oz)	140	0	0
Shen Essentials	1 bottle (14 oz)	140	0	0

FOOD	PORTION	CALS.	SAT. FAT	FAT
Sustacal				
Vanilla	8 oz	240	1	6
Sweet Success				
Chewy Bar Chocolate Brownie	1 (1.6 oz)	120	2	4
Chewy Bar Chocolate Peanut Butter	1 (1.6 oz)	120	2	4
Chewy Bar Chocolate Raspberry	1 (1.6 oz)	120	2	4
Chewy Bar Chocolate Chip	1 (1.6 oz)	120	2	4
Chewy Bar Oatmeal Raisin	1 (1.6 oz)	120	2	4
Chocolate Raspberry Truffle	1 can (10 fl oz)	200	1	3
Chocolate Raspberry as prep w/ skim milk	9 fl oz	180	1	1
Chocolate Mocha Supreme	1 can (10 fl oz)	200	1	3
Chocolate Mocha Supreme as prep w/ skim milk	9 fl oz	180	1	tr
Classic Chocolate Chip as prep w/ skim milk	9 fl oz	180	2	1
Creamy Milk Chocolate	1 carton (12 fl oz)	220	1	2
Creamy Milk Chocolate	1 can (10 fl oz)	200	1	3
Creamy Milk Chocolate as prep w/ skim milk	9 fl oz	180	1	1
Creamy Vanilla Delight as prep w/ skim milk	9 fl oz	180	1	tr
Dark Chocolate Fudge	1 can (10 fl oz)	200	1	3
Dark Chocolate Fudge	1 carton (12 fl oz)	220	1	2
Dark Chocolate Fudge as prep w/ skim milk	9 fl oz	180	1	1
Rich Chocolate Almond	1 carton (12 fl oz)	220	1	2
Rich Chocolate Almond	1 can (10 fl oz)	200	1	3
Rich Chocolate Almond as prep w/ skim milk	9 fl oz	180	1	tr
Smooth Vanilla Creme	1 can (10 fl oz)	200	1	3
The Pumper				
Body Building Milkshake Banana	1 serv (13.5 oz)	390	1	2
Body Building Milkshake Chocolate	1 serv (13.5 oz)	390	1	2
Think!				
Apple Spice	1 bar (2 oz)	205	1	3
Chocolate Almond Coconut Raisin	1 bar (2 oz)	243	2	7
Chocolate Fruit Harvest	1 bar (2 oz)	217	1	3

FOOD	PORTION	CALS.	SAT. FAT	FAT
Ultra Slim-Fast				
Cafe Mocha as prep w/ skim milk	8 oz	200	—	tr
Chocolate Royale as prep w/ skim milk	8 oz	200	—	1
Crunch Bar Cocoa Almond	1	110	—	3
Crunch Bar Cocoa Raspberry	1	100	—	3
Crunch Bar Vanilla Almond	1	110	—	4
Dutch Chocolate as prep w/ water	8 oz	220	—	tr
French Vanilla as prep w/ skim milk	8 oz	190	—	tr
French Vanilla as prep w/ water	8 oz	220	—	tr
Fruit Juice Mix as prep w/ fruit juice	8 oz	200	—	tr
Nutrition Bar Dutch Chocolate	1	130	—	4
Nutrition Bar Peanut Butter	1	140	—	6
Pina Colada as prep w/ skim milk	8 oz	180	—	tr
Ready-To-Drink Chocolate Royale	12 oz	250	—	1
Ready-To-Drink Chocolate Royale	11 oz	230	—	3
Ready-To-Drink French Vanilla	11 oz	230	—	5
Ready-To-Drink French Vanilla	12 oz	220	—	tr
Ready-To-Drink Strawberry Supreme	12 oz	220	—	1
Strawberry Supreme as prep w/ water	8 oz	220	—	tr
Strawberry as prep w/ skim milk	8 oz	190	—	1
Viactiv				
Calcium Chews	1	20	—	1
Vita-J				
Apple Juice	11.5 fl oz	8	0	0
Fruit Punch	11.5 fl oz	8	0	0
Grapefruit Cocktail w/ Raspberry	11.5 fl oz	8	0	0
Orange Juice	11.5 fl oz	8	0	0

NUTS MIXED
(see also INDIVIDUAL NAMES)

FOOD	PORTION	CALS.	SAT. FAT	FAT
dry roasted w/ peanuts	1 oz	169	2	15
dry roasted w/ peanuts salted	1 oz	169	2	15
oil roasted w/ peanuts	1 oz	175	2	16

FOOD	PORTION	CALS.	SAT. FAT	FAT
oil roasted w/ peanuts salted	1 oz	175	2	16
oil roasted w/o peanuts	1 oz	175	3	16
oil roasted w/o peanuts salted	1 oz	175	3	16
Estee				
Fruit & Nut Mix	¼ cup	210	7	12
Fisher				
Mixed Deluxe Lightly Salted	1 oz	180	3	16
Mixed Deluxe Salted	1 oz	180	3	16
Mixed Oil Roasted 25% More Cashews Lightly Salted	1 oz	180	3	16
Mixed Oil Roasted 25% More Cashews Salted	1 oz	180	3	16
Nut & Fruit Pina Colada	1 oz	150	2	10
Nut & Fruit Raisin Cranberry	1 oz	150	2	10
Nut & Fruit Tropical Fruit	1 oz	140	1	8
Nut Toppings Oil Roasted With Peanuts	1 oz	190	3	17
Peanuts Cashews	1 oz	170	2	13
Guy's				
Mixed With Peanuts	1 oz	180	—	16
Tasty Mix	1 oz	130	—	7
Planters				
Cashews & Peanuts Honey Roasted	1 oz	150	2	12
Deluxe Oil Roasted	1 oz	170	2	16
Dry Roasted	1 oz	170	2	14
Honey Roasted	1 oz	140	2	13
Lightly Salted Oil Roasted	1 oz	170	2	15
No Brazils Lightly Salted Oil Roasted	1 oz	170	2	15
No Brazils Oil Roasted	1 oz	170	2	15
Oil Roasted	1 oz	170	3	15
Select Mix Cashews Almonds & Macadamias Oil Roasted	1 oz	170	3	16
Select Mix Cashews Almonds & Pecans Oil Roasted	1 oz	170	2	15
Unsalted Oil Roasted	1 oz	170	2	15

OCTOPUS

fresh steamed	3 oz	140	tr	2

OHELOBERRIES

fresh	1 cup	39	—	tr

OIL

(see also FAT)

FOOD	PORTION	CALS.	SAT. FAT	FAT
almond	1 cup	1927	1	218
almond	1 tbsp	120	1	14
apricot kernel	1 cup	1927	14	218
apricot kernel	1 tbsp	120	1	14
avocado	1 tbsp	124	2	14
butter oil	1 tbsp	112	8	13
butter oil	1 cup	1795	127	204
canola	1 tbsp	124	2	14
coconut	1 tbsp	117	12	14
corn	1 tbsp	120	2	14
corn	1 cup	1927	28	218
cottonseed	1 cup	1927	56	218
cottonseed	1 tbsp	120	4	14
cupu assu	1 tbsp	120	7	14
grapeseed	1 tbsp	120	1	14
hazelnut	1 cup	1927	1	218
hazelnut	1 tbsp	120	1	14
mustard	1 tbsp	124	2	14
oat	1 tbsp	120	3	14
olive	1 tbsp	119	2	14
olive	1 cup	1909	26	216
palm	1 tbsp	120	7	14
palm	1 cup	1927	107	218
palm kernel	1 tbsp	117	11	14
peanut	1 tbsp	119	2	14
peanut	1 cup	1909	36	216
poppyseed	1 tbsp	120	2	14
rice bran	1 tbsp	120	3	14
safflower	1 tbsp	120	1	14
safflower	1 cup	1927	20	218
sesame	1 tbsp	120	2	14
sheanut	1 tbsp	120	6	14
soybean	1 tbsp	120	2	14
soybean	1 cup	1927	31	218
sunflower	1 cup	1927	23	218
sunflower	1 tbsp	120	1	14
teaseed	1 tbsp	120	3	14
tomatoseed	1 tbsp	120	3	14
vegetable soybean & cottonseed	1 cup	1927	2	218
vegetable soybean & cottonseed	1 tbsp	120	2	14
walnut	1 cup	1927	20	218
walnut	1 tbsp	120	1	14
wheat germ	1 tbsp	120	3	14

FOOD	PORTION	CALS.	SAT. FAT	FAT
Arrowhead				
Flax Seed	1 tbsp (0.5 fl oz)	120	1	14
Hazelnut	1 tbsp (0.5 fl oz)	120	1	14
Bertolli				
Classico	1 tbsp	120	—	14
Extra Light	1 tbsp	120	—	14
Extra Virgin	1 tbsp	120	—	14
Crisco				
Corn Canola	1 tbsp (0.5 fl oz)	120	2	14
Oil	1 tbsp (0.5 fl oz)	120	2	14
Puritan Canola	1 tbsp (0.5 fl oz)	120	1	14
Eden				
Hot Pepper Sesame	1 tbsp (0.5 oz)	130	2	14
Safflower	1 tbsp (0.5 oz)	120	1	14
Sesame	1 tbsp (0.5 oz)	140	2	15
Toasted Sesame	1 tbsp (0.5 oz)	130	2	14
Hain				
All Blend	1 tbsp	120	2	14
Almond	1 tbsp	120	1	14
Apricot Kernel	1 tbsp	120	1	14
Avocado	1 tbsp	120	1	14
Canola	1 tbsp	120	1	14
Canola Organic	1 tbsp	120	1	14
Coconut	1 tbsp	120	12	14
Corn	1 tbsp	120	2	14
Garlic & Oil	1 tbsp	120	3	14
Olive	1 tbsp	120	2	14
Peanut	1 tbsp	120	2	14
Rice Bran	1 tbsp	120	3	14
Safflower	1 tbsp	120	1	14
Safflower Hi-Oleic	1 tbsp	120	1	14
Safflower Organic	1 tbsp	120	1	14
Sesame	1 tbsp	120	2	14
Soy	1 tbsp	120	2	14
Sunflower	1 tbsp	120	2	14
Sunflower Organic	1 tbsp	120	2	14
Walnut	1 tbsp	120	2	14
Hollywood				
Canola	1 tbsp	120	1	14
Peanut	1 tbsp	120	4	14
Safflower	1 tbsp	120	1	14
Soy	1 tbsp	120	3	14
Sunflower	1 tbsp	120	2	14
House Of Tsang				
Hot Chili Sesame	1 tsp (5 g)	45	1	5

FOOD	PORTION	CALS.	SAT. FAT	FAT
House Of Tsang (CONT.)				
Mongolian Fire	1 tsp (5 g)	45	1	5
Pure Sesame	1 tsp (5 g)	45	1	5
Singapore Curry	1 tsp (5 g)	45	1	5
Wok Oil	1 tbsp (0.5 oz)	130	3	14
Italica				
Olive Oil	1 tbsp	120	2	9
Orville Redenbacher's				
Oil	1 tbsp	120	2	14
Pam				
Butter	⅓ sec spray (0.3 g)	0	0	0
Cooking Spray	⅓ sec spray (0.3 g)	0	0	0
Olive Oil	⅓ sec spray (0.3 g)	0	0	0
Planters				
Peanut	1 tbsp (0.5 oz)	120	3	14
Popcorn	1 tbsp (0.5 oz)	120	3	14
Pompeian				
Olive	1 tbsp	130	—	14
Progresso				
Olive Extra Light	1 tbsp	119	2	14
Olive Extra Mild	1 tbsp (0.5 oz)	120	2	14
Olive Extra Virgin	1 tbsp (0.5 oz)	120	2	14
Olive Riviera Blend	1 tbsp (0.5 oz)	120	2	14
Smart Beat				
Canola	1 tbsp	120	1	14
Oil	1 tbsp	120	1	14
Tree Of Life				
Almond	1 tbsp (0.5 g)	130	1	14
Apricot Kernel	1 tbsp (0.5 g)	130	1	14
Avocado	1 tbsp (0.5 g)	130	3	14
Macadamia Nut	1 tbsp (0.5 g)	130	2	14
Olive Extra Virgin Organic	1 tbsp (0.5 g)	130	1	14
Sesame	1 tbsp (0.5 g)	130	2	14
Toasted Sesame	1 tbsp (0.5 oz)	130	2	14
Weight Watchers				
Butter Spray	⅓ sec spray	0	0	0
Cooking Spray	⅓ sec spray	0	0	0
Wesson				
Canola	1 tbsp	120	1	14
Cooking Spray Lite	0.5 sec spray	0	—	0
Corn	1 tbsp	120	2	14
Olive	1 tbsp	120	2	14
Sunflower	1 tbsp	120	2	14
Vegetable	1 tbsp	120	2	14

FOOD	PORTION	CALS.	SAT. FAT	FAT
FISH OIL				
cod liver	1 tbsp	123	3	14
herring	1 tbsp	123	3	14
menhaden	1 tbsp	123	4	14
salmon	1 tbsp	123	3	14
sardine	1 tbsp	123	4	14
shark	3½ oz	945	—	100
whale	3½ oz	945	—	100
Hain				
Cod Liver	1 tbsp	120	—	14
Cod Liver Cherry	1 tbsp	120	—	14
Cod Liver Mint	1 tbsp	120	—	14
OKRA				
CANNED				
Allen				
Cut	½ cup (4.4 oz)	25	0	0
McIlhenny				
Pickled	2 pieces (1 oz)	7	tr	tr
Trappey				
Cocktail Hot	2 pieces (1 oz)	8	tr	tr
Cocktail Mild	1 piece (1 oz)	9	tr	tr
Creole Gumbo	½ cup (4.2 oz)	35	0	0
Cut	½ cup (4.4 oz)	25	0	0
FRESH				
raw	8 pods	36	tr	tr
raw sliced	½ cup	19	tr	tr
sliced cooked	½ cup	25	tr	tr
sliced cooked	8 pods	27	tr	tr
FROZEN				
sliced cooked	1 pkg (10 oz)	94	tr	1
sliced cooked	½ cup	34	tr	tr
Birds Eye				
Cut	¾ cup (2.9 oz)	25	0	0
Whole	9 pods (3 oz)	25	0	0
Fresh Like				
Cut	3.5 oz	26	—	tr
Whole	3.5 oz	32	—	tr
Hanover				
Cut	½ cup	25	—	0
Whole	½ cup	35	—	0
OLIVES				
green	3 extra lg	15	tr	2
green	4 med	15	tr	2
ripe	1 sm	4	tr	tr

FOOD	PORTION	CALS.	SAT. FAT	FAT
ripe	1 lg	5	tr	tr
ripe	1 jumbo	7	tr	1
ripe	1 colossal	12	tr	1
spanish stuffed	5 (0.5 oz)	15	0	1
Italia In Tavola				
Black Olives Paste	1 tbsp (0.5 oz)	20	—	2
Progresso				
Oil Cured	6 (0.5 oz)	80	1	6
Olive Salad (drained)	2 tbsp (0.8 oz)	25	0	3
Tee Pee				
Spanish Green	2 oz	98	—	10

ONION
CANNED
FOOD	PORTION	CALS.	SAT. FAT	FAT
chopped	½ cup	21	tr	tr
whole	1 (2.2 oz)	12	tr	tr
Boar's Head				
Sweet Vidalia In Sauce	1 tbsp	10	0	0
Vlasic				
Lightly Spiced Cocktail Onions	1 oz	4	0	0
Watkins				
Liquid Spice	1 tbsp (0.5 oz)	120	2	14
DRIED				
flakes	1 tbsp	16	tr	tr
powder	1 tsp	7	—	tr
Watkins				
Flakes	¼ tsp (1 g)	0	0	0
FRESH				
chopped cooked	½ cup	47	tr	tr
raw chopped	1 tbsp	4	tr	tr
scallions raw chopped	1 tbsp	2	tr	tr
welsh raw	3½ oz	34	tr	tr
Antioch Farms				
Vidalia	1 med	60	—	0
Dole				
Green Chopped	1 tbsp	2	—	tr
Medium	1	60	—	0
FROZEN				
chopped cooked	1 tbsp	4	tr	tr
chopped cooked	½ cup	30	tr	tr
rings	7 (2.5 oz)	285	6	19
rings cooked	2 (0.7 oz)	81	2	5
whole cooked	3½ oz	28	0	tr
Birds Eye				
Diced	⅔ cup (3 oz)	30	0	0
Pearl Onions In Cream Sauce	½ cup (4.4 oz)	60	1	2

FOOD	PORTION	CALS.	SAT. FAT	FAT
Fresh Like				
Diced	3.5 oz	29	—	0
Whole	3.5 oz	37	—	tr
Kineret				
Rings	6 (3 oz)	200	3	10
Mrs. Paul's				
Crispy Onion Rings	2½ oz	190	—	12
Ore Ida				
Chopped	¾ cup (3 oz)	25	0	0
Onion Ringers	6 pieces (3 oz)	240	3	14
Southland				
Chopped	2 oz	15	—	0
TAKE-OUT				
fried	½ cup (7.5 oz)	176	6	11
rings breaded & fried	8 to 9	275	7	16

OPOSSUM

FOOD	PORTION	CALS.	SAT. FAT	FAT
roasted	3 oz	188	—	9

ORANGE

FOOD	PORTION	CALS.	SAT. FAT	FAT
CANNED				
Del Monte				
Mandarin In Heavy Syrup	½ cup (4.4 oz)	80	0	0
Dole				
Mandarin Segments	½ cup	70	—	tr
Pineapple Mandarin Segments	½ cup	80	—	tr
FRESH				
california navel	1	65	tr	tr
california valencia	1	59	tr	tr
florida	1	69	tr	tr
peel	1 tbsp	6	tr	tr
sections	1 cup	85	tr	tr
Dole				
Orange	1	50	—	0

ORANGE EXTRACT

FOOD	PORTION	CALS.	SAT. FAT	FAT
Virginia Dare				
Virginia Dare	1 tsp	22	—	0

ORANGE JUICE

FOOD	PORTION	CALS.	SAT. FAT	FAT
canned	1 cup	104	tr	tr
chilled	1 cup	110	tr	1
fresh	1 cup	111	tr	tr
orange drink	6 oz	94	0	0
After The Fall				
Juice	1 bottle (10 oz)	110	0	0

FOOD	PORTION	CALS.	SAT. FAT	FAT
Big Juicy				
Drink	8 oz	110	0	0
Bright & Early				
Chilled	8 fl oz	120	0	0
Frozen	8 fl oz	120	0	0
Capri Sun				
Drink	1 pkg (7 oz)	100	0	0
Del Monte				
Juice	8 fl oz	110	0	0
Everfresh				
Juice	1 can (8 oz)	100	0	0
Ruby Red Orange Drink	1 can (8 oz)	130	0	0
Fresh Samantha				
Juice	1 cup (8 oz)	109	0	1
Hi-C				
Box	8.45 fl oz	130	0	0
Drink	8 fl oz	130	0	0
Drink	1 can (11.5 fl oz)	180	0	0
Hood				
From Concentrate	1 cup (8 oz)	120	0	0
Select	1 cup (8 oz)	120	0	0
With Calcium	1 cup (8 oz)	120	0	0
Kool-Aid				
Drink Mix Orange as prep	1 serv (8 oz)	60	0	0
Orange Drink as prep w/ sugar	1 serv (8 oz)	100	0	0
Libby				
Juice	6 fl oz	80	0	0
Minute Maid				
Box	8.45 fl oz	120	0	0
Calcium Rich Chilled	8 fl oz	120	0	0
Calcium Rich frzn	8 fl oz	120	0	0
Chilled	8 fl oz	110	0	0
Country Style Chilled	8 fl oz	110	0	0
Country Style frzn	8 fl oz	110	0	0
Juices To Go	1 can (11.5 fl oz)	160	0	0
Juices To Go	1 bottle (16 fl oz)	110	0	0
Juices To Go	1 bottle (10 fl oz)	140	0	0
Orange Punch Box	8.45 fl oz	130	0	0
Premium Choice Chilled	8 fl oz	110	0	0
Pulp Free Chilled	8 fl oz	110	0	0
Pulp Free frzn	8 fl oz	110	0	0
Reduced Acid frzn	8 fl oz	110	0	0
Mott's				
From Concentrate	10 fl oz	130	0	1

FOOD	PORTION	CALS.	SAT. FAT	FAT
Nantucket Nectars				
100% Juice	8 oz	120	0	0
NutraShake				
Fourtified	1 pkg (4 oz)	50	0	0
Ocean Spray				
100% Juice	8 oz	120	0	0
Odwalla				
Juice	8 fl oz	110	—	1
Shasta Plus				
Orange Drink	1 can (11.5 oz)	160	0	0
Sippin' Pak				
100% Pure	8.45 fl oz	110	0	0
Snapple				
Juice	10 fl oz	130	0	0
Orangeade	8 fl oz	120	0	0
Tang				
Orange Drink as prep	1 serv (8 oz)	90	0	0
Sugar Free Orange as prep	1 serv (8 oz)	5	0	0
Tree Of Life				
Juice	8 fl oz	110	0	0
Tropicana				
Double Vitamin C	8 fl oz	110	0	0
Juice	8 oz	110	0	0
Ruby Red	8 oz	110	0	0
Season's Best	8 oz	110	0	0
Season's Best Homestyle	8 fl oz	110	0	0
Tropical	8 oz	110	0	0
With Calcium	8 fl oz	110	0	0
Veryfine				
100% Juice	1 bottle (10 oz)	150	0	0
Chillers Artric Orange	8 fl oz	130	0	0
Juice Blend	1 can (11.5 oz)	160	0	0
Orange Drink	1 bottle (10 oz)	160	0	0

OREGANO

FOOD	PORTION	CALS.	SAT. FAT	FAT
ground	1 tsp	5	tr	tr
Watkins				
Liquid Spice	1 tbsp (0.5 oz)	120	2	14

ORGAN MEATS

(see BRAINS, GIBLETS, GIZZARD, HEART, KIDNEY, LIVER, SWEETBREADS)

ORIENTAL FOOD

(see ASIAN FOOD, EGG ROLLS, DINNER, NOODLES, RICE, SUSHI)

OSTRICH

FOOD	PORTION	CALS.	SAT. FAT	FAT
ostrich	3 oz	127	—	3

FOOD	PORTION	CALS.	SAT. FAT	FAT
OYSTERS				
CANNED				
eastern	1 cup	170	2	6
eastern	3 oz	58	1	2
Bumble Bee				
Whole	½ cup (3.5 oz)	100	1	4
FRESH				
eastern cooked	6 med	58	1	2
eastern cooked	3 oz	117	1	4
eastern raw	6 med	58	1	2
eastern raw	1 cup	170	2	6
pacific raw	3 oz	69	tr	2
pacific raw	1 med	41	tr	1
steamed	1 med	41	tr	1
TAKE-OUT				
battered & fried	6 (4.9 oz)	368	5	18
breaded & fried	6 (4.9 oz)	368	5	18
eastern breaded & fried	6 med (88 g)	173	3	11
eastern breaded & fried	3 oz	167	3	11
oysters rockefeller	3 oysters	66	—	2
PANCAKES				
FROZEN				
buttermilk	1 4 in diam (1.3 ox)	83	tr	1
plain	1 4 in diam (1.3 oz)	83	tr	1
Aunt Jemima				
Blueberry	3 (3.4 oz)	210	1	4
Buttermilk	3 (3 oz)	180	1	3
Lowfat	3 (3.4 oz)	130	0	2
Original	3 (3.4 oz)	200	1	3
Downyflake				
Blueberry	3	290	—	9
Buttermilk	3	280	—	9
Pancakes And Sausages	1 pkg (5.5 oz)	430	—	23
Regular	3	280	—	9
Eggo				
Buttermilk	3 (4.1 oz)	270	2	8
Jimmy Dean				
Flapstick	1 (2.5 oz)	240	4	14
Flapstick Blueberry	1 (2.5 oz)	260	4	15
Quaker				
Lite Pancakes & Lite Links	1 pkg (6 oz)	310	—	10
Lite Pancakes & Lite Syrup	1 pkg (6 oz)	260	—	3
Pancakes & Sausages	1 pkg (6 oz)	420	—	16

FOOD	PORTION	CALS.	SAT. FAT	FAT
HOME RECIPE				
plain	1 (4 in diam)	86	1	4
MIX				
buckwheat	1 (4 in diam)	62	1	2
buttermilk	1 4 in diam (1.3 oz)	74	tr	1
plain	1-4 in diam (1.3 oz)	74	tr	1
sugar free low sodium	1 (3 in diam)	44	tr	tr
whole wheat	1 (4 in diam)	92	1	3
Arrowhead				
Multigrain Pancake & Waffle Mix	¼ cup (1.2 oz)	120	0	1
Aunt Jemima				
Buckwheat Pancake & Waffle Mix	¼ cup (1.4 oz)	120	0	1
Buttermilk Pancake & Waffle Mix	⅓ cup (1.9 oz)	190	1	2
Original Pancake & Waffle Mix	⅓ cup (1.6 oz)	150	0	1
Pancake & Waffle Mix Regular	⅓ cup (1.9 oz)	190	1	2
Pancake & Waffle Mix Whole Wheat	¼ cup (1.4 oz)	130	0	1
Betty Crocker				
Buttermilk as prep	3	200	1	3
Original as prep	3	200	1	3
Bisquick				
Shake 'N Pour Blueberry as prep	3	210	1	4
Shake 'N Pour as prep	3	200	4	5
Shake 'N Pour as prep	3	210	1	4
Estee				
Pancake Mix as prep	4 (4 in diam)	180	0	0
Fast Shake				
Blueberry	1 serv (2.5 oz)	251	—	3
Buttermilk	1 serv (2.5 oz)	258	—	3
Original	1 serv (2.5 oz)	266	—	4
Hodgson Mill				
Buckwheat	⅓ cup (1.8 oz)	160	0	1
Hungry Jack				
Potato as prep	3 (3 in diam)	90	0	2
Robin Hood				
Buttermilk as prep	3	230	2	6
Stone-Buhr				
Buckwheat	¼ cup (1.4 oz)	130	0	1
Oat Bran	¼ cup (1.4 oz)	130	0	0
Whole Wheat	¼ cup (1.4 oz)	120	0	1

FOOD	PORTION	CALS.	SAT. FAT	FAT
Wanda's				
Blue Corn	⅓ cup mix per serv (1.7 oz)	170	0	2
TAKE-OUT				
blueberry	1 (4 in diam)	84	1	4
buckwheat	1 (4 in diam)	55	1	2
w/ butter & syrup	2 (8.1 oz)	520	6	14

PANCAKE/WAFFLE SYRUP

(see also SYRUP)

FOOD	PORTION	CALS.	SAT. FAT	FAT
low calorie	1 tbsp	12	0	0
maple	1 cup (11.1 oz)	824	—	1
maple	1 tbsp (0.8 oz)	52	—	0
pancake syrup	1 tbsp (0.7 oz)	57	0	0
pancake syrup	1 cup (11 oz)	903	0	0
pancake syrup light	1 oz	46	—	0
pancake syrup w/ butter	1 tbsp (0.7 oz)	59	tr	tr
pancake syrup w/ butter	1 cup (11 oz)	933	3	5
Aunt Jemima				
Butter Rich	¼ cup (2.8 oz)	210	0	0
Butterlite	¼ cup (2.5 oz)	100	0	0
Lite	¼ cup (2.5 oz)	100	0	0
Syrup	¼ cup (2.8 oz)	210	0	0
Brer Rabbit				
Dark	2 tbsp	120	0	0
Light	2 Tbsp	120	0	0
Estee				
Maple	¼ cup	80	0	0
Log Cabin				
Country Kitchen	1 oz	103	0	0
Lite	1 oz	49	0	0
Mrs. Butter-worth's				
Original	¼ cup (2 oz)	230	0	0
Mrs. Richardson's				
Lite	¼ cup (2.5 oz)	100	0	0
Original Recipe	¼ cup (2.8 oz)	210	0	0
Red Wing				
Lite	¼ cup (2 oz)	100	0	0
Syrup	¼ cup (2 oz)	210	0	0
Tree Of Life				
Maple	¼ cup (2.1 oz)	200	0	0

PANCREAS

(see SWEETBREADS)

FOOD	PORTION	CALS.	SAT. FAT	FAT
PAPAYA				
fresh	1	117	tr	tr
fresh cubed	1 cup	54	tr	tr
Sonoma				
Dried Pieces	2 pieces (2 oz)	200	0	4
PAPAYA JUICE				
nectar	1 cup	142	tr	tr
Everfresh				
Premium Drink	1 can (8 oz)	140	0	0
Goya				
Nectar	6 oz	110	—	0
Kern's				
Nectar	6 fl oz	110	0	0
Libby				
Nectar	1 can (11.5 fl oz)	210	0	0
Nantucket Nectars				
Cocktail	8 oz	120	0	0
PAPRIKA				
paprika	1 tsp	6	tr	tr
Watkins				
Ground	¼ tsp (0.5 oz)	0	0	0
PARSLEY				
dry	1 tsp	1	—	tr
dry	1 tbsp	1	—	tr
fresh chopped	½ cup	11	tr	tr
Dole				
Chopped	1 tbsp	10	—	tr
PARSNIPS				
fresh cooked	1 (5.6 oz)	130	tr	tr
fresh sliced cooked	½ cup	63	tr	tr
raw sliced	½ cup	50	tr	tr
PASSION FRUIT				
purple fresh	1	18	—	tr
PASSION FRUIT JUICE				
purple	1 cup	126	—	tr
yellow	1 cup	149	—	tr
Snapple				
Passion Supreme	10 fl oz	160	0	0
PASTA				
(see also NOODLES, PASTA DINNERS, PASTA SALAD)				

FOOD	PORTION	CALS.	SAT. FAT	FAT
DRY				
corn cooked	1 cup (4.9 oz)	176	tr	1
elbows	1 cup	389	tr	2
elbows cooked	1 cup (4.9 oz)	197	tr	1
shells small cooked	1 cup (4 oz)	162	tr	1
shells small protein fortified cooked	1 cup (4 oz)	189	tr	tr
spaghetti cooked	1 cup (4.9 oz)	197	tr	1
spaghetti protein fortified cooked	1 cup (4.9 oz)	230	tr	tr
spinach spaghetti cooked	1 cup (4.9 oz)	182	tr	1
spirals cooked	1 cup (4.7 oz)	189	tr	tr
vegetable cooked	1 cup (4.7 oz)	172	tr	tr
whole wheat cooked	1 cup (4.9 oz)	174	tr	tr
whole wheat spaghetti cooked	1 cup (4.9 oz)	174	tr	1
Anthony				
Pasta	2 oz	210		1
Barilla				
Conchiglie Rigate	1 cup (2 oz)	200	0	1
Gemelli as prep	1 cup (2 oz)	200	0	1
Pennette Rigate	1⅓ cups (2 oz)	200	0	1
Bella Via				
Angel Hair	2 oz	200	0	0
Artichoke Angel Hair as prep	⅔ cup	200	0	0
Artichoke Spaghetti as prep	⅔ cup	200	0	0
Elbows	2 oz	200	0	0
Fettucini as prep	⅔ cup	200	0	0
Linguini	2 oz	200	0	0
Penne as prep	⅔ cup	200	0	0
Rotelli	2 oz	200	0	0
Shells	2 oz	200	0	0
Spaghetti	2 oz	200	0	0
Ziti	2 oz	200	0	0
Classico				
Gnocchi Di Toscana	1 cup (2 oz)	210	0	1
Creamette				
Elbow Macaroni not prep	2 oz	210	—	1
Linguini Egg	2 oz	221	—	3
Rotelle	2 oz	210	—	1
Rotini Rainbow	2 oz	210	—	1
Spaghetti Egg	2 oz	221	—	3
Spaghetti Thin	2 oz	210	—	1
Spaghetti not prep	2 oz	210	—	1
Spinach Ribbons not prep	2 oz	210	—	1
Ziti	2 oz	210	—	1

FOOD	PORTION	CALS.	SAT. FAT	FAT
Cuore				
Capellini cooked	1⅓ cup (2 oz)	190	0	1
Fusilli cooked	1⅓ cup (2 oz)	190	0	1
Tortiglioni cooked	1⅓ cup (2 oz)	190	0	1
De Bole's				
Whole Wheat Organic Elbows	2 oz	210	0	2
DeCecco				
Whole Wheat Linguine cooked	2 oz	180	0	2
DeFino				
Lasagna No Boil	1 oz	102	—	tr
Ribbons No Boil	2 oz	204	—	2
Delverde				
Spaghetti Whole Wheat	2 oz	206	1	1
Eden				
Elbows Whole Wheat Organic	2 oz	210	0	2
Elbows Whole Wheat Vegetable Organic	2 oz	210	0	2
Kudzu And Sweet Potato Pasta	2 oz	190	0	0
Kudzu Kiri Pasta	2 oz	190	0	0
Mung Bean Pasta Harusame	2 oz	190	0	0
Organic Endless Tubes	½ cup (1.9 oz)	210	0	1
Ribbons Durum Wheat Curry Organic	2 oz	220	0	1
Ribbons Durum Wheat Organic	2 oz	220	0	1
Ribbons Durum Wheat Paella Organic	2 oz	220	0	1
Ribbons Durum Wheat Parsley Garlic Organic	2 oz	220	0	1
Ribbons Durum Wheat Pesto Organic	2 oz	220	0	1
Ribbons Whole Wheat Spinach Organic	2 oz	200	0	2
Rice Pasta Bifun	2 oz	200	0	1
Shells Durum Wheat Vegetable Organic	2 oz	210	0	1
Soba	2 oz	200	0	2
Soba 100% Buckwheat	2 oz	200	0	0
Soba Lotus Root	2 oz	190	0	1
Soba Mugwort	2 oz	190	0	1
Soba Wild Yam Jinenjo	2 oz	190	0	1
Somen	2 oz	200	0	2
Spaghetti Durum Wheat Organic	2 oz	210	0	1
Spaghetti Kamut Organic	2 oz	210	0	2

	PORTION	CALS.	SAT. FAT	FAT
a (CONT.)				
oni Spicy Italian Sausage Bell Pepper	1 cup (3.6 oz)	330	4	10
s Hair	1 cup	160	0	2
Roasted Garlic Tortellini	1 cup	340	4	11
cine	1 cup	200	0	2
heese Raviolo	1 cup	350	9	15
inguine	1 cup	200	0	2
Sausage Ravioli In	1¼ cup	350	6	12
n Bell Pepper Pasta				
Chicken Tortellini In	1 cup	270	3	5
cked Black Pepper Pasta				
heese Ravioli	1 cup	280	4	7
e	1 cup	200	0	2
rella Garlic Tortelloni	1 cup	300	5	8
Tortelloni	1 cup	320	5	8
ello Mushroom Tortelloni	1 cup	310	5	7
ll Pepper Fettuccine	1 cup	200	0	2
h Fettuccine	1 cup	190	0	2
ied Tomato Ravioli	1⅓ cup	380	8	14
heese Tortellini	¾ cup	250	4	7
ne Bell Pepper Basil	2 oz	220	0	2
ne Parsley Garlic	2 oz	220	0	2
e Spinach	2 oz	220	0	2
s Vegetable	2 oz	220	0	2
s Whole Wheat	2 oz	200	0	2
Mixed Vegetable	2 oz	210	0	1
Mixed Vegetable	2 oz	210	0	1
Cracked Pepper Garlic	1 cup (4.3 oz)	340	5	9
se				
CIPE				
egg cooked	2 oz	71	tr	1
w/ egg cooked	2 oz	74	tr	1
DINNERS				
DINNER, PASTA SALAD)				
ee				
1,2,3's In Cheese	7.5 oz	180	tr	1
Sauce				
1,2,3's w/ Mini	7.5 oz	260	4	11
alls				

FOOD	PORTION	CALS.	SAT. FAT	FAT
Eden (CONT.)				
Spaghetti Pasley Garlic Organic	2 oz	210	0	1
Spaghetti Whole Wheat Organic	2 oz	210	0	2
Spirals Durum Wheat Vegetable Organic	2 oz	210	0	1
Spirals Kamut Organic	2 oz	210	0	2
Spirals Sesame Rice Organic	2 oz	200	0	2
Spirals Whole Wheat Vegetable Organic	2 oz	210	0	2
Udon	2 oz	200	0	2
Udon Brown Rice	2 oz	200	0	2
Ensemble				
Elbow	2 oz	190	0	1
Fettucine	2 oz	190	0	1
Gioia				
Pasta	2 oz	210	0	1
Hanover				
Spaghetti Wheels	½ cup	90	—	0
Hodgson Mill				
Spaghetti Whole Wheat Spinach not prep	2 oz	190	1	2
Veggie Bows not prep	2 oz	200	0	1
Veggie Rotini not prep	2 oz	200	0	1
Veggie Wagon Wheels not prep	2 oz	200	0	1
Whole Wheat Spirals not prep	2 oz	190	1	1
La Molisana				
Radiatori	2 oz	230	—	1
Lupini				
Elbow uncooked	½ cup (2 oz)	190	0	2
Spaghetti Light uncooked	½ cup (2 oz)	190	0	2
Spaghetti With Triticale	½ pkg (2 oz)	190	1	3
Luxury				
Pasta	2 oz	210	0	1
Merlino's				
Pasta	2 oz	210	0	1
Noodles By Leonardo				
Capellini	2 oz	200	0	1
Elbows not prep	½ cup (2 oz)	200	0	1
Fettucini	2 oz	200	0	1
Linguine not prep	½ cup (2 oz)	200	0	1
Rigatoni	2 oz	200	0	1
Rotini	2 oz	200	0	1

FOOD	PORTION	CALS.	SAT. FAT	FAT
Noodles By Leonardo (CONT.)				
Shells not prep	½ cup (2 oz)	200	0	1
Spaghetti not prep	½ cup (2 oz)	200	0	1
Spaghettini	2 oz	200	0	1
Vermicelli not prep	½ cup (2 oz)	200	0	1
Penn Dutch				
Pasta	2 oz	210	0	1
Pomi				
Capellini	2 oz	210	—	1
Prince				
Egg	2 oz	221	1	3
Pasta	2 oz	210	0	1
Rainbow	2 oz	210	0	1
Spinach Egg	2 oz	220	—	3
Pritikin				
Spaghetti Whole Wheat	⅓ box (2 oz)	190	0	1
Spiral	⅔ cup (2 oz)	190	0	1
Red Cross				
Pasta	2 oz	210	0	1
Ronco				
Pasta	2 oz	210	0	1
Ronzoni				
Elbows	¾ cup (2 oz)	210	—	1
Fettucini	¾ cup (2 oz)	210	—	1
Fusilli	¾ cup (2 oz)	210	—	1
Lasagne	¾ cup (2 oz)	210	—	1
Manicotti	¾ cup (2 oz)	210	—	1
Mostaccioli	¾ cup (2 oz)	210	—	1
Rigatoni	¾ cup (2 oz)	210	—	1
Rotelle uncooked	¾ cup (2 oz)	210	—	1
Rotini uncooked	¾ cup (2 oz)	210	—	1
Shells uncooked	¾ cup (2 oz)	210	—	1
Shells Jumbo	¾ cup (2 oz)	210	—	1
Spaghetti not prep	¾ cup (2 oz)	210	—	1
Tubettini	¾ cup (2 oz)	210	—	1
San Giorgio				
Bowties Egg	2 oz	210	—	3
Capellini	2 oz	210	—	1
Elbow Macaroni	2 oz	210	—	1
Fettuccine Egg	2 oz	210	—	3
Fettuccini Florentine	2 oz	210	—	3
Lasagne	2 oz	210	—	1
Linguini	2 oz	210	—	1
Mostaccioli Rigati	2 oz	210	—	1

FOOD	PORTION
San Giorgio (CONT.)	
Rigatoni	2 oz
Rotini	2 oz
Shells	2 oz
Spaghetti	2 oz
Spaghetti Thin	2 oz
Vermicelli	2 oz
Ziti Cut	2 oz
Tree Of Life	
Cajun as prep	⅝ cup (4.9 oz)
Confetti as prep	⅝ cup (4.9 oz)
Garlic & Parsley as prep	⅝ cup (4.9 oz)
Jamaican Spice as prep	⅝ cup (4.9 oz)
Lemon Pepper as prep	⅝ cup (4.9 oz)
Spinach as prep	⅝ cup (4.9 oz)
Tex Mex as prep	⅝ cup (4.9 oz)
Thai as prep	⅝ cup (4.9 oz)
Tomato Basil as prep	⅝ cup (4.9 oz)
Vimco	
Pasta	2 oz
FRESH	
cooked	2 oz
spinach cooked	2 oz
Contadina	
Angel's Hair	1¼ cup (2.8 oz)
Fettuccine	1¼ cup (2.9 oz)
Fettuccine Cholesterol Free	1 cup (2.9 oz)
Light Ravioli Cheese	1 cup (3.1 oz)
Light Ravioli Garden Vegetable	1¼ cup (3.8 oz)
Light Tortellini Garlic & Cheese	1 cup (3.6 oz)
Linguine	1¼ cup (3 oz)
Linguine Cholesterol Free	1¼ cup (3.1 oz)
Ravioli Beef And Garlic	1¼ cup (4 oz)
Ravioli Cheese	1 cup (3.1 oz)
Ravioli Chicken And Rosemary	1¼ cup (4 oz)
Tagliatelli Spinach	1¼ cup (3.1 oz)
Tortellini Spianch Three Cheese	¾ cup (3.1 oz)
Tortelloni Cheese	¾ cup (3 oz)
Tortelloni Cheese And Basil	1 cup (4 oz)
Tortelloni Chicken And Prosciutto	1 cup (3.8 oz)
Tortelloni Chicken And Vegetable	¾ cup (2.9 oz)

FOOD
Contadi
Torte
F
Di Giorr
Ange
Beef
Fett
Four
Hert
Italia
G
Lem
C
Ligh
Ling
Mo
Pes
Por
Rec
Spi
Sun
Thr
Herb's
Fett
Fett
Fett
Ribb
Ribb
Roti
Shell
Trios
Ravi
Ch
HOME
made w
plain ma
PASTA
(see a
CANNE
Chef Boy
ABC's
Fla
ABC's
Me

FOOD	PORTION	CALS.	SAT. FAT	FAT
Chef Boyardee (CONT.)				
Beef Ravioli	7.5 oz	190	2	4
Beef Ravioli 99% Fat Free	1 cup (8.6 oz)	210	0	1
Beefaroni	7.5 oz	220	1	7
Cheese Ravioli In Meat Sauce	7.5 oz	200	—	3
Dinosaurs In Cheese Flavor Sauce	7.5 oz	180	tr	1
Dinosaurs w/ Meatballs	7.5 oz	240	3	9
Elbows In Beef Sauce	7.5 oz	210	—	7
Lasagna	7.5 oz	230	—	9
Lasagna In Garden Vegetable Sauce	7.5 oz	170	tr	1
Macaroni & Cheese	7.5 oz	180	tr	5
Pasta Rings & Meatballs	7.5 oz	220	3	8
Rigatoni	7.5 oz	210	—	6
Rings & Franks	7.5 oz	190	2	5
Shells In Meat Sauce	7.5 oz	210	—	6
Shells In Mushroom Sauce	7.5 oz	170	tr	1
Spaghetti & Meat Balls	7.5 oz	230	—	7
Tic Tac Toes In Cheese Flavor Sauce	7.5 oz	170	tr	1
Tic Tac Toes w/ Mini Meatballs	7.5 oz	250	3	10
Turtles In Sauce	7.5 oz	160	—	1
Turtles w/ Meatballs	7.5 oz	210	3	8
Franco-American				
Beef RavioliO's In Meat Sauce	½ can (7½ oz)	250	—	8
CircusO's Pasta In Tomato & Cheese Sauce	½ can (7⅜ oz)	170	—	2
CircusO's Pasta With Meatballs In Tomato Sauce	½ can (7⅜ oz)	210	—	8
Macaroni & Cheese	½ can (7⅜ oz)	170	—	6
Spaghetti In Tomato Sauce w/ Cheese	½ can (7⅜ oz)	180	—	2
Spaghetti w/ Meatballs In Tomato Sauce	½ can (7⅜ oz)	220	—	8
SpaghettiO's With Meatballs	½ can (7⅜ oz)	220	—	9
SpaghettiO's With Sliced Franks	½ can (7⅜ oz)	220	—	9
SpaghettiO's In Tomato & Cheese Sauce	½ can (7⅜ oz)	170	—	2
SportyO's In Tomato & Cheese Sauce	½ can (7½ oz)	170	—	2
SportyO's Pasta With Meatballs In Tomato Sauce	½ can (7⅜ oz)	210	—	8

FOOD	PORTION	CALS.	SAT. FAT	FAT
Franco-American (CONT.)				
TeddyO's In Tomato & Cheese Sauce	½ can (7½ oz)	170	—	2
TeddyO's Pasta With Meatballs	½ can (7⅝ oz)	210	—	8
Hormel				
Spaghetti & Meatballs	1 can (7½ oz)	210	4	7
Kid's Kitchen				
Microwave Meals Cheezy Mac & Beef	1 cup (7½ oz)	260	3	7
Microwave Meals Noodle Rings & Chicken	1 cup (7½ oz)	150	2	4
Microwave Meals Spaghetti Rings & Franks	1 cup (7½ oz)	240	4	9
Progresso				
Beef Ravioli	1 cup (9.1 oz)	260	2	5
Cheese Ravioli	1 cup (9.1 oz)	220	1	2
Van Camp's				
Spaghetti Weenee	1 can (8 oz)	230	2	8
FROZEN				
Amy's Organic				
Macaroni & Cheese	1 pkg (9 oz)	390	8	14
Macaroni & Soy Cheese	1 pkg (9 oz)	360	1	14
Pasta Primavera	1 pkg (9.5 oz)	320	7	12
Ravioli w/ Sauce	1 pkg (9.5 oz)	340	3	12
Tofu Vegetable Lasagna	1 pkg (9.5 oz)	300	1	10
Vegetable Lasagna	1 pkg (9.5 oz)	300	4	10
Whole Meals Cannelloni	1 pkg (9 oz)	260	5	11
Armour				
Classics Chicken Fettucini	1 meal (10 oz)	230	4	8
Banquet				
Family Entree Lasagna w/ Meat Sauce	1 serv (8 oz)	240	3	7
Family Entree Macaroni & Beef	1 serv (8 oz)	230	3	7
Family Entree Macaroni & Cheese	1 serv (8 oz)	300	5	10
Family Entree Noodles & Chicken	1 serv (8 oz)	210	3	9
Family Entree Noodles & Beef	1 serv (7.47 oz)	140	2	4
Birds Eye				
Easy Recipe Meal Starter Cheesy Cheese	1 serv	280	2	8
Easy Recipe Meal Starter Chicken Primavera as prep	1 serv	280	2	8

FOOD	PORTION	CALS.	SAT. FAT	FAT
Birds Eye (CONT.)				
Easy Recipe Meal Starter Chicken Alfredo as prep	1 serv	280	2	8
Pasta Secrets Creamy Peppercorn	2⅓ cups (6.6 oz)	300	6	15
Pasta Secrets Italian Pesto	2⅓ cups (6.4 oz)	240	2	9
Pasta Secrets Primavera	2⅓ cups (6.6 oz)	230	3	10
Pasta Secrets Three Cheese	2 cups (6.1 oz)	230	3	8
Pasta Secrets White Cheddar	2 cups (6.3 oz)	240	3	10
Pasta Secrets Zesty Garlic	2 cups (5.9 oz)	240	3	10
Budget Gourmet				
Cheese Ravioli	1 meal (9.5 oz)	290	6	13
Lasagna Italian Sausage	1 meal (10 oz)	430	—	23
Lasagna Vegetable	1 meal (10.5 oz)	390	5	10
Lasagne Three Cheese	1 meal (10 oz)	390	—	17
Lasagne With Meat Sauce	1 meal (9.4 oz)	290	4	11
Linguini With Shrimp & Clams	1 meal (9.5 oz)	280	5	10
Linguini With Shrimp And Clams	1 meal (10 oz)	270	—	9
Macaroni & Cheese	1 meal (5.75 oz)	230	—	12
Macaroni & Cheese With Cheddar & Parmesan	1 meal (10.5 oz)	330	4	8
Manicotti Cheese	1 meal (10 oz)	440	—	24
Pasta Alfredo With Broccoli	1 meal (5.5 oz)	210	—	10
Penne Pasta With Chunky Tomato Sauce & Italian Sausage	1 meal (10 oz)	320	2	9
Rigatoni In Cream Sauce With Broccoli & Chicken	1 meal (10.8 oz)	290	3	7
Spaghetti With Chunky Tomato & Meat Sauce	1 meal (10 oz)	300	2	8
Tortellini Cheese	1 meal (5.5 oz)	200	—	8
Ziti In Marinara Sauce	1 meal (6.25 oz)	200	—	9
Dining Light				
Cheese Cannelloni	9 oz	310	—	9
Ensemble				
Cheese Ravioli & Marinara Sauce	1 pkg (9.9 oz)	250	3	5
Fettucine Alfredo	1 pkg (9.9 oz)	330	4	9
Fettucine Primavera	1 pkg (9.9 oz)	270	3	7
Four Cheese Lasagna	1 pkg (9.9 oz)	270	2	4
Linguine Marinara	1 pkg (9.9 oz)	290	3	7
Mac 'n Cheese	1 pkg (9.9 oz)	320	3	8

FOOD	PORTION	CALS.	SAT. FAT	FAT
Formagg				
Penne Pasta Alfredo	⅔ cup (5 oz)	190	0	2
Penne Pasta Primavera	⅔ cup (5 oz)	190	0	2
Vegetable Pasta & Caesar Italian Garden	⅔ cup (5 oz)	190	0	2
Green Giant				
Create A Meal Creamy Alfredo as prep	1¼ cups (10 oz)	380	5	12
Create A Meal Creamy Cheddar as prep	1½ cups (10 oz)	290	6	10
Create A Meal Creamy Chicken Noodle as prep	1¼ cups (10 oz)	350	5	11
Pasta Accents Alfredo	2 cups (5.6 oz)	210	3	5
Pasta Accents Creamy Cheddar	2⅓ cups (6.7 oz)	250	3	8
Pasta Accents Florentine	2 cups (7.3 oz)	310	3	9
Pasta Accents Garden Herb Seasoning	2 cups (6.8 oz)	230	4	7
Pasta Accents Garlic Seasoning	2 cups (6.6 oz)	260	5	10
Pasta Accents Primavera	2¼ cups (7 oz)	320	5	12
Pasta Accents White Cheddar Sauce	1¾ cups (5.6 oz)	300	4	12
Healthy Choice				
Beef Macaroni Casserole	1 meal (8.5 oz)	200	1	1
Cheese Ravioli Parmigiana	1 meal (9 oz)	250	2	4
Chicken Broccoli Alfredo	1 meal (12.1 oz)	370	3	8
Chicken Fettucini Alfredo	1 meal (8.5 oz)	250	1	3
Classics Pasta Shells Marinara	1 meal (12 oz)	360	2	3
Classics Turkey Fettuccine Alla Crema	1 meal (12.5 oz)	350	2	4
Fettucini Alfredo	1 meal (8 oz)	240	2	5
Lasagna Roma	1 meal (13.5 oz)	390	2	5
Macaroni & Cheese	1 meal (9 oz)	290	2	5
Spaghetti Bolognese	1 meal (10 oz)	260	1	3
Three Cheese Manicotti	1 meal (11 oz)	310	5	9
Vegetable Pasta Italiano	1 meal (10 oz)	220	0	1
Zucchini Lasagna	1 meal (14 oz)	330	1	2
Kid Cuisine				
Macaroni & Cheese	1 pkg (10.6 oz)	420	5	12
Mini Cheese Ravioli	1 pkg (9.82 oz)	320	2	5
Le Menu				
Entree LightStyle Garden Vegetables Lasagna	10½ oz	260	—	8

FOOD	PORTION	CALS.	SAT. FAT	FAT
Le Menu (CONT.)				
Entree LightStyle Lasagna With Meat Sauce	10 oz	290	—	8
Entree LightStyle Meat Sauce & Cheese Tortellini	8 oz	250	—	8
Entree LightStyle Spaghetti With Beef Sauce And Mushrooms	9 oz	280	—	6
LightStyle 3-Cheese Stuffed Shells	10 oz	280	—	8
LightStyle Cheese Tortellini	10 oz	230	—	6
Manicotto With Three Cheeses	11¾ oz	390	—	15
Lean Cuisine				
Alfredo Pasta Primavera	1 pkg (10 oz)	290	3	7
Angel Hair Pasta	1 pkg (10 oz)	220	1	3
Bow Tie Pasta & Creamy Tomato Sauce	1 pkg (9.5 oz)	260	2	6
Cafe Classics Bow Tie Pasta & Chicken	1 pkg (9.5 oz)	250	1	5
Cafe Classics Cheese Lasagna w/ Chicken Scaloppini	1 pkg (10 oz)	290	2	8
Cheddar Bake With Pasta	1 pkg (9 oz)	220	3	6
Cheese Cannelloni	1 pkg (9.1 oz)	230	2	4
Cheese Lasagna Casserole	1 pkg (10 oz)	270	3	6
Cheese Ravioli	1 pkg (8.5 oz)	270	3	7
Cheese Stuffed Shells	1 serv (8.9 oz)	230	3	5
Chicken Fettucini	1 pkg (9.25 oz)	280	2	6
Chicken Lasagna	1 pkg (10 oz)	270	3	8
Classic Cheese Lasagna	1 pkg (11.5 oz)	270	3	5
Fettucini Alfredo	1 pkg (9 oz)	300	3	7
Fettucini Primavera	1 pkg (10 oz)	270	3	7
Five Cheese Lasagna	1 serv (8 oz)	210	2	4
Lasagne With Meat Sauce	1 pkg (10.5 oz)	290	4	6
Macaroni & Beef	1 pkg (10 oz)	270	2	4
Macaroni & Cheese	1 pkg (10 oz)	290	4	7
Penne Pasta Bolognese	1 pkg (9.5 oz)	270	3	6
Penne Pasta w/ Tomato Basil Sauce	1 pkg (10 oz)	270	1	4
Spaghetti w/ Meat Sauce	1 pkg (11.5 oz)	290	2	5
Spaghetti w/ Meatballs	1 pkg (9.5 oz)	280	2	6
Vegetable Lasagna	1 pkg (10.5 oz)	260	3	7
Life Choice				
Linguini Roma	1 meal (13.2 oz)	230	0	1
Sun Dried Tomato Manicotti	1 meal (11.65 oz)	220	1	3
Vegetable Lasagna Primavera	1 meal (11.2 oz)	170	1	1

FOOD	PORTION	CALS.	SAT. FAT	FAT
Lulgino's				
& Pomodoro Sauc With Meatballs	1 pkg (9 oz)	320	4	11
& Pomodoro Sauce With Meatballs	1 cup (6.3 oz)	270	3	9
Cheese Ravioli & Alfredo With Broccoli Sauce	1 pkg (8.5 oz)	420	13	25
Cheese Tortellini & Alfredo Sauce With Broccoli	1 pkg (8 oz)	390	12	24
Fettuccine Alfredo	1 cup (7.5 oz)	330	4	11
Fettuccine Alfredo	1 pkg (9.4 oz)	390	5	14
Fettuccine Alfredo With Broccoli	1 pkg (9.2 oz)	360	8	16
Fettuccine Carbonara	1 pkg (9 oz)	360	4	13
Lasagna Alfredo	1 pkg (9 oz)	360	6	20
Lasagna Alfredo	1 cup (6.3 oz)	300	5	17
Lasagna Pollo	1 pkg (9 oz)	320	5	14
Lasagna With Meat Sauce	1 pkg (9 oz)	290	4	10
Lasagna With Meat Sauce	1 cup (7.2 oz)	240	3	8
Lasagna With Vegetables	1 pkg (9 oz)	290	3	10
Linguini With Clams & Sauce	1 pkg (9 oz)	270	2	6
Linguini With Red Sauce &	1 pkg (9 oz)	260	1	6
Linguini With Seafood	1 pkg (9 oz)	290	2	8
Macaroni & Cheese	1 pkg (9 oz)	370	6	15
Macaroni & Cheese	1 cup (7.2 oz)	310	7	12
Marinara Sauce Penne Pasta Italian Sausage & Peppers	1 pkg (9 oz)	350	4	17
Marinara Sauce Penne Pasta Italian Sausage & Peppers	1 cup (7.4 oz)	290	3	14
Meat Ravioli & Pomodoro Sauce	1 pkg (8.5 oz)	320	5	13
Minestrone With Penne Pasta	1 cup (6.3 oz)	180	1	6
Penne Pollo	1 pkg (9 oz)	330	5	14
Penne Primavera	1 pkg (9 oz)	350	4	10
Rigatoni Pomodoro Italiano	1 pkg (9 oz)	290	2	8
Shells & Cheese With Jalapenos	1 pkg (8.5 oz)	360	6	15
Spaghetti Bolognese	1 pkg (9 oz)	270	3	8
Spaghetti Marinara	1 pkg (10 oz)	250	1	2
Spinach Ravioli & Primavera Sauce	1 pkg (8.5 oz)	360	8	17
Morton				
Macaroni & Cheese	1 serv (8 oz)	220	3	6

FOOD	PORTION	CALS.	SAT. FAT	FAT
Mrs. Paul's				
Entrees Light Seafood Lasagne	9½ oz	290	—	8
Entrees Light Seafood Rotini	9 oz	240	—	6
Seafood Rotini	9 oz	240	2	6
Palmazone				
Macaroni 'n Cheese	½ pkg (6 oz)	260	—	7
Pasta Favorites				
Chicken Pasta Primavera	1 pkg (10.5 oz)	330	5	13
Fettuccini Alfredo	1 pkg (10.5 oz)	370	8	18
Italian Sausage & Peppers	1 pkg (10.5 oz)	340	4	13
Lasagna	1 pkg (10.5 oz)	290	2	9
Macaroni & Cheese	1 pkg (10.5 oz)	350	4	12
Pasta Primavera	1 pkg (10.5 oz)	320	6	14
Spaghetti w/ Meatballs	1 pkg (10.5 oz)	370	5	16
Vegetable Lasagna	1 pkg (10.5 oz)	260	2	6
White Cheddar & Rotini	1 pkg (10.5 oz)	350	5	12
Senor Felix's				
Lasagna Southwestern	1 serv (6 oz)	160	4	7
Stouffer's				
Cheddar Pasta w/ Beef & Tomatoes	1 pkg (11 oz)	450	10	19
Cheese Manicotti	1 pkg (9 oz)	380	9	17
Cheese Ravioli	1 pkg (10.6 oz)	380	6	13
Chicken Lasagna	1 serv (7.8 oz)	320	5	17
Fettucini Alfredo	1 pkg (10 oz)	520	16	28
Fettucini Primavera	1 pkg (10 oz)	430	12	20
Five Cheese Lasagna	1 pkg (10.75 oz)	360	7	13
Grilled Chicken & Angel Hair Pasta	1 pkg (10.9 oz)	380	4	13
Homestyle Chicken Fettucini	1 pkg (10.5 oz)	390	4	15
Homestyle Chicken Parmigiana w/ Spaghetti	1 pkg (12 oz)	460	4	16
Homestyle Veal Parmigiana w/ Spaghetti	1 pkg (11.9 oz)	430	5	17
Lasagna Bake	1 pkg (10.25 oz)	370	5	12
Lasagna w/ Meat Sauce	1 pkg (10.5 oz)	370	7	14
Macaroni & Cheese	1 cup (6 oz)	320	7	16
Macaroni & Cheese w/ Broccoli	1 pkg (10.5 oz)	360	8	17
Macaroni & Beef	1 pkg (11.5 oz)	420	8	20
Noodles Romanoff	1 pkg (12 oz)	490	6	25
Pasta Shells w/ American Cheese	1 cup (6 oz)	260	4	10
Salisbury Steak w/ Macaroni & Cheese	1 serv (11.3 oz)	410	8	19

FOOD	PORTION	CALS.	SAT. FAT	FAT
Stouffer's (CONT.)				
Spaghetti w/ Meat Sauce	1 pkg (10 oz)	350	4	12
Spaghetti w/ Meatballs	1 pkg (12.6 oz)	440	5	15
Tuna Noodle Casserole	1 pkg (10 oz)	320	4	10
Turkey Tettrazini	1 pkg (10 oz)	360	7	17
Vegetable Lasagna	1 pkg (10.5 oz)	440	8	20
Swanson				
Homestyle Lasagne With Meat Sauce	10½ oz	400	—	15
Homestyle Macaroni & Cheese	10 oz	390	—	19
Homestyle Spaghetti With Italian Style Meatballs	13 oz	490	—	18
Macaroni & Cheese	12¼ oz	370	—	15
Macaroni & Cheese	7 oz	200	—	8
Spaghetti & Meatballs	12½ oz	390	—	17
Tabatchnick				
Macaroni & Cheese	7.5 oz	280	6	12
Ultra Slim-Fast				
Pasta Primavera	12 oz	340	—	9
Spaghetti With Beef & Mushroom Sauce	12 oz	370	—	10
Weight Watchers				
Garden Lasagna	1 pkg (11 oz)	270	4	7
Homestyle Macaroni & Cheese	1 pkg (9 oz)	290	3	7
Smart Ones Angel Hair Pasta	1 pkg (9 oz)	180	0	2
Smart Ones Bowtie Pasta & Mushrooms Marsala	1 pkg (9.65 oz)	270	4	7
Smart Ones Chicken Fettucini	1 pkg (10 oz)	300	2	9
Smart Ones Creamy Rigatoni w/ Broccoli & Chicken	1 pkg (9 oz)	230	1	2
Smart Ones Fettucini Alfredo w/ Broccoli	1 pkg (8.5 oz)	230	4	6
Smart Ones Lasagna Florentine	1 pkg (10 oz)	200	0	2
Smart Ones Lasagna Alfredo	1 pkg (9 oz)	300	4	7
Smart Ones Lasagna w/ Meat Sauce	1 pkg (10.25 oz)	270	4	6
Smart Ones Lasagna w/ Meat Sauce	1 pkg (9 oz)	240	1	2
Smart Ones Macaroni & Cheese	1 pkg (9 oz)	220	1	2
Smart Ones Pasta & Spinach Romano	1 pkg (10.4 oz)	260	3	8
Smart Ones Pasta w/ Tomato Basil Sauce	1 pkg (9.6 oz)	260	3	7
Smart Ones Penne Pasta w/ Sun-Dried Tomatoes	1 pkg (10 oz)	280	5	8

FOOD	PORTION	CALS.	SAT. FAT	FAT
Weight Watchers (CONT.)				
Smart Ones Penne Pollo	1 pkg (10 oz)	290	3	6
Smart Ones Ravioli Florentine	1 pkg (8.5 oz)	220	1	2
Smart Ones Spaghetti Marinara	1 pkg (9 oz)	280	2	7
Smart Ones Spaghetti w/ Meat Sauce	1 pkg (10 oz)	280	2	6
Smart Ones Spicy Penne & Ricotta	1 pkg (10.2 oz)	280	2	6
Smart Ones Tuna Noodle Casserole	1 pkg (9.5 oz)	270	3	7
Smart Ones Zita Mozzarella	1 pkg (9 oz)	290	2	7
HOME RECIPE				
macaroni & cheese	1 cup	430	10	22
spaghetti w/ meatballs & tomato sauce	1 cup	330	4	12
MIX				
Casbah				
Pasta Fasul	1 pkg (1.6 oz)	150	0	1
Hain				
Pasta & Sauce Creamy Parmesan	¼ pkg	150	—	3
Pasta & Sauce Creamy Swiss	¼ pkg	170	—	4
Pasta & Sauce Fettuccine Alfredo	¼ pkg	180	—	4
Pasta & Sauce Italian Herb	¼ pkg	110	—	2
Pasta & Sauce Primavera	¼ pkg	140	—	4
Pasta & Sauce Tangy Cheddar	¼ pkg	180	—	6
Hamburger Helper				
Ravioli as prep	1 cup	280	4	10
Ravioli w/ White Cheese Topping as prep	1 cup	310	4	10
Kraft				
Deluxe Macaroni & Cheese Four Cheese Blend as prep	1 cup (6.2 oz)	320	7	10
Deluxe Macaroni & Cheese Original as prep	1 cup (6.1 oz)	320	6	10
Light Deluxe Macaroni & Cheese as prep	1 cup (6.5 oz)	290	3	5
Macaroni & Cheese All Shapes as prep	1 cup (6.9 oz)	410	5	18
Macaroni & Cheese Original as prep	1 cup (6.9 oz)	410	5	18
Macaroni & Cheese Original as prep light recipe	1 cup (6.4 oz)	290	2	6

FOOD	PORTION	CALS.	SAT. FAT	FAT
Kraft (CONT.)				
Premium Macaroni & Cheese Cheesy Alfredo as prep	1 cup (6.9 oz)	410	5	19
Premium Macaroni & Cheese Mild White Cheddar as prep	1 cup (6.8 oz)	410	4	19
Premium Macaroni & Cheese Thick 'N Creamy as prep	1 cup (7.6 oz)	420	5	19
Premium Macaroni & Cheese Three Cheese as prep	1 cup (6.9 oz)	410	4	18
Spaghetti Classics Mild Italian as prep	1 cup (9.1 oz)	240	1	3
Spaghetti Classics Tangy Italian as prep	1 cup (8.9 oz)	240	1	2
Spaghetti Classics Zesty Cheese as prep	1 cup (8.6 oz)	240	1	2
Spaghetti Classics w/ Meat Sauce as prep	1 cup (8.2 oz)	330	4	10
Lipton				
Pasta & Sauce Angel Hair Chicken Broccoli as prep	1 cup	260	1	8
Pasta & Sauce Angel Hair Parmesan as prep	1 cup	280	3	11
Pasta & Sauce Bow Tie Chicken Primavera as prep	1 cup	290	4	10
Pasta & Sauce Bow Tie Italian Cheese as prep	1 cup	300	5	12
Pasta & Sauce Butter & Herbs as prep	1 cup	270	3	10
Pasta & Sauce Cheddar Broccoli as prep	1 cup	340	4	11
Pasta & Sauce Chicken Herb Parmesan as prep	1 cup	80	2	9
Pasta & Sauce Chicken Stir-Fry as prep	1 cup	270	1	8
Pasta & Sauce Creamy Garlic as prep	1 cup	350	5	13
Pasta & Sauce Creamy Mushroom as prep	1 cup	320	4	11
Pasta & Sauce Garlic & Butter Linguine as prep	1 cup	260	2	9
Pasta & Sauce Mild Cheddar Cheese as prep	1 cup	290	4	10
Pasta & Sauce Roasted Garlic Chicken as prep	1 cup	290	3	10

FOOD	PORTION	CALS.	SAT. FAT	FAT
Lipton (CONT.)				
Pasta & Sauce Roasted Garlic & Olive Oil w/ Tomato as prep	1 cup	270	2	9
Pasta & Sauce Rotini Primavera as prep	1 cup	320	5	12
Pasta & Sauce Savory Herb w/ Garlic as prep	1 cup	280	3	9
Pasta & Sauce Three Cheese Rotini as prep	1 cup	320	5	12
Melting Pot				
Terrazza Black Beans & Penne	1 cup	180	0	1
Terrazza Florentine Red Beans & Fusilli	1 cup	220	0	1
Terrazza Red Lentils & Bow Ties	1 cup	240	1	2
Terrazza Tuscan White Beans & Gemell	1 cup	220	0	1
Nile Spice				
Pasta'n Sauce Mediterranean	1 pkg	210	3	5
Pasta'n Sauce Parmesan	1 pkg	200	2	3
Pasta'n Sauce Primavera	1 pkg	200	3	4
Ultra Slim-Fast				
Macaroni & Cheese	2.3 oz	230	—	3
Uncle Ben				
Country Inn Pasta & Sauce Angel Hair Parmesan	1 serv (2.2 oz)	245	—	5
Country Inn Pasta & Sauce Broccoli & White Cheddar	1 serv (2.2 oz)	240	—	5
Country Inn Pasta & Sauce Butter & Herb	1 serv (2 oz)	230	—	6
Country Inn Pasta & Sauce Creamy Garlic	1 serv (2.4 oz)	261	—	5
Country Inn Pasta & Sauce Fettuccine Alfredo	1 serv (2.2 oz)	310	—	6
Country Inn Pasta & Sauce Herb Linguine	1 serv (2.2 oz)	240	—	3
Country Inn Pasta & Sauce Mushroom Fettuccine	1 serv (2.2 oz)	250	—	6
Country Inn Pasta & Sauce Vegetable Alfredo	1 serv (2.2 oz)	240	—	5
Velveeta				
Rotini & Cheese w/ Broccoli as prep	1 cup (7.2 oz)	400	10	16
Shells & Cheese Bacon as prep	1 cup (6.8 oz)	360	8	14

FOOD	PORTION	CALS.	SAT. FAT	FAT
Velveeta (CONT.)				
Shells & Cheese Original as prep	1 cup (6.6 oz)	360	8	13
Shells & Cheese Salsa as prep	1 cup (7.5 oz)	380	9	14
READY-TO-EAT				
Tyson				
Rosemary Penne	1 pkg (12.5 oz)	330	2	5
SHELF-STABLE				
Chef Boyardee				
Microwave Main Meal Beans & Pasta	10.5 oz	200	tr	1
Microwave Main Meal Beef Ravioli Suprema	10.5 oz	290	—	4
Microwave Main Meal Cheese Ravioli Suprema	10.5 oz	290	—	4
Microwave Main Meal Fettuccine	10.5 oz	290	4	9
Microwave Main Meal Lasagna	10.5 oz	290	—	8
Microwave Main Meal Meat Tortellini	10.5 oz	220	2	4
Microwave Main Meal Noodles w/ Chicken	10.5 oz	170	—	1
Microwave Main Meal Peas & Pasta	10.5 oz	190	tr	2
Microwave Main Meal Spaghetti Suprema	10.5 oz	200	—	7
Microwave Main Meal Zesty Macaroni	10.5 oz	290	—	8
Microwave Main Meal Ziti In Sauce	10.5 oz	210	tr	tr
Hormel				
Microcup Meals Lasagna	1 cup (7.5 oz)	250	7	14
Microcup Meals Macaroni & Cheese	1 cup (7.5 oz)	260	6	11
Microcup Meals Ravioli w/ Tomato Sauce	1 cup (7.5 oz)	220	2	6
Microcup Meals Spaghetti & Meatballs	1 cup (7.5 oz)	220	4	7
Kid's Kitchen				
Microwave Meals Beefy Macaroni	1 cup (7.5 oz)	190	3	6
Microwave Meals Macaroni & Cheese	1 cup (7.5 oz)	260	6	11
Microwave Meals Mini Ravioli	1 cup (7.5 oz)	240	3	7
Microwave Meals Spaghetti & Meatballs	1 cup (7.5 oz)	220	4	7

FOOD	PORTION	CALS.	SAT. FAT	FAT
Kid's Kitchen (CONT.)				
Microwave Meals Spaghetti Ring & Meatballs	1 cup (7.5 oz)	250	3	7
Lunch Bucket				
Beef Ravioli In Tomato Sauce	1 pkg (7.5 oz)	180	2	4
Italian Pasta w/ Chicken	1 pkg (7.5 oz)	130	1	2
Lasagna 'n Meatsauce	1 pkg (7.5 oz)	160	2	3
Light'n Healthy Pasta'n Garden Vegetables	1 pkg (7.5 oz)	150	—	1
Macaroni 'n Beef in Meatsauce	1 pkg (7.5 oz)	180	2	5
Macaroni'n Cheese	1 pkg (7.5 oz)	190	5	7
Pasta'n Chicken	1 pkg (7.5 oz)	150	2	5
Spaghetti'n Meatsauce	1 pkg (7.5 oz)	160	2	3
My Own Meal				
Cheese Tortellini	1 pkg (10 oz)	340	3	10
TAKE-OUT				
macaroni & cheese	1 cup	230	5	10

PASTA MACHINE MIX
Wanda's

FOOD	PORTION	CALS.	SAT. FAT	FAT
Dried Tomato	⅓ cup mix per serv (1.9 oz)	202	0	1
Durum & Semolina	⅓ cup mix per serv (1.9 oz)	199	0	1
Semolina Blend	⅓ cup mix per serv (1.9 oz)	202	0	1
Spinach	⅓ cup mix per serv (1.9 oz)	202	0	1
Whole Wheat & Semolina	⅓ cup mix per serv (1.9 oz)	198	0	1

PASTA SALAD
MIX
Kraft

FOOD	PORTION	CALS.	SAT. FAT	FAT
Herb & Garlic as prep	¾ cup (4.9 oz)	280	2	14
Pasta Salad Classic Ranch w/ Bacon as prep	¾ cup (4.7 oz)	350	4	22
Pasta Salad Creamy Ceasar as prep	¾ cup (4.8 oz)	340	4	21
Pasta Salad Garden Primavera as prep	¾ cup (5 oz)	240	2	8
Pasta Salad Italian 97% Fat Free as prep	¾ cup (4.9 oz)	190	1	2
Pasta Salad Parmesan Peppercorn as prep	¾ cup (4.9 oz)	360	4	23

FOOD	PORTION	CALS.	SAT. FAT	FAT
Suddenly Salad				
Classic Pasta	¾ cup	250	1	8
Classic Pasta Reduced Fat Recipe	¾ cup	210	1	4
Garden Italian 98% Fat Free	¾ cup	140	0	1
TAKE-OUT				
elbow macaroni salad	3.5 oz	160	2	5
italian style pasta salad	3.5 oz	140	1	7
mustard macaroni salad	3.5 oz	190	1	10
pasta salad w/ vegetables	3.5 oz	140	3	4

PASTRY

(see BROWNIE, CAKE, DANISH PASTRY)

PATE

FOOD	PORTION	CALS.	SAT. FAT	FAT
antipasto pate	1 can (2.25 oz)	110	2	9
chicken liver canned	1 tbsp (13 g)	109	—	2
chicken liver canned	1 oz	238	—	4
duck pate	1 oz	96	—	8
fish pate	1 oz	76	—	7
goose liver smoked canned	1 oz	131	—	12
goose liver smoked canned	1 tbsp (13 g)	60	—	6
liver canned	1 oz	90	—	8
liver canned	1 tbsp (13 g)	41	—	4
mushroom anchovy pate	1 can (2.25 oz)	130	2	11
pate foie gras	1 oz	127	3	13
pork pate	1 oz	107	4	10
pork pate en croute	1 oz	91	3	7
rabbit pate	1 oz	66	3	5
salmon pate	1 can (2.25 oz)	140	2	10
shrimp	1 can (2.25 oz)	140	2	10
smoked turkey	1 can (2.25 oz)	170	3	13
Sells				
Liver	2.08 oz	190	—	16

PEACH
CANNED

FOOD	PORTION	CALS.	SAT. FAT	FAT
halves in heavy syrup	1 half	60	tr	tr
halves in light syrup	1 half	44	tr	tr
halves juice pack	1 half	34	tr	tr
halves water pack	1 half	18	tr	tr
spiced in heavy syrup	1 cup	180	tr	tr
spiced in heavy syrup	1 fruit	66	tr	tr
Del Monte				
Halves Cling In Heavy Syrup	½ cup (4.5 oz)	100	0	0
Halves Cling Lite	½ cup (4.4 oz)	60	0	0

FOOD	PORTION	CALS.	SAT. FAT	FAT
Del Monte (CONT.)				
Halves Cling Melba In Heavy Syrup	½ cup (4.5 oz)	100	0	0
Halves Freestone In Heavy Syrup	½ cup (4.5 oz)	100	0	0
Sliced Cling Fruit Naturals	½ cup (4.4 oz)	60	0	0
Sliced Cling In Heavy Syrup	½ cup (4.5 oz)	100	0	0
Sliced Cling Lite	½ cup (4.4 oz)	60	0	0
Sliced Freestone In Heavy Syrup	½ cup (4.5 oz)	100	0	0
Sliced Freestone Lite	½ cup (4.4 oz)	60	0	0
Snack Cups Diced Fruit Naturals	1 serv (4.5 oz)	60	0	0
Snack Cups Diced Fruit Naturals EZ-Open Lid	1 serv (4.2 oz)	60	0	0
Snack Cups Diced In Heavy Syrup	1 serv (4.5 oz)	100	0	0
Snack Cups Diced In Heavy Syrup EZ-Open Lid	1 serv (4.2 oz)	90	0	0
Snack Cups Diced Lite	1 serv (4.5 oz)	60	0	0
Snack Cups Diced Lite EZ-Open Lid	1 serv (4.2 oz)	60	0	0
Whole Cling In Heavy Syrup	½ cup (4.2 oz)	100	0	0
Hunt's				
Halves	½ cup (4.5 oz)	100	0	0
Slices	½ cup (4.5 oz)	100	0	0
Libby				
Halves Yellow Cling Lite	½ cup (4.4 oz)	60	0	0
Sliced Yellow Cling Lite	½ cup (4.4 oz)	60	0	0
DRIED				
halves	10	311	tr	1
halves cooked w/ sugar	½ cup	139	tr	tr
halves cooked w/o sugar	½ cup	99	tr	tr
Del Monte				
Sun Dried	⅓ cup (1.4 oz)	90	0	0
Mariani				
Peaches	¼ cup	140	—	0
Sonoma				
Pieces	3-5 pieces (1.4 oz)	120	0	0
FRESH				
peach	1	37	tr	tr
sliced	1 cup	73	tr	tr
Dole				
Peach	2	70		0

FOOD	PORTION	CALS.	SAT. FAT	FAT
FROZEN				
slices sweetened	1 cup	235	tr	tr
Big Valley				
Freestone	⅔ cup (4.9 oz)	50	0	0
PEACH JUICE				
nectar	1 cup	134	tr	tr
Goya				
Nectar	6 oz	110	—	0
Kern's				
Nectar	6 fl oz	110	0	0
Libby				
Nectar	1 can (11.5 fl oz)	210	0	0
Mott's				
Fruit Basket Orchard Peach Juice Cocktail as prep	8 fl oz	130	0	0
Nantucket Nectars				
The Original	8 oz	120	0	0
Snapple				
Dixie Peach	10 fl oz	140	0	0
PEANUT BUTTER				
chunky	1 cup	1520	25	129
chunky	2 tbsp	188	3	16
smooth	2 tbsp	188	3	16
smooth	1 cup	1517	25	128
Arrowhead				
Creamy	2 tbsp (1.1 oz)	200	3	15
Crunchy	2 tbsp (1.1 oz)	200	3	15
BAMA				
Creamy	2 tbsp	200	—	17
Crunchy	2 tbsp	200	—	17
Jelly & Peanut Butter	2 tbsp	150	—	7
Crazy Richard's				
Natural Creamy	2 tbsp (1.1 oz)	190	2	16
Estee				
Creamy Low Sodium	2 tbsp (1 oz)	190	3	15
Hollywood				
Creamy	1 tbsp	35	0	3
Crunchy	1 tbsp	35	0	3
Unsalted	1 tbsp	35	0	3
Jif				
Creamy	2 tbsp (1.1 oz)	190	3	16
Extra Crunchy	2 tbsp (1.1 oz)	190	3	16
Reduced Fat	2 tbsp (1.3 oz)	190	3	12

FOOD	PORTION	CALS.	SAT. FAT	FAT
Jif (CONT.)				
Simply Creamy	2 tbsp (1.1 oz)	190	3	16
Simply Extra Crunchy	2 tbsp (1.1 oz)	190	3	16
Peter Pan				
Creamy	2 tbsp	190	2	16
Creamy Salt Free	2 tbsp	190	2	17
Crunchy	2 tbsp	190	2	16
Crunchy Salt Free	2 tbsp	190	2	17
Red Wing				
Creamy	2 tbsp (1.1 oz)	200	3	16
Crunchy	2 tbsp (1.1 oz)	200	3	16
Reese's				
Peanut Butter Chips	1 tbsp (0.5 oz)	80	4	4
Skippy				
Reduced Fat Creamy	2 tbsp	190	3	12
Tree Of Life				
Creamy	2 tbsp (1 oz)	190	4	15
Creamy No Salt	2 tbsp (1 oz)	190	4	15
Creamy Organic	2 tbsp (1 oz)	190	4	16
Creamy Organic No Salt	2 tbsp (1 oz)	190	4	16
Crunchy	2 tbsp (1 oz)	190	4	15
Crunchy No Salt	2 tbsp (1 oz)	190	4	15
Crunchy Organic	2 tbsp (1 oz)	190	4	16
Crunchy Organic No Salt	2 tbsp (1 oz)	190	4	16
Peanut Wonder 78% Less Fat	2 tbsp (1 oz)	100	1	4
PEANUTS				
chocolate coated	10 (1.4 oz)	208	6	13
chocolate coated	1 cup (5.2 oz)	773	22	50
cooked	½ cup	102	1	7
virginia oil roasted	1 oz	161	2	14
virginia oil roasted	1 cup	826	9	70
Beer Nuts				
Peanuts	1 pkg (1 oz)	180	—	14
Estee				
Candy Coated	¼ cup	200	4	9
Fisher				
Party Peanuts	1 oz	160	—	14
Salted-In-Shell shelled	1 oz	170	2	14
Spanish Roasted	1 oz	180	3	16
Frito Lay				
Honey Roasted	1 serv (1.5 oz)	270	4	21
Hot	1 serv (1.1 oz)	190	3	16
Salted	1 oz	200	4	16

FOOD	PORTION	CALS.	SAT. FAT	FAT
Guy's				
Dry Roasted	1 oz	170	—	14
Spanish Salted	1 oz	170	—	14
Lance				
Honey Toasted	1 pkg (1⅜ oz)	220	3	15
Roasted	1 pkg (1¼ oz)	190	3	14
Salted	1 pkg (1⅛ oz)	200	3	15
Salted Long Tube	¼ cup (1 oz)	180	3	14
Little Debbie				
Salted	¼ cup (1 oz)	160	2	14
Pennant				
Oil Roasted	1 oz	170	2	14
Planters				
Cocktail Lightly Salted Oil Roasted	1 oz	170	2	15
Cocktail Oil Roasted	1 oz	170	2	14
Cocktail Unsalted Oil Roasted	1 oz	170	2	14
Dry Roasted	1 oz	160	2	13
Fun Size! Oil Roasted	2 pkg (1 oz)	170	2	15
Heat Hot Spicy Oil Roasted	1 pkg (1.7 oz)	290	4	25
Heat Hot Spicy Oil Roasted	1 oz	160	2	14
Heat Hot Spicy Oil Roasted	1 pkg (2 oz)	330	4	29
Heat Mild Spicy Oil Roasted	1 oz	160	2	14
Honey Roasted	1 oz	160	2	13
Honey Roasted Dry Roasted	1 pkg (1.7 oz)	260	3	19
Lightly Salted Dry Roasted	1 oz	160	2	14
Lightly Salted Dry Roasted	1 pkg (1.75 oz)	290	3	25
Lightly Salted Oil Roasted	1 pkg (1.8 oz)	300	4	27
Munch'N Go Singles Heat Hot Spicy Oil Roasted	1 pkg (2.5 oz)	410	5	36
Reduced Fat Honey Roasted	⅓ cup (1 oz)	130	1	7
Salted Oil Roasted	1 pkg (1 oz)	170	2	15
Spanish Oil Roasted	1 oz	170	3	14
Spanish Raw	1 oz	150	3	13
Sweet N Crunchy	1 oz	140	1	7
Unsalted Dry Roasted	1 oz	160	2	14
Weight Watchers				
Honey Roasted	1 pkg (0.7 oz)	100	1	5

PEAR
CANNED

FOOD	PORTION	CALS.	SAT. FAT	FAT
halves in heavy syrup	1 cup	188	tr	tr
halves in heavy syrup	1 half	68	tr	tr
halves in light syrup	1 half	45	tr	tr

FOOD	PORTION	CALS.	SAT. FAT	FAT
halves juice pack	1 cup	123	tr	tr
halves water pack	1 half	22	tr	tr
Del Monte				
Halves Fruit Naturals	½ cup (4.4 oz)	60	0	0
Halves In Heavy Syrup	½ cup (4.5 oz)	100	0	0
Halves Lite	½ cup (4.4 oz)	60	0	0
Sliced In Heavy Syrup	½ cup (4.5 oz)	100	0	0
Sliced Lite	½ cup (4.4 oz)	60	0	0
Snack Cups Diced In Heavy Syrup	1 serv (4.5 oz)	100	0	0
Snack Cups Diced In Heavy Syrup EZ-Open Lid	1 serv (4.2 oz)	90	0	0
Snack Cups Diced Lite	1 serv (4.5 oz)	60	0	0
Snack Cups Diced Lite EZ-Open Lid	1 serv (4.2 oz)	60	0	0
Libby				
Halves Lite	½ cup (4.3 oz)	60	0	0
Sliced Lite	½ cup (4.3 oz)	60	0	0
DRIED				
halves	10	459	tr	1
halves	1 cup	472	tr	1
halves cooked w/ sugar	½ cup	196	tr	tr
halves cooked w/o sugar	½ cup	163	tr	tr
Mariani				
Pears	¼ cup	150	—	0
Sonoma				
Pieces	3-4 pieces (1.4 oz)	120	0	0
FRESH				
asian	1 (4.3 oz)	51	tr	tr
pear	1	98	tr	1
Dole				
Pear	1	100	—	1
PEAR JUICE				
nectar	1 cup	149	tr	tr
Goya				
Nectar	6 oz	120	—	0
Kern's				
Nectar	6 fl oz	120	0	0
Libby				
Nectar	1 can (11.5 fl oz)	220	0	0
PEAS				
CANNED				
green	½ cup	59	tr	tr

FOOD	PORTION	CALS.	SAT. FAT	FAT
Allen				
Crowder	½ cup (4.5 oz)	110	1	1
Purple Hull	½ cup (4.4 oz)	120	1	1
Crest Top				
Early June	½ cup (4.5 oz)	100	0	1
Del Monte				
Sweet	½ cup (4.4 oz)	60	0	0
Sweet 50% Less Salt	½ cup (4.4 oz)	60	0	0
Sweet No Salt Added	½ cup (4.4 oz)	60	0	0
Sweet Very Young	½ cup (4.4 oz)	60	0	0
East Texas Fair				
Cream Peas	½ cup (4.4 oz)	120	1	1
Crowder	½ cup (4.5 oz)	110	1	1
Lady Peas With Snaps	½ cup (4.3 oz)	100	1	1
Peas 'n Pork	½ cup (4.5 oz)	110	1	2
Pepper Peas	½ cup (4.5 oz)	120	1	1
Purple Hull	½ cup (4.4 oz)	120	1	1
White Acre	½ cup (4.3 oz)	100	1	1
Green Giant				
Sweet	½ cup (4.3 oz)	60	0	0
Sweet 50% Less Sodium	½ cup (4.3 oz)	60	0	0
Homefolks				
Crowder	½ cup (4.5 oz)	110	1	1
Purple Hull	½ cup (4.4 oz)	120	1	1
LeSueur				
Early Peas	½ cup (4.2 oz)	60	0	0
Early Peas 50% Less Sodium	½ cup (4.2 oz)	60	0	0
Sweet	½ cup (4.2 oz)	60	0	0
Sweet 50% Less Sodium	½ cup (4.2 oz)	60	0	0
Owatonna				
Early June or Sweet	½ cup	70	—	0
Seneca				
Natural Pack	½ cup	60	0	0
Peas	½ cup	50	0	0
Sunshine				
Field Peas	½ cup (4.4 oz)	120	1	1
Lady Peas	½ cup (4.3 oz)	100	1	1
Trappey				
Field Peas With Bacon	½ cup (4.5 oz)	90	1	1
Field Peas With Snaps And Bacon	½ cup (4.5 oz)	110	1	1
DRIED				
split cooked	1 cup	231	tr	1
Bascom's				
Yellow Split as prep	½ cup	110	0	0

FOOD	PORTION	CALS.	SAT. FAT	FAT
Hurst				
HamBeens Green Split Peas w/ Ham	1 serv	120	0	1
FRESH				
green cooked	½ cup	67	tr	tr
green raw	½ cup	58	tr	tr
snap peas cooked	½ cup	34	tr	tr
snap peas raw	½ cup	30	tr	tr
Dole				
Sugar Peas	½ cup	30	—	tr
FROZEN				
green cooked	½ cup	63	tr	tr
snap peas cooked	½ cup	42	tr	tr
snap peas cooked	1 pkg (10 oz)	132	tr	1
Birds Eye				
Baby Pea Blend	¾ cup (2.6 oz)	40	0	0
Baby Sweet	⅔ cup (3.1 oz)	70	0	1
Field Peas w/ Snaps	⅔ cup (3.4 oz)	130	0	1
Purple Hull Peas	½ cup (2.8 oz)	110	0	1
Chun King				
Snow Pea Pods	½ pkg (3 oz)	35	0	2
Fresh Like				
Green	3.5 oz	85	—	1
Tiny Green	3.5 oz	63	—	tr
Green Giant				
Butter Sauce	¾ cup (4 oz)	100	2	2
Butter Sauce LeSueur Baby Peas	¾ cup (4 oz)	100	2	2
Harvest Fresh LeSueur Baby	⅔ cup (3.2 oz)	70	0	0
Harvest Fresh Sugar Snap	⅔ cup (3.2 oz)	50	0	0
Harvest Fresh Sweet	⅔ cup (3.3 oz)	60	0	0
LaSueur Baby Sweet	⅔ cup (2.8 oz)	60	0	0
LaSueur Early June	⅔ cup (2.8 oz)	80	0	0
LaSueur Early June w/ Mushrooms	¾ cup (3 oz)	60	0	0
Select Sugar Snap	¾ cup (2.8 oz)	35	0	0
Sweet	⅔ cup (3.1 oz)	70	0	0
Hanover				
Petite	½ cup	70	—	0
Snow Peas	½ cup	35	—	0
Sweet	½ cup	70	—	0
Tree Of Life				
Peas	⅔ cup (3.1 oz)	70	0	0

FOOD	PORTION	CALS.	SAT. FAT	FAT
PECANS				
dry roasted	1 oz	187	1	18
dry roasted salted	1 oz	187	1	18
oil roasted	1 oz	195	2	20
oil roasted salted	1 oz	195	2	20
Planters				
Chips	1 pkg (2 oz)	390	3	40
Gold Measure Halves	1 pkg (2 oz)	390	3	40
Halves	1 oz	190	2	20
Honey Roasted	1 oz	180	2	16
Pieces	1 oz	190	2	20
Pieces	1 pkg (2 oz)	390	3	40
PECTIN				
powder	1 pkg (1.75 oz)	163	—	tr
powder	¼ pkg (0.4 oz)	39	0	0
Slim Set				
Packet	1 pkg	208	0	0
Powder	1 tbsp	3	0	0
Sure Jell				
For Lower Sugar Recipes	¼ tsp (0.7 g)	5	0	0
Pectin	¼ tsp (0.9 g)	5	0	0
PEPEAO				
pepeao dried	½ cup	36	—	tr
pepeao raw sliced	1 cup	25	—	tr
PEPPER				
black	1 tsp	5	tr	tr
cayenne	1 tsp	6	tr	tr
red	1 tsp	6	tr	tr
white	1 tsp	7	—	tr
Ac'cent				
Lemon	½ tsp	0	0	0
Seasoned	½ tsp	0	0	0
Lawry's				
Lemon	1 tsp	6	—	tr
Watkins				
Black	¼ tbsp (0.5 g)	0	0	0
Cajun	¼ tbsp (0.5 g)	0	0	0
Cracked Black	¼ tbsp (0.5 g)	0	0	0
Dijon	¼ tbsp (0.5 g)	0	0	0
Garlic Peppercorn Blend	¼ tbsp (1 g)	0	0	0
Herb	¼ tbsp (0.5 g)	0	0	0
Italian	¼ tbsp (0.5 g)	0	0	0
Lemon	¼ tbsp (1 g)	0	0	0

FOOD	PORTION	CALS.	SAT. FAT	FAT
Watkins (CONT.)				
Mexican	¼ tbsp (0.5 g)	0	0	0
Red Pepper Flakes	¼ tsp (0.5 oz)	0	0	0
Royal Pepper Blend	¼ tbsp (0.5 g)	0	0	0
PEPPERS				
CANNED				
chili green	1 cup (5.5 oz)	29	tr	tr
chili green hot chopped	½ cup	17	tr	tr
chili red hot	1 (2.6 oz)	18	tr	tr
chili red hot chopped	½ cup	17	tr	tr
green halves	½ cup	13	tr	tr
jalapeno chopped	½ cup	17	tr	tr
red halves	½ cup	13	tr	tr
Chi-Chi's				
Chilies Diced Green	2 tbsp (1.2 oz)	10	0	0
Chilies Green Whole	¾ pepper (1 oz)	10	0	0
Del Monte				
Chilpotle In Spice Sauce	2 tbsp (1.1 oz)	20	0	1
Hot Chili	4 (1 oz)	10	0	0
Jalapeno Nacho Pickled Sliced	2 tbsp (1 oz)	5	0	0
Jalapeno Pickled Sliced	2 tbsp (1.1 oz)	5	0	0
Jalapeno Pickled Whole	2 tbsp (1.1 oz)	5	0	0
Jalapeno Whole	1 (0.7 oz)	3	0	0
Hebrew National				
Filet	¼ pepper (1 oz)	9	0	0
Hot Cherry	⅓ pepper (1 oz)	11	0	0
Red Filet	¼ pepper (1 oz)	9	0	0
McIlhenny				
Jalapeno Nacho Slices	12 slices (1.1 oz)	7	tr	tr
Old El Paso				
Green Chilies Chopped	2 tbsp (1 oz)	5	0	0
Green Chilies Whole	1 (1.2 oz)	10	0	0
Jalapenos Peeled	3 (1 oz)	10	0	0
Jalapenos Pickled	2 (0.9 oz)	5	0	0
Jalapenos Slices	2 tbsp (1.1 oz)	15	0	0
Progresso				
Cherry (drained)	2 tbsp (0.9 oz)	30	0	2
Fried (drained)	2 tbsp (0.9 oz)	60	1	5
Hot Cherry	1 (1 oz)	15	0	0
Pepper Salad (drained)	2 tbsp (0.9 oz)	25	0	2
Roasted	½ piece (1 oz)	10	0	0
Tuscan (drained)	3 (1 oz)	10	0	0
Rosoff's				
Sweet	¼ pepper (1 oz)	9	0	0

FOOD	PORTION	CALS.	SAT. FAT	FAT
Schorr's				
Filet Peppers	1 oz	9	0	0
Trappey				
Banana Mild	3 peppers (1 oz)	6	tr	tr
Banana Sliced Rings	21 slices (1 oz)	6	tr	tr
Cherry Hot	2 peppers (1 oz)	7	tr	tr
Cherry Mild	2 peppers (1 oz)	10	tr	tr
Dulcito Italian Pepperoncini	4 peppers (1 oz)	8	tr	tr
In Vinegar Hot	15 peppers (1 oz)	9	tr	tr
Jalapeno Hot Sliced	21 slices (1 oz)	4	tr	tr
Jalapeno Whole	2 peppers (1 oz)	11	tr	0
Serano	7 peppers (1 oz)	7	tr	tr
Tempero Golden Greek Pepperoncini	4 peppers (1 oz)	7	tr	tr
Torrido Santa Fe Grande	3 peppers (1 oz)	10	tr	tr
Vlasic				
Hot Banana Pepper Rings	1 oz	4	0	0
Hot Cherry	1 oz	10	0	0
Jalapeno Mexican Hot	1 oz	8	0	0
Mexican Tiny Hot	1 oz	6	0	0
Mild Cherry	1 oz	8	0	0
Mild Greek Pepperoncini Salad Peppers	1 oz	4	0	0
DRIED				
ancho	1 (0.6 oz)	48	tr	1
green	1 tbsp	1	tr	tr
pasilla	1 (7 g)	24	—	1
red	1 tbsp	1	tr	tr
FRESH				
banana raw	1 cup (4.4 oz)	33	tr	1
banana raw	1 (4 in) (1.2 oz)	9	tr	tr
chili green hot raw	1	18	tr	tr
chili green hot raw chopped	½ cup	30	tr	tr
chili red hot raw	1 (1.6 oz)	18	tr	tr
chili red raw chopped	½ cup	30	tr	tr
green chopped cooked	½ cup	19	tr	tr
green cooked	1 (2.6 oz)	20	tr	tr
green raw	1 (2.6 oz)	20	tr	tr
green raw chopped	½ cup	13	tr	tr
hungarian raw	1 (0.9 oz)	8	tr	tr
jalapeno raw	1 (0.5 oz)	4	tr	tr
jalapeno raw sliced	1 cup (3.2 oz)	27	tr	1
red chopped cooked	½ cup	19	tr	tr
red cooked	1 (2.6 oz)	20	tr	tr
red raw	1 (2.6 oz)	20	tr	tr

FOOD	PORTION	CALS.	SAT. FAT	FAT
red raw chopped	½ cup	13	tr	tr
serrano raw	1 (6 g)	2	0	tr
serrano raw chopped	1 cup (3.7 oz)	34	tr	tr
yellow raw	1 (6.5 oz)	50	—	tr
yellow raw	10 strips	14	—	tr
Dole				
Medium	1	25	—	1
FROZEN				
green chopped not prep	1 oz	6	tr	tr
red chopped	1 oz	6	tr	tr
Birds Eye				
Diced Green	¾ cup (2.9 oz)	20	0	0
Southland				
Green Diced	2 oz	10	—	0
Sweet Red & Green Cut	2 oz	15	—	0

PERCH
FRESH

FOOD	PORTION	CALS.	SAT. FAT	FAT
cooked	3 oz	99	tr	1
cooked	1 fillet (1.6 oz)	54	tr	1
ocean perch atlantic cooked	3 oz	103	tr	2
ocean perch atlantic cooked	1 fillet (1.8 oz)	60	tr	1
ocean perch atlantic raw	3 oz	80	tr	1
raw	3 oz	77	tr	1
FROZEN				
Gorton's				
Fishmarket Fresh Ocean Perch	5 oz	140	—	3
Van De Kamp's				
Battered Fillets	2 (4 oz)	300	3	20

PERSIMMONS

FOOD	PORTION	CALS.	SAT. FAT	FAT
dried japanese	1	93	—	tr
fresh	1	32	—	tr
fresh japanese	1	118	—	tr
Sonoma				
Dried	6-8 pieces (1.4 oz)	140	0	0

PHEASANT

FOOD	PORTION	CALS.	SAT. FAT	FAT
breast w/o skin raw	½ breast (6.4 oz)	243	2	6
leg w/o skin raw	1 (3.6 oz)	143	2	5
roasted	3.5 oz	215	3	9
w/ skin raw	½ pheasant (14 oz)	723	11	37
w/o skin raw	½ pheasant (12.4 oz)	470	4	13

PHYLLO DOUGH

FOOD	PORTION	CALS.	SAT. FAT	FAT
phyllo dough	1 oz	85	tr	2
sheet	1	57	tr	1

FOOD	PORTION	CALS.	SAT. FAT	FAT
Ekizian				
Sheets	½ lb	865	7	17
PICANTE				
(see SALSA)				
PICKLES				
dill	1 (2.3 oz)	12	tr	tr
quick sour	1 (1.2 oz)	4	tr	tr
sweet	1 (1.2 oz)	41	tr	tr
sweet gherkin	1 sm (½ oz)	20	tr	tr
Claussen				
Bread 'N Butter Slices	1 slice	7	—	tr
Dill Spears	1 spear	4	—	tr
Kosher Halves	1 half	9	—	tr
Kosher Slices	1 slice	1	—	tr
Kosher Whole	1	9	—	tr
No Garlic Dills	1	17	—	tr
Del Monte				
Dill Halves	¼ pickle (1 oz)	5	0	0
Dill Hamburger Chips	5 pieces (1 oz)	5	0	0
Dill Sweet Chips	5 pieces (1 oz)	40	0	0
Dill Sweet Gherkin	2 pickles (1 oz)	40	0	0
Dill Sweet Midgets	3 pickles (1 oz)	40	0	0
Dill Sweet Whole	2 pickles (1 oz)	40	0	0
Dill Tiny Kosher	1½ pickle (1 oz)	5	0	0
Dill Whole Pickles	1½ pickle (1 oz)	5	0	0
Hebrew National				
Half Sour	½ pickle (1 oz)	4	0	0
Kosher	⅓ pickle (1 oz)	4	0	0
Kosher Barrel Cured Dill	1 pkg	23	0	0
Kosher Barrel Cured Hot Dill	1 pkg	23	0	0
Kosher Chips	3 slices (1 oz)	4	0	0
Kosher Halves	⅓ pickle (1 oz)	4	0	0
Kosher Large	⅕ pickle (1 oz)	4	0	0
Kosher Spears	½ spear (1 oz)	4	0	0
Sour Garlic	⅓ pickle (1 oz)	3	0	0
McIlhenny				
Hot N' Sweet	4 (1 oz)	42	tr	tr
Rosoff's				
Half Sour	⅓ pickle (1 oz)	4	0	0
Half Sour Spears	½ spear (1 oz)	4	0	0
Kosher	⅓ pickle (1 oz)	4	0	0
Kosher Halves	⅓ pickle (1 oz)	4	0	0

FOOD	PORTION	CALS.	SAT. FAT	FAT
Schorr's				
Garlic	⅓ pickle (1 oz)	3	0	0
Half Sour	½ spear (1 oz)	4	0	0
Half Sour	⅓ pickle (1 oz)	4	0	0
Kosher Deli	½ pickle (1 oz)	4	0	0
Kosher Halves	⅓ pickle (1 oz)	4	0	0
Kosher Spears	½ spear (1 oz)	4	0	0
Kosher Whole	⅓ pickle (1 oz)	4	0	0
Vlasic				
Bread & Butter Chips	1 oz	30	0	0
Bread & Butter Chunks	1 oz	25	0	0
Bread & Butter Stixs	1 oz	18	0	0
Deli Bread & Butter	1 oz	25	0	0
Deli Dill Halves	1 oz	4	0	0
Half-The-Salt Hamburger Dill Chips	1 oz	2	0	0
Half-The-Salt Kosher Crunchy Dills	1 oz	4	0	0
Half-The-Salt Kosher Dill Spears	1 oz	4	0	0
Half-The-Salt Sweet Butter Chips	1 oz	30	0	0
Hot & Spicy Garden Mix	1 oz	4	0	0
Kosher Baby Dills	1 oz	4	0	0
Kosher Crunchy Dills	1 oz	4	0	0
Kosher Dill Gherkins	1 oz	4	0	0
Kosher Dill Spears	1 oz	4	0	0
Kosher Snack Chunks	1 oz	4	0	0
No Garlic Dill Spears	1 oz	4	0	0
Original Dills	1 oz	2	0	0
Polish Snack Chunk Dills	1 oz	4	0	0
Zesty Crunchy Dills	1 oz	4	0	0
Zesty Dill Snack Chunks	1 oz	4	0	0
Zesty Dill Spears	1 oz	4	0	0
PIE				
(see also PIE CRUST)				
FILLING				
apple	⅙ can (2.6 oz)	74	tr	tr
apple	1 can (21 oz)	599	tr	1
cherry	⅙ can (2.6 oz)	85	tr	tr
cherry	1 can (21 oz)	683	tr	1
pumpkin pie mix	1 cup	282	tr	tr
Comstock				
MoreFruit Light Cherry	⅓ cup (2.9 oz)	60	0	0

FOOD	PORTION	CALS.	SAT. FAT	FAT
Libby				
Pumpkin Pie Mix	½ cup	100	—	0
None Such				
Mincemeat Condensed	¼ pkg	220	—	2
Mincemeat Ready-to-Use	⅓ cup	200	—	1
Mincemeat Ready-to-Use With Brandy & Rum	⅓ cup	220	—	2
FROZEN				
apple	⅛ of 9 in pie (4.4 oz)	297	3	14
blueberry	⅛ of 9 in pie (4.4 oz)	289	2	13
cherry	⅛ of 9 in pie (4.4 oz)	325	3	14
chocolate creme	⅙ of 8 in pie (4 oz)	344	6	22
coconut creme	⅙ of 7 in pie (2.2 oz)	191	5	11
lemon meringue	⅙ of 8 in pie (4.5 oz)	303	2	10
peach	⅙ of 8 in pie (4.1 oz)	261	2	12
Amy's Organic				
Apple	1 serv (8 oz)	280	—	12
Banquet				
Apple	⅕ pie (4 oz)	300	6	13
Banana Cream	⅓ pie (4.7 oz)	350	5	21
Cherry	⅕ pie (4 oz)	290	6	14
Chocolate Cream	⅓ pie (4.7 oz)	360	5	20
Coconut Cream	⅓ pie (4.7 oz)	350	6	20
Lemon Cream	⅓ pie (4.7 oz)	360	5	20
Mincemeat	⅕ pie (4 oz)	310	6	13
Peach	⅕ pie (4 oz)	260	5	12
Pumpkin	⅙ pie (4 oz)	250	3	8
Kineret				
Apple Homestyle	⅙ pie (4 oz)	313	4	16
McMillin's				
Apple	4 oz	430	—	23
Berry	4 oz	430	—	23
Cherry	4 oz	430	—	24
Chocolate Pudding	4 oz	420	—	21
Coconut Pudding	4 oz	450	—	26
Lemon	4 oz	450	—	25
Peach	4 oz	430	—	24
Strawberry	4 oz	400	—	20
Mrs. Smith's				
Apple	⅛ of 8 in pie (4.3 oz)	270	2	11
Apple	⅛ of 9 in pie (4.6 oz)	370	4	18
Apple	⅒ of 10 in pie (4.6 oz)	280	3	12
Apple Cranberry	⅛ of 8 in pie (4.3 oz)	280	2	11

FOOD	PORTION	CALS.	SAT. FAT	FAT
Mrs. Smith's (CONT.)				
Apple Lattice Ready To Serve	⅕ of 8 in pie (4.6 oz)	310	3	13
Banana Cream	¼ of 8 in pie (3.4 oz)	250	3	9
Berry	⅙ of 8 in pie (4.3 oz)	280	2	11
Blackberry	⅙ of 8 in pie (4.3 oz)	280	2	11
Blueberry	⅙ of 8 in pie	260	2	11
Boston Cream	⅛ of 8 in pie (2.4 oz)	170	2	5
Cherry	⅒ of 10 in pie (4.6 oz)	410	—	18
Cherry	⅙ of 8 in pie	270	2	11
Cherry	⅛ of 9 in pie (4.6 oz)	320	3	13
Cherry Lattice Ready To Serve	⅕ of 8 in pie (4.6 oz)	320	3	13
Chocolate Cream	¼ of 8 in pie (3.4 oz)	290	4	14
Coconut Cream	¼ of 8 in pie (3.4 oz)	280	4	14
Coconut Custard	⅕ of 8 in pie (5 oz)	280	5	12
Dutch Apple	⅒ of 10 in pie (4.6 oz)	320	3	12
Dutch Apple	⅙ of 8 in pie	310	3	13
Dutch Apple	⅛ of 9 in pie (4.5 oz)	300	3	12
French Silk Cream	⅕ of 8 in pie (4.8 oz)	410	6	21
Hearty Pumpkin	⅕ of 8 in pie (5.2 oz)	280	3	10
Lemon Cream	¼ of 8 in pie (3.4 oz)	270	3	13
Lemon Meringue	⅕ of 8 in pie (4.8 oz)	300	2	8
Mince	⅙ of 8 in pie (4.3 oz)	300	2	11
Peach	⅙ of 8 in pie	260	2	11
Peach	⅛ of 9 in pie (4.6 oz)	310	3	13
Pecan	⅛ of 10 in pie (4.5 oz)	500	4	23
Pumpkin	⅛ of 10 in pie (5.1 oz)	250	2	8
Pumpkin	⅕ of 8 in pie (5.2 oz)	270	2	8
Red Raspberry	⅙ of 8 in pie (4.3 oz)	280	2	11
Strawberry Rhubarb	⅙ of 8 in pie (4.3 oz)	280	2	11
Strawberry Rhubarb	⅕ of 8 in pie (4.8 oz)	520	4	23
Pet-Ritz				
Apple	⅙ pie (4.33 oz)	330	—	12
Banana Cream	⅙ pie (2.33 oz)	170	—	9
Blueberry	⅙ pie (4.33 oz)	370	—	12
Cherry	⅙ pie (4.33 oz)	300	—	12
Chocolate Cream	⅙ pie (2.33 oz)	190	—	8
Coconut Cream	⅙ pie (2.33 oz)	190	—	8
Egg Custard	⅙ pie (4.0 oz)	200	—	8
Lemon Cream	⅙ pie (2.33 oz)	190	—	9
Mince	⅙ pie (4.33 oz)	280	—	9
Neapolitan Cream	⅙ pie (2.33 oz)	180	—	10
Peach	⅙ pie (4.33 oz)	320	—	12

FOOD	PORTION	CALS.	SAT. FAT	FAT
Pet-Ritz (CONT.)				
Pumpkin Custard	⅙ pie (4.33 oz)	250	—	9
Strawberry Cream	⅙ pie (2.33 oz)	170	—	9
Sweet Potato	⅙ pie (3.33 oz)	150	—	7
Sara Lee				
Chocolate Silk	⅕ pie (4.8 oz)	500	16	32
Coconut Cream	⅕ pie (4.8 oz)	480	14	31
Fruit's Of The Forest	⅛ pie (4.6 oz)	340	5	19
Homestyle Apple	⅛ pie (4.6 oz)	340	4	16
Homestyle Blueberry	⅛ pie (4.6 oz)	360	4	15
Homestyle Cherry	⅛ pie (4.6 oz)	330	4	15
Homestyle Dutch Apple	⅛ pie (4.6 oz)	350	3	15
Homestyle Mince	⅛ pie (4.6 oz)	390	4	17
Homestyle Peach	⅛ pie (4.6 oz)	330	3	13
Homestyle Pecan	⅛ pie (4.2 oz)	520	5	24
Homestyle Pumpkin	⅛ pie (4.6 oz)	260	3	11
Homestyle Raspberry	⅛ pie (4.6 oz)	380	5	19
Lemon Meringue	⅙ pie (5 oz)	350	3	11
Slice Lemon Icebox	1 (3.5 oz)	260	2	9
Slice Southern Pecan	1 (4 oz)	470	4	23
Weight Watchers				
Mississippi Mud	1 piece (2.45 oz)	160	2	5
HOME RECIPE				
pecan	⅛ of 9 in pie (4.3 oz)	502	5	27
pumpkin	⅛ of 9 in pie (5.4 oz)	316	5	14
MIX				
banana cream no-bake	⅛ of 9 in pie (3.2 oz)	231	6	12
chocolate mousse no-bake	⅛ of 9 in pie (3.3 oz)	247	8	15
coconut creme no-bake	⅛ of 9 in pie (3.3 oz)	259	10	17
Jell-O				
No Bake Chocolate Silk as prep	⅛ pie (4.4 oz)	320	6	16
Royal				
Key Lime Pie Filling	mix for 1 serv	50	0	0
Lemon Pie Filling	mix for 1 serv	50	0	0
Lemon Meringue No-Bake	⅛ pie	210	—	5
READY-TO-EAT				
Entenmann's				
Apple Homestyle	1 serv (2.1 oz)	140	—	7
Coconut Custard	1 serv (1.8 oz)	140	—	8
SNACK				
apple	1 (3 oz)	266	7	14
apple fried	1 (6.4 oz)	404	3	21
blueberry fried	1 (6.4 oz)	404	3	21
cherry	1 (3 oz)	266	7	14

FOOD	PORTION	CALS.	SAT. FAT	FAT
cherry fried	1 (6.4 oz)	404	3	21
lemon	1 (3 oz)	266	7	14
lemon fried	1 (6.4 oz)	404	3	21
peach fried	1 (6.4 oz)	404	3	21
strawberry fried	1 (6.4 oz)	404	3	21
Dolly Madison				
Apple	1 (4.5 oz)	480	9	22
Blueberry	1 (4.5 oz)	480	10	21
Cherry	1 (4.5 oz)	470	11	22
Chocolate Pudding	1 (4.5 oz)	530	11	25
Lemon	1 (4.5 oz)	500	11	24
Peach	1 (4.5 oz)	480	10	21
Pecan	1 (3 oz)	360	8	19
Pecan Fried	1 (4.5 oz)	530	9	21
Pineapple	1 (4.5 oz)	460	10	21
Hostess				
Apple	1 (4.5 oz)	480	9	22
Blackberry	1 (4.5 oz)	520	11	21
Blueberry	1 (4.5 oz)	480	10	21
Cherry	1 (4.5 oz)	470	11	22
French Apple	1 (4.5 oz)	480	9	22
Lemon	1 (4.5 oz)	500	11	24
Peach	1 (4.5 oz)	480	10	21
Pineapple	1 (4.5 oz)	460	10	21
Strawberry	1 (4.5 oz)	510	9	23
Lance				
Pecan	1 (3 oz)	350	4	17
Tastykake				
Apple	1 (4 oz)	270	1	11
Blueberry	1 (4 oz)	300	1	11
Cherry	1 (4 oz)	290	1	11
Coconut Creme	1 (4 oz)	370	4	21
French Apple	1 (4.2 oz)	310	1	11
Lemon	1 (4 oz)	300	2	13
Peach	1 (4 oz)	280	1	11
Pineapple	1 (4 oz)	290	1	12
Pineapple Cheese	1 (4 oz)	320	3	12
Pumpkin	1 (4 oz)	340	2	14
Strawberry	1 (3.5 oz)	320	1	12
Tastyklair	1 (4 oz)	400	3	20
TAKE-OUT				
apple	⅙ of 9 in pie (5.4 oz)	411	5	19
banana cream	⅙ of 9 in pie (5.2 oz)	398	6	20
blueberry	⅙ of 9 in pie (5.2 oz)	360	4	18
butterscotch	⅙ of 9 in pie (4.5 oz)	355	5	18

FOOD	PORTION	CALS.	SAT. FAT	FAT
cherry	⅛ of 9 in pie (6.3 oz)	486	5	22
coconut creme	⅛ of 9 in pie (4.7 oz)	396	8	21
coconut custard	⅛ of 8 in pie (3.6 oz)	271	6	14
custard	⅛ of 9 in pie (4.5 oz)	262	4	11
lemon meringue	⅛ of 9 in pie (4.5 oz)	362	4	16
mince	⅛ of 9 in pie (5.8 oz)	477	4	18
pecan	⅛ of 8 in pie (4 oz)	452	4	21
pumpkin	⅛ of 8 in pie (3.8 oz)	229	2	10
vanilla cream	⅛ of 9 in pie (4.4 oz)	350	5	18
PIE CRUST				
(*see also* PIE)				
FROZEN				
baked	⅛ of 9 in pie (0.6 oz)	82	2	5
baked	9 in shell (4.4 oz)	647	13	41
puff pastry baked	1 shell (1.4 oz)	223	2	15
Oronoque				
Deep Dish	⅙ pie (1.41 oz)	200	—	13
Pie Crust	⅙ pie (1.23 oz)	170	—	12
Pepperidge Farm				
Puff Pastry Sheets	⅙ sheet (1.4 oz)	170	3	11
Puff Pastry Shell	1 (1.6 oz)	190	4	13
Puff Pastry Squares	1 sq (2 oz)	240	5	16
Pet-Ritz				
Deep Dish	⅛ pie (0.7 oz)	90	2	5
Regular	⅛ pie (0.6 oz)	80	2	5
Tart Shells	1 (1 oz)	130	2	8
HOME RECIPE				
9-inch crust	1	900	15	60
baked	9 in shell (6.3 oz)	949	15	62
baked	⅛ of 9 in crust (0.8 oz)	119	2	8
MIX				
as prep	9 in crust (5.6 oz)	801	12	49
as prep	⅛ of 9 in pie (0.7 oz)	100	2	6
Betty Crocker				
Pie Crust	⅛ crust	110	2	8
Flako				
Mix	¼ cup (0.9 oz)	130	3	8
Jiffy				
As prep	⅐ crust	180	4	10
READY-TO-EAT				
chocolate cookie crumb baked	⅛ of 9 in pie (1 oz)	139	2	9
chocolate cookie crumb baked	9 in crust (7.7 oz)	1130	15	69
chocolate cookie crumb chilled	9 in crust (7.8 oz)	1127	15	69

FOOD	PORTION	CALS.	SAT. FAT	FAT
chocolate cookie crumb chilled	⅛ of 9 in pie (1 oz)	142	2	9
graham cracker baked	⅛ of 9 in pie (1 oz)	148	2	8
graham cracker baked	9 in crust (8.4 oz)	1181	12	60
graham cracker chilled	⅛ of 9 in pie (1 oz)	150	2	8
graham cracker chilled	9 in crust (8.6 oz)	1182	12	60
vanilla wafer cracker crumbs baked	9 in crust (6.1 oz)	937	13	64
vanilla wafer cracker crumbs baked	⅛ of 9 in pie (0.8 oz)	119	2	8
vanilla wafer cracker crumbs chilled	⅛ of 9 in pie (0.8 oz)	117	2	8
vanilla wafer cracker crumbs chilled	9 in crust (6.2 oz)	934	13	64
Generic Label				
Graham	⅛ pie (0.7 oz)	110	3	5
Honey Maid				
Graham	⅛ crust (1 oz)	140	2	7
Nabisco				
Nilla	⅛ crust (1 oz)	140	2	8
Oreo				
Crumb Crust	⅛ crust (1 oz)	140	2	11
REFRIGERATED				
All Ready				
Crust	⅛ pie (0.9 oz)	120	3	7

PIEROGI
Empire				
Potato Cheese	3 (4.6 oz)	260	3	6
Potato Onion	3 (4.6 oz)	250	1	5
Golden				
Potato Cheese	3 (4 oz)	250	2	8
Potato Onion	3 (4 oz)	210	2	6
Mrs. T's				
Potato And Cheddar Cheese	1 (1.3 oz)	60	—	tr
Potato And Onion	1 (1.3 oz)	50	—	tr
Sauerkraut	1	60	—	0

PIGEON
w/ skin & bone	3.5 oz	169	—	10

PIGEON PEAS
dried cooked	½ cup	102	tr	tr
dried cooked	1 cup	204	tr	1

PIGNOLIA
(see PINE NUTS)

FOOD	PORTION	CALS.	SAT. FAT	FAT
PIG'S EARS AND FEET				
ear simmered	1	184	4	12
feet pickled	1 oz	58	2	5
feet pickled	1 lb	921	25	73
feet simmered	3 oz	165	4	11
Hormel				
Pickled Feet	2 oz	80	2	6
Pickled Hocks	2 oz	110	3	8
PIKE				
northern cooked	3 oz	96	tr	1
northern cooked	½ fillet (5.4 oz)	176	tr	1
northern raw	3 oz	75	tr	1
roe raw	3½ oz	130	—	2
walleye baked	3 oz	101	tr	1
PILLNUTS				
pillnuts-canarytree dried	1 oz	204	9	23
PIMIENTOS				
canned	1 tbsp	3	tr	tr
Dromedary				
Peeled	½ tsp (4 g)	0	0	0
Unpeeled	½ tsp (4 g)	0	0	0
PINE NUTS				
pignolia dried	1 tbsp	51	1	5
pignolia dried	1 oz	146	2	14
pinyon dried	1 oz	161	3	17
Progresso				
Pignoli	1 jar (1 oz)	170	1	13
PINEAPPLE				
CANNED				
chunks in heavy sirup	1 cup	199	tr	tr
chunks juice pack	1 cup	150	tr	tr
crushed in heavy syrup	1 cup	199	tr	tr
slices in heavy syrup	1 slice	45	tr	tr
slices in light syrup	1 slice	30	tr	tr
slices juice pack	1 slice	35	tr	tr
slices water pack	1 slice	19	tr	tr
tidbits in heavy syrup	1 cup	199	tr	tr
tidbits in juice	1 cup	150	tr	tr
tidbits in water	1 cup	79	tr	tr
Del Monte				
Chunks In Heavy Syrup	½ cup (4.3 oz)	90	0	0
Chunks In Its Own Juice	½ cup (4.4 oz)	70	0	0

FOOD	PORTION	CALS.	SAT. FAT	FAT
Del Monte (CONT.)				
Crushed In Heavy Syrup	½ cup (4.4 oz)	90	0	0
Crushed In Its Own Juice	½ cup (4.3 oz)	70	0	0
Sliced In Heavy Syrup	½ cup (4.1 oz)	90	0	0
Sliced In Its Own Juice	½ cup (4 oz)	60	0	0
Snack Cups Tidbits In Juice	1 serv (4.5 oz)	70	0	0
Snack Cups Tidbits In Juice EZ-Open Lid	1 serv (4.2 oz)	60	0	0
Spears In Its Own Juice	½ cup (4.3 oz)	70	0	0
Tidbits In Its Own Juice	½ cup (4.3 oz)	70	0	0
Wedges In Its Own Juice	½ cup (4.3 oz)	70	0	0
Dole				
All Cuts Juice Pack	½ cup	70	—	tr
All Cuts Syrup Pack	½ cup	90	0	0
Libby				
Crushed	1 cup with juice	140	0	0
Sliced In Unsweetened Juice	1 cup with juice	140	0	0
DRIED				
Sonoma				
Pieces	2 pieces (1.4 oz)	140	0	2
FRESH				
diced	1 cup	77	tr	tr
slice	1 slice	42	tr	tr
Dole				
Pineapple	2 slices	90	—	1
FROZEN				
chunks sweetened	½ cup	104	tr	tr
PINEAPPLE JUICE				
canned	1 cup	139	tr	tr
frzn as prep	1 cup	129	tr	tr
frzn not prep	6 oz	387	tr	tr
After The Fall				
Mandarin Pineapple	1 can (12 oz)	150	0	0
Bright & Early				
Frozen	8 fl oz	120	0	0
Del Monte				
Juice	1 serv (11.5 oz)	190	0	0
Juice	6 fl oz	80	0	0
Juice	8 fl oz	110	0	0
Dole				
Chilled	8 oz	130	0	0
Minute Maid				
Box	8.45 fl oz	130	0	0
Frozen	8 fl oz	110	0	0

FOOD	PORTION	CALS.	SAT. FAT	FAT
PINK BEANS				
CANNED				
Goya				
Spanish Style	7.5 oz	140	—	tr
DRIED				
cooked	1 cup	252	tr	1
PINTO BEANS				
CANNED				
pinto	1 cup	186	tr	1
Allen				
Pinto Beans	½ cup (4.5 oz)	110	0	1
Brown Beauty				
Pinto Beans	½ cup (4.5 oz)	110	0	1
Chi-Chi's				
Pinto Beans	½ cup (4.3 oz)	100	0	1
East Texas Fair				
Pinto Beans	½ cup (4.5 oz)	110	0	1
Eden				
Organic	½ cup (4.6 oz)	100	0	0
Organic Spicy w/ Jalapeno & Red Peppers	½ cup (4.6 oz)	125	0	0
Gebhardt				
Pinto Beans	4 oz	100	—	tr
Goya				
Spanish Style	7.5 oz	140	—	1
Green Giant				
Pinto Beans	½ cup (4.4 oz)	110	0	1
Old El Paso				
Pinto Beans	½ cup (4.6 oz)	110	0	1
Progresso				
Pinto Beans	½ cup (4.6 oz)	110	0	1
Trappey				
Jalapinto With Bacon	½ cup (4.5 oz)	120	1	1
With Bacon	½ cup (4.5 oz)	120	1	1
DRIED				
cooked	1 cup	235	tr	1
Arrowhead				
Dried	¼ cup (1.5 oz)	150	0	1
Bean Cuisine				
Dried	½ cup	115	—	1
Hurst				
HamBeens w/ Ham	3 tbsp (1.2 oz)	120	0	1
FROZEN				
cooked	3 oz	152	tr	tr

FOOD	PORTION	CALS.	SAT. FAT	FAT
PINYON				
(see PINE NUTS)				
PISTACHIOS				
dry roasted	1 oz	172	2	15
dry roasted salted	1 oz	172	2	15
dry roasted salted	1 cup	776	9	68
Dole				
Shelled	1 oz	163	—	14
Shells On	1 oz	90	—	7
Fisher				
Red Tint	1 oz	170	3	15
Lance				
Pistachios	1 pkg (1⅛ oz)	90	1	7
Planters				
Munch'N Go Singles Shelled Dry Roasted	1 pkg (2 oz)	330	4	29
Red Salted Dry Roasted	1 pkg	160	2	14
Uncolored Dry Roasted	½ cup	160	2	14
Sonoma				
Salted Shelled	¼ cup (1 oz)	190	2	14
PITANGA				
fresh	1 cup	57	—	1
fresh	1	2	—	tr
PIZZA				
(see also PIZZA DOUGH, PIZZA SAUCE)				
Amy's Organic				
Cheese	1 (13 oz)	310	4	11
Pocket Sandwich Cheese Pizza	1 (4.5 oz)	290	4	9
Pocket Sandwich Veggie Pepperoni Pizza	1 (4.5 oz)	220	3	7
Roasted Vegetable	1 (12 oz)	270	1	8
Spinach	1 (14 oz)	320	4	11
Appian Way				
Pizza Mix Thick Crust	⅓ pie (4.2 oz)	290	2	5
Celeste				
Italian Bread Deluxe	1 (5.1 oz)	290	3	11
Italian Bread Garlic & Herb Zesty Chicken	1 (5 oz)	260	2	8
Italian Bread Pepperoni	1 (5 oz)	320	4	13
Italian Bread Zesty Four Cheese	1 (4.6 oz)	300	6	12
Large Cheese	¼ pie (4.4 oz)	320	8	16
Large Deluxe	¼ pie (5.5 oz)	350	6	18
Large Pepperoni	¼ pie (4.7 oz)	350	7	20

FOOD	PORTION	CALS.	SAT. FAT	FAT
Celeste (CONT.)				
Large Suprema With Meat	⅕ pie (4.6 oz)	290	5	16
Large Zesty Four Cheese	¼ pie (4.4 oz)	330	8	16
Small Cheese	1 (7.5 oz)	540	13	25
Small Deluxe	1 (8.2 oz)	540	10	29
Small Hot & Zesty Four Cheese	1 (7 oz)	530	13	27
Small Original Four Cheese	1 (7 oz)	540	12	30
Small Pepperoni	1 (6.7 oz)	520	10	27
Small Sausage	1 (7.5 oz)	530	9	27
Small Suprema Vegetable	1 (7.5 oz)	480	8	23
Small Suprema With Meat	1 (9 oz)	580	10	31
Small Zesty Four Cheese	1 (7 oz)	530	13	27
Croissant Pocket				
Stuffed Sandwich Pepperoni Pizza	1 piece (4.5 oz)	350	5	15
Di Giorno				
Rising Crust 12 inch Four Cheese	⅙ pie (4.9 oz)	320	6	11
Rising Crust 12 inch Italian Sausage	⅙ pie (5.3 oz)	360	7	14
Rising Crust 12 inch Pepperoni	⅙ pie (5.2 oz)	370	8	16
Rising Crust 12 inch Supreme	⅙ pie (5.8 oz)	380	8	17
Rising Crust 12 inch Three Meat	⅙ pie (5.4 oz)	380	8	16
Rising Crust 12 inch Vegetable	⅙ pie (5.6 oz)	310	5	10
Rising Crust 8 inch Chicken Supreme	⅓ pie (4.8 oz)	270	5	9
Rising Crust 8 inch Four Cheese	⅓ pie (4 oz)	260	5	9
Rising Crust 8 inch Italian Sausage	⅓ pie (4.4 oz)	300	6	12
Rising Crust 8 inch Pepperoni	⅓ pie (4.2 oz)	300	6	13
Rising Crust 8 inch Spinach	⅓ pie (4.3 oz)	250	4	8
Rising Crust 8 inch Supreme	⅓ pie (4.7 oz)	310	6	14
Rising Crust 8 inch Three Meat	⅓ pie (4.4 oz)	310	6	13
Rising Crust 8 inch Vegetable	⅓ pie (4.6 oz)	250	4	8
Empire				
3 Pack	1 (3 oz)	210	4	9
Bagel	1 (2 oz)	150	3	5
English Muffin	1 (2 oz)	130	3	5
Pizza	½ pie (5 oz)	340	7	13
Healthy Choice				
French Bread Cheese	1 (5.6 oz)	310	2	4
French Bread Pepperoni	1 (6 oz)	360	4	9

FOOD	PORTION	CALS.	SAT. FAT	FAT
Healthy Choice (CONT.)				
French Bread Sausage	1 (6 oz)	330	2	4
French Bread Supreme	1 (6.35 oz)	340	2	6
Hot Pocket				
Stuffed Sandwich Pepperoni & Sausage Pizza	1 (4.5 oz)	340	6	16
Stuffed Sandwich Pepperoni Pizza	1 (4.5 oz)	350	8	17
Jack's				
Great Combinations 12 inch Bacon Cheeseburger	¼ pie (4.7 oz)	360	9	18
Great Combinations 12 inch Double Cheese	¼ pie (4.9 oz)	380	11	19
Great Combinations 12 inch Pepperoni	¼ pie (5.2 oz)	410	9	19
Great Combinations 12 inch Pepperoni & Mushrooms	¼ pie (4.8 oz)	340	7	16
Great Combinations 12 inch Sausage	¼ pie (5.4 oz)	390	8	18
Great Combinations 12 inch Sausage & Mushroom	¼ pie (4.9 oz)	310	7	15
Great Combinations 12 inch Sausage & Pepperoni	¼ pie (4.8 oz)	350	8	19
Great Combinations 12 inch Supreme	¼ pie (5.2 oz)	350	8	18
Great Combinations 9 inch Double Cheese	½ pie (5.5 oz)	430	12	21
Great Combinations 9 inch Pepperoni & Sausage	½ pie (5.1 oz)	380	8	18
Naturally Rising 12 inch Bacon Cheeseburger	⅙ pie (5 oz)	350	7	15
Naturally Rising 12 inch Canadian Bacon	⅙ pie (4.9 oz)	280	5	9
Naturally Rising 12 inch Cheese	⅙ pie (4.5 oz)	290	6	10
Naturally Rising 12 inch & Combination w/ Sausage Pepperoni	⅙ pie (5.2 oz)	360	8	17
Naturally Rising 12 inch Pepperoni	⅙ pie (4.9 oz)	350	8	16
Naturally Rising 12 inch Pepperoni Supreme	⅙ pie (5.1 oz)	340	8	16
Naturally Rising 12 inch Sausage	⅙ pie (5.1 oz)	340	7	15

FOOD	PORTION	CALS.	SAT. FAT	FAT
Jack's (CONT.)				
Naturally Rising 12 inch Spicy Italian Sausage	⅙ pie (5.1 oz)	330	7	14
Naturally Rising 12 inch The Works	⅙ pie (5.3 oz)	330	7	14
Naturally Rising 9 inch Cheese	⅓ pie (4.7 oz)	300	6	10
Naturally Rising 9 inch & Combination w/ Sausage Pepperoni	¼ pie (4.2 oz)	300	7	14
Naturally Rising 9 inch Pepperoni	⅓ pie (5.2 oz)	360	8	16
Naturally Rising 9 inch Sausage	⅓ pie (5.4 oz)	360	7	16
Naturally Rising 9 inch The Works	¼ pie (4.5 oz)	280	6	12
Original 12 inch Canadian Bacon	¼ pie (4.4 oz)	280	5	10
Original 12 inch Cheese	⅓ pie (5 oz)	360	7	13
Original 12 inch Hamburger	¼ pie (4.4 oz)	300	7	14
Original 12 inch Pepperoni	¼ pie (4.3 oz)	330	7	15
Original 12 inch Sausage	¼ pie (4.3 oz)	300	7	14
Original 12 inch Spicy Italian Sausage	¼ pie (4.3 oz)	290	6	13
Original 9 inch Pepperoni	½ pie (5 oz)	380	8	18
Original 9 inch Sausage	½ pie (5.1 oz)	360	7	16
Pizza Bursts Combination Sausage & Pepperoni	6 pieces (3 oz)	250	4	12
Pizza Bursts Pepperoni	6 pieces (3 oz)	260	5	14
Pizza Bursts Sausage	6 pieces (3 oz)	250	4	12
Pizza Bursts Supercheese	6 pieces (3 oz)	250	5	12
Pizza Bursts Supreme	6 pieces (3 oz)	250	4	13
Kid Cuisine				
Cheese	1 (8 oz)	430	3	11
Hamburger	1 (8.30 oz)	400	4	11
Kineret				
Bagel Pizza	2 (4 oz)	300	6	10
Slice	1 (4.9 oz)	490	4	9
Lean Cuisine				
French Bread Cheese	1 pkg (6 oz)	300	3	5
French Bread Deluxe	1 pkg (6.1 oz)	300	3	6
French Bread Pepperoni	1 pkg (5.25 oz)	310	3	7
Lean Pockets				
Stuffed Sandwich Pizza Deluxe	1 (4.5 oz)	270	3	8
Old El Paso				
Pizza Burrito Cheese	1 (3.5 oz)	320	4	9

FOOD	PORTION	CALS.	SAT. FAT	FAT
Old El Paso (CONT.)				
Pizza Burrito Pepperoni	1 (3.5 oz)	260	5	10
Pizza Burrito Sausage	1 (3.5 oz)	260	4	9
Pepperidge Farm				
Gourmet Crust Cheese	1 (4.4 oz)	390	7	20
Gourmet Crust Pepperoni	1 (4.5 oz)	420	9	23
Small World				
Four Cheese	1 (4 oz)	240	3	6
Special Delivery				
Organic	⅓ pizza (5.3 oz)	320	5	9
Organic Soy Kaas	⅓ pizza (5.3 oz)	320	2	7
Stouffer's				
French Bread Bacon Cheddar	1 piece (5.7 oz)	430	7	21
French Bread Cheese	1 piece (5.2 oz)	370	6	16
French Bread Cheeseburger	1 piece (6 oz)	420	6	20
French Bread Deluxe	1 piece (6.2 oz)	430	7	21
French Bread Double Cheese	1 piece (5.9 oz)	400	7	16
French Bread Pepperoni	1 piece (5.6 oz)	430	8	20
French Bread Pepperoni & Mushroom	1 piece (6.1 oz)	440	7	20
French Bread Sausage	1 piece (6 oz)	420	7	18
French Bread Sausage & Pepperoni	1 piece (6.25 oz)	470	8	23
French Bread Three Meat	1 piece (6.25 oz)	460	8	21
French Bread Vegetable Deluxe	1 piece (6.4 oz)	380	6	16
French Bread White Pizza	1 piece (5.1 oz)	460	7	23
Tombstone				
Double Top Pepperoni	⅙ pie (4.5 oz)	340	9	19
Double Top Sausage	⅙ pie (4.6 oz)	320	9	17
Double Top Sausage & Pepperoni	⅙ pie (4.6 oz)	340	9	19
Double Top Supreme	⅙ pie (4.7 oz)	330	9	18
Double Top Two Cheese	⅙ pie (5.2 oz)	380	11	19
For One ½ Less Fat Cheese	1 pie (6.5 oz)	460	5	10
For One ½ Less Fat Vegetable	1 pie (7.2 oz)	360	4	9
For One Extra Cheese	1 pie (6.9 oz)	520	13	28
For One Pepperoni	1 pie (6.9 oz)	550	14	32
For One Supreme	1 pie (7.5 oz)	550	14	32
Light Supreme	⅕ pie (4.8 oz)	270	4	9
Light Vegetable	⅕ pie (4.6 oz)	240	3	7
Original 12 inch Canadian Bacon	¼ pie (5.5 oz)	350	7	14
Original 12 inch Deluxe	⅕ pie (4.8 oz)	310	6	14
Original 12 inch Extra Cheese	¼ pie (5.1 oz)	350	8	15
Original 12 inch Hamburger	⅕ pie (4.4 oz)	310	7	15

FOOD	PORTION	CALS.	SAT. FAT	FAT
Tombstone (CONT.)				
Original 12 inch Pepperoni	¼ pie (5.3 oz)	400	9	21
Original 12 inch Sausage	⅕ pie (4.4 oz)	300	6	14
Original 12 inch Sausage & Mushroom	⅕ pie (4.6 oz)	300	6	14
Original 12 inch Sausage & Pepperoni	⅕ pie (4.4 oz)	320	7	16
Original 12 inch Supreme	⅕ pie (5.1 oz)	320	7	16
Original 9 inch Deluxe	⅓ pie (4.4 oz)	280	6	13
Original 9 inch Extra Cheese	½ pie (5.6 oz)	380	8	19
Original 9 inch Hamburger	⅓ pie (4 oz)	280	6	13
Original 9 inch Pepperoni	⅓ pie (4 oz)	300	7	15
Original 9 inch Pepperoni & Sausage	⅓ pie (4.1 oz)	300	7	15
Original 9 inch Sausage	⅓ pie (4 oz)	280	6	13
Original 9 inch Supreme	⅓ pie (4.4 oz)	310	7	16
Oven Rising Italian Sausage	⅙ pie (5.1 oz)	320	6	13
Oven Rising Pepperoni	⅙ pie (4.9 oz)	340	7	15
Oven Rising Supreme	⅙ pie (5.1 oz)	320	6	14
Oven Rising Three Cheese	⅙ pie (4.8 oz)	320	8	13
Oven Rising Three Meat	⅙ pie (5.1 oz)	340	7	15
Thin Crust Four Meat Combo	¼ pie (5 oz)	380	10	23
Thin Crust Italian Sausage	¼ pie (5 oz)	370	10	22
Thin Crust Pepperoni	¼ pie (4.8 oz)	400	11	25
Thin Crust Supreme	¼ pie (5 oz)	380	10	22
Thin Crust Supreme Taco	¼ pie (5.1 oz)	370	11	23
Thin Crust Three Cheese	¼ pie (4.7 oz)	360	11	21
Weight Watchers				
Smart Ones Deluxe Combo	1 (6.57 oz)	380	6	11
Smart Ones Pepperoni	1 (5.56 oz)	390	4	12
TAKE-OUT				
cheese	12 in pie	1121	12	26
cheese	⅛ of 12 in pie	140	2	3
cheese deep dish individual	1 (5.5 oz)	460	9	24
cheese meat & vegetables	⅛ of 12 in pie	184	2	5
cheese meat & vegetables	12 in pie	1472	12	43
pepperoni	12 in pie	1445	18	56
pepperoni	⅛ of 12 in pie	181	2	7
PIZZA DOUGH				
Boboli				
Shell + Sauce	⅛ lg shell (2.6 oz)	170	1	3
Shell + Sauce	⅛ sm shell (2.6 oz)	170	1	3
House of Pasta				
Frozen	⅛ of 14 in pie (1.9 oz)	140	0	1

FOOD	PORTION	CALS.	SAT. FAT	FAT
Jiffy				
As prep	¼ crust	180	3	3
Pillsbury				
Crust	⅕ crust (2 oz)	150	0	2
Robin Hood				
Crust	¼ crust	160	1	2
Sassafras				
Cornmeal Pizza Crust	1 slice (1.4 oz)	140	0	0
Italian Pizza Crust Mix	1 slice (1.4 oz)	140	0	0
Wanda's				
Crust Mix Oregano & Basil	⅒ pie (1.4 oz)	149	0	0
Crust Mix Oregano & Basil Whole Wheat	⅒ pie (1.4 oz)	141	0	1
Watkins				
Crust Mix	⅛ pkg (1.8 oz)	180	0	1
PIZZA SAUCE				
Boboli				
Sauce	¼ cup (2.5 oz)	40	0	0
Sauce	1 pkg (1.2 oz)	20	0	0
Contadina				
Flavored With Pepperoni	¼ cup	40	1	2
Pizza Sauce	¼ cup	35	—	2
Squeeze	¼ cup	35	—	2
With Italian Cheeses	¼ cup	40	—	2
Eden				
Pizza Pasta Sauce	½ cup (4.4 oz)	80	0	3
Muir Glen				
Organic	¼ cup (2.2 oz)	40	—	1
Progresso				
Pizza Sauce	¼ cup (2.2 oz)	35	0	1
Ragu				
Quick Traditional	3 tbsp (1.7 oz)	35	—	2
Tree Of Life				
Sauce	¼ cup (1.9 oz)	30	—	1
PLANTAINS				
fresh uncooked	1 (6.3 oz)	218	—	1
sliced cooked	½ cup	89	—	tr
Chifles				
Plantain Chips	1 pkg (2 oz)	170	2	11
PLUMS				
CANNED				
purple in heavy syrup	3	119	tr	tr
purple in heavy syrup	1 cup	320	tr	tr

FOOD	PORTION	CALS.	SAT. FAT	FAT
purple in light syrup	1 cup	158	tr	tr
purple in light syrup	3	83	tr	tr
purple juice pack	3	55	tr	tr
purple juice pack	1 cup	146	tr	tr
purple water pack	1 cup	102	tr	tr
purple water pack	3	39	tr	tr
FRESH				
plum	1	36	tr	tr
sliced	1 cup	91	tr	1
Dole				
Plums	2	70	—	1
POI				
poi	½ cup	134	tr	tr
POKEBERRY SHOOTS				
cooked	½ cup	16	—	tr
raw	½ cup	18	—	tr
Allen				
Pokeberry Shoots	½ cup (4.1 oz)	35	0	1
POLENTA				
(see CORNMEAL)				
Aurora				
Ready-To-Use	½ cup (5 oz)	110	0	0
Frieda's				
Dried Tomato	4 oz	80	0	0
Italian Herb	4 oz	80	0	0
Mexicana	4 oz	80	0	0
Original	4 oz	80	0	0
Wild Mushroom	4 oz	80	0	0
Melissa's				
Original	4 oz	80	0	0
POLLACK				
atlantic baked	3 oz	100	tr	1
Mrs. Paul's				
Fillets Light frzn	1 fillet (4.5 oz)	240	—	11
POMEGRANATE JUICE				
Cortas				
Concentrated Juice	1 tbsp (0.6 oz)	40	0	0
POMEGRANATES				
pomegranate	1	104	—	tr
POMPANO				
florida cooked	3 oz	179	4	10
florida raw	3 oz	140	3	8

FOOD	PORTION	CALS.	SAT. FAT	FAT
POPCORN				
(see also CHIPS, POPCORN CAKES, PRETZELS, SNACKS)				
air-popped	1 cup (0.3 oz)	31	tr	tr
air-popped	1 oz	108	tr	1
caramel coated	1 oz	122	1	4
caramel coated	1 cup (1.2 oz)	152	1	5
carmel coated w/ peanuts	⅔ cup (1 oz)	114	tr	2
cheese	1 cup (0.4 oz)	58	1	4
cheese	1 oz	149	2	9
oil popped	1 oz	142	1	8
oil popped	1 cup (0.4 oz)	55	1	3
Barrel O' Fun				
Baked Curl	1 oz	150	2	9
Caramel Corn	1 oz	115	0	1
Corn Pop	1 oz	190	1	16
Popcorn	1 oz	160	1	12
White Cheddar Pops	1 oz	170	1	13
Chester's				
Butter	3 cups	160	2	12
Caramel Craze	¾ cup	130	0	2
Cheddar Cheese	3 cups	190	3	13
Microwave Butter	5 cups	200	2	12
Cracker Jack				
Fat Free Butter Toffee	¾ cup	110	0	0
Fat Free] Caramel	¾ cup	110	0	0
Original	½ cup	120	0	2
Estee				
Caramel	1 cup	120	0	2
Greenfield				
Caramel	1 cup (1 oz)	120	tr	2
Herr's				
Regular	3 cups (1 oz)	140	2	11
Jiffy Pop				
Bag Butter	3 cups	90	1	5
Bag Lite	3 cups	70	tr	3
Bag Regular	3 cups	100	1	6
Glazed Popcorn Clusters	1 oz	120	tr	2
Microwave Butter	4 cup	140	—	7
Microwave Regular	4 cup	140	—	7
Pan Butter	4 cup	130	—	6
Pan Regular	4 cup	130	—	6
Jolly Time				
America's Best 94% Fat Free	1 cup	20	0	0
Blast O Butter	1 cup	45	1	3
Blast O Butter Light	1 cup	30	0	2

FOOD	PORTION	CALS.	SAT. FAT	FAT
Jolly Time (CONT.)				
Butter Licious	1 cup	35	0	2
Butter Licious Light	1 cup	30	0	2
Crispy & White	1 cup	40	1	3
Crispy & White Light	1 cup	25	0	1
Healthy Pop 94% Fat Free	1 cup	20	0	0
White Air Popped	5 cups	100	0	1
Yellow Air Popped	5 cups	100	0	1
Lance				
Cheese	1 pkg (0.6 oz)	90	2	5
Plain	1 pkg (0.5 oz)	70	1	3
White Cheddar	1 pkg (0.6 oz)	100	2	8
White Cheddar	1 pkg (0.9 oz)	150	3	11
Louise's				
Fat-Free Apple Cinnamon	1 oz	100	0	0
Fat-Free Buttery Toffee	1 oz	100	0	0
Fat-Free Caramel	1 oz	100	0	0
Newman's Own				
Microwave Butter Flavor	3½ cups	170	2	11
Microwave Light Butter	3½ cups	110	1	3
Microwave Light Natural	3½ cups	110	1	3
Microwave Natural	3½ cups	170	2	11
Popcorn unpopped	3 tbsp	110	0	2
Orville Redenbacher's				
Gourmet Hot Air	3 cups	40	—	tr
Gourmet Original	3 cups	80	—	4
Gourmet White	3 cups	80	—	4
Microwave Gourmet	3 cups	100	1	6
Microwave Gourmet Butter	3 cups	100	1	6
Microwave Gourmet Butter Toffee	2½ cups	210	3	12
Microwave Gourmet Caramel	2½ cups	240	3	14
Microwave Gourmet Cheddar Cheese	3 cups	130	2	8
Microwave Gourmet Frozen	3 cups	100	1	6
Microwave Gourmet Frozen Butter	3 cups	100	1	6
Microwave Gourmet Light	3 cups	70	1	3
Microwave Gourmet Light Butter	3 cups	70	1	3
Microwave Gourmet Salt Free	3 cups	100	1	6
Microwave Gourmet Salt Free Butter	3 cups	100	1	6
Microwave Gourmet Sour Cream 'n Onion	3 cups	160	3	12

FOOD	PORTION	CALS.	SAT. FAT	FAT
Planters				
Fiddle Faddle Caramel Fat Free	1 cup (1 oz)	110	0	0
Pop Secret				
94% Fat Free Butter	1 cup (5 g)	20	0	0
94% Fat Free Natural	1 cup (5 g)	20	0	0
Butter	1 cup (7 g)	35	1	3
Cheddar Cheese	1 cup (6 g)	30	1	2
Jumbo Pop Butter	1 cup (7 g)	40	1	3
Jumbo Pop Movie Theater Butter	1 cup (7 g)	40	1	3
Light Butter	1 cup (5 g)	20	0	1
Light Movie Theater Butter	1 cup (5 g)	25	0	1
Light Natural	1 cup (5 g)	25	0	1
Movie Theater Butter	1 cup (7 g)	40	1	3
Nacho Cheese	1 cup (6 g)	30	1	2
Natural	1 cup (6 g)	35	1	3
Pop Chips	1½ cups (1 oz)	130	1	4
Real Butter	1 cup (7 g)	35	1	3
Smartfood				
Butter	3 cups	150	2	9
Low Fat Toffee Crunch	¾ cup	110	0	1
Reduced Fat Golden Butter	3⅓ cups	130	1	4
Reduced Fat White Cheddar	3 cups	140	2	6
White Cheddar	2 cups	190	3	12
Snyder's of Hanover				
Butter	1 oz	140	—	9
Ultra Slim-Fast				
Lite N' Tasty	0.5 oz	60	—	2
Utz				
Au Natural	3 cups (1 oz)	120	0	1
Butter	2 cups (1 oz)	170	2	12
Cheese	2 cups (1 oz)	150	2	10
Hulless Puff'N Corn	2 cups (1 oz)	180	3	15
Hulless Puff'N Corn Hot Cheese	1 pkg (1.75 oz)	290	3	22
Hulless Pull'N Corn Cheese	2 cups (1 oz)	170	2	12
White Cheddar	2 cups (1 oz)	150	2	9
Weight Watchers				
Butter	1 pkg (0.66 oz)	90	0	3
Butter Toffee	1 pkg (0.9 oz)	110	1	3
Caramel	1 pkg (0.9 oz)	100	0	1
Microwave	1 pkg (1 oz)	100	0	1
White Cheddar Cheese	1 pkg (0.66 oz)	90	1	4
Wise				
Tender Eating	0.5 oz	70	—	6

FOOD	PORTION	CALS.	SAT. FAT	FAT
Wise (CONT.)				
With Real Premium White Cheddar Cheese	0.5 oz	70	—	5

POPCORN CAKES

FOOD	PORTION	CALS.	SAT. FAT	FAT
popcorn cake	1 (0.3 oz)	38	tr	tr
Lundberg				
Organic Lightly Salted	1	60	—	1
Organic Unsalted	1	60	—	1
Rye With Caraway Lightly Salted	1	59	0	0
Mother's				
Butter Flavor	1 (0.3 oz)	35	0	0
Unsalted	1 (0.3 oz)	35	0	0
Orville Redenbacher's				
Chocolate Peanut Crunch Mini	6 pieces (0.5 oz)	60	0	1
Peanut Caramel Crunch	6 (0.5 oz)	60	0	1
Quaker				
Blueberry Crunch	1 (0.5 oz)	50	0	0
Butter Mini	6 (0.5 oz)	50	—	1
Butter Popped	1 (0.3 oz)	35	0	0
Caramel	1 (0.5 oz)	50	0	0
Caramel Mini	5 (0.5 oz)	50	—	1
Cheddar Cheese Mini	6 (0.5 oz)	50	—	1
Lightly Salted Mini	7 (0.5 oz)	50	—	1
Monterey Jack	1 (0.4 oz)	40	0	0
Strawberry Crunch	1 (0.5 oz)	50	0	0
White Cheddar	1 (0.4 oz)	40	0	0

POPOVER

FOOD	PORTION	CALS.	SAT. FAT	FAT
home recipe as prep w/ 2% milk	1 (1.4 oz)	87	1	3
home recipe as prep w/ whole milk	1 (1.4 oz)	90	1	3
mix as prep	1 (1.2 oz)	67	tr	2

POPPY SEEDS

FOOD	PORTION	CALS.	SAT. FAT	FAT
poppy seeds	1 tsp	15	tr	1

PORK

(see also BACON, BACON SUBSTITUTES, CANADIAN BACON, DELI MEATS/COLD CUTS, HAM, PORK DISHES, SAUSAGE)

FOOD	PORTION	CALS.	SAT. FAT	FAT
CANNED				
Hormel				
Pickled Tidbits	2 oz	100	3	8
FRESH				
boston blade roast lean & fat cooked	3 oz	229	6	16

FOOD	PORTION	CALS.	SAT. FAT	FAT
boston blade steak lean & fat cooked	3 oz	220	5	14
center loin roast lean bone in cooked	3 oz	169	3	8
center loin chop lean bone in cooked	3 oz	172	3	7
center rib chop lean & fat bone in cooked	3 oz	213	5	13
center rib roast lean & fat bone in cooked	3 oz	217	5	13
fresh ham rump lean roasted	3 oz	175	2	7
fresh ham rump lean & fat roasted	3 oz	214	4	12
fresh ham shank lean roasted	3 oz	183	3	9
fresh ham shank lean & fat roasted	3 oz	246	6	17
fresh ham whole lean roasted	3 oz	179	3	8
fresh ham whole lean roasted diced	1 cup	285	4	13
fresh ham whole lean & fat roasted	3 oz	232	6	15
fresh ham whole lean & fat roasted diced	1 cup	369	9	24
ground cooked	3 oz	252	7	18
leg loin & shoulder lean only roasted	3 oz	198	—	11
loin chop lean bone in braised	3 oz	191	4	11
loin chop lean bone in broiled	3 oz	199	4	12
loin roast lean bone in roasted	3 oz	210	5	13
loin whole lean & fat braised	3 oz	203	4	12
loin whole lean & fat broiled	3 oz	206	4	12
loin whole lean & fat roasted	3 oz	211	5	12
lungs braised	3 oz	84	1	3
pancreas cooked	3 oz	186	3	9
ribs country style lean & fat braised	3 oz	252	7	18
shoulder arm picnic lean & fat roasted	3 oz	269	7	20
shoulder whole lean & fat roasted	3 oz	248	7	18
shoulder whole lean & fat roasted diced	1 cup	394	11	29
shoulder whole lean roasted	3 oz	196	4	12
shoulder whole lean roasted diced	1 cup	311	6	18
sirloin chop lean & fat bone in braised	3 oz	208	5	13

FOOD	PORTION	CALS.	SAT. FAT	FAT
sirloin roast lean & fat bone in cooked	3 oz	222	5	14
spareribs braised	3 oz	338	10	26
spleen braised	3 oz	127	1	3
tail simmered	3 oz	336	11	30
tenderloin lean roasted	3 oz	139	1	4
top loin chop boneless lean & fat cooked	3 oz	198	4	11
top loin roast boness lean & fat cooked	3 oz	192	4	10
Oscar Mayer				
Sweet Morsel Smoked Boneless Pork Shoulder Butt	3 oz	180	5	15
READY-TO-EAT				
Tyson				
Pork Pattie	1 (3.8 oz)	200	4	11

PORK DISHES

Jimmy Dean

FOOD	PORTION	CALS.	SAT. FAT	FAT
BBQ Pork Rib Sandwich	1 (5.4 oz)	440	7	23
TAKE-OUT				
pork roast	2 oz	70	1	3
tourtiere	1 piece (4.9 oz)	451	10	34

POSOLE

(see HOMINY)

POT PIE

Amy's Organic

FOOD	PORTION	CALS.	SAT. FAT	FAT
Broccoli	1 (7.5 oz)	430	10	22
Country Vegetable	1 (7.5 oz)	370	9	16
Shepard's	1 (8 oz)	160	0	4
Vegetable	1 (7.5 oz)	360	11	18
Vegetable Non-Dairy	1 (7.5 oz)	320	1	9
Award Brand				
Beef	1 (7 oz)	350	8	18
Chicken	1 (7 oz)	350	8	19
Banquet				
Family Entree Chicken Pie	1 serv (8 oz)	450	12	30
Macaroni & Cheese	1 pkg (6.5 oz)	200	2	3
Vegetable & Cheese	1 (7 oz)	390	8	18
Vegetable Pie w/ Beef	1 (7 oz)	330	7	15
Vegetable Pie w/ Chicken	1 (7 oz)	350	7	18
Vegetable Pie w/ Turkey	1 (7 oz)	370	8	20

FOOD	PORTION	CALS.	SAT. FAT	FAT
Empire				
Chicken	1 (8.1 oz)	440	5	21
Turkey	1 (8.1 oz)	470	5	23
Great Value				
Beef	1 (7 oz)	390	8	19
Chicken	1 (7 oz)	380	8	20
Turkey	1 (7 oz)	400	8	22
Lean Cuisine				
Chicken Pie	1 pkg (9.5 oz)	290	3	9
Turkey & Country Vegetable	1 pkg (9.5 oz)	320	3	9
Morton				
Beef	1 (7 oz)	310	8	17
Chicken	1 (7 oz)	320	7	18
Macaroni & Cheese	1 (6 oz)	160	2	3
Turkey	1 (7 oz)	300	9	18
Mrs. Paterson's				
Aussie Pie Chicken	1 (5.5 oz)	460	8	25
Aussie Pie Chicken Low Fat	1 (5.5 oz)	380	6	17
Aussie Pie Philly Steak	1 (5.5 oz)	420	8	24
Ozark Valley				
Chicken	1 (7 oz)	330	7	19
Macaroni & Cheese	1 (6.5 oz)	160	2	3
Turkey	1 (7 oz)	280	6	16
Stouffer's				
Beef Pie	1 pkg (10 oz)	450	9	26
Chicken Pie	1 pkg (10 oz)	540	10	33
Turkey	1 pkg (10 oz)	530	9	33
Swanson				
Beef	7 oz	370	—	19
Beef Hungry Man	16 oz	610	—	31
Chicken	7 oz	380	—	22
Chicken Homestyle	8 oz	410	—	21
Hungry Man Chicken	16 oz	630	—	35
Hungry Man Turkey	16 oz	650	—	36
Turkey	7 oz	380	—	21
TAKE-OUT				
beef	1/3 of 9 in pie (7.4 oz)	515	8	30
chicken	1/3 of 9 in pie (8.1 oz)	545	10	31

POTATO

(see also CHIPS, KNISH, PANCAKES)

CANNED

potatoes	1/2 cup	54	tr	tr

FOOD	PORTION	CALS.	SAT. FAT	FAT
Allen				
Refried Potatoes	½ cup (4.5 oz)	150	1	3
Butterfield				
Diced	⅔ cup (5.7 oz)	100	0	0
Sliced	½ cup (5.7 oz)	100	0	0
Whole	2½ pieces (5.6 oz)	90	0	0
Del Monte				
New Sliced	⅔ cup (5.4 oz)	60	0	0
New Whole	⅔ cup (5.5 oz)	60	0	0
Hormel				
Au Gratin & Bacon	1 can (7.5 oz)	250	5	14
Seneca				
Potatoes	½ cup	80	0	0
Sunshine				
Whole	2½ pieces (5.6 oz)	90	0	0
FRESH				
baked w/ skin	1 (6.5 oz)	220	tr	tr
boiled	½ cup	68	tr	tr
microwaved	1 (7 oz)	212	tr	tr
microwaved w/o skin	½ cup	78	tr	tr
raw w/o skin	1 (3.9 oz)	88	tr	tr
PurelyIdaho				
Oven Roasts	1 serv (3 oz)	70	0	0
Yukon Gold				
Fresh	1 (5.3 oz)	110	—	0
FROZEN				
french fries	10 strips	111	2	4
french fries thick cut	10 strips	109	2	4
hashed brown	½ cup	170	4	9
potato puffs	½ cup	138	3	7
potato puffs as prep	1	16	tr	1
Birds Eye				
Whole	3 (2.6 oz)	50	0	0
Budget Gourmet				
Baked With Broccoli And Cheese	1 pkg (10.5 oz)	300	4	10
Cheddared Potatoes	1 pkg (5.5 oz)	260	—	16
Cheddared Potatoes With Broccoli	1 pkg (5 oz)	150	—	7
Three Cheese Potatoes	1 pkg (5.75 oz)	220	—	11
Empire				
Crinkle Cut French Fries	½ cup (3 oz)	90	1	2
Latkes Potato Pancakes	1 (2 oz)	80	2	2
Latkes Mini Potato Pancakes	2 (2 oz)	90	1	3

FOOD	PORTION	CALS.	SAT. FAT	FAT
Golden				
Potato Pancakes	1 (1.33 oz)	71	0	3
Healthy Choice				
Cheddar Broccoli Potatoes	1 meal (10.5 oz)	310	2	5
Garden Potato Casserole	1 meal (9.25 oz)	200	2	4
Kineret				
Crinkle Cut	18 pieces (3 oz)	120	1	4
Kugel	1 piece (2.5 oz)	150	2	10
Latkes	1 (1.5 oz)	90	—	5
Latkes Mini	10 (3 oz)	160	1	9
Lean Cuisine				
Deluxe Cheddar	1 pkg (10.4 oz)	270	4	7
Roasted Potatoes w/ Broccoli & Cheddar Cheese Sauce	1 pkg (10.25 oz)	260	4	6
MicroMagic				
French Fries Low Fat	1 pkg (3 oz)	130	1	3
Oh Boy!				
Stuffed With Cheddar Cheese	1 (6 oz)	130	—	4
Stuffed With Real Bacon	1 (6 oz)	120	—	3
Ore Ida				
Cheddar Browns	1 patty (3 oz)	90	1	3
Cottage Fries	14 pieces (3 oz)	130	1	4
Crispers!	17 pieces (3 oz)	220	2	13
Crispers! Nacho	10 pieces (3 oz)	170	3	9
Crispers! Texas	3 oz	170	3	10
Crispy Crowns!	12 pieces (3 oz)	100	2	11
Crispy Crunchies	12 pieces (3 oz)	160	2	9
Deep Fries Crinkle Cuts	18 pieces (3 oz)	160	1	7
Deep Fries French Fries	22 pieces (3 oz)	160	1	7
Dinner Fries Country Style	8 pieces (3 oz)	110	1	3
Fast Fries	23 pieces (3 oz)	140	2	6
Fast Fries Ranch	22 pieces (3 oz)	150	2	7
Golden Crinkles	16 pieces (3 oz)	120	1	4
Golden Fries	16 pieces (3 oz)	120	1	4
Golden Patties	1 (2.5 oz)	140	2	7
Golden Twirls	28 pieces (3 oz)	160	1	7
Hash Browns Country Style	1 cup (2.6 oz)	60	0	0
Hash Browns Shredded	1 patty (3 oz)	70	0	0
Hash Browns Southern Style	¾ cup (3 oz)	70	0	0
Hot Tots	9 pieces (3 oz)	150	1	6
Mashed Natural Butter	½ cup (2.1 oz)	80	1	2
Microwave Crinkle Cuts	1 pkg (3.5 oz)	180	2	8
Microwave Hash Browns	1 patty (2 oz)	110	2	6
Microwave Tater Tots	1 pkg (3.75 oz)	190	3	10
O'Brien Potatoes	¾ cup (3 oz)	60	0	0

FOOD	PORTION	CALS.	SAT. FAT	FAT
Ore Ida (CONT.)				
Pixie Crinkles	33 pieces (3 oz)	140	1	5
Shoestrings	38 pieces (3 oz)	150	1	5
Snackin' Fries	1 pkg (5 oz)	180	4	20
Snackin' Fries Extra Zesty	1 pkg (5 oz)	180	4	20
Tater ABC's	10 pieces (3 oz)	190	5	11
Tater Tots	9 pieces (3 oz)	160	2	8
Tater Tots Bacon	9 pieces (3 oz)	150	2	7
Tater Tots Onion	9 pieces (3 oz)	150	2	7
Toaster Hash Browns	2 patties (3.5 oz)	190	2	12
Topped Broccoli & Cheese	½ (6 oz)	150	2	4
Topped Salsa & Cheese	½ (5.5 oz)	160	2	5
Topped Vegetable Primavera	1 (6.13 oz)	160	2	5
Twice Baked Butter	1 (5 oz)	200	3	9
Twice Baked Cheddar Cheese	1 (5 oz)	190	3	8
Twice Baked Ranch	1 (5 oz)	180	2	6
Twice Bakes Sour Cream & Chives	1 (5 oz)	180	2	6
Waffle Fries	15 pieces (3 oz)	140	2	5
Wedges With Skin	9 pieces (3 oz)	110	1	3
Zesties!	12 pieces (3 oz)	160	2	9
Stouffer's				
Au Gratin	½ cup (5.75 oz)	130	3	6
Scalloped	½ cup (5.75 oz)	140	1	6
Weight Watchers				
Smart Ones Baked Broccoli & Cheese	1 pkg (10 oz)	250	4	6
HOME RECIPE				
au gratin	½ cup	160	6	9
mashed w/ whole milk & margarine	⅓ cup	66	tr	tr
scalloped	½ cup	105	3	5
MIX				
au gratin as prep	4½ oz	127	4	6
instant mashed flakes as prep w/ whole milk & butter	½ cup	118	4	6
instant mashed flakes not prep	½ cup	78	tr	tr
instant mashed granules as prep w/ whole milk & butter	½ cup	114	3	5
scalloped as prep	4½ oz	127	4	6
Barbara's				
Mashed not prep	⅓ cup (0.8 oz)	70	0	0
Betty Crocker				
Au Gratin Low Fat Recipe	½ cup	110	1	1

FOOD	PORTION	CALS.	SAT. FAT	FAT
Betty Crocker (CONT.)				
Au Gratin as prep	½ cup	150	2	6
Cheddar & Bacon	½ cup	150	2	6
Cheddar & Bacon Low Fat Recipe	½ cup	120	1	3
Cheddar & Sour Cream	½ cup	130	1	3
Chicken & Vegetable	⅔ cup	140	1	4
Chicken & Vegetable Low Fat Recipe	⅔ cup	120	1	3
Hash Browns	½ cup	190	2	8
Homestyle Broccoli Au Gratin	½ cup	140	2	6
Homestyle Broccoli Au Gratin Low Fat Recipe	½ cup	110	1	3
Homestyle Cheddar Cheese	½ cup	120	1	3
Homestyle Cheddar Cheese Stove Top Recipe	½ cup	140	2	5
Homestyle Cheesy Scalloped	½ cup	140	2	6
Homestyle Cheesy Scalloped Low Fat Recipe	½ cup	110	1	3
Julienne	½ cup	150	2	6
Mashed Butter & Herb	½ cup	160	3	8
Mashed Butter & Herb Reduced Fat Recipe	½ cup	130	2	5
Mashed Chicken & Herb	½ cup	150	2	7
Mashed Chicken & Herb Reduced Fat Recipe	½ cup	120	1	4
Mashed Four Cheese	½ cup	150	2	7
Mashed Four Cheese Reduced Fat Recipe	½ cup	120	1	4
Mashed Potato Buds	⅔ cup	160	2	8
Mashed Potato Buds Reduced Fat Recipe	⅔ cup	120	1	4
Mashed Roasted Garlic	½ cup	150	2	8
Mashed Roasted Garlic Reduced Fat Recipe	½ cup	130	1	5
Mashed Sour Cream & Chives	½ cup	150	2	7
Mashed Sour Cream & Chives Reduced Fat Recipe	½ cup	120	1	4
Potato Shakers Original	⅔ cup	140	1	4
Potato Shakers Original Low Fat Recipe	⅔ cup	120	0	2
Ranch	½ cup	160	2	6
Scalloped	½ cup	150	2	6
Scalloped Low Fat Recipe	⅔ cup	110	0	1

FOOD	PORTION	CALS.	SAT. FAT	FAT
Betty Crocker (CONT.)				
Sour Cream'n Chive	½ cup	160	2	7
Three Cheese	½ cup	150	2	6
Twice Baked Cheddar & Bacon Low Fat Recipe	⅔ cup	130	1	3
Twice Baked Cheddar & Bacon as prep	⅔ cup	210	3	11
Country Store				
Mashed not prep	⅓ cup	70	0	0
Hungry Jack				
Au Gratin as prep	½ cup	150	3	5
Cheddar & Bacon as prep	½ cup	150	3	5
Chessy Scalloped as prep	½ cup	150	3	5
Creamy Scalloped as prep	½ cup	150	3	5
Mashed Butter Flavored as prep	½ cup	150	2	7
Mashed Flakes as prep	½ cup	160	2	7
Mashed Garlic Flavored as prep	½ cup	150	2	7
Mashed Parsley Butter as prep	½ cup	150	2	7
Mashed Sour Cream 'n Chives as prep	½ cup	150	2	7
Sour Cream & Chives as prep	½ cup	160	4	6
Idaho				
Mashed Potato Flakes as prep	½ cup	150	2	6
Mashed Potato Granules as prep	½ cup	160	2	7
Shake 'N Bake				
Perfect Potatoes Crispy Cheddar	⅙ pkg (7 g)	30	2	2
Perfect Potatoes Herb & Garlic	⅙ pkg (7 g)	20	0	0
Perfect Potatoes Home Fries	⅙ pkg (7 g)	20	0	0
Perfect Potatoes Parmesan Peppercorn	⅙ pkg (7 g)	25	1	1
Perfect Potatoes Savory Onion	⅙ pkg (7 g)	20	0	0
REFRIGERATED				
Simply Potatoes				
Au Gratin	¼ pkg (3 oz)	130	—	8
Hash Browns	⅕ pkg (4 oz)	100	—	tr
Hash Browns Onion	⅕ pkg (4 oz)	120	—	tr
Hash Browns Southwest Style	⅕ pkg (4 oz)	100	—	tr
Mashed	⅕ pkg (4 oz)	90	—	2
Scalloped	¼ pkg (3 oz)	100	—	5

FOOD	PORTION	CALS.	SAT. FAT	FAT
SHELF-STABLE				
Lunch Bucket				
Scalloped w/ Ham Chunks	1 pkg (7.5 oz)	170	3	7
Micro Cup Meals				
Microcup Meals Scalloped Potatoes w/ Ham	1 cup (7.5 oz)	240	6	14
TAKE-OUT				
baked topped w/ cheese sauce	1	475	11	29
baked topped w/ cheese sauce & bacon	1	451	10	26
baked topped w/ cheese sauce & broccoli	1	402	9	14
baked topped w/ cheese sauce & chili	1	481	13	22
baked topped w/ sour cream & chives	1	394	10	22
french fries	1 reg	235	4	12
french fries	1 lg	355	6	19
hash brown	½ cup (2.5 oz)	151	4	9
indian yogurt potatoes	1 serv	315	4	9
mashed	½ cup	111	1	4
mustard potato salad	3.5 oz	120	0	6
o'brien	1 cup	157	2	3
potato pancakes	1 (1.3 oz)	101	1	7
potato salad	½ cup	179	2	10
potato salad w/ vegetables	3.5 oz	120	1	3

PRESERVE
(see JAM/JELLY/PRESERVE)

PRETZELS
(see also CHIPS, POPCORN, SNACKS)

FOOD	PORTION	CALS.	SAT. FAT	FAT
chocolate covered	1 (0.4 oz)	50	1	2
chocolate covered	1 oz	130	2	5
dutch twist	4 (2.1 oz)	229	tr	2
pretzels	1 oz	108	tr	1
rods	4 (2 oz)	229	tr	2
sticks	10	10	tr	tr
sticks	120 (2 oz)	229	tr	2
twist	1 (½ oz)	65	tr	1
twists	10 (2.1 oz)	229	tr	2
whole wheat	2 sm (1 oz)	103	tr	1
whole wheat	2 med (2 oz)	205	tr	2
Bachman				
Thin'n Right	12 (1 oz)	120	0	1

FOOD	PORTION	CALS.	SAT. FAT	FAT
Barrel O' Fun				
Mini	1 oz	110	0	1
Sticks	1 oz	110	0	1
Twists	1 oz	110	0	1
Estee				
Chocolate Covered	7	130	4	6
Dutch	2 (1.1 oz)	130	0	1
Unsalted	23 (1 oz)	120	0	1
Formagg				
Pretzel Nuts	1 oz	120	1	4
Gardetto's				
Mustard	1 pkg (0.5 oz)	50	0	1
Herr's				
Hard Sourdough	1 (1 oz)	100	0	0
Lance				
Pretzels	1 pkg (1.25 oz)	140	0	1
Little Debbie				
Mini Twists	1 pkg (1.2 oz)	140	0	1
Manischewitz				
Bagel Pretzels Original	4 (1 oz)	110	0	0
Mister Salty				
Chips	16 (1 oz)	110	0	3
Dutch	2 (1.1 oz)	120	0	1
Fat Free Chips	16 (1 oz)	100	0	0
Mini	22 (1 oz)	110	0	1
Sticks Fat Free	47 (1 oz)	110	0	0
Twist Fat Free	9 (1 oz)	110	0	0
Mr. Phipps				
Chips Lower Sodium	16 (1 oz)	120	0	3
Chips Original	16 (1 oz)	120	0	3
Chips Original Fat Free	16 (1 oz)	100	0	0
Nabisco				
Air Crisps Fat Free	23 pieces (1 oz)	110	0	0
Nestle				
Flipz Milk Chocolate Covered	9 pieces (1 oz)	130	4	5
Flipz White Fudge Covered	9 pieces (1 oz)	130	5	6
Newman's Own				
Salted Rounds Organic	1 pkg (1.4 oz)	150	0	2
Planters				
Twists	1 oz	100	0	1
Twists	1 pkg (1.5 oz)	160	0	1
Quinlan				
Beers	1 oz	110	1	2
Hard Sourdough	1 oz	110	1	2
Logs	1 oz	110	1	2

FOOD	PORTION	CALS.	SAT. FAT	FAT
Quinlan (CONT.)				
Nuggets	1 oz	110	1	2
Rods	1 oz	110	1	2
Sticks	1 oz	110	1	2
Thins	1 oz	110	1	2
Rold Gold				
Crispy's Thins	4 (1 oz)	110	0	2
Fat Free Cheddar Cheese	17 (1 oz)	110	0	0
Fat Free Honey Mustard	17 (1 oz)	110	0	0
Fat Free Sticks	48 (1 oz)	110	0	0
Fat Free Thins	12 pieces (1 oz)	110	0	0
Fat Free Tiny Twists	18 pieces (1 oz)	110	0	0
Honey Mustard	16 (1 oz)	110	0	1
Rods	3 (1 oz)	110	0	1
Sour Dough Nuggets	11 (1 oz)	110	0	0
Seyfart's				
Butter Rods	1 oz	110	—	1
Snyder's of Hanover				
Dips White Fudge	1 oz	130	4	6
Logs	1 oz	310	0	0
Minis	1 oz	310	0	0
Minis Unsalted	1 oz	310	0	0
Nibblers	1 oz	310	0	0
Oat Bran	1 oz	120	—	1
Old Fashioned Hard	1 oz	111	0	0
Old Fashioned Hard Unsalted	1 oz	100	0	0
Old Tyme	1 oz	310	0	0
Old Tyme Unsalted	1 oz	110	0	0
Rods	1 oz	310	0	0
Snaps	24 (1 oz)	120	0	1
Sourdough Hard Buttermilk Ranch	1 oz	130	1	5
Sourdough Hard Cheddar Cheese	1 oz	160	1	7
Sourdough Hard Honey Mustard & Onion	1 oz	130	1	5
Stix	1 oz	310	0	0
Very Thins	1 oz	310	0	0
Ultra Slim-Fast				
Lite N' Tasty	1 oz	100	—	tr
Utz				
Country Store Stix	5 (1 oz)	110	0	1
Fat Free Hard	1 (0.8 oz)	90	0	0
Fat Free Hard No Salt Added	1 (0.8 oz)	90	0	0
Fat Free Sour Dough Nuggets	10 (1 oz)	100	0	0

FOOD	PORTION	CALS.	SAT. FAT	FAT
Utz (CONT.)				
Fat Free Stix	14 (1 oz)	100	0	0
Fat Free Thin	10 (1 oz)	100	0	0
Honey Mustard & Onion	⅓ cup (1 oz)	130	1	6
Rods	3 (1 oz)	120	0	1
Specials	5 (1 oz)	110	0	1
Specials Extra Dark	5 (1 oz)	110	0	1
Specials Unsalted	5 (1 oz)	110	0	1
Wheels	20 (1 oz)	100	0	1
Weight Watchers				
Oat Bran Nuggets	1 pkg (1.5 oz)	170	0	3

PRICKLYPEAR
fresh	1	42	—	1

PRUNE JUICE
Del Monte				
Juice	8 fl oz	170	0	0

PRUNES
CANNED				
in heavy syrup	5	90	tr	tr
in heavy syrup	1 cup	245	tr	tr
DRIED				
cooked w/ sugar	½ cup	147	tr	tr
cooked w/o sugar	½ cup	113	tr	tr
dried	10	201	tr	tr
Del Monte				
Pitted	¼ cup (1.4 oz)	120	0	0
Unpitted	⅓ cup (1.4 oz)	110	0	0
Mariani				
Pitted	¼ cup	140	—	1
Whole	¼ cup	140	—	1
Sonoma				
Pitted	¼ cup (1.4 oz)	120	0	0
Sunsweet				
Orange Essence Pitted Prunes	6 (1.4 oz)	100	0	0

PUDDING
(see also CUSTARD, PUDDING POPS)

HOME RECIPE				
bread pudding	1 recipe 6 serv (26.4 oz)	1266	17	44
chocolate as prep w/ whole milk	½ cup (5.5 oz)	221	3	6
cornstarch	½ cup (4.4 oz)	137	3	5
rice	½ cup (5.3 oz)	217	3	4

FOOD	PORTION	CALS.	SAT. FAT	FAT
MIX				
banana as prep w/ 2% milk	½ cup (4.9 oz)	142	1	2
banana as prep w/ whole milk	½ cup (4.9 oz)	157	3	4
chocolate as prep w/ 2% milk	½ cup (5 oz)	150	2	3
chocolate as prep w/ whole milk	½ cup (5 oz)	158	3	5
coconut cream as prep w/ 2% milk	½ cup (4.9 oz)	148	3	4
coconut cream as prep w/ whole milk	½ cup (4.9 oz)	160	3	4
instant banana as prep w/ 2% milk	½ cup (5.2 oz)	152	1	3
instant banana as prep w/ whole milk	½ cup (5.2 oz)	167	3	4
instant chocolate as prep w/ 2% milk	½ cup (5.2 oz)	149	2	3
instant chocolate as prep w/ whole milk	½ cup (5.2 oz)	164	3	5
instant coconut cream as prep w/ 2% milk	½ cup (5.2 oz)	157	2	3
instant coconut cream as prep w/ whole milk	½ cup (5.2 oz)	172	3	5
instant lemon as prep w/ 2% milk	½ cup (5.2 oz)	155	1	4
instant lemon as prep w/ whole milk	½ cup (5.2 oz)	169	3	4
instant vanilla as prep w/ 2% milk	½ cup (5 oz)	147	1	2
instant vanilla as prep w/ whole milk	½ cup (5 oz)	181	2	4
lemon	½ cup (5.1 oz)	163	1	2
rice as prep w/ 2% milk	½ cup (5.1 oz)	161	1	2
rice as prep w/ whole milk	½ cup (5.1 oz)	175	3	4
tapioca as prep w/ 2% milk	½ cup (5 oz)	147	1	2
tapioca as prep w/ whole milk	½ cup (5 oz)	161	3	4
vanilla as prep w/ 2% milk	½ cup (4.9 oz)	141	1	2
vanilla as prep w/ whole milk	½ cup (4.9 oz)	155	3	4
Emes				
Dietetic as prep w/ skim milk	½ cup (4 fl oz)	71	—	1
Jell-O				
Americana Rice as prep w/ skim milk	½ cup (5.2 oz)	140	0	0
Americana Tapioca as prep w/ skim milk	½ cup (5.1 oz)	130	0	0
Banana Cream as prep w/ 2% milk	½ cup (5.1 oz)	140	2	3
Butterscotch as prep w/ 2% milk	½ cup (5.2 oz)	160	2	3
Chocolate as prep w/ 2% milk	½ cup (5.2 oz)	150	2	3

FOOD	PORTION	CALS.	SAT. FAT	FAT
Jell-O (CONT.)				
Chocolate Fudge as prep w/ 2% milk	½ cup (5.2 oz)	150	2	3
Coconut Cream as prep w/ 2% milk	½ cup (5.1 oz)	150	4	5
Fat Free Chocolate as prep w/ skim milk	½ cup (5.2 oz)	130	0	0
Fat Free Vanilla as prep w/ skim milk	½ cup (5.1 oz)	130	0	0
Instant Banana Cream as prep w/ 2% milk	½ cup (5.2 oz)	150	2	3
Instant Butterscotch as prep w/ 2% milk	½ cup (5.2 oz)	150	2	3
Instant Chocolate as prep w/ 2% milk	½ cup (5.2 oz)	160	2	3
Instant Chocolate Fudge as prep w/ 2% milk	½ cup (4.2 oz)	160	2	3
Instant Coconut Cream as prep w/ 2% milk	½ cup (4.2 oz)	160	4	5
Instant French Vanilla as prep w/ 2% milk	½ cup (4.2 oz)	150	2	3
Instant Lemon as prep w/ 2% milk	½ cup (4.2 oz)	150	2	3
Instant Pistachio as prep w/ 2% milk	½ cup (4.2 oz)	160	2	3
Instant Vanilla as prep w/ 2% milk	½ cup (4.2 oz)	150	2	3
Instant Fat Free Chocolate as prep w/ skim milk	½ cup (5.3 oz)	140	0	0
Instant Fat Free Devil's Food as prep w/ skim milk	½ cup (5.3 oz)	140	0	0
Instant Fat Free Sugar Free Banana as prep w/ skim milk	½ cup (4.6 oz)	70	0	0
Instant Fat Free Sugar Free Butterscotch as prep w/ skim milk	½ cup (4.6 oz)	70	0	0
Instant Fat Free Sugar Free Chocolate Fudge as prep w/ skim milk	½ cup (4.7 oz)	80	0	0
Instant Fat Free Sugar Free Chocolate as prep w/ skim milk	½ cup (4.6 oz)	80	0	0
Instant Fat Free Sugar Free Vanilla as prep w/ skim milk	½ cup (4.6 oz)	70	0	0

FOOD	PORTION	CALS.	SAT. FAT	FAT
Jell-O (CONT.)				
Instant Fat Free Sugar Free White Chocolate as prep w/ skim milk	½ cup (4.6 oz)	70	0	0
Instant Fat Free Vanilla as prep w/ skim milk	½ cup (5.2 oz)	140	0	0
Instant Fat Free White Chocolate as prep w/ skim milk	½ cup (5.2 oz)	140	0	0
Lemon as prep	½ cup (4.4 oz)	140	1	2
Milk Chocolate as prep w/ 2% milk	½ cup (5.2 oz)	150	2	3
Sugar Free Chocolate as prep w/ 2% milk	½ cup (4.6 oz)	90	2	3
Sugar Free Vanilla as prep w/ 2% milk	½ cup (4.5 oz)	80	2	3
Vanilla as prep w/ 2% milk	½ cup (5.1 oz)	140	2	3
Louisiana Purchase				
Bread	1 serv (1.3 oz)	150	3	3
My*T*Fine				
Butterscotch	mix for 1 serv	90	0	0
Chocolate	mix for 1 serv	100	0	0
Chocolate Almond	mix for 1 serv	100	0	1
Chocolate Fudge	mix for 1 serv	100	0	0
Lemon	mix for 1 serv	90	0	0
Vanilla	mix for 1 serv	90	0	0
Vanilla Tapioca	mix for 1 serv	80	0	0
Royal				
Banana Cream	mix for 1 serv	80	0	0
Banana Cream Instant	mix for 1 serv	90	0	0
Butterscotch	mix for 1 serv	90	0	0
Butterscotch Instant	mix for 1 serv	90	0	0
Cherry Vanilla Instant	mix for 1 serv	90	0	0
Chocolate	mix for 1 serv	90	0	0
Chocolate Almond Instant	mix for 1 serv	120	—	1
Chocolate Chocolate Chip Instant	mix for 1 serv	110	0	1
Chocolate Instant	mix for 1 serv	110	0	0
Chocolate Peanut Butter Instant	mix for 1 serv	110	0	1
Chocolate Sugar Free Instant	mix for 1 serv	50	—	0
Dark 'n Sweet Chocolate	mix for 1 serv	90	0	0
Dark'N Sweet Instant	mix for 1 serv	110	0	0
Lemon Instant	mix for 1 serv	90	0	0

FOOD	PORTION	CALS.	SAT. FAT	FAT
Royal (CONT.)				
Pistachio Instant	mix for 1 serv	90	0	1
Strawberry Instant	mix for 1 serv	100	0	0
Toasted Coconut Instant	mix for 1 serv	100	—	2
Vanilla	mix for 1 serv	80	0	0
Vanilla Chocolate Chip Instant	mix for 1 serv	90	0	1
Vanilla Instant	mix for 1 serv	90	0	0
READY-TO-EAT				
banana	1 pkg (5 oz)	180	1	5
chocolate	1 pkg (5 oz)	189	1	6
lemon	1 pkg (5 oz)	177	1	4
rice	1 pkg (5 oz)	231	2	11
tapioca	1 pkg (5 oz)	169	1	5
vanilla	1 pkg (4 oz)	146	1	4
Del Monte				
Snack Cups Banana	1 serv (4 oz)	140	1	4
Snack Cups Butterscotch	1 serv (4 oz)	140	1	4
Snack Cups Chocolate	1 serv (4 oz)	160	1	4
Snack Cups Chocolate Fudge	1 serv (4 oz)	150	1	4
Snack Cups Chocolate Peanut Butter	1 serv (4 oz)	160	1	4
Snack Cups Lite Chocolate	1 serv (4 oz)	100	0	1
Snack Cups Lite Vanilla	1 serv (4 oz)	90	0	1
Snack Cups Tapioca	1 serv (4 oz)	140	1	4
Snack Cups Vanilla	1 serv (4 oz)	150	1	4
Handi-Snacks				
Banana	1 serv (3.5 oz)	120	1	4
Butterscotch	1 serv (3.5 oz)	120	1	4
Chocolate	1 serv (3.5 oz)	130	1	4
Chocolate Fudge	1 serv (3.5 oz)	130	1	4
Fat Free Chocolate	1 serv (3.5 oz)	90	0	0
Fat Free Vanilla	1 serv (3.5 oz)	90	0	0
Tapioca	1 serv (3.5 oz)	120	1	4
Vanilla	1 serv (3.5 oz)	120	1	4
Hunt's				
Snack Pack Banana	1 (4 oz)	158	2	6
Snack Pack Butterscotch	1 (4 oz)	153	2	6
Snack Pack Chocolate	1 (4 oz)	167	2	6
Snack Pack Chocolate Fudge	1 (4 oz)	167	1	6
Snack Pack Chocolate Marshmallow	1 (4 oz)	155	2	6
Snack Pack Fat Free Chocolate	1 (4 oz)	96	0	tr
Snack Pack Fat Free Tapioca	1 (4 oz)	95	0	tr
Snack Pack Fat Free Vanilla	1 (4 oz)	93	0	tr

FOOD	PORTION	CALS.	SAT. FAT	FAT
Hunt's (CONT.)				
Snack Pack Lemon	1 (4 oz)	162	1	3
Snack Pack Swirl Chocolate Caramel	1 (4 oz)	168	1	6
Snack Pack Swirl Chocolate Peanut Butter	1 (4 oz)	166	2	6
Snack Pack Swirl Milk Chocolate	1 (4 oz)	164	1	6
Snack Pack Swirl Smores	1 (4 oz)	154	2	6
Snack Pack Tapioca	1 (4 oz)	151	1	6
Snack Pack Vanilla	1 (4 oz)	163	1	6
Imagine Foods				
Lemon Dream	1 (4 oz)	120	0	0
Jell-O				
Chocolate	1 serv (4 oz)	160	2	5
Chocolate Marshmallow	1 serv (4 oz)	160	2	5
Chocolate Vanilla Swirls	1 serv (4 oz)	160	2	5
Free Chocolate	1 serv (4 oz)	100	0	0
Free Chocolate Vanilla Swirl	1 serv (4 oz)	100	0	0
Free Devil's Food	1 serv (4 oz)	100	0	0
Free Rocky Road	1 serv (4 oz)	100	0	0
Free Vanilla	1 serv (4 oz)	100	0	0
Tapioca	1 serv (4 oz)	140	2	4
Tapioca	1 serv (4 oz)	100	0	0
Vanilla	1 serv (4 oz)	160	2	5
Kozy Shack				
Banana	1 pkg (4 oz)	130	2	3
Chocolate	1 pkg (4 oz)	140	2	4
Light Chocolate	1 pkg (4 oz)	110	1	1
Light Vanilla	1 pkg (4 oz)	110	0	1
Rice	1 pkg (4 oz)	130	2	3
Tapioca	1 pkg (4 oz)	140	2	3
Vanilla	1 pkg (4 oz)	130	2	3
NutraBalance				
Low Lactose All Flavors	1 serv (4 oz)	225	—	8
Snack Pack				
Banana	4.25 oz	145	1	6
Butterscotch	4.25 oz	170	1	6
Chocolate	4.25 oz	170	1	6
Chocolate Marshmallow	4.25 oz	165	1	6
Chocolate Fudge	4.25 oz	165	1	6
Lemon	4.25 oz	150	1	4
Light Chocolate	4.25 oz	100	tr	2
Light Tapioca	4.25 oz	100	tr	2

FOOD	PORTION	CALS.	SAT. FAT	FAT
Snack Pack (CONT.)				
Tapioca	4.25 oz	150	1	5
Vanilla	4.25 oz	170	1	6
Swiss Miss				
Butterscotch	4 oz	180	1	6
Chocolate	4 oz	180	1	6
Chocolate Fudge	4 oz	220	2	6
Chocolate Sundae	4 oz	220	2	7
Fat Free Vanilla	1 serv (3.5 oz)	90	0	0
Light Chocolate	4 oz	100	tr	1
Light Chocolate Fudge	4 oz	100	tr	1
Light Vanilla Chocolate Parfait	4 oz	100	tr	1
Tapioca	4 oz	160	1	5
Vanilla	4 oz	190	1	7
Vanilla Parfait	4 oz	180	1	6
Vanilla Sundae	4 oz	200	2	7
Ultra Slim-Fast				
Butterscotch	4 oz	100	—	tr
Chocolate	4 oz	100	—	tr
Vanilla	4 oz	100	—	tr
TAKE-OUT				
bread pudding	½ cup (4.4 oz)	212	3	7
chocolate	½ cup (5.5 oz)	206	2	4
tapioca	½ cup (5.3 oz)	189	—	7
vanilla	½ cup (4.3 oz)	130	3	4

PUDDING POPS

(*see also* ICE CREAM AND FROZEN DESSERTS, YOGURT FROZEN)

chocolate	1 (1.6 oz)	72	—	2
vanilla	1 (1.6 oz)	75	—	2

PUMMELO

fresh	1	228	—	tr
sections	1 cup	71	—	tr

PUMPKIN

CANNED

pumpkin	½ cup	41	tr	tr
Libby				
Solid Pack	½ cup	60	—	1
Owatonna				
Pumpkin	½ cup	40	—	1
FRESH				
cooked mashed	½ cup	24	tr	tr
flowers cooked	½ cup	10	tr	tr
flowers raw	1	0	0	0

FOOD	PORTION	CALS.	SAT. FAT	FAT
leaves cooked	½ cup	7	tr	tr
leaves raw	½ cup	4	tr	tr
raw cubed	½ cup	15	tr	tr
SEEDS				
dried	1 oz	154	2	13
roasted	1 oz	148	2	12
roasted	1 cup	1184	18	96
salted & roasted	1 oz	148	2	12
salted & roasted	1 cup	1184	18	96
whole roasted	1 oz	127	1	6
whole roasted	1 cup	285	2	12
whole salted roasted	1 oz	127	1	6
whole salted roasted	1 cup	285	2	12
PURSLANE				
cooked	1 cup	21	—	tr
raw	1 cup	7	—	tr
QUAHOGS				
(see CLAM)				
QUAIL				
breast w/o skin raw	1 (2 oz)	69	tr	2
w/ skin raw	1 quail (3.8 oz)	210	4	13
w/o skin raw	1 quail (3.2 oz)	123	1	4
QUICHE				
TAKE-OUT				
lorraine	⅛ of 8 in pie	600	23	48
QUINCE				
fresh	1	53	tr	tr
QUINOA				
quinoa not prep	1 cup (6 oz)	636	1	10
Arrowhead				
Quinoa	¼ cup (1.4 oz)	140	0	2
Eden				
Not Prep	¼ cup (1.6 oz)	170	0	3
RABBIT				
domestic w/o bone roasted	3 oz	167	2	7
wild w/o bone stewed	3 oz	147	1	3
RACCOON				
roasted	3 oz	217	—	12
RADICCHIO				
leaf	3.5 oz	18	tr	tr
raw shredded	½ cup	5	—	tr

FOOD	PORTION	CALS.	SAT. FAT	FAT
RADISHES				
DRIED				
chinese	½ cup	157	tr	tr
daikon	½ cup	157	tr	tr
FRESH				
chinese raw	1 (12 oz)	62	tr	tr
chinese raw sliced	½ cup	8	tr	tr
chinese sliced cooked	½ cup	13	tr	tr
daikon raw	1 (12 oz)	62	tr	tr
daikon raw sliced	½ cup	8	tr	tr
daikon sliced cooked	½ cup	13	tr	tr
red raw	10	7	tr	tr
red sliced	½ cup	10	tr	tr
white icicle raw	1 (½ oz)	2	tr	tr
Dole				
Radishes	7	20	—	0
TAKE-OUT				
moo namul saengche korean salad	1 serv (3.7 oz)	34	tr	tr
RAISINS				
chocolate coated	10 (0.4 oz)	39	1	2
chocolate coated	1 cup (6.7 oz)	741	17	28
seedless	1 tbsp	27	tr	tr
Cinderella				
Seedless	½ cup	250	—	0
Del Monte				
Golden	¼ cup (1.4 oz)	130	0	0
Raisins	1 box (1.5 oz)	140	0	0
Raisins	1 box (1 oz)	90	0	0
Raisins	1 box (0.5 oz)	45	0	0
Raisins	¼ cup (1.4 oz)	130	0	0
Yogurt Raisins Strawberry	1 pkg (0.9 oz)	110	3	3
Yogurt Raisins Vanilla	1 pkg (0.9 oz)	110	3	3
Yogurt Raisins Vanilla	1 pkg (1 oz)	120	3	3
Yogurt Raisins Vanilla	3 tbsp (1 oz)	130	3	3
Dole				
CinnaRaisins	1 pkg (1 oz)	95	0	0
Golden	½ cup	250	0	0
Seedless	½ cup	250	0	0
Estee				
Chocolate Covered	¼ cup	180	5	6
Sonoma				
Monukka Thompson	¼ cup (1.4 oz)	130	0	0

FOOD	PORTION	CALS.	SAT. FAT	FAT
Tree Of Life				
Organic	¼ cup (1.4 oz)	130	0	0
RASPBERRIES				
CANNED				
in heavy syrup	½ cup	117	tr	tr
FRESH				
raspberries	1 cup	61	tr	1
raspberries	1 pint	154	tr	2
Dole				
Raspberries	1 cup	45	—	0
FROZEN				
sweetened	1 cup	256	tr	tr
sweetened	1 pkg (10 oz)	291	tr	tr
Big Valley				
Raspberries	⅔ cup (4.9 oz)	80	0	0
Birds Eye				
Red	½ cup (4.4 oz)	90	0	0
RASPBERRY JUICE				
Crystal Geyser				
Juice Squeeze Mountain Raspberry	1 bottle (12 fl oz)	135	0	0
Crystal Light				
Raspberry Ice Drink	1 serv (8 oz)	5	0	0
Raspberry Ice Drink Mix as prep	1 serv (8 oz)	5	0	0
Dole				
Country Raspberry	8 fl oz	140	0	0
Fresh Samantha				
Raspberry Dream Smoothie	1 cup (8 oz)	120	0	1
Kool-Aid				
Drink Mix as prep	1 serv (8 oz)	60	0	0
Raspberry Drink as prep w/ sugar	1 serv (8 oz)	100	0	0
Splash Blue Raspberry Drink	1 serv (8 oz)	120	0	0
RED BEANS				
CANNED				
Allen				
Red Beans	½ cup (4.5 oz)	160	0	1
Green Giant				
Red Beans	½ cup (4.5 oz)	100	0	1
Hunt's				
Small	½ cup (4.5 oz)	89	0	1

FOOD	PORTION	CALS.	SAT. FAT	FAT
Van Camp's				
Red Beans	½ cup (4.6 oz)	90	0	0
DRIED				
Bean Cuisine				
Dried	½ cup	115	—	1
MIX				
Pasta & Beans Barcelona Red With Radiatore	½ cup	170	1	4
Mahatma				
Red Beans & Rice	1 cup	190	0	1

RED KIDNEY BEANS
DRIED
Hurst

FOOD	PORTION	CALS.	SAT. FAT	FAT
HamBeens w/ Ham	1 serv	120	0	1

RELISH

FOOD	PORTION	CALS.	SAT. FAT	FAT
cranberry orange	½ cup	246	—	tr
piccalilli	1.4 oz	13	—	tr
Claussen				
Pickle Relish	1 tbsp	14	—	tr
Del Monte				
Hamburger	1 tbsp (0.5 oz)	20	0	0
Hot Dog	1 tbsp (0.5 oz)	15	0	0
Sweet Pickle	1 tbsp (0.5 oz)	20	0	0
Green Giant				
Corn	1 tbsp (0.6 oz)	20	0	0
Old El Paso				
Jalapeno	1 tbsp (0.5 oz)	5	0	0
Vlasic				
Dill	1 oz	2	0	0
Hamburger	1 oz	40	0	0
Hot Dog	1 oz	40	—	1
Hot Piccalilli	1 oz	35	0	0
India	1 oz	30	0	0
Sweet	1 oz	30	0	0

RENNIN

FOOD	PORTION	CALS.	SAT. FAT	FAT
tablet	1 (0.9 g)	1	—	0

RHUBARB

FOOD	PORTION	CALS.	SAT. FAT	FAT
fresh	½ cup	13	—	tr
frzn	½ cup	60	—	tr
frzn as prep w/ sugar	½ cup	139	—	tr

RICE
(see also BRAN, CEREAL, FLOUR, RICE CAKES, WILD RICE)

FOOD	PORTION	CALS.	SAT. FAT	FAT
brown long grain cooked	1 cup (6.8 oz)	216	tr	2
brown medium grain cooked	1 cup (6.8 oz)	218	tr	2
glutinous cooked	1 cup (6.1 oz)	169	tr	tr
white long grain cooked	1 cup (5.5 oz)	205	tr	tr
white long grain instant cooked	1 cup (5.8 oz)	162	tr	tr
white medium grain cooked	1 cup (6.5 oz)	242	tr	tr
white short grain cooked	1 cup (6.5 oz)	242	tr	tr
Arrowhead				
Basmati Brown	¼ cup (1.5 oz)	150	0	1
Basmati White	¼ cup (1.5 oz)	150	0	0
Brown Quick Regular	⅓ cup (1.5 oz)	150	0	1
Brown Quick Spanish Style	¼ pkg (1.4 oz)	150	0	1
Brown Quick Vegetable Herb	¼ pkg (1.4 oz)	150	0	1
Brown Quick Wild Rice & Herb	¼ pkg (1.3 oz)	140	0	1
Birds Eye				
Rice & Broccoli In Cheese Sauce	1 pkg (10 oz)	290	3	9
White & Wild	1 cup (6.6 oz)	180	2	4
Budget Gourmet				
Oriental Rice With Vegetables	1 pkg (5.75 oz)	230	—	12
Rice Pilaf With Green Beans	1 pkg (5.5 oz)	230	—	11
Carolina				
Red Beans & Rice as prep	¼ pkg	190	0	1
Casbah				
Basmati as prep	1 cup	158	—	tr
Jambalaya	1 pkg (1.4 oz)	130	0	0
La Fiesta	1 pkg (1.59 oz)	170	0	1
Nutted Pilaf as prep	1 cup	220	0	3
Pilaf as prep	1 cup	200	0	tr
Spanish Pilaf as prep	1 cup	200	0	1
Thai Yum	1 pkg (1.7 oz)	180	0	3
Chun King				
Fried Rice	1 pkg (8 oz)	290	2	6
Fried Rice With Chicken	1 pkg (8 oz)	270	2	6
Goodman's				
Rice & Vermicelli For Beef	¾ cup	160	0	1
Rice & Vermicelli For Chicken	¾ cup	160	0	1
Goya				
Arroz Amarillo	¼ cup (1.6 oz)	170	0	0
Green Giant				
Rice & Broccoli	1 pkg (10 oz)	320	4	12
Rice Medley	1 pkg (10 oz)	240	2	3
Rice Pilaf	1 pkg (10 oz)	230	2	3
White & Wild	1 pkg (10 oz)	250	1	5

FOOD	PORTION	CALS.	SAT. FAT	FAT
Hain				
Almondine	½ cup	130	—	5
Oriental 3-Grain Goodness	½ cup	120	—	5
Kikkoman				
Fried Rice Seasoning Mix	1 oz pkg	91	—	tr
Kitchen Del Sol				
Mediterranean Paella Costa Brave as prep	½ cup (1.2 oz)	130	tr	2
Mediterranean Sunny Lemon Pilaf as prep	½ cup (1.2 oz)	110	0	1
Mediterranean Tomato & Basil With Pine Nuts	½ cup (1 oz)	110	1	4
Lipton				
Golden Saute Onion Mushroom	½ cup (2.1 oz)	240	2	4
Oriental Stir Fry as prep	1 cup	270	1	8
Rice & Sauce Alfredo Broccoli as prep	1 cup	320	5	12
Rice & Sauce Beef as prep	1 cup	270	1	8
Rice & Sauce Cajun Style as prep	1 cup	270	1	7
Rice & Sauce Cajun Style w/ Beans as prep	1 cup	310	1	8
Rice & Sauce Cheddar Broccoli as prep	1 cup	280	3	9
Rice & Sauce Chicken & Parmesan Risotto as prep	1 cup	270	2	9
Rice & Sauce Chicken Broccoli as prep	1 cup	280	2	9
Rice & Sauce Chicken Flavor as prep	1 cup	280	2	9
Rice & Sauce Creamy Chicken as prep	1 cup	290	3	11
Rice & Sauce Herb & Butter as prep	1 cup	280	4	11
Rice & Sauce Medley as prep	1 cup	270	2	9
Rice & Sauce Mushroom as prep	1 cup	270	1	8
Rice & Sauce Mushroom & Herb as prep	1 cup	290	2	8
Rice & Sauce Oriental as prep	1 cup	280	1	8
Rice & Sauce Pilaf as prep	1 cup	260	1	11
Rice & Sauce Scampi Style as prep	1 cup	270	2	9
Rice & Sauce Spanish as prep	1 cup	270	1	8

FOOD	PORTION	CALS.	SAT. FAT	FAT
Lipton (CONT.)				
Rice & Sauce Teriyaki as prep	1 cup	270	1	8
Roasted Chicken as prep	1 cup	260	1	8
Salsa Style as prep	1 cup	220	1	7
Southwestern Chicken Flavor as prep	1 cup	260	1	11
Luigino's				
Fried Rice Chicken	1 pkg (8 oz)	250	2	5
Fried Rice Pork	1 pkg (8 oz)	250	3	7
Fried Rice Pork & Shrimp	1 pkg (8 oz)	250	2	5
Fried Rice Shrimp	1 pkg (8 oz)	220	2	4
Risotto Parmesano	1 pkg (8 oz)	360	6	20
Mahatma				
Broccoli & Cheese	1 cup	200	1	2
Jambalaya	1 cup (2 oz)	190	0	1
Long Grain & Wild	1 cup (2 oz)	190	0	1
Pilaf	1 cup (2 oz)	190	0	0
Spanish	1 cup (2 oz)	180	0	1
Yellow Rice Mix	1 cup	190	0	0
Melting Pot				
Risotto Melanese w/ Saffron	1 cup	210	0	0
Risotto Primavera	1 cup	200	0	1
Risotto Sun-Dried Tomatoes & Peas	1 cup	200	0	1
Risotto Three Cheese	1 cup	200	1	2
Risotto Wild Mushroom	1 cup	200	0	1
Minute				
Boil-In-Bag White as prep	1 cup (5.7 oz)	190	0	0
Instant Brown as prep	1 cup (5.2 oz)	170	0	2
Instant White as prep	1 cup (5.7 oz)	160	0	0
Long Grain & Wild Seasoned w/ Herbs as prep	1 cup (7.8 oz)	230	0	1
Near East				
Barley Pilaf as prep	1 cup	220	1	4
Beef Pilaf as prep	1 cup	220	1	5
Curry Rice as prep	1 cup	220	1	4
Lentil Pilaf as prep	1 cup	210	1	4
Long Grain & Wild as prep	1 cup	220	1	5
Pilaf Brown Rice as prep	1 cup	220	1	5
Pilaf Chicken as prep	1 cup	220	1	5
Pilaf Kosher as prep	1 cup	220	1	5
Spanish Pilaf as prep	1 cup	230	1	6
Old El Paso				
Mexican	½ cup (4 oz)	410	1	2
Spanish	1 cup (8.6 oz)	130	—	1

FOOD	PORTION	CALS.	SAT. FAT	FAT
Pritikin				
Mexican	⅓ cup (2 oz)	200	0	2
Oriental	⅓ cup (2 oz)	190	0	2
Success				
Beef Oriental	½ cup	190	0	1
Broccoli & Cheese	½ cup	200	1	2
Brown & Wild	½ cup	190	0	1
Classic Chicken	½ cup	150	0	1
Long Grain & Wild	½ cup	190	0	0
Pilaf	½ cup	200	0	0
Spanish	½ cup	190	0	1
Ultra Slim-Fast				
Oriental Style	2.3 oz	240	—	1
Rice & Chicken Sauce	2.3 oz	240	—	1
Uncle Ben				
Boil-In-Bag	1 serv (0.9 oz)	94	—	tr
Brown	1 serv (1.6 oz)	158	—	1
Brown & Wild Fast Cooking	1 serv (1.3 oz)	120	—	1
Country Inn Broccoli Almondine	1 serv (1.2 oz)	124	—	2
Country Inn Broccoli & White Cheddar	1 serv (1.2 oz)	131	—	3
Country Inn Broccoli Au Gratin	1 serv (1.1 oz)	116	—	2
Country Inn Chicken Stock	1 serv (1.2 oz)	123	—	1
Country Inn Chicken With Wild Rice	1 serv (1.1 oz)	108	—	1
Country Inn Creamy Chicken & Mushroom	1 serv (1.3 oz)	138	—	3
Country Inn Creamy Chicken & Wild Rice	1 serv (1.3 oz)	135	—	1
Country Inn Green Bean Almondine	1 serv (1.2 oz)	128	—	2
Country Inn Herbed Au Gratin	1 serv (1.2 oz)	119	—	2
Country Inn Homestyle Chicken & Vegetables	1 serv (1.3 oz)	139	—	3
Country Inn Rice Florentine	1 serv (1.2 oz)	212	—	2
Country Inn Vegetable Pilaf	1 serv (1.2 oz)	115	—	1
In An Instant	1 serv (1.1 oz)	111	—	tr
Long Grain & Wild Chicken Stock Sauce	1 serv (1.3 oz)	133	—	2
Long Grain & Wild Fast Cooking	1 serv (1 oz)	101	—	tr
Long Grain & Wild Garden Vegetable Blend	1 serv (1.3 oz)	128	—	1
Long Grain & Wild Original	1 serv (1 oz)	96	—	tr
White Converted	1 serv (1.2 oz)	123	—	tr

FOOD	PORTION	CALS.	SAT. FAT	FAT
Van Camp's				
Spanish	1 cup (9 oz)	180	1	3
Watkins				
Brown & Wild	¼ cup (1.6 oz)	160	0	0
Calico Medley	¼ cup (1.6 oz)	160	0	0
East/West Medley	¼ cup (1.6 oz)	160	0	0
Heartland Medley	¼ cup (1.6 oz)	160	0	0
Minnesota Medley	¼ cup (1.6 oz)	160	0	0
White & Wild	¼ cup (1.6 oz)	160	0	0
TAKE-OUT				
nasi goreng indonesian rice & vegetables	1 cup (4.9 oz)	130	0	0
paella	1 serv (7 oz)	308	3	16

RICE CAKES
(see also POPCORN CAKES*)*

FOOD	PORTION	CALS.	SAT. FAT	FAT
brown rice	1 (0.3 oz)	35	tr	tr
brown rice & buckwheat	1 (0.3 oz)	34	tr	tr
brown rice & buckwheat unsalted	1 (0.3 oz)	34	tr	tr
brown rice & corn	1 (0.3 oz)	35	tr	tr
brown rice & rye	1 (0.3 oz)	35	tr	tr
brown rice & sesame seed	1 (0.3 oz)	35	tr	tr
brown rice multigrain	1 (0.3 oz)	35	tr	tr
brown rice multigrain unsalted	1 (0.3 oz)	35	tr	tr
brown rice unsalted	1 (0.3 oz)	35	tr	tr
Estee				
Banana Nut	5	60	0	1
Cinnamon Spice	5	60	0	0
Granny Smith Apple	5	60	0	0
Mixed Berry	5	60	0	0
Peanut Butter Crunch	5	60	0	0
Hain				
5-Grain	1	40	—	tr
Mini Apple Cinnamon	½ oz	60	—	tr
Mini Barbeque	½ oz	70	—	3
Mini Cheese	½ oz	60	—	2
Mini Honey Nut	½ oz	60	—	tr
Mini Nacho Cheese	½ oz	70	—	2
Mini Plain	½ oz	60	—	tr
Mini Plain No Salt Added	½ oz	60	—	tr
Mini Ranch	½ oz	70	—	3
Mini Teriyaki	½ oz	50	—	tr
Plain	1	40	—	tr
Plain No Salt Added	1	40	—	tr
Sesame	1	40	—	tr
Sesame No Salt	1	40	—	tr

FOOD	PORTION	CALS.	SAT. FAT	FAT
Lundberg				
Organic Lightly Salted	1	60	—	1
Organic Unsalted	1	60	—	1
Premium Lightly Salted	1	60	—	1
Premium Unsalted	1	60	—	1
Sesame Lightly Salted	1	59	0	0
Mother's				
Mini Apple	5 (0.5 oz)	50	0	0
Mini Caramel	5 (0.5 oz)	50	0	0
Mini Cinnamon	5 (0.5 oz)	50	0	0
Mini Plain Unsalted	7 (0.5 oz)	60	0	0
Multigrain Lightly Salted	1 (0.3 oz)	35	0	0
Rye Unsalted	1 (0.3 oz)	35	0	0
Wheat Unsalted	1 (0.3 oz)	35	0	0
Pritikin				
Mini Apple Crisp	5 (0.5 oz)	50	0	0
Multigrain	1 (0.3 oz)	35	0	0
Multigrain Unsalted	1 (0.3 oz)	35	0	0
Plain	1 (0.3 oz)	35	0	0
Plain Unsalted	1 (0.3 oz)	35	0	0
Sesame Low Sodium	1 (0.3 oz)	35	0	0
Sesame Unsalted	1 (0.3 oz)	35	0	0
Quaker				
Apple Cinnamon	1 (0.5 oz)	50	0	0
Banana Crunch	1 (0.5 oz)	50	0	0
Cinnamon Crunch	1 (0.5 oz)	50	0	0
Mini Apple Cinnamon	5 (0.5 oz)	50	0	0
Mini Banana Nut	5 (0.5 oz)	50	0	0
Mini Butter Popped Corn	6 (0.5 oz)	50	0	0
Mini Caramel Corn	5 (0.5 oz)	50	0	0
Mini Chocolate Crunch	5 (0.5 oz)	50	0	0
Mini Cinnamon Crunch	5 (0.5 oz)	50	0	0
Mini Honey Nut	5 (0.5 oz)	50	0	0
Mini Monterey Jack	6 (0.5 oz)	50	0	0
Mini White Cheddar	6 (0.5 oz)	50	0	0
Salt-Free	1 (0.3 oz)	35	0	0
Salted	1 (0.3 oz)	35	0	0
Tree Of Life				
Fat Free Mini Apple Cinnamon	15	60	0	0
Fat Free Mini Caramel	15	60	0	0
Fat Free Mini Honey Nut	15	60	0	0
Fat Free Mini Jalapeno	15	60	0	0
Fat Free Mini Plain	15	50	0	0
Weight Watchers				
Apple Cinnamon	1 oz	110	0	1

FOOD	PORTION	CALS.	SAT. FAT	FAT
Weight Watchers (CONT.)				
Butter	1 oz	110	0	2
Caramel	1 oz	110	0	1
White Cheddar	1 oz	100	0	1
ROCKFISH				
pacific cooked	1 fillet (5.2 oz)	180	1	3
pacific cooked	3 oz	103	tr	2
pacific raw	3 oz	80	tr	1
ROE				
(see also INDIVIDUAL FISH NAMES)				
fish	3.5 oz	39	tr	2
fresh baked	1 oz	58	1	2
ROLL				
(see also BISCUIT, CROISSANT, ENGLISH MUFFIN, MUFFIN, POPOVER, SCONE)				
FROZEN				
New York				
Garlic	1 (2 oz)	210	2	10
Sara Lee				
Deluxe Cinnamon Rolls w/ Icing	1 (2.7 oz)	370	9	15
Deluxe Cinnamon Rolls w/o Icing	1 (2.7 oz)	320	9	15
HOME RECIPE				
dinner as prep w/ 2% milk	1 (2½ in)	111	1	3
dinner as prep w/ whole milk	1 (2½ in)	112	1	3
raisin & nut	1 (2 oz)	196	1	7
MIX				
Dromedary				
Hot Roll Mix	2	239	—	5
Natural Ovens				
German Hard	1 (2.1 oz)	138	0	1
Gourmet Dinner	1 (1 oz)	50	0	1
Hearty Sandwich	1 (1.8 oz)	110	0	1
READY-TO-EAT				
brioche sweet roll	1 (3.5 oz)	410	14	23
brown & serve	1 (1 oz)	85	tr	2
cheese	1 (2.3 oz)	238	4	12
cinnamon raisin	1 (2¾ in)	223	3	10
dinner	1 (1 oz)	85	tr	2
egg	1 (2½ in)	107	1	2
french	1 (1.3 oz)	105	tr	2
hamburger	1 (1.5 oz)	123	1	2
hamburger multi-grain	1 (1.5 oz)	113	1	2
hamburger reduced calorie	1 (1.5 oz)	84	tr	1

FOOD	PORTION	CALS.	SAT. FAT	FAT
hard	1 (3½ in)	167	tr	2
hotdog	1 (1.5 oz)	123	1	2
hotdog multi-grain	1 (1.5 oz)	113	1	2
hotdog reduced calorie	1 (1.5 oz)	84	tr	1
kaiser	1 (3½ in)	167	tr	2
oat bran	1 (1.2 oz)	78	tr	tr
rye	1 (1 oz)	81	tr	1
submarine	1 (4.7 oz)	155	tr	2
wheat	1 (1 oz)	77	tr	2
whole wheat	1 (1 oz)	75	tr	1
Alvarado St. Bakery				
Burger Buns	1 (2.2 oz)	140	0	2
Hot Dog Buns	1 (2.2 oz)	140	0	2
Arnold				
8-inch Francisco	1 (2.5 oz)	210	—	3
Augusto Pan Cubano	1	230	—	3
Bakery Light	1 (1.5 oz)	80	0	<2
Bran'nola Buns	1 (1.5 oz)	100	0	1
Deli Kaiser	1	170	—	2
Deli Onion	1	170	—	2
Dinner Plain	1 (0.7 oz)	50	0	1
Dinner Sesame	1 (0.7 oz)	50	0	1
Dutch Egg	1	130	tr	3
French Francisco	1 (2.5 oz)	210	—	3
French Mini Francisco	1	130	—	2
Hamburger	1	120	—	2
Hot Dog	1 (1.5 oz)	110	tr	2
Hot Dog Bran'nola	1 (1.5 oz)	110	tr	2
Hot Dog New England Style	1	110	—	2
Italian 8-inch Savoni	1	210	tr	3
Onion Premium	1 (2.6 oz)	180	—	1
Party Petite	2	70	tr	2
Potato	1	140	—	2
Sandwich Soft Sesame	1	130	—	3
Sourdough Brown N' Serve	1 (1 oz)	100	—	1
Sourdough Francisco	1 (1 oz)	100	—	1
Wheat Old Fashioned	2	80	—	3
August Bros.				
Dinner	1	90	—	1
Kaiser	1	170	—	1
Onion	1	160	—	1
Sesame Cubano	1	170	—	1
Bread Du Jour				
Cracked Wheat	1 (1.2 oz)	100	0	1

FOOD	PORTION	CALS.	SAT. FAT	FAT
Bread Du Jour (CONT.)				
Italian	1 (1.2 oz)	90	0	1
Sourdough	1 (1.2 oz)	90	0	1
Country Kitchen				
Frankfurt	1	120	—	2
Dicarlo's				
Extra Sourdough	1 (1.6 oz)	100	0	1
French	1 (1 oz)	70	0	1
Frelhofer's				
Brown 'N Serve	1 (1 oz)	80	0	2
Home Pride				
Dinner Wheat	1 (1.9 oz)	160	1	4
Hamburger Potato Bun	1 (1.9 oz)	130	0	2
Hot Dog Potato Bun	1 (1.9 oz)	130	0	2
Sandwich Roll Wheat	1 (1.9 oz)	160	1	4
White	2 (1.6 oz)	130	1	4
Levy				
Sub Old Country	1	180	—	2
Martin's				
Big Marty Poppy	1	170	—	2
Big Marty Sesame	1	170	—	2
Hoagie	1	240	—	3
Hoagie Sesame	1	240	—	3
Potato Dinner	1	100	—	1
Potato Long	1	140	—	1
Potato Party	1	50	—	1
Potato Sandwich	1	140	—	1
Sandwich Whole Wheat 100% Stoneground	1	160	—	2
Pepperidge Farm				
Brown & Serve Club	1 (1.6 oz)	120	0	1
Parker House	1 (0.9 oz)	80	1	2
Roman Meal				
Brown & Serve	2 (2 oz)	140	tr	3
Dinner	2 (2 oz)	136	tr	2
Hamburger	1 (1.6 oz)	111	tr	2
Hotdog	1 (1.5 oz)	103	tr	2
Sandwich	1 (2.7 oz)	181	tr	3
Sandwich	1 (2.7 oz)	181	tr	3
San Francisco				
Sourdough	1 (1.8 oz)	180	0	0
Stroehmann				
Hamburger	1 (1.4 oz)	100	0	2
Hamburger Potato	1 (1.9 oz)	140	0	2

FOOD	PORTION	CALS.	SAT. FAT	FAT
Stroehmann (CONT.)				
Hot Dog	1 (1.4 oz)	100	0	2
Hot Dog Potato	1 (1.9 oz)	140	0	2
The Baker				
Honey Cinnamon Raisin	1 (2 oz)	150	0	2
Wonder				
Brown & Serve	1 (1 oz)	80	1	2
Brown & Serve Sourdough	1 (1 oz)	70	0	2
Brown & Serve Wheat	1 (1 oz)	80	0	2
Bun	1 (3 oz)	220	1	3
Club French	1 (1.6 oz)	120	1	2
Club Grain	1 (1.6 oz)	120	0	2
Club Sourdough	1 (1.6 oz)	120	0	2
Dinner	2 (1.6 oz)	130	0	1
Dinner Honey Rich	1 (1.3 oz)	100	0	2
Dinner Wheat	2 (1.6 oz)	140	0	3
Hamburger	1 (2.5 oz)	190	1	3
Hamburger	1 (2 oz)	150	0	3
Hamburger	1 (2.5 oz)	180	0	3
Hamburger	1 (1.5 oz)	110	0	2
Hamburger Wheat	1 (1.9 oz)	140	0	2
Hamburger Wheat	1 (1.5 oz)	120	1	2
Hoagie French	1 (3 oz)	220	1	3
Hoagie Grain	1 (3 oz)	220	1	3
Hoagie Sourdough	1 (3 oz)	220	1	3
Hot Dog	1 (2 oz)	160	1	3
Kaiser	1 (2.2 oz)	180	1	3
Kaiser Hoagie	1 (3 oz)	220	1	3
Multigrain	1 (1.8 oz)	140	1	2
Potato Bun	1 (1.5 oz)	110	0	1
Steak	1 (2.5 oz)	190	1	3
REFRIGERATED				
cinnamon w/ frosting	1	109	1	4
crescent	1 (1 oz)	98	1	4
Pillsbury				
Apple Cinnamon	1 (1.5 oz)	150	2	6
Caramel	1 (1.7 oz)	170	2	7
Cinnamon w/ Icing	1 (1.5 oz)	150	2	6
Cinnamon w/ Icing Reduced Fat	1 (1.5 oz)	140	1	4
Cinnamon Raisin w/ Icing	1 (1.7 oz)	170	2	6
Cornbread Twists	1 (1.4 oz)	140	2	6
Crecents Reduced Fat	1 (1 oz)	100	1	5
Crescent	1 (1 oz)	110	2	6
Dinner	1 (1.4 oz)	110	0	2

FOOD	PORTION	CALS.	SAT. FAT	FAT
Pillsbury (CONT.)				
Dinner Wheat	1 (1.4 oz)	110	0	2
Orange Sweet Roll w/ Icing	1 (1.7 oz)	150	2	7
ROSELLE				
fresh	1 cup	28	—	tr
ROSEMARY				
dried	1 tsp	4	—	tr
ROUGHY				
orange baked	3 oz	75	tr	1
RUTABAGA				
cooked mashed	½ cup	41	tr	tr
raw cubed	½ cup	25	tr	tr
Sunshine				
Diced	½ cup (4.2 oz)	30	0	0
SABLEFISH				
baked	3 oz	213	3	17
smoked	3 oz	218	4	17
smoked	1 oz	72	1	6
SAFFLOWER				
seeds dried	1 oz	147	1	11
SAFFRON				
saffron	1 tsp	2	—	tr
SAGE				
ground	1 tsp	2	tr	tr
Watkins				
Sage	¼ tsp (0.5 g)	0	0	0
SALAD				
(see also LETTUCE, PASTA SALAD)				
MIX				
Dole				
All American Toss	2 cups (3.5 oz)	50	0	1
American Blend	1½ cups (3 oz)	15	0	0
Classic	1½ cups (3 oz)	15	0	0
Classic Romaine Blend	1½ cups (3 oz)	15	0	0
Coleslaw	1½ cups (3 oz)	25	0	0
European Special Blend	2 cups (3 oz)	15	0	0
Family Greener	1½ cups (3 oz)	15	0	0
Garlice Caesar Complete w/ Dressing	1½ cups (3.5 oz)	180	3	15
Greek Marinade	1½ cups (3.5 oz)	100	2	8

FOOD	PORTION	CALS.	SAT. FAT	FAT
Dole (CONT.)				
Light Caesar Complete w/ Dressing	1½ cups (3.5 oz)	60	0	1
Light Herb Ranch Complete w/ Dressing	1½ cups (3.5 oz)	50	1	1
Light Roasted Garlic Caesar Complete w/ Dressing	1½ cups (3.5 oz)	60	0	1
Light Zesty Italian Complete w/ Dressing	1½ cups (3.5 oz)	50	0	1
Mediterranean Marinade	2 cups (3.5 oz)	90	1	8
Oriental Complete w/ Dressing	1½ cups (3.5 oz)	120	1	6
Romano Complete w/ Dressing	1½ cups (3.5 oz)	150	2	12
Salad-In-A-Minute Spinach	3.5 oz	180	2	9
Sunflower Ranch Complete w/ Dressing	1½ cups (3.5 oz)	160	2	16
Tomato & Mozzarella Medley	2 cups (3.5 oz)	60	1	2
Triple Cheese Toss	2 cups (3.5 oz)	80	3	5
Fresh Express				
American Salad	1½ cups (3 oz)	20	0	0
Caesar Salad	1½ cups (3 oz)	140	1	11
European Salad	1½ cups (3 oz)	20	0	0
Fancy Field Greens	1½ cups (3 oz)	15	0	0
Garden Salad	1½ cups (3 oz)	20	0	0
Italian Salad	1½ cups (3 oz)	20	0	0
Oriental Salad	1½ cups (3 oz)	120	1	8
Original Iceberg Garden w/ Zip	1½ cups (3 oz)	15	0	0
Riviera Salad	1½ cups (3 oz)	10	0	0
Spinach Salad	1½ cups (3 oz)	130	0	3
Veggie Lover's	1½ cups (3 oz)	20	0	0
Suddenly Salad				
Caesar	¾ cup	220	2	9
Caesar Low Fat Recipe	¾ cup	170	0	3
Italian Pepperoni	1 cup	190	1	4
Italian Pepperoni Low Fat Recipe	1 cup	180	0	2
Ranch & Bacon	¾ cup	330	3	20
Ranch & Bacon Low Fat Recipe	¾ cup	180	0	2
Weight Watchers				
Caesar Salad	1 serv (3.5 oz)	60	0	0
Caesar Salad w/ Cookies	1 pkg (4.3 oz)	160	1	3
European Salad	1 serv (3.5 oz)	60	0	0

FOOD	PORTION	CALS.	SAT. FAT	FAT
Weight Watchers (CONT.)				
European Salad w/ Cookies	1 pkg (4.3 oz)	160	1	3
Garden Salad	1 serv (3.5 oz)	60	0	0
Garden Salad w/ Cookies	1 pkg (4 oz)	120	1	2
TAKE-OUT				
caesar	2 cups (5 oz)	235	2	20
tossed w/o dressing	1½ cups	32	0	tr
tossed w/o dressing	¾ cup	16	0	0
tossed w/o dressing w/ cheese & egg	1½ cups	102	3	6
tossed w/o dressing w/ chicken	1½ cups	105	tr	2
tossed w/o dressing w/ pasta & seafood	1½ cups (14.6 oz)	380	3	21
tossed w/o dressing w/ shrimp	1½ cups	107	tr	2

SALAD DRESSING
HOME RECIPE

FOOD	PORTION	CALS.	SAT. FAT	FAT
french	1 tbsp	88	2	10
vinegar & oil	1 tbsp	72	2	8
MIX				
Et Tu				
Caesar Salad Kit	1 serv	140	1	12
Good Seasons				
Cheese Garlic as prep	2 tbsp (1 oz)	140	3	16
Fat Free Honey Mustard as prep	2 tbsp (1.2 oz)	20	0	0
Fat Free Italian as prep	2 tbsp (1.1 oz)	10	0	0
Fat Free Ranch as prep	2 tbsp (1.2 oz)	20	0	0
Fat Free Zesty Herb as prep	2 tbsp (1.1 oz)	10	0	0
Garlic & Herbs as prep	2 tbsp (1 oz)	140	2	15
Gourmet Caesar as prep	2 tbsp (1.1 oz)	150	3	16
Gourmet Parmesan Italian as prep	2 tbsp (1.1 oz)	150	3	16
Honey French as prep	2 tbsp (1.2 oz)	160	2	15
Honey Mustard as prep	2 tbsp (1.1 oz)	150	2	15
Italian as prep	2 tbsp (1 oz)	140	2	15
Mexican Spice as prep	2 tbsp (1.1 oz)	140	3	15
Mild Italian as prep	2 tbsp (1.1 oz)	150	3	15
Oriental Sesame as prep	2 tbsp (1.1 oz)	150	3	16
Reduced Calorie Italian as prep	2 tbsp (1 oz)	50	1	5
Reduced Calorie Zesty Italian as prep	2 tbsp (1 oz)	50	1	5
Roasted Garlic as prep	2 tbsp (1.1 oz)	150	2	15
Zesty Italian as prep	2 tbsp (1 oz)	140	2	15

FOOD	PORTION	CALS.	SAT. FAT	FAT
Hain				
No Oil 1000 Island	1 tbsp	12	—	0
No Oil Bleu Cheese	1 tbsp	14	—	1
No Oil Buttermilk	1 tbsp	11	—	tr
No Oil Caesar	1 tbsp	6	—	tr
No Oil French	1 tbsp	12	—	0
No Oil Garlic & Cheese	1 tbsp	6	—	tr
No Oil Herb	1 tbsp	2	—	0
No Oil Italian	1 tbsp	2	—	0
READY-TO-EAT				
blue cheese	1 tbsp	77	2	8
french	1 tbsp	67	2	6
french reduced calorie	1 tbsp	22	tr	1
italian	1 tbsp	69	1	7
italian reduced calorie	1 tbsp	16	tr	2
russian	1 tbsp	76	1	8
russian reduced calorie	1 tbsp	23	tr	1
sesame seed	1 tbsp	68	1	7
thousand island	1 tbsp	59	1	6
thousand island reduced calorie	1 tbsp	24	tr	2
Benecol				
Creamy Italian	2 tbsp	100	2	10
Ranch	2 tbsp	130	2	13
Thousand Island	2 tbsp	130	2	12
Estee				
Creamy French	2 tbsp (1 oz)	10	0	0
Italian	2 tbsp	5	0	0
Hain				
1000 Island	1 tbsp	50	—	5
Canola Garden Tomato	1 tbsp	60	—	6
Canola Italian	1 tbsp	50	—	5
Canola Spicy French Mustard	1 tbsp	50	—	5
Canola Tangy Citrus	1 tbsp	50	—	5
Creamy Caesar	1 tbsp	60	—	6
Creamy Caesar Low Salt	1 tbsp	60	—	6
Creamy French	1 tbsp	60	—	6
Creamy Italian	1 tbsp	80	—	8
Creamy Italian No Salt Added	1 tbsp	80	—	8
Cucumber Dill	1 tbsp	80	—	8
Dijon Vinaigrette	1 tbsp	50	—	5
Garlic & Sour Cream	1 tbsp	70	—	7
Honey & Sesame	1 tbsp	60	—	5
Italian Cheese Vinaigrette	1 tbsp	55	—	6
Old Fashioned Buttermilk	1 tbsp	70	—	7

FOOD	PORTION	CALS.	SAT. FAT	FAT
Hain (CONT.)				
Poppyseed Rancher's	1 tbsp	60	—	7
Savory Herb No Salt Added	1 tbsp	90	—	10
Swiss Cheese Vinaigrette	1 tbsp	60	—	7
Traditional Italian	1 tbsp	80	—	8
Traditional Italian No Salt Added	1 tbsp	60	—	6
Hollywood				
Caesar	1 tbsp	70	1	7
Creamy French	1 tbsp	70	1	7
Creamy Italian	1 tbsp	90	1	9
Dijon Vinaigrette	1 tbsp	60	1	6
Italian	1 tbsp	90	1	9
Italian Cheese	1 tbsp	80	1	8
Old Fashion Buttermilk	1 tbsp	75	1	8
Poppy Seed Rancher's	1 tbsp	75	1	8
Thousand Island	1 tbsp	60	1	6
Kraft				
⅓ Less Fat Catalina	2 tbsp (1.2 oz)	80	1	5
⅓ Less Fat Cucumber Ranch	2 tbsp (1.1 oz)	60	1	5
⅓ Less Fat Italian	2 tbsp (1.1 oz)	70	1	7
⅓ Less Fat Ranch	2 tbsp (1.1)	110	2	11
⅓ Less Fat Thousand Island	2 tbsp (1.2 oz)	70	1	5
Bacon & Tomato	2 tbsp (1.1 oz)	140	3	14
Buttermilk Ranch	2 tbsp (1.1 oz)	150	3	16
Caesar Italian	2 tbsp (1.1 oz)	100	2	10
Caesar Ranch	2 tbsp (1.1 oz)	110	2	11
Catalina	2 tbsp (1.1 oz)	120	2	10
Catalina With Honey	2 tbsp (1.1 oz)	130	2	11
Classic Caesar	2 tbsp (1.1 oz)	110	2	11
Coleslaw	2 tbsp (1.1 oz)	130	2	11
Creamy French	2 tbsp (1.1 oz)	160	3	15
Creamy Garlic	2 tbsp (1.1 oz)	110	2	11
Creamy Italian	2 tbsp (1.1 oz)	110	2	11
Cucumber Ranch	2 tbsp (1.1 oz)	140	2	15
Free Blue Cheese	2 tbsp (1.2 oz)	45	0	0
Free Caesar Italian	2 tbsp (1.2 oz)	25	0	0
Free Catalina	2 tbsp (1.2 oz)	35	0	0
Free Classic Caesar	2 tbsp (1.2 oz)	45	0	0
Free Creamy Italian	2 tbsp (1.2 oz)	50	0	0
Free French	2 tbsp (1.2 oz)	45	0	0
Free Garlic Ranch	2 tbsp (1.2 oz)	45	0	0
Free Honey Dijon	2 tbsp (1.2 oz)	45	0	0
Free Italian	2 tbsp (1.2 oz)	20	0	0
Free Peppercorn Ranch	2 tbsp (1.2 oz)	45	0	0

FOOD	PORTION	CALS.	SAT. FAT	FAT
Kraft (CONT.)				
Free Ranch	1 tbsp (1.2 oz)	50	0	0
Free Red Wine Vinegar	2 tbsp (1.1 oz)	15	0	0
Free Thousand Island	2 tbsp (1.2 oz)	40	0	0
Garlic Ranch	2 tbsp (1 oz)	180	3	19
Herb Vinaigrette	2 tbsp (1.1 oz)	140	2	15
Honey Dijon	2 tbsp (1.1 oz)	110	2	10
Honey Mustard	2 tbsp (1.1 oz)	110	2	10
House Italian w/ Olive Oil Blend	2 tbsp (1.1 oz)	120	2	12
Peppercorn Ranch	2 tbsp (1 oz)	170	3	18
Pesto Italian	2 tbsp (1.1 oz)	90	2	9
Ranch	2 tbsp (1 oz)	170	3	18
Roka Blue Cheese	2 tbsp (1.1 oz)	130	3	13
Russian	2 tbsp (1.2 oz)	130	2	10
Sour Cream & Onion Ranch	2 tbsp (1 oz)	170	3	18
Thousand Island	2 tbsp (1.1 oz)	110	2	10
Thousand Island With Bacon	2 tbsp (1.1 oz)	130	2	12
Tomato & Herb Italian	2 tbsp (1.1 oz)	100	1	9
Zesty Italian	2 tbsp (1.1 oz)	110	1	11
Marzetti				
Bacon Spinach Salad	2 tbsp	80	2	15
Blue Cheese	2 tbsp	160	3	17
Buttermilk & Herb	2 tbsp	180	3	20
Buttermilk Bacon Ranch	2 tbsp	180	3	19
Buttermilk Blue Cheese	2 tbsp	160	3	18
Buttermilk Parmesan Pepper	2 tbsp	170	3	18
Buttermilk Parmesan Ranch	2 tbsp	160	3	17
Buttermilk Ranch	2 tbsp	180	3	20
Buttermilk Veggie Dip	2 tbsp	170	3	18
Caesar	2 tbsp	150	3	16
Caesar Ranch	2 tbsp	190	3	20
California French	2 tbsp	160	2	13
Celery Seed	2 tbsp	160	2	13
Chunky Blue Cheese	2 tbsp	150	3	16
Classic Caesar Ranch	2 tbsp	190	3	20
Country French	2 tbsp	150	2	13
Cracked Peppercorn	2 tbsp	140	3	14
Creamy Garlic Italian	2 tbsp	160	3	17
Creamy Italian	2 tbsp	150	3	16
Crispy Celery Seed	2 tbsp	160	2	13
Dijon Honey Mustard	2 tbsp	140	2	13
Dijon Ranch	2 tbsp	170	3	18
Dutch Sweet'N Sour	2 tbsp	160	2	13
Fat Free California French	2 tbsp	45	0	0

FOOD	PORTION	CALS.	SAT. FAT	FAT
Marzetti (CONT.)				
Fat Free Honey Dijon	2 tbsp	60	0	0
Fat Free Honey French	2 tbsp	45	0	0
Fat Free Italian	2 tbsp	15	0	0
Fat Free Peppercorn Ranch	2 tbsp	30	0	0
Fat Free Ranch	2 tbsp	30	0	0
Fat Free Raspberry	2 tbsp	70	0	0
Fat Free Slaw	2 tbsp	45	0	0
Fat Free Sweet & Sour	2 tbsp	45	0	0
Fat Free Thousand Island	2 tbsp	35	0	0
Garden Ranch	2 tbsp	180	3	19
Gusto Italian	2 tbsp	120	2	13
Honey Dijon	2 tbsp	140	2	13
Honey Dijon Ranch	2 tbsp	150	3	15
Honey French	2 tbsp	160	2	14
Honey French Blue Cheese	2 tbsp	160	2	13
House Caesar	2 tbsp	150	3	16
Italian With Olive Oil	2 tbsp	120	2	13
Light Blue Cheese	2 tbsp	60	2	6
Light Buttermilk Ranch	2 tbsp	90	2	9
Light California French	2 tbsp	80	1	6
Light Chunky Blue Cheese	2 tbsp	80	2	7
Light French	2 tbsp	40	0	2
Light French	2 tbsp	40	0	2
Light Honey French	2 tbsp	80	1	4
Light Italian	2 tbsp	60	1	5
Light Ranch	2 tbsp	90	2	8
Light Red Wine Vinegar & Oil	2 tbsp	20	0	1
Light Slaw	2 tbsp	60	1	7
Light Sweet & Sour	2 tbsp	100	1	6
Light Thousand Island	2 tbsp	70	1	5
Old Fashioned Poppyseed	2 tbsp	140	2	11
Olde Venice Italain	2 tbsp	130	2	13
Olde World Caesar	2 tbsp	150	3	16
Parmesan Pepper	2 tbsp	160	3	17
Peppercorn Ranch	2 tbsp	180	3	19
Poppyseed	2 tbsp	160	2	13
Potato Salad Dressing	2 tbsp	120	2	13
Ranch	2 tbsp	180	3	20
Red Wine Vinegar & Oil	2 tbsp	130	2	14
Romano Cheese Caesar	2 tbsp	150	3	16
Romano Italian	2 tbsp	160	3	17
Savory Italian	2 tbsp	110	2	12
Slaw	2 tbsp	170	3	16

FOOD	PORTION	CALS.	SAT. FAT	FAT
Marzetti (CONT.)				
Southern Slaw	2 tbsp	100	2	11
Sweet & Saucy	2 tbsp	140	2	12
Sweet & Sour	2 tbsp	160	2	13
Thousand Island	2 tbsp	150	2	15
Vintage Champagne	2 tbsp	150	2	16
Wilde Raspberry	2 tbsp	150	2	12
Nasoya				
Creamy Dill	2 tbsp (1 oz)	63	tr	5
Creamy Italian	2 tbsp (1 oz)	60	0	5
Garden Herb	2 tbsp (1 oz)	61	tr	5
Sesame Garlic	2 tbsp (1 oz)	63	tr	5
Thousand Island	2 tbsp (1 oz)	62	tr	4
Newman's Own				
Balsamic Vinaigrette	2 tbsp (1.1 oz)	90	1	9
Caesar	2 tbsp (1.1 oz)	150	2	16
Light Italian	2 tbsp (1.1 oz)	20	0	1
Olive Oil & Vinegar	2 tbsp (1 oz)	150	3	16
Ranch	2 tbsp (1 oz)	180	3	19
Pfeiffer				
1000 Island	2 tbsp	140	2	14
California French	2 tbsp	140	2	12
French	2 tbsp	150	2	13
Honey Dijon	2 tbsp	140	2	13
Lite Italian	2 tbsp	50	1	5
Ranch	2 tbsp	180	3	20
Savory Italian	2 tbsp	110	2	12
Pritikin				
Dijon Balsamic Vinaigrette	2 tbsp (1 oz)	3	0	0
French	2 tbsp (1 oz)	35	0	0
Honey Dijon	2 tbsp (1 oz)	45	0	0
Honey French	2 tbsp (1 oz)	40	0	0
Italian	2 tbsp (1 oz)	20	0	0
Raspberry Vinaigrette	2 tbsp (1 oz)	45	0	0
Red Wing				
"K" Dressing	1 tbsp (0.5 oz)	70	1	7
Chunky Blue Cheese	2 tbsp (1 oz)	130	2	13
Creamy Ranch	2 tbsp (1 oz)	150	2	15
French Traditional	2 tbsp (1 oz)	130	2	11
Italian Traditional	2 tbsp (1 oz)	100	2	11
Spicy Sweet French	2 tbsp (1 oz)	130	2	11
Thousand Island Thick & Rich	2 tbsp (1 oz)	110	2	9
Russell Stover				
French	2 tbsp (0.8 oz)	130	2	11

FOOD	PORTION	CALS.	SAT. FAT	FAT
Seven Seas				
⅓ Less Fat Creamy Italian	2 tbsp (1.1 oz)	60	1	5
⅓ Less Fat Italian w/ Olive Oil Blend	2 tbsp (1.1 oz)	45	0	4
⅓ Less Fat Ranch	2 tbsp (1.1 oz)	100	2	9
⅓ Less Fat Red Wine Vinegar & Oil	2 tbsp (1.1 oz)	45	0	4
⅓ Less Fat Viva Italian	2 tbsp (1.1 oz)	45	0	4
2 Cheese Italian	2 tbsp (1.1 oz)	70	1	7
Chunky Blue Cheese	2 tbsp (1.1 oz)	130	3	13
Classic Caesar	2 tbsp (1.1 oz)	100	2	10
Creamy Italian	2 tbsp (1.1 oz)	120	2	12
Free Ranch	2 tbsp (1.2 oz)	45	0	0
Free Red Wine Vinegar	2 tbsp (1.1 oz)	15	0	0
Free Sour Cream & Onion Ranch	2 tbsp (1.2 oz)	50	0	0
Free Viva Italian	2 tbsp (1.1 oz)	10	0	0
Green Goddess	2 tbsp (1.1 oz)	130	2	13
Herbs & Spices	2 tbsp (1.1 oz)	90	1	9
Ranch	2 tbsp (1.1 oz)	160	3	17
Red Wine Vinegar & Oil	2 tbsp (1.1 oz)	90	1	9
Viva Italian	2 tbsp (1.1 oz)	90	1	9
Viva Russian	2 tbsp (1.1 oz)	150	3	16
Tree Of Life				
Cafe Venice	2 tbsp (1 oz)	100	1	12
Fat Free Blue Cheese	2 tbsp (1 oz)	15	—	1
Fat Free Honey French	2 tbsp (1 oz)	35	0	0
Fat Free Italian Garlic	2 tbsp (1 oz)	20	0	0
Fat Free Oriental Ginger	2 tbsp (1 oz)	15	0	0
Frisco's Raspberry	2 tbsp (1 oz)	120	1	11
Maison Caesar	2 tbsp (1 oz)	70	1	6
Shanghai Palace	2 tbsp (1 oz)	80	0	7
Ultra Slim-Fast				
French	1 tbsp	20	—	tr
Italian	1 tbsp	6	—	tr
W.J. Clark				
Ginger Orange Vinaigrette	1 tbsp	73	1	7
Herbs & Romano	1 tbsp	67	tr	6
Lemon Peppercorn	1 tbsp	72	1	7
Lime Cilantro Vinaigrette	1 tbsp	73	1	8
Poppy Seed	1 tbsp	75	tr	6
Sweet Pepper Basil	1 tbsp	69	tr	7
Tarragon Honey Mustard	1 tbsp	66	tr	6

FOOD	PORTION	CALS.	SAT. FAT	FAT
Walden Farms				
Fat Free Balsamic Vinaigrette	2 tbsp (1 oz)	15	0	0
Fat Free Bleu Cheese	2 tbsp (1 oz)	25	0	0
Fat Free Caesar	2 tbsp (1 oz)	25	0	0
Fat Free Creamy Italian With Parmesan	1 tbsp (1 oz)	25	0	0
Fat Free French Style	2 tbsp (1 oz)	25	0	0
Fat Free Honey Dijon	2 tbsp (1 oz)	25	0	0
Fat Free Italian	2 tbsp (1 oz)	10	0	0
Fat Free Ranch	2 tbsp (1 oz)	25	0	0
Fat Free Raspberry Vinaigrette	2 tbsp (1 oz)	20	0	0
Fat Free Russian	2 tbsp (1 oz)	30	0	0
Fat Free Sodium Free Italian	2 tbsp (1 oz)	10	0	0
Fat Free Sugar Free Italian	2 tbsp (1 oz)	0	0	0
Fat Free Thousand Island	2 tbsp (1 oz)	35	0	0
Italian With Sun Dried Tomato	2 tbsp (1 oz)	15	0	0
Ranch With Sun Dried Tomato	2 tbsp (1 oz)	25	0	0
Weight Watchers				
Fat Free Caesar	1 pkg (0.75 oz)	5	0	0
Fat Free Caesar	2 tbsp	10	0	0
Fat Free Creamy Italian	2 tbsp	30	0	0
Fat Free French Style	2 tbsp	40	0	0
Fat Free Honey Dijon	2 tbsp	45	0	0
Fat Free Italian	2 tbsp	10	0	0
Fat Free Ranch	1 pkg (0.75 oz)	25	0	0
Fat Free Ranch	2 tbsp	35	0	0
Wishbone				
Caesar	2 tbsp (1 oz)	90	2	10
Chunky Blue Cheese	2 tbsp (1 oz)	150	3	17
Classic House Italian	2 tbsp (1 oz)	140	2	14
Classic Olive Oil Italian	2 tbsp (1 oz)	60	1	5
Creamy Caesar	2 tbsp (1 oz)	180	3	18
Creamy Italian	2 tbsp (1 oz)	110	2	10
Creamy Roasted Garlic	2 tbsp (1 oz)	110	2	10
Deluxe French	2 tbsp (1 oz)	120	2	11
Fat Free Chunky Blue Cheese	2 tbsp (1 oz)	35	0	0
Fat Free Chunky Blue Cheese	2 tbsp	35	0	0
Fat Free Creamy Italian	2 tbsp (1 oz)	35	0	0
Fat Free Creamy Roasted Garlic	2 tbsp (1 oz)	40	0	0
Fat Free Deluxe French	2 tbsp (1 oz)	30	0	0
Fat Free Honey Dijon	2 tbsp (1 oz)	45	0	0
Fat Free Italian	2 tbsp (1 oz)	10	0	0
Fat Free Parmesan & Onion	2 tbsp (1 oz)	45	0	0
Fat Free Ranch	2 tbsp (1 oz)	40	0	0

FOOD	PORTION	CALS.	SAT. FAT	FAT
Wishbone (CONT.)				
Fat Free Red Wine Vinaigrette	2 tbsp (1 oz)	35	0	0
Fat Free Sweet N' Spicy French	2 tbsp (1 oz)	30	0	0
Fat Free Thousand Island	2 tbsp (1 oz)	35	0	0
Italian	2 tbsp (1 oz)	80	1	8
Lite French	2 tbsp (1 oz)	50	1	2
Lite Italian	2 tbsp (1 oz)	15	0	1
Lite Ranch	2 tbsp (1 oz)	100	1	8
Olive Oil Vinaigrette	2 tbsp (1 oz)	60	1	5
Oriental	2 tbsp (1 oz)	70	1	5
Parmesan & Onion	2 tbsp (1 oz)	110	2	10
Ranch	2 tbsp (1 oz)	160	3	17
Red Wine Vinaigrette	2 tbsp (1 oz)	80	1	5
Robusto Italian	2 tbsp (1 oz)	90	1	8
Russian	2 tbsp (1 oz)	110	1	6
Sweet N' Spicy French	2 tbsp (1 oz)	140	2	12
Thousand Island	2 tbsp (1 oz)	140	2	12
SALMON				
CANNED				
chum w/ bone	1 can (13.9 oz)	521	5	20
chum w/ bone	3 oz	120	1	5
pink w/ bone	1 can (15.9 oz)	631	7	27
pink w/ bone	3 oz	118	1	5
sockeye w/ bone	1 can (12.9 oz)	566	6	27
sockeye w/ bone	3 oz	130	1	6
Bumble Bee				
Keta	3.5 oz	160	2	8
Pink	3.5 oz	160	2	8
Pink Skinless & Boneless	3.25 oz	120	1	5
Red	3.5 oz	180	2	10
Red Skinless & Boneless	3.25 oz	130	1	6
Libby				
Keta	½ can (3.8 oz)	140	—	6
Pink	½ can (3.8 oz)	150	—	7
FRESH				
atlantic baked	3 oz	155	1	7
chinook baked	3 oz	196	3	11
chum baked	3 oz	131	1	4
coho cooked	3 oz	157	1	6
coho cooked	½ fillet (5.4 oz)	286	2	12
coho raw	3 oz	124	1	5
pink baked	3 oz	127	1	4
roe raw	3.5 oz	207	—	10

FOOD	PORTION	CALS.	SAT. FAT	FAT
sockeye cooked	½ fillet (5.4 oz)	334	3	17
sockeye cooked	3 oz	183	2	9
sockeye raw	3 oz	143	1	7
SMOKED				
chinook	1 oz	33	tr	1
chinook	3 oz	99	1	4
Nathan's				
Nova	2 oz	80	1	3
TAKE-OUT				
roulette w/ spinach stuffing	1 serv (4 oz)	160	2	6

SALSA

(see also KETCHUP, SAUCE, SPANISH FOOD)

FOOD	PORTION	CALS.	SAT. FAT	FAT
Casa Fiesta				
Chili Salsa	1 oz	9	—	tr
Picante Mild	1 oz	9	—	tr
Chi-Chi's				
Con Queso	2 tbsp (1.1 oz)	90	3	7
Hot	2 tbsp (1 oz)	10	0	0
Medium	2 tbsp (1 oz)	10	0	0
Mild	2 tbsp (1 oz)	10	0	0
Picante Hot	2 tbsp (1 oz)	10	0	0
Picante Medium	2 tbsp (1 oz)	10	0	0
Picante Mild	2 tbsp (1 oz)	10	0	0
Verde Medium	2 tbsp (1.2 oz)	15	0	0
Verde Mild	2 tbsp (1.2 oz)	15	0	0
Del Monte				
Mexicana	2 tbsp (1.1 oz)	5	0	0
Taquera	2 tbsp (1.1 oz)	5	0	0
Verde	2 tbsp (1.1 oz)	10	0	0
Guiltless Gourmet				
Roasted Red Pepper	2 tbsp (1 oz)	10	0	0
Southwestern Grill	2 tbsp (1 oz)	10	0	0
Hain				
Hot	¼ cup	22	0	0
Mild	¼ cup	20	0	0
Heluva Good Cheese				
Cheese & Salsa	2 tbsp (1.1 oz)	80	5	6
Thick & Chunky Hot	2 tbsp (1.2 oz)	10	0	0
Thick & Chunky Mild	2 tbsp (1.2 oz)	10	0	0
Hot Cha Cha				
Medium	2 tbsp (1 oz)	5	0	0
Hunt's				
Alfresco Medium	2 tbsp (1.1 oz)	10	tr	tr
Alfresco Mild	2 tbsp (1.1 oz)	10	tr	tr

FOOD	PORTION	CALS.	SAT. FAT	FAT
Hunt's (CONT.)				
Hot	2 tbsp (1.1 oz)	27	0	tr
Medium	2 tbsp (1.1 oz)	27	0	tr
Mild	2 tbsp (1.1 oz)	27	0	tr
Picante Medium	2 tbsp (1.1 oz)	11	0	tr
Picante Mild	2 tbsp (1.1 oz)	11	0	tr
Louise's				
Fat Free BBQ Black Bean	1 oz	10	0	0
Fat Free Black Bean	1 oz	10	0	0
Fat Free Medium	1 oz	10	0	0
Fat Free Mild	1 oz	10	0	0
Fat Free Nacho Queso	1 oz	15	0	0
Muir Glen				
Organic Fat Free Hot	2 tbsp (1.1 oz)	10	—	0
Organic Fat Free Medium	2 tbsp (1.1 oz)	10	—	0
Organic Fat Free Mild	2 tbsp (1.1 oz)	10	—	0
Newman's Own				
Bandito Hot	2 tbsp (1.1 oz)	10	0	0
Bandito Medium	2 tbsp (1.1 oz)	10	0	0
Bandito Mild	2 tbsp (1.1 oz)	10	0	0
Peach	2 tbsp (1.1 oz)	25	0	0
Pineapple	2 tbsp (1.1 oz)	15	0	0
Roasted Garlic	2 tbsp (1.1 oz)	10	0	0
Old El Paso				
Green Chili Medium	2 tbsp (1 oz)	10	0	0
Homestyle	2 tbsp (1 oz)	5	0	0
Homestyle Mild	2 tbsp (1 oz)	5	0	0
Picante Hot	2 tbsp (1 oz)	10	0	0
Picante Medium	2 tbsp (1 oz)	10	0	0
Picante Mild	2 tbsp (1 oz)	10	0	0
Picante Thick'n Chunky Hot	2 tbsp (1 oz)	10	0	0
Picante Thick'n Chunky Medium	2 tbsp (1 oz)	10	0	0
Picante Thick'n Chunky Mild	2 tbsp (1 oz)	10	0	0
Pico De Gallo Hot	2 tbsp (1 oz)	5	0	0
Pico De Gallo Medium	1 tbsp (1 oz)	5	0	0
Salsa Verde	2 tbsp (1 oz)	10	0	0
Thick'n Chunky Hot	2 tbsp (1 oz)	10	0	0
Thick'n Chunky Medium	2 tbsp (1 oz)	10	0	0
Thick'n Chunky Mild	2 tbsp (1 oz)	10	0	0
Ortega				
Hot Green Chili	1 tbsp	6	0	0
Medium Green Chili	1 tbsp	6	0	0
Mild Green Chili	1 tbsp	8	0	0

FOOD	PORTION	CALS.	SAT. FAT	FAT
Pace				
Picante	2 tbsp (1 fl oz)	7	0	0
Thick & Chunky	2 tbsp (1 fl oz)	12	0	0
Progresso				
Italian Hot	2 tbsp (1 oz)	30	0	0
Italian Medium	2 tbsp (1 oz)	10	0	0
Italian Mild	2 tbsp (1 oz)	10	0	0
Rosarita				
Chunky Hot	3 tbsp (1.5 oz)	25	—	tr
Chunky Medium	3 tbsp (1.5 oz)	25	—	tr
Chunky Mild	3 tbsp (1.5 oz)	25	—	tr
Taco Salsa Chunky Medium	3 tbsp (1.5 oz)	25	—	tr
Taco Salsa Chunky Mild	3 tbsp (1.5 oz)	25	—	tr
Tabasco				
Picante	2 tbsp (1.5 oz)	17	tr	tr
Taco Bell				
Smooth 'N Zesty Picante Medium	2 tbsp (1.1 oz)	15	0	0
Smooth 'N Zesty Picante Mild	2 tbsp (1.1 oz)	15	0	0
Thick 'N Chunky Salsa Hot	2 tbsp (1.1 oz)	15	0	0
Thick 'N Chunky Salsa Medium	2 tbsp (1.1 oz)	15	0	0
Thick 'N Chunky Salsa Mild	2 tbsp (1.1 oz)	15	0	0
Tostitos				
Con Queso	2.3 oz	80	2	5
Hot	2.3 oz	30	0	0
Low Fat Con Queso	2.5 oz	80	2	3
Medium	2.3 oz	30	0	0
Mild	2.3 oz	30	0	0
Restaurant Style	2.2 oz	30	0	0
Ultimate Garden	2.4 oz	30	0	0
Tree Of Life				
Hot	2 tbsp (1 oz)	10	0	0
Medium	2 tbsp (1 oz)	10	0	0
Mild	2 tbsp (1 oz)	10	0	0
No Salt	2 tbsp (1 oz)	10	0	0
Utz				
Chunky	2 tbsp (1 fl oz)	60	0	0
Watkins				
Salsa Seasoning Blend	⅛ tsp (0.5 g)	0	0	0
Tropical	2 tbsp (1 oz)	60	0	0
Wise				
Picante	2 tbsp	12	0	0
SALSIFY				
fresh sliced cooked	½ cup	46	—	tr
raw sliced	½ cup	55	—	tr

FOOD	PORTION	CALS.	SAT. FAT	FAT
SALT/SEASONED SALT				
(see also SALT SUBSTITUTES)				
salt	1 tbsp (18 g)	0	0	0
salt	1 tsp (6 g)	0	0	0
Hain				
Sea Salt	1 tsp	0	0	0
Sea Salt Iodized	1 tsp	0	0	0
Morton				
Garlic	1 tsp	3	—	tr
Iodized	1 tsp	tr	—	0
Kosher	1 tsp	0	—	0
Lite	¼ tsp (1.4 g)	tr	—	0
Nature's Season Seasoning Blend	1 tsp	3	—	tr
Non-Iodized	1 tsp	0	—	0
Seasoned	1 tsp	4	—	tr
Watkins				
Bacon Cheese Salt	¼ tbsp (1 g)	0	0	0
Butter Salt	¼ tbsp (1 g)	0	0	0
Cheese Salt	¼ tbsp (1 g)	0	0	0
Garlic Salt	¼ tsp (1 g)	0	0	0
Salt & Vinegar Seasoning	¼ tsp (1 g)	0	0	0
Seasoning Salt	¼ tsp (1 g)	0	0	0
Sour Cream & Onion Salt	¼ tbsp (1 g)	0	0	0
SALT SUBSTITUTES				
Cardia				
Salt Alternative	1 pkg (0.6 g)	0	0	0
Estee				
Salt-It	¼ tsp	0	0	0
Morton				
Salt Substitute	¼ tsp (1.2 g)	tr	0	0
Mrs. Dash				
Onion & Herb	⅛ tsp (0.02 oz)	2	—	0
NoSalt				
Salt Alternative	1 pkg (0.75 g)	0	0	0
Papa Dash				
Lite Salt	½ tsp (1 g)	0	0	0
SANDWICH				
TAKE-OUT				
chicken fillet plain	1	515	9	29
chicken fillet w/ cheese lettuce mayonnaise & tomato	1	632	12	39
croque monsieur	1 (12.4 oz)	765	26	46
fish fillet w/ tartar sauce	1	431	5	55

FOOD	PORTION	CALS.	SAT. FAT	FAT
fish fillet w/ tartar sauce & cheese	1	524	8	29
fried egg w/ cheese	1	340	7	19
fried egg w/ cheese & ham	1	348	7	16
ham w/ cheese	1	353	6	15
roast beef submarine sandwich w/ tomato lettuce & mayonnaise	1	411	7	13
roast beef w/ cheese	1	402	9	18
roast beef plain	1	346	4	14
steak w/ tomato lettuce salt & mayonnaise	1	459	4	14
submarine w/ salami ham cheese lettuce tomato onion & oil	1	456	7	19
tuna salad submarine sandwich w/ lettuce & oil	1	584	5	28

SAPODILLA
fresh	1	140	—	2
fresh cut up	1 cup	199	—	3

SAPOTES
fresh	1	301	—	1

SARDINES
CANNED
atlantic in oil w/ bone	2	50	tr	3
atlantic in oil w/ bone	1 can (3.2 oz)	192	1	11
pacific in tomato sauce w/ bone	1	68	1	5
pacific in tomato sauce w/ bone	1 can (13 oz)	658	11	44
Del Monte				
In Tomato Sauce	1 fish (1.4 oz)	50	1	3
Port Clyde				
In Louisiana Hot Sauce	1 can (3.75 oz)	170	2	9
In Mustard Sauce	1 can (3.75 oz)	150	2	9
In Soybean Oil Select Small	1 can (3.3 oz)	220	4	17
In Soybean Oil With Hot Chilies	1 can (3.3 oz)	155	2	9
In Soybean Oil drained	1 can (3.3 oz)	220	4	17
In Spring Water	1 can (3.3 oz)	170	4	10
In Tomato Sauce	1 can (3.75 oz)	150	2	9
Underwood				
Brisling In Olive Oil	3.75 oz	260	—	20
In Mustard Sauce	3.75 oz	220	—	16
In Sild Oil drained	3.75 oz	460	—	42
In Soya Oil drained	3 oz	230	—	18

FOOD	PORTION	CALS.	SAT. FAT	FAT
Underwood (CONT.)				
In Tomato Sauce	3.75 oz	220	—	16
With Tabasco Pepper Sauce drained	3 oz	220	—	16
Viking's Delight				
Brisling In Olive Oil	1 can (3.75 oz)	460	—	42
Brisling In Olive Oil drained	1 can (3.75 oz)	260	—	20

SAUCE
(see also BARBECUE SAUCE, GRAVY, PIZZA SAUCE, SALSA, SPAGHETTI SAUCE, TOMATO)

FOOD	PORTION	CALS.	SAT. FAT	FAT
JARRED				
teriyaki	1 tbsp	15	0	0
teriyaki	1 oz	30	0	0
Armour				
Chili Hot Dog	¼ cup (2.2 oz)	120	4	9
Meatless Sloppy Joe Sauce	¼ cup (2.2 oz)	30	0	0
Boar's Head				
Ham Glaze Brown Sugar & Spice	2 tbsp (1.4 oz)	120	0	0
Casa Fiesta				
Taco Mild	1 oz	9	—	tr
Cheez Whiz				
Cheese	2 tbsp (1.2 oz)	90	5	7
Cheese Jalapeno Pepper	2 tbsp (1.2 oz)	90	5	7
Cheese Mild Salsa	2 tbsp (1.2 oz)	100	5	7
Chi-Chi's				
Enchilada	¼ cup (2.1 oz)	30	1	2
Taco	1 tbsp (0.5 oz)	10	0	0
Contadina				
Sweet 'n Sour	2 tbsp	40	—	1
Del Monte				
Cocktail	¼ cup (2.7 oz)	100	0	0
Sloppy Joe Hickory Flavor	¼ cup (2.4 oz)	70	0	0
Sloppy Joe Italian Style	¼ cup (2.4 oz)	70	0	0
Sloppy Joe Original	¼ cup (2.4 oz)	70	0	0
El Molino				
Taco Red Mild	2 tbsp	10	0	0
Escoffier				
Diable	1 tbsp	20	0	0
Fritos				
Texas-Style Chili Hearty Topping	2.3 oz	50	1	2
Ultimate Taco Hearty Topping	2.3 oz	50	1	2
Gebhardt				
Enchilada Sauce	3 tbsp (1.5 oz)	25	1	1

FOOD	PORTION	CALS.	SAT. FAT	FAT
Gebhardt (CONT.)				
Hot Dog Chili Sauce	2 tbsp	30	tr	1
Hot Sauce	½ tsp	tr	—	tr
Green Giant				
Sloppy Joe	¼ cup (2.6 oz)	50	0	0
Sloppy Joe as prep w/ meat	1 serv (4.4 oz)	200	4	11
Heinz				
Worcestershire	1 tbsp	6	0	0
Heluva Good Cheese				
Cocktail	¼ cup (1.6 oz)	40	0	0
Hormel				
Not-So-Sloppy-Joe Sauce	¼ cup (2.2 oz)	70	0	0
House Of Tsang				
Bangkok Padang	1 tbsp (0.6 oz)	45	1	3
Hoisin	1 tsp (6 g)	15	0	0
Mandarin Marinade	1 tbsp (0.6 oz)	25	0	0
Saigon Sizzle	1 tbsp (0.6 oz)	40	0	1
Spicy Brown Bean	1 tsp (6 g)	15	0	0
Stir Fry Classic	1 tbsp (0.6 oz)	25	0	1
Stir Fry Sweet & Sour	1 tbsp (0.6 oz)	30	0	0
Stir Fry Szechuan Spicy	1 tbsp (0.6 oz)	20	0	1
Sweet & Sour Concentrate	1 tsp (6 g)	10	0	0
Teriyaki Korean	1 tbsp (0.6 oz)	30	0	1
Hunt's				
Chicken Sensations Barbecue Flavor	1 tbsp (0.5 oz)	35	tr	3
Chicken Sensations Italian Garlic	1 tbsp (0.5 oz)	30	tr	3
Chicken Sensations Lemon Herb	1 tbsp (0.5 oz)	31	tr	3
Chicken Sensations South Westren	1 tbsp (0.5 oz)	27	tr	3
Pepper Sauce Original	1 tsp (5.2 g)	1	0	tr
Steak	1 tbsp (0.6 oz)	10	0	tr
Just Rite				
Hot Dog	2 oz	60	1	3
Kraft				
Cocktail	¼ cup (2.3 oz)	60	0	1
Fat Free Tartar Sauce	2 tbsp (1.1 oz)	25	0	0
Lemon & Herb Tartar Sauce	2 tbsp (1 oz)	150	3	16
Reduced Fat Sandwich Spread	1 tbsp (0.5 oz)	35	0	3
Sandwich Spread	1 tbsp (0.5 oz)	50	1	4
Sweet'n Sour	2 tbsp (1.2 oz)	60	0	0
Tartar	2 tbsp (1.1 oz)	90	2	9

FOOD	PORTION	CALS.	SAT. FAT	FAT
Lawry's				
Marinade Lemon Pepper	1 tbsp (0.5 oz)	10	—	1
Teriyaki Marinade	2 tbsp	72	tr	tr
Lea & Perrins				
Steak	1 oz	40	—	tr
Manwich				
Bold	¼ cup (2.2 oz)	62	0	1
Burrito	¼ cup (2.2 oz)	25	0	tr
Mexican	¼ cup (2.2 oz)	27	0	tr
Original	¼ cup (2.2 oz)	32	0	tr
Taco	¼ cup (2.2 oz)	31	0	tr
Thick & Chunky	¼ cup (2.3 oz)	44	0	tr
Marzetti				
Teriyaki Stir-Fry	2 tbsp	80	0	2
McIlhenny				
Tabasco	1 tsp	1	tr	tr
Mrs. Dash				
Steak	1 tbsp (0.4 oz)	17	—	tr
Newman's Own				
Spicy Simmer Sauce Diavolo	½ cup (4.4 oz)	70	0	3
Old El Paso				
Enchilada Hot	¼ cup (2 oz)	30	—	2
Enchilada Mild	¼ cup (2 oz)	25	—	1
Green Chili Enchilada Sauce	¼ cup (2.1 oz)	30	—	2
Taco Hot	1 tbsp (0.5 oz)	5	0	0
Taco Medium	1 tbsp (0.5 oz)	5	0	0
Taco Mild	1 tbsp (0.5 oz)	5	0	0
Taco Sauce	1 tbsp (0.5 oz)	5	0	0
Taco Sauce Extra Chunky Medium	1 tbsp (0.5 oz)	5	0	0
Taco Sauce Extra Chunky Mild	1 tbsp (0.5 oz)	5	0	0
Ortega				
Taco Thick & Smooth Hot	1 tbsp	8	0	0
Taco Thick & Smooth Mild	1 tbsp	8	0	0
Taco Western Style	1 oz	8	—	0
Progresso				
Alfredo	½ cup (4.4 oz)	310	15	27
Red Wing				
Chili Sauce	1 tbsp (0.6 oz)	20	0	0
Seafood Cocktail	¼ cup (2 oz)	90	0	1
Sauce Arturo				
Original	¼ cup (2.2 fl oz)	50	0	1
Simmer Chef				
Golden Honey Mustard	½ cup (4 fl oz)	150	0	2
Hearty Onion & Mushroom	½ cup (4 fl oz)	50	0	1

FOOD	PORTION	CALS.	SAT. FAT	FAT
Snow's				
Newburg With Sherry	⅓ cup	120	—	8
Welsh Rarebit Cheese	½ cup	170	—	11
Tabasco				
Caribbean Steak Sauce	1 tbsp (0.6 oz)	15	0	0
Garlic Basting Sauce	1 tbsp (0.6 oz)	20	0	0
Habanero Sauce	1 tsp (0.2 oz)	5	0	0
Hot Sauce w/ Garlic	1 tsp (0.2 oz)	0	0	0
Jalapeno Pepper Sauce	1 tbsp	15	0	0
New Orleans Steak Sauce	1 tbsp (0.6 oz)	15	0	0
Pepper Sauce	1 tsp (0.2 oz)	0	0	0
Taco Bell				
Taco Sauce Medium	2 tbsp (1.1 oz)	15	0	0
Taco Sauce Mild	2 tbsp (1.1 oz)	15	0	0
The Restaurant Hot Sauce	1 tsp (5 g)	0	0	0
Tostitos				
Beef Fiesta Nacho	2.4 oz	120	3	8
Chicken Quesadilla Topping	2.5 oz	90	2	6
Watkins				
Inferno Hot Pepper Sauce	2 tbsp (1 oz)	35	0	0
Steak Sauce	1 tbsp (0.5 oz)	20	0	0
MIX				
bearnaise as prep w/ milk & butter	1 cup	701	42	68
cheese as prep w/ milk	1 cup	307	9	17
curry as prep w/ milk	1 cup	270	6	15
mushroom as prep w/ milk	1 cup	228	5	10
sourcream as prep w/ milk	1 cup	509	16	30
stroganoff as prep	1 cup	271	7	11
sweet & sour as prep	1 cup	294	tr	tr
teriyaki as prep	1 cup	131	tr	1
white as prep w/ milk	1 cup	241	6	13
Cajun King				
Etoufee Seasoning Mix	3.5 oz	383	—	6
Jambalaya Seasoning Mix	3.5 oz	375	—	9
Durkee				
A La King as prep	1 cup	60	1	4
Cheese as prep	¼ cup	25	1	2
Hollandaise as prep	2 tbsp	10	0	0
White as prep	¼ cup	20	0	1
French's				
Cheese as prep	¼ cup	25	0	1
Hollandaise as prep	2 tbsp	10	0	0
Kikkoman				
Marinade For Meat	1 oz pkg	64	—	tr

FOOD	PORTION	CALS.	SAT. FAT	FAT
Kikkoman (CONT.)				
Sweet & Sour	2⅛ oz pkg	228	—	tr
Teriyaki	1½ oz pkg	125	—	tr
Watkins				
Beef Marinade	¼ tbsp (2 g)	5	0	0
Calypso Hot Pepper Sauce	1 tsp (5 g)	10	0	0
Caribbean Red Pepper Sauce	1 tsp (5 g)	10	0	0
Chicken & Pork Marinade	¼ tbsp (2 g)	5	0	0
Fish & Seafood Marinade	¼ tbsp (2 g)	10	0	0
Meat Magic	1 tsp (6 g)	10	0	0
SHELF-STABLE				
Cheez Whiz				
Cheese Sqeezable	2 tbsp (1.2 oz)	100	4	8
Fresh Gourmet				
Stir 'n Sauce Italian	1 tbsp (0.5 oz)	30	—	1
TAKE-OUT				
bearnaise	1 oz	177	12	19
SAUERKRAUT				
canned	½ cup	22	tr	tr
Boar's Head				
Sauerkraut	2 tbsp (1 oz)	5	0	0
Claussen				
Canned	½ cup	17	—	tr
Del Monte				
Canned	½ cup (4.2 oz)	15	0	0
Hebrew National				
Gallon Kraut	½ cup	25	0	0
New Kraut	½ cup (3.1 oz)	50	—	1
Rosoff's				
Sauerkraut	½ cup (3.2 oz)	50	—	1
Schorr's				
New Kraut	½ cup (3.2 oz)	50	—	1
Seneca				
Canned	2 tbsp	5	0	0
Vlasic				
Old Fashioned	1 oz	4	0	0
SAUSAGE				
(see also HOT DOG, SAUSAGE SUBSTITUTES)				
bierschinken	3.5 oz	174	—	11
bierwurst	3.5 oz	258	—	21
bockwurst	3.5 oz	276	—	25
bockwurst pork & veal raw	1 link (2.3 oz)	200	7	18
bratwurst pork cooked	1 link (3 oz)	256	8	22
brotwurst pork	1 oz	92	3	8

FOOD	PORTION	CALS.	SAT. FAT	FAT
brotwurst pork & beef	1 link (2.5 oz)	226	7	19
chipolata	3.5 oz	342	12	32
chorizo	3.5 oz	499	17	45
fleischwurst	3.5 oz	305	—	29
italian pork cooked	1 (2.4 oz)	216	6	17
italian pork cooked	1 (3 oz)	268	8	21
jagdwurst	3.5 oz	211	—	16
kielbasa pork	1 oz	88	3	8
knockwurst pork & beef	1 oz	87	3	8
knockwurst pork & beef	1 (2.4 oz)	209	7	19
polish pork	1 (8 oz)	739	23	65
polish pork	1 oz	92	3	8
pork & beef cooked	1 patty (1 oz)	107	4	10
pork & beef cooked	1 link (½ oz)	52	2	5
pork cooked	1 link (½ oz)	48	1	4
pork cooked	1 patty (1 oz)	100	3	8
smoked beef cooked	1 sausage (1.4 oz)	134	—	12
smoked pork & beef	1 link (2.4 oz)	229	7	21
smoked pork & beef	1 sm link (½ oz)	54	2	5
vienna canned	1 (½ oz)	45	1	4
vienna canned	7 (4 oz)	315	10	28
zungenwurst (tongue)	3.5 oz	285	—	24
Aidells				
Andouille Cajun Cooked	1 (3.5 oz)	220	8	17
Burmese Curry Cooked	1 (3.5 oz)	220	5	15
Chicken & Apple Fresh	1 (1.9 oz)	110	2	8
Chicken & Apple Smoked	1 (3.5 oz)	220	5	16
Chicken & Turkey New Mexico Smoked	1 (3.5 oz)	220	5	16
Chicken & Turkey Thai Fresh	1 (3.5 oz)	200	5	16
Chicken & Turkey Thai Smoked	1 (3.5 oz)	220	5	16
Chicken & Turkey With Sun-Dried Tomatoes & Basil Fresh	1 (3.5 oz)	200	6	15
Chicken & Turkey With Sun-Dried Tomatoes & Basil Smoked	1 (3.5 oz)	200	5	14
Creole Hot Cooked	1 (3.5 oz)	220	7	16
Duck & Turkey Smoked	1 (3.5 oz)	220	4	16
Hunter's Cooked	1 (3.5 oz)	240	5	19
Italian Hot Fresh	1 (3.5 oz)	230	6	18
Italian Mild Fresh	1 (3.5 oz)	230	6	18
Lamb & Beef With Rosemary Fresh	1 (3.5 oz)	220	6	16

FOOD	PORTION	CALS.	SAT. FAT	FAT
Aidells (CONT.)				
Lemon Chicken Cooked	1 (3.5 oz)	220	5	16
Mexican Chorizo Beef Fresh	1 (3.5 oz)	400	14	37
Whiskey Fennel Cooked	1 (3.5 oz)	230	7	18
Armour				
Vienna Sausage 25% Less Fat	3 (1.9 oz)	130	4	11
Vienna Sausage 50% Less Fat	3 (1.9 oz)	90	3	7
Vienna Sausage Chicken & Beef	3 (1.9 oz)	120	4	10
Vienna Sausage Hot'n Spicy	3 (2.1 oz)	150	5	13
Vienna Sausage In BBQ Sauce	3 (2.1 oz)	150	5	13
Vienna Sausage In Beef Stock	3 (1.9 oz)	150	6	14
Vienna Sausage Jalapeno In Beef Stock	3 (1.9 oz)	170	6	16
Banner				
Sausage Stomachs	2 oz	90	3	5
Sausage Tripe	2 oz	90	3	5
Bilinski's				
Chicken & Vegetable	1 (3 oz)	80	1	2
Chicken Italian With Peppers & Onions	1 (3 oz)	120	1	4
Boar's Head				
Bratwurst	1 (4 oz)	300	11	25
Hot Smoked	1 (3.2 oz)	280	10	25
Kielbasa	2 oz	120	4	10
Knockwurst	1 (4 oz)	310	11	27
Golden Brown				
Beef	1	80	—	7
Mild	1	100	—	10
Spicy	1	100	—	9
Healthy Choice				
Low Fat Smoked	2 oz	70	1	2
Low Fat Smoked Polska Kielbasa	2 oz	70	1	2
Hebrew National				
Beef Knocks	1 (3 oz)	260	—	25
Polish Beef	1 link	240	—	22
Hillshire				
Beer Bratwurst	1 (2 oz)	190	—	17
Bratwurst Fresh	1 (2 oz)	190	—	17
Bratwurst Light Fresh	1 (2 oz)	150	—	11
Bratwurst Spicy	1 (2 oz)	180	—	17
Flavorseal Kielbasa Polska	2 oz	190	—	17
Flavorseal Kielbasa Polska Beef	2 oz	190	—	17
Flavorseal Kielbasa Polska Lite	2 oz	130	—	11

FOOD	PORTION	CALS.	SAT. FAT	FAT
Hillshire (CONT.)				
Flavorseal Kielbasa Polska Mild	2 oz	190	—	17
Flavorseal Kielbasa Polska Turkey	2 oz	90	—	5
Flavorseal Smoked	2 oz	190	—	17
Flavorseal Smoked Beef	2 oz	180	—	16
Flavorseal Smoked Beef & Cheddar	2 oz	190	—	15
Flavorseal Smoked Country Recipe	2 oz	180	—	16
Flavorseal Smoked Hot	2 oz	180	—	16
Flavorseal Smoked Lite	2 oz	130	—	11
Flavorseal Smoked Turkey	2 oz	90	—	5
Flavorseal Smoked w/ Italian Seasoning	2 oz	200	—	18
Italian Mild	1 (2 oz)	190	—	17
Italian Mild Light	1 (2 oz)	150	—	11
Italian Hot	1 (2 oz)	180	—	17
Italian Hot Light	1 (2 oz)	150	—	11
Kielbasa Fresh Polska	1 (2 oz)	190	—	17
Kielbasa Fresh Polska Lower Fat	1 (2 oz)	150	—	11
Links 80% Fat Free Cheddar Hots	2 oz	150	—	12
Links 80% Fat Free Kielbasa	2 oz	130	—	10
Links 80% Fat Free Smokies	2 oz	130	—	10
Links Brats Fully Cooked	2 oz	170	—	16
Links Bratwurst Smoked	2 oz	190	—	17
Links Bun Size Cheddarwurst	2 oz	200	—	18
Links Bun Size Kielbasa	2 oz	180	—	16
Links Bun Size Smoked	2 oz	180	—	16
Links Bun Size Smoked Beef	2 oz	180	—	16
Links Cheddarwurst	2 oz	190	—	17
Links Cheddarwurst Lite	1 link (2.7 oz)	190	—	15
Links Hot	2 oz	190	—	16
Links Hot Beef	2 oz	190	—	17
Links Hot Lite	1 link (2.7 oz)	190	—	15
Links Kielbasa Polska	2 oz	190	—	17
Links Kielbasa Polska Lite	1 link (2.7 oz)	190	—	15
Links Knockwurst Lite	2 oz	180	—	16
Links Lit'l Polskas	2 oz	180	—	16
Links Lit'l Smokies	2 oz	180	—	16
Links Lit'l Smokies Beef	2 oz	180	—	16
Links Lit'l Smokies Cheddar	2 oz	180	—	16

FOOD	PORTION	CALS.	SAT. FAT	FAT
Hillshire (CONT.)				
Links Lit'l Smokies Light	2 oz	120	—	8
Links Polish	2 oz	190	—	17
Links Smoked	2 oz	190	—	18
Mexican Style	1 (2 oz)	190	—	17
Mexican Style Lower Fat	1 (2 oz)	150	—	11
Hormel				
Kielbasa	2 oz	150	5	13
Light & Lean 97 Dinner Smoked	2 oz	60	1	2
Pickled Hot	6 (2 oz)	140	5	11
Pickled Smoked	6 (2 oz)	140	5	11
Smoked Summer	2 oz	200	8	18
Vienna	2 oz	140	5	14
Vienna Chicken	2 oz	110	3	9
Jimmy Dean				
Brick Sausage	2.5 oz	270	9	25
Bulk	2.5 oz	300	10	28
Hickory Smoked Dinner Sausage	2 oz	170	5	14
Pattie Pre-Cooked	1 (1.9 oz)	230	8	22
Polska Kielbaska	2 oz	170	5	15
Sage Pattie	1 (2 oz)	200	7	19
Sausage Pattie Raw	1 (2 oz)	200	6	19
Skinless Link	2 (2 oz)	200	7	19
Skinless Link	4 (2 oz)	200	7	19
Little Sizzlers				
Brown & Serve	3 links (2.1 oz)	190	8	22
Brown & Serve	2 patties (1.8 oz)	190	6	18
Cooked	2 patties (1.8 oz)	230	8	22
Cooked	3 links (1.8 oz)	230	8	22
Heat & Serve Pork cooked	3 links (1.8 oz)	230	8	22
Louis Rich				
Polska Kielbasa	2 oz	90	2	5
Turkey Hot	2.5 oz	120	3	8
Turkey Original	2.5 oz	120	3	8
Turkey Smoked	2 oz	90	2	5
Mr. Turkey				
Breakfast	2.5 oz	130	—	9
Hearty Blend Polish Kielbasa	1 oz	70	—	6
Hearty Blend Smoked	1 oz	70	—	6
Hot Smoked	1 oz	45	—	3
Italian Smoked	1 oz	45	—	3
Polish Kielbasa	1 oz	45	—	3
Smoked	1 oz	45	—	3

FOOD	PORTION	CALS.	SAT. FAT	FAT
Old Smokehouse				
Summer Sausage	2 oz	200	8	18
Oscar Mayer				
Pork cooked	2 links (1.7 oz)	170	5	15
Smokies Beef	1 (1.5 oz)	120	5	11
Smokies Cheese	1 (1.5 oz)	130	5	12
Smokies Link	1 (1.5 oz)	130	4	12
Smokies Little	6 (2 oz)	170	6	15
Smokies Little Cheese	6 (2 oz)	180	6	16
Perdue				
Breakfast Links Turkey Cooked	2 links (2 oz)	100	2	6
Hot Italian Turkey Cooked	1 link (2.4 oz)	110	2	6
Sweet Italian Turkey Cooked	1 link (2.4 oz)	110	2	6
Rudy's Farm				
Italian Hot	2.5 oz	240	7	22
Italian Mild	2.5 oz	240	7	22
Italian Mild Natural Casing	1 (2 oz)	190	6	17
Morning Right Link	3 (2.9 oz)	150	4	10
Morning Right Pattie	2 (2.9 oz)	150	4	10
Pattie Pre-Cooked	1 (1.4 oz)	100	2	6
Smoked	4 (2.1 oz)	200	6	18
Sweet Link	1 (3.9 oz)	380	12	35
Shady Brook				
Turkey Breakfast	2 oz	80	2	4
Turkey Hot Italian	2 oz	100	2	5
Turkey Old World Style	4 oz	190	3	11
Turkey Sweet Italian	2 oz	100	2	5
Shofar				
Knockwurst Beef	1 (3 oz)	260	9	23
Turkey Store				
Breakfast	2 links (2 oz)	140	3	11
Wampler				
Breakfast Turkey	2 (2.4 oz)	110	2	6
Italian Turkey	1 (2.7 oz)	120	2	6
TAKE-OUT				
pork	1 patty (1 oz)	100	3	8
pork	1 link (0.5 oz)	48	1	4

SAUSAGE DISHES

Jimmy Dean				
Italian Sausage & Mozzarella Sandwich	1 (4.5 oz)	380	9	22
Wampler Longacre				
Italian Sausage w/ Peppers & Onions	1 cup	210	—	11

FOOD	PORTION	CALS.	SAT. FAT	FAT
SAUSAGE SUBSTITUTES				
GardenSausage				
Patty	1 (2.5 oz)	140	2	3
Knox Mountain Farm				
No-So-Sausage	1 serv (⅒ pkg)	120	—	1
Lightlife				
Gimme Lean	2 oz	70	0	0
Lean Link Breakfast	1 (1.2 oz)	60	1	3
Lean Link Italian	1 (1.4 oz)	60	1	2
Light	2 (2.4 oz)	80	0	0
Loma Linda				
Linketts	1 (1.2 oz)	70	1	5
Little Links	2 (1.6 oz)	90	1	6
Morningstar Farms				
Breakfast Links	2 (1.6 oz)	60	1	3
Breakfast Patties	1 (1.3 oz)	70	1	3
Grillers	1 patty (2.2 oz)	140	2	7
Sausage Style Recipe Crumbles	⅔ cup (1.9 oz)	90	0	3
Natural Touch				
Vegan Sausage Crumbles	½ cup (1.9 oz)	60	0	0
White Wave				
Meatless Healthy Links	2 (1.6 oz)	140	2	10
Worthington				
Leanies	1 link (1.4 oz)	110	2	8
Prosage Links	2 (1.6 oz)	60	1	3
Saucettes	1 link (1.3 oz)	90	1	6
Super Links	1 (1.7 oz)	110	1	8
Veja Links	1 (1.1 oz)	50	1	3
SAVORY				
ground	1 tsp	4	—	tr
SCALLOP				
FRESH				
raw	3 oz	75	tr	1
FROZEN				
Mrs. Paul's				
Fried	2 oz	160	—	7
HOME RECIPE				
breaded & fried	2 lg	67	1	3
TAKE-OUT				
breaded & fried	6 (5 oz)	386	5	19
SCONE				
apricot scone	1	232	—	7

FOOD	PORTION	CALS.	SAT. FAT	FAT
Finnegan's				
Cranberry	1 (2.7 oz)	90	0	2
Irish Raisin	1 (2.7 oz)	90	0	2
Health Valley				
Apple Kiwi	1	180	0	0
Cinnamon Raisin	1	180	0	0
Cranberry Orange	1	180	0	0
Mountain Blueberry	1	180	0	0
Pineapple Banana	1	180	0	0
TAKE-OUT				
orange poppy	1 (3 oz)	260	4	6
raisin	1 (3 oz)	270	4	6

SCROD

Gorton's				
Microwave Entree Baked	1 pkg	320	4	18

SCUP

fresh baked	3 oz	115	—	3

SEA BASS
(see BASS)

SEA TROUT
(see TROUT)

SEAWEED

agar dried	1 oz	87	tr	tr
agar fresh	1 oz	tr	tr	tr
irishmoss fresh	1 oz	14	tr	tr
kelp fresh	1 oz	12	tr	tr
kombu fresh	1 oz	12	tr	tr
laver fresh	1 oz	10	tr	tr
nori fresh	1 oz	10	tr	tr
spirulina dried	1 oz	83	1	2
spirulina fresh	1 oz	7	tr	tr
tangle fresh	1 oz	12	tr	tr
wakame fresh	1 oz	13	tr	tr
Eden				
Agar Agar Bars	1 tbsp (2.5 oz)	10	0	0
Agar Agar Flakes	1 tbsp (2.5 oz)	10	0	0
Arame	½ cup (0.3 oz)	30	0	0
Hiziki	½ cup (0.3 oz)	30	0	0
Kombu	3.5 in piece (3.3 g)	10	0	0
Nori	1 sheet (2.5 g)	10	0	0
Sushi Nori	1 sheet (2.5 g)	10	0	0

FOOD	PORTION	CALS.	SAT. FAT	FAT
Eden (CONT.)				
Wakame	½ cup (0.3 oz)	25	0	0
Wakame Flakes	½ cup (0.3 oz)	25	0	0
Maine Coast				
Alaria	⅓ cup (7 g)	18	0	0
Dulse	⅓ cup (7 g)	18	0	0
Dulse Flakes	1 oz	75	—	1
Kelp	⅓ cup (7 g)	17	0	0
Kelp Crunch	1 bar (1 oz)	129	1	6
Kelp Crunch Peanut-Raisin	1 bar (1 oz)	129	1	6
Laver	⅓ cup (7 g)	22	0	0
Sea Seasoning Dulse	1 g	3	0	0
Sea Seasoning Dulse With Celery	1 g	3	0	0
Sea Seasoning Dulse With Garlic	1 g	3	0	0
Sea Seasoning Dulse With Sesame	1 g	3	0	0
Sea Seasoning Kelp	1 g	3	0	0
Sea Seasoning Kelp With Cayenne	1 g	3	0	0
Sea Seasoning Nori	1 g	3	0	0
Sea Seasoning Nori With Ginger	1 g	3	0	0

SEITAN
(see WHEAT)

SEMOLINA
dry	1 cup (5.9 oz)	601	tr	2

SESAME
seeds	1 tsp	16	—	2
seeds dried	1 tbsp	52	1	5
seeds dried	1 cup	825	10	72
seeds roasted & toasted	1 oz	161	2	14
sesame butter	1 tbsp	95	1	8
sesame crunch candy	1 oz	146	1	9
sesame crunch candy	20 pieces (1.2 oz)	181	2	12
sesame sticks	1 oz	153	2	10
sesame sticks unsalted	1 oz	153	2	10
tahini from roasted & toasted kernels	1 tbsp	89	1	8
tahini from stone ground kernels	1 tbsp	86	1	7
tahini from unroasted kernels	1 tbsp	85	1	8

FOOD	PORTION	CALS.	SAT. FAT	FAT
Arrowhead				
Sesame Tahini	1 oz	170	—	17
Casbah				
Tahini Sauce Mix as prep	¼ cup	160	0	13
Eden				
Sesame Shake	½ tsp (1.5 g)	10	0	1
Sesame Shake Garlic	½ tsp (1.5 g)	10	0	1
Sesame Shake Organic Seaweed	½ tsp (1.5 g)	10	0	1
Joyva				
Tahini	2 tbsp (1 oz)	200	3	18
Planters				
Nut Mix	1 oz	150	2	12
Stone-Buhr				
Seeds Raw	4 tsp (1 oz)	180	3	16
SESBANIA				
flower	1	1	0	0
flowers	1 cup	5	—	tr
flowers cooked	1 cup	23	—	tr
SHAD				
american baked	3 oz	214	—	15
roe baked w/ butter & lemon	3.5 oz	126	—	3
roe raw	3½ oz	130	—	2
SHALLOTS				
dried	1 tbsp	3	0	0
raw chopped	1 tbsp	7	tr	tr
SHARK				
batter-dipped & fried	3 oz	194	3	12
raw	3 oz	111	1	4
SHEEPSHEAD FISH				
cooked	3 oz	107	tr	1
cooked	1 fillet (6.5 oz)	234	1	3
raw	3 oz	92	1	2
SHELLFISH				
(see INDIVIDUAL NAMES, SHELLFISH SUBSTITUTES)				
SHELLFISH SUBSTITUTES				
crab imitation	3 oz	87	—	1
scallop imitation	3 oz	84	—	tr
shrimp imitation	3 oz	86	—	1
surimi	3 oz	84	—	1
surimi	1 oz	28	—	tr

FOOD	PORTION	CALS.	SAT. FAT	FAT
Louis Kemp				
Crab Delights	½ cup (3 oz)	90	0	0
Lobster Delights	½ cup (3 oz)	80	0	0
Scallop Delights	13 pieces (3 oz)	80	0	0
Ocean Magic				
Imitation King Crab	3 oz	80	—	tr
SHELLIE BEANS				
canned	½ cup	37	tr	tr
SHERBET				
(see also ICES AND ICE POPS)				
orange	½ cup (4 fl oz)	132	1	2
orange	½ gal	2158	19	31
orange	1 bar (2.75 fl oz)	91	1	1
orange home recipe	½ cup	120	—	2
Borden				
Orange	½ cup	110	—	1
Breyers				
Fat Free Orange	½ cup (3 oz)	110	0	0
Fat Free Rainbow	½ cup (3 oz)	110	0	0
Fat Free Raspberry	½ cup (3 oz)	120	0	0
Fat Free Tropical	½ cup (3 oz)	110	0	0
Orange	½ cup (3 oz)	120	1	1
Rainbow	½ cup (3 oz)	120	1	2
Raspberry	½ cup (3 oz)	120	1	2
Tropical	½ cup (3 oz)	120	1	1
Hood				
Lime Orange Lemon	½ cup (3.1 oz)	120	1	1
Orange	½ cup (3.1 oz)	120	1	1
Rainbow Swirl	½ cup (3.1 oz)	120	1	1
Raspberry Orange Lime	½ cup (3.1 oz)	120	1	1
Sealtest				
Lime	½ cup (3 oz)	130	0	1
Orange	½ cup (3 oz)	130	1	1
Rainbow Orange Red Raspberry Lime	½ cup (3 oz)	130	1	1
Red Raspberry	½ cup (3 oz)	130	1	1
SHRIMP				
CANNED				
canned	3 oz	102	tr	2
canned	1 cup	154	tr	3
Robinson				
Canned Shrimp	2 oz	58	—	1

FOOD	PORTION	CALS.	SAT. FAT	FAT
FRESH				
cooked	4 large	22	tr	tr
cooked	3 oz	84	tr	1
raw	3 oz	90	tr	1
raw	4 large	30	tr	tr
FROZEN				
Cajun Cookin'				
Shrimp Creole	12 oz	390	—	11
Shrimp Etouffee	17 oz	360	—	9
Shrimp Jambalaya	12 oz	450	—	20
Gorton's				
Butterfly Shrimp	4 oz	160	—	tr
Microwave Crunchy Shrimp	5 oz	380	3	20
Microwave Entree Shrimp Scampi	1 pkg	390	—	30
Shrimp Crisps	4 oz	280	—	15
Mrs. Paul's				
Entrees Light Seafood & Clams With Linguini	10 oz	240	2	5
Van De Kamp's				
Breaded Butterfly	7 (4 oz)	280	3	14
Breaded Popcorn	20 (4 oz)	270	2	13
Breaded Whole	7 (4 oz)	240	2	10
TAKE-OUT				
breaded & fried	3 oz	206	2	10
breaded & fried	6 to 8 (6 oz)	454	5	25
SMELT				
rainbow cooked	3 oz	106	tr	3
rainbow raw	3 oz	83	tr	2
SNACKS				
(see also CHIPS, FRUIT SNACKS, NUTS MIXED, POPCORN, POPCORN CAKES, PRETZELS, RICE CAKES)				
cheese puffs	1 oz	157	2	10
corn puffs cheese	1 bag (8 oz)	1256	15	78
corn twists cheese	1 bag (8 oz)	1256	15	78
corn twists cheese	1 oz	157	2	10
oriental mix	1 oz	155	—	12
pork skins	1 oz	154	3	9
pork skins barbecue	1 oz	152	3	9
trail mix	1 oz	131	2	8
trail mix	1 cup (5.3 oz)	693	8	44
trail mix tropical	1 oz	115	2	5
trail mix w/ chocolate chips	1 oz	137	2	9
trail mix w/ chocolate chips	1 cup (5.1 oz)	707	9	47

FOOD	PORTION	CALS.	SAT. FAT	FAT
Baken-ets				
BBQ	9 (0.5 oz)	70	2	5
Hot N'Spicy	7 (0.5 oz)	70	2	5
Hot N'Spicy Cracklins	8 (0.5 oz)	80	2	5
Regular	9 (0.5 oz)	80	3	5
Regular Cracklins	8 (0.5 oz)	40	2	6
Barbara's				
Cheese Puffs Bakes	1½ cups (1 oz)	160	2	11
Cheese Puffs Jalapeno	¾ cup (1 oz)	150	2	9
Cheese Puffs Original	¾ cup (1 oz)	150	2	10
Big Dipper				
Bagel Chips Lowfat Barbeque	12 (1 oz)	110	0	2
Bagel Chips Lowfat Garlic	12 (1 oz)	120	0	2
Bagel Chips Lowfat Original	12 (1 oz)	110	0	2
Bugles				
Baked Cheddar Cheese	1½ cups (1 oz)	130	1	4
Baked Original	1½ cups (1 oz)	130	1	4
Baked Original	1 pkg (1.4 oz)	170	1	5
Nacho	1⅓ cups (1 oz)	160	7	9
Nacho	1 pkg (0.9 oz)	130	6	7
Original	1 pkg (1.5 oz)	230	11	13
Original	1⅓ cups (1 oz)	160	8	9
Ranch	1⅓ cups (1 oz)	160	8	9
Smokin BBQ	1⅓ cups (1 oz)	150	7	8
Sour Cream & Onion	1⅓ cups (1 oz)	160	8	9
Cheetos				
Crunchy	21 pieces (1 oz)	160	3	10
Curls	15 pieces (1 oz)	150	3	10
Curls	15 pieces (1 oz)	150	—	9
Flamin' Hot	21 pieces (1 oz)	160	2	10
Nacho Cheese	23 pieces (1 oz)	160	3	10
Puffed Balls	38 pieces (1 oz)	150	3	10
Puffs	29 pieces (1 oz)	160	3	10
Zig Zags	17 pieces (1 oz)	170	3	11
Cheez Doodles				
Crunchy	1 oz	160	—	10
Puffed	1 oz	150	—	9
Cheez Waffies				
Snacks	1 oz	140	—	8
Chex Mix				
Bold'n Zesty	1 pkg (1.7 oz)	230	2	9
Cheddar Cheese	1 pkg (1.7 oz)	220	2	9
Hot'n Spicy	⅔ cup (1 oz)	130	1	5
Hot'n Spicy	1 pkg (1.7 oz)	210	2	7
Traditional	1 pkg (1.7 oz)	210	1	7

FOOD	PORTION	CALS.	SAT. FAT	FAT
Combos				
Cheddar Cheese Cracker	1 pkg (1.7 oz)	250	3	13
Cheddar Cheese Cracker	1 oz	140	2	8
Cheddar Cheese Pretzel	1 oz	130	1	5
Cheddar Cheese Pretzel	1 pkg (1.8 oz)	240	2	9
Chili Cheese w/ Corn Shell	1 oz	140	1	6
Chili Cheese w/ Corn Shell	1 pkg (1.7 oz)	230	2	11
Mustard Pretzel	1 pkg (1.8 oz)	230	1	8
Mustard Pretzel	1 oz	130	1	4
Nacho Cheese Pretzel	1 pkg (1.7 oz)	230	2	8
Nacho Cheese Pretzel	1 oz	130	1	5
Nacho Cheese w/ Tortilla Shell	1 oz	140	1	6
Nacho Cheese w/ Tortilla Shell	1 pkg (1.7 oz)	230	2	11
Peanut Butter Cracker	1 oz	140	2	8
Pepperoni & Cheese Pizza	1 oz	140	1	7
Pepperoni & Cheese Pizza	1 pkg (1.7 oz)	240	2	11
Pizzeria Pretzel	1 pkg (1.8 oz)	230	2	8
Pizzeria Pretzel	1 oz	130	1	5
Tortilla Ranch	1 bag (1.7 oz)	240	3	12
Tortilla Ranch	1 oz	140	2	7
Cornnuts				
Barbecue	1 oz	120	tr	4
Nacho Cheese	1 oz	120	tr	4
Original	1 oz	120	tr	4
Original	1 pkg (2 oz)	260	2	8
Picante	1 oz	120	tr	4
Ranch	1 oz	120	tr	4
Dakota Gourmet				
Amazing Corn Classic	1 pkg (1 oz)	360	1	7
Amazing Corn Cool Ranch	1 pkg (1 oz)	367	1	9
Amazing Corn Mesquite BBQ	1 pkg (1 oz)	369	1	8
Heart Smart Toasted Corn	⅓ cup (1 oz)	110	0	2
Toasted Corn Heart Smart	1 pkg (1.75 oz)	177	tr	3
Trail Mix Heart Smart	1 pkg (1.75 oz)	172	0	0
Doo Dads				
Snacks	1 oz	130	1	6
Energy Food Factory				
Poprice Cheddar Cheese	½ oz	60	—	3
Poprice Herb & Garlic	½ oz	50	—	2
Poprice Lite	½ oz	50	—	2
Poprice Original No Salt	½ oz	45	0	0
Frito Lay				
Funyuns	13 (1 oz)	140	2	7
Munchos	16 (1 oz)	160	2	10
Munchos BBQ	14 (1 oz)	160	2	10

FOOD	PORTION	CALS.	SAT. FAT	FAT
Hapi				
Chili Bits	½ cup (1 oz)	110	0	0
Health Valley				
Cheddar Lites Green Onion	1¾ cups	120	—	3
Cheddar Lites Original	1¾ cups	120	—	3
Corn Puffs Caramel	2 cups	120	—	2
Low Fat Potato Puffs Cheddar Cheese	1½ cups	110	—	3
Low Fat Potato Puffs Garlic w/ Cheese	1½ cups	260	—	3
Low Fat Potato Puffs Zesty Ranch	1½ cups	110	—	3
Innovative Foods				
Roasted Sweet Corn	1 pkg (0.8 oz)	76	0	0
Lance				
Cheese Balls	1 pkg (1 oz)	150	2	8
Crunchy Cheese Twists	1 pkg (1.25 oz)	190	—	4
Gold-N-Chees	1 pkg (1 oz)	130	2	5
Onion Rings	1 pkg (0.9 oz)	100	2	8
Pork Skins	1 pkg (0.4 oz)	65	2	4
Pork Skins BBQ	1 pkg (0.4 oz)	60	2	4
Mr. Peanut				
Peanut Butter Crisps Graham	12 pieces (1.1 oz)	150	2	8
Pita Puffs				
Barbeque	35 (1 oz)	120	0	3
Lowfat Garlic	35 (1 oz)	110	0	1
Lowfat Original	35 (1 oz)	110	0	1
Lowfat Salsa	35 (1 oz)	110	0	1
Pizza	35 (1 oz)	120	0	2
Ranch	35 (1 oz)	120	0	2
Planters				
Cheez Balls	1 oz	150	2	10
Cheez Balls	1 pkg (1 oz)	150	2	10
Cheez Curls	1 pkg (1.2 oz)	190	3	12
Cheez Mania Original	42 pieces (1 oz)	150	2	10
Heat Snack Mix	1 oz	140	1	8
Robert's American Gourmet				
Pirate's Booty Puffed Rice & Corn w/ Cheddar	1 oz	120	0	3
Snyder's of Hanover				
Cheddar Cheese Twists	1 oz	150	—	8
Kruncheez	1 oz	160	—	10
Nibblers Garlic Bread	13 pieces (1 oz)	130	1	3
Onion Toasters	1 oz	150	—	8

FOOD	PORTION	CALS.	SAT. FAT	FAT
Snyder's of Hanover (CONT.)				
Snack Mix	1 oz	170	1	8
Sopaipillas Apple & Cinnamon	1 oz	150	1	8
Splurge				
Snack Mix Fat Free Original	⅔ cup (1 oz)	100	0	0
Ultra Slim-Fast				
Lite N' Tasty Cheese Curls	1 oz	110	—	3
Utz				
Caramel Corn Clusters	1⅛ cups (1 oz)	120	0	2
Cheese Balls	50 (1 oz)	150	3	9
Cheese Curls	18 (1 oz)	150	3	9
Cheese Curls Crunchy	30 (1 oz)	160	2	10
Cheese Curls Reduced Fat	32 (1 oz)	140	1	6
Onion Rings	41 (1 oz)	140	1	7
Party Mix	¾ cup (1 oz)	140	1	6
Pork Cracklins	0.5 oz	90	3	7
Pork Cracklins Hot & Spicy	0.5 oz	80	2	5
Pork Rinds	0.5 oz	80	2	5
Pork Rinds BBQ	0.5 oz	80	2	5
Weight Watchers				
Cheese Curls	1 pkg (0.5 oz)	70	1	3

SNAIL

cooked	3 oz	233	tr	1
raw	3 oz	117	tr	tr

SNAPPER

cooked	3 oz	109	tr	1
cooked	1 fillet (6 oz)	217	1	3
raw	3 oz	85	tr	1

SODA

(see also DRINK MIXERS, SPORTS DRINKS, WATER)

club	12 oz	0	0	0
cola	12 oz	151	—	tr
cream	12 oz	191	0	0
diet cola	12 oz	2	0	0
diet cola w/ equal	12 oz	2	0	0
diet cola w/ saccharin	12 oz	2	0	0
ginger ale	12 oz can	124	—	0
grape	12 oz	161	0	0
lemon lime	12 oz	149	0	0
orange	12 oz	177	0	0
pepper type	12 oz	151	—	tr
quinine	12 oz	125	0	0

FOOD	PORTION	CALS.	SAT. FAT	FAT
root beer	12 oz	152	0	0
tonic water	12 oz	125	0	0
7 Up				
Cherry	1 oz	13	—	0
Cherry Diet	1 oz	tr	—	0
Diet	1 oz	tr	—	0
Gold	1 oz	13	—	0
Gold Diet	1 oz	tr	—	0
Original	1 oz	12	—	0
After The Fall				
Raspberry Ginger Ale	1 can (12 oz)	150	0	0
Barrelhead				
Root Beer	8 fl oz	110	0	0
Barritts				
Ginger Beer	1 bottle (12 oz)	200	0	0
Best Health				
Root Beer	1 bottle (12 oz)	165	0	0
Vanilla Cream	1 bottle (12 oz)	170	0	0
Burst				
Cola Strawberry	8 fl oz	117	0	0
Canada Dry				
Birch Beer Brown	8 fl oz	110	0	0
Birch Beer Clear	8 fl oz	110	0	0
Black Cherry Wishniak	8 fl oz	130	0	0
Cactus Cooler	8 fl oz	110	0	0
California Strawberry	8 fl oz	110	0	0
Club	8 fl oz	0	0	0
Club Sodium Free	8 fl oz	0	0	0
Concord Grape	8 fl oz	120	0	0
Diet Ginger Ale	8 fl oz	0	0	0
Diet Ginger Ale Cherry	8 fl oz	0	0	0
Diet Ginger Ale Cranberry	8 fl oz	0	0	0
Diet Ginger Ale Lemon	8 fl oz	5	0	0
Diet Tonic Water	8 fl oz	0	0	0
Diet Tonic Water Twist Of Lime	8 fl oz	0	0	0
Ginger Ale	8 fl oz	100	0	0
Ginger Ale Cherry	8 fl oz	110	0	0
Ginger Ale Cranberry	8 fl oz	100	0	0
Ginger Ale Golden	8 fl oz	100	0	0
Ginger Ale Lemon	8 fl oz	100	0	0
Half & Half	8 fl oz	110	0	0
Hi-Spot	8 fl oz	110	0	0
Island Lime	8 fl oz	140	0	0

FOOD	PORTION	CALS.	SAT. FAT	FAT
Jamaica Cola	8 fl oz	110	0	0
Lemon Sour	8 fl oz	100	0	0
Peach	8 fl oz	120	0	0
Pina Pineapple	8 fl oz	110	0	0
Seltzer	8 fl oz	0	0	0
Seltzer Cherry	8 fl oz	0	0	0
Seltzer Cranberry Lime	8 fl oz	0	0	0
Seltzer Grapefruit	8 fl oz	0	0	0
Seltzer Lemon Lime	8 fl oz	0	0	0
Seltzer Mandarin Orange	8 fl oz	0	0	0
Seltzer Peach	8 fl oz	0	0	0
Seltzer Raspberry	8 fl oz	0	0	0
Seltzer Strawberry	8 fl oz	0	0	0
Seltzer Tropical	8 fl oz	0	0	0
Sunripe Orange	8 fl oz	140	0	0
Tahitian Treat	8 fl oz	150	0	0
Tonic Water	8 fl oz	100	0	0
Tonic Water Twist Of Lime	8 fl oz	100	0	0
Vanilla Cream	8 fl oz	120	0	0
Vichy Water	8 fl oz	0	0	0
Wild Cherry	8 fl oz	110	0	0
Clearly 2				
Black Cherry	8 fl oz	2	—	0
Key Lime	8 fl oz	2	—	0
Clearly Canadian				
Alpine Fruit & Berries	8 fl oz	90	—	0
Boysenberry Mist	8 fl oz	2	—	0
Coastal Cranberry	8 fl oz	90	—	0
Country Raspberry	8 fl oz	80	—	0
Green Apple	8 fl oz	80	—	0
Mountain Blackberry	8 fl oz	100	—	0
Orchard Peach Strawberry	8 fl oz	90	—	0
Soda	8 fl oz	0	0	0
Summer Strawberry	8 fl oz	80	—	0
Western Longanberry	8 fl oz	80	—	0
Wild Cherry	8 fl oz	90	—	0
Coca-Cola				
Cherry	8 fl oz	104	0	0
Classic	8 fl oz	97	0	0
Classic Caffeine-Free	8 fl oz	97	0	0
Coke II	8 fl oz	105	0	0
Diet	8 fl oz	1	0	0
Diet Cherry	8 fl oz	1	0	0
Diet Coke Caffeine-free	8 fl oz	1	0	0

FOOD	PORTION	CALS.	SAT. FAT	FAT
Cott				
Cola	8 fl oz	110	0	0
Ginger Ale	8 fl oz	90	0	0
Grape	8 fl oz	130	0	0
Orange	8 fl oz	140	0	0
Pineapple	8 fl oz	130	0	0
Punch	8 fl oz	130	0	0
Seltzer	8 fl oz	0	0	0
Crush				
Cherry	8 fl oz	140	0	0
Grape	8 fl oz	110	0	0
Orange	8 fl oz	140	0	0
Orange Diet	8 fl oz	0	0	0
Pineapple	8 fl oz	140	0	0
Strawberry	8 fl oz	130	0	0
Tropical Fruit Punch	1 can (11.5 fl oz)	200	0	0
Tropical Fruit Punch	1 bottle (10 fl oz)	180	0	0
Diet Rite				
Black Cherry Salt/Sodium Free	8 fl oz	2	0	0
Cola	8 fl oz	1	0	0
Cola Caffeine/Sugar Free	8 fl oz	1	0	0
Cola Salt/Sodium Free	8 fl oz	1	0	0
Fruit Punch Salt/Sodium Free	8 fl oz	2	0	0
Golden Peach Salt/Sodium Free	8 fl oz	2	0	0
Key Lime Salt/Sodium Free	8 fl oz	7	0	0
Pink Grapefruit Salt/Sodium Free	8 fl oz	2	0	0
Red Raspberry Salt/Sodium Free	8 fl oz	3	0	0
Tangerine Salt/Sodium Free	8 fl oz	2	0	0
White Grape Salt/Sodium Free	8 fl oz	1	0	0
Dr Pepper				
Diet	1 oz	tr	—	0
Free	1 oz	12	—	0
Free Diet	1 oz	tr	—	0
Original	1 oz	13	—	0
Dr. Nehi				
Soda	8 fl oz	100	0	0
Fanta				
Ginger Ale	8 fl oz	86	0	0
Grape	8 fl oz	117	0	0
Orange	8 fl oz	118	0	0
Root Beer	8 fl oz	111	0	0

FOOD	PORTION	CALS.	SAT. FAT	FAT
Fresca				
Soda	8 fl oz	3	0	0
Health Valley				
Ginger Ale	1 bottle	160	0	0
Rootbeer Old Fashioned	1 bottle	160	0	0
Sarsaparilla Rootbeer	1 bottle	160	0	0
Hires				
Cream	8 fl oz	130	0	0
Cream Soda Diet	8 fl oz	0	0	0
Original Mocha	8 fl oz	100	0	0
Original Mocha Diet	8 fl oz	5	0	0
Root Beer	8 fl oz	130	0	0
Root Beer Diet	8 fl oz	0	0	0
IBC				
Root Beer	8 oz	110	0	0
Kick				
Soda	8 fl oz	120	0	0
Like				
Cola	1 oz	13	—	0
Cola Sugar Free	1 oz	tr	—	0
Mello Yellow				
Diet	8 fl oz	4	0	0
Soda	8 fl oz	119	0	0
Minute Maid				
Berry	8 fl oz	111	0	0
Diet Orange	8 fl oz	2	0	0
Fruit Punch	8 fl oz	117	0	0
Grape	8 fl oz	121	0	0
Grapefruit	8 fl oz	108	0	0
Orange	8 fl oz	118	0	0
Peach	8 fl oz	110	0	0
Pineapple	8 fl oz	109	0	0
Raspberry	8 fl oz	111	0	0
Soda	8 fl oz	110	0	0
Strawberry	8 fl oz	122	0	0
Mountain Dew				
Diet	8 fl oz	2	0	0
Soda	8 fl oz	118	0	0
Mr. PiBB				
Diet	8 fl oz	1	0	0
Soda	6 oz	97	0	0
Mug				
Cream	8 fl oz	122	0	0
Diet Cream	8 fl oz	2	0	0

FOOD	PORTION	CALS.	SAT. FAT	FAT
Mug (CONT.)				
Diet Root Beer	8 fl oz	1	0	0
Root Beer	8 fl oz	141	0	0
Nehi				
Cream	8 fl oz	120	0	0
Fruit Punch	8 fl oz	120	0	0
Ginger Ale	8 fl oz	90	0	0
Grape	8 fl oz	120	0	0
Orange	8 fl oz	130	0	0
Peach	8 fl oz	130	0	0
Pineapple	8 fl oz	130	0	0
Quinine Water	8 fl oz	90	0	0
Root Beer	8 fl oz	120	0	0
Strawberry	8 fl oz	120	0	0
Wild Red	8 fl oz	120	0	0
Old Colony				
Grape	8 fl oz	140	0	0
Orangina				
Sparkling Citrus	6 fl oz	80	0	0
Pepsi				
Caffeine Free	8 fl oz	105	0	0
Diet	8 fl oz	1	0	0
Diet Caffeine Free	8 fl oz	1	0	0
Regular	8 fl oz	105	0	0
Ramblin' Root Beer				
Ramblin' Root Beer	8 fl oz	120	0	0
Razing Razberry				
Cola	8 fl oz	117	0	0
Royal Crown				
Caffeine Free Cola	8 fl oz	110	0	0
Cherry	8 fl oz	110	0	0
Cola	8 fl oz	100	0	0
Diet	8 fl oz	1	0	0
Diet Caffeine Free	8 fl oz	1	0	0
Diet Cranberry Apple Salt/ Sodium Free	8 fl oz	2	0	0
Diet Cranberry Salt/Sodium Free	8 fl oz	2	0	0
Royal Mistic				
'N Juice Black Cherry	12 fl oz	146	0	0
'N Juice Peach Vanilla	12 fl oz	146	0	0
'N Juice Tangerine Orange	12 fl oz	146	0	0
'N Juice Tropical Supreme	12 fl oz	152	0	0
'N Juice Wild Berry	12 fl oz	156	0	0

FOOD	PORTION	CALS.	SAT. FAT	FAT
Royal Mistic (CONT.)				
Caribbean Fruit Punch	16 fl oz	230	0	0
Grape Strawberry	16 fl oz	230	0	0
Sparkling Diet With Lime Kiwi	11.1 fl oz	0	0	0
Sparkling Diet With Raspberry Boysenberry	11.1 fl oz	0	0	0
Sparkling Diet With Royal Peach	11.1 fl oz	0	0	0
Sparkling Diet With Wild Cherry	11.1 fl oz	0	0	0
Sparkling With Lime Kiwi	11.1 fl oz	112	0	0
Sparkling With Mandarin Orange Pineappple	11.1 fl oz	120	0	0
Sparkling With Mango Passion	11.1 fl oz	112	0	0
Sparkling With Raspberry Boysenberry	11.1 fl oz	112	0	0
Sparkling With Royal Peach	11.1 fl oz	112	0	0
Sparkling With Wild Cherry	11.1 fl oz	112	0	0
Saranac				
Diet Root Beer	1 bottle (12 oz)	35	0	0
Ginger Beer	1 bottle (12 oz)	160	0	0
Root Beer	1 bottle (12 oz)	180	0	0
Schweppes				
Bitter Lemon	8 fl oz	110	0	0
Club	8 fl oz	0	0	0
Club Sodium Free	8 fl oz	0	0	0
Diet Ginger Ale	8 fl oz	0	0	0
Diet Ginger Ale Dry Grape	8 fl oz	2	0	0
Diet Ginger Ale Raspberry	8 fl oz	0	0	0
Ginger Ale	8 fl oz	90	0	0
Ginger Ale Dry Grape	8 fl oz	100	0	0
Ginger Ale Raspberry	8 fl oz	100	0	0
Ginger Beer	8 fl oz	100	0	0
Grape	8 fl oz	130	0	0
Grapefruit	8 fl oz	110	0	0
Lemon Sour	8 fl oz	110	0	0
Lemon-Lime	8 fl oz	100	0	0
Seltzer Black Berry	8 fl oz	0	0	0
Seltzer Lemon	8 fl oz	0	0	0
Seltzer Lemon Lime	8 fl oz	0	0	0
Seltzer Lime	8 fl oz	0	0	0
Seltzer Orange	8 fl oz	0	0	0
Seltzer Peaches & Cream	8 fl oz	0	0	0
Seltzer Raspberry	8 fl oz	0	0	0
Tonic Citrus	8 fl oz	90	0	0

FOOD	PORTION	CALS.	SAT. FAT	FAT
Schweppes (CONT.)				
Tonic Cranberry	8 fl oz	90	0	0
Tonic Raspberry	8 fl oz	90	0	0
Tonic Water Diet	8 fl oz	0	0	0
Shasta				
Black Cherry	1 can (12 oz)	170	0	0
Caffeine Free Cola	1 can (12 oz)	160	0	0
Cherry Cola	1 can (12 oz)	160	0	0
Club Soda	1 can (12 oz)	0	0	0
Cola	1 can (12 oz)	170	0	0
Creme	1 can (12 oz)	190	0	0
Diet Black Cherry	1 can (12 oz)	0	0	0
Diet Caffeine Free Cola	1 can (12 oz)	0	0	0
Diet Cherry Cola	1 can (12 oz)	0	0	0
Diet Cola	1 can (12 oz)	0	0	0
Diet Creme	1 can (12 oz)	0	0	0
Diet Doc Shasta	1 can (12 oz)	0	0	0
Diet Ginger Ale	1 can (12 oz)	0	0	0
Diet Grape	1 can (12 oz)	0	0	0
Diet Grapefruit	1 can (12 oz)	0	0	0
Diet Grapefruit	1 can (12 oz)	0	0	0
Diet Kiwi-Strawberry	1 can (12 oz)	0	0	0
Diet Lemon-Lime Twist	1 can (12 oz)	0	0	0
Diet Orange	1 can (12 oz)	0	0	0
Diet Pineapple-Orange	1 can (12 oz)	0	0	0
Diet Raspberry Creme	1 can (12 oz)	0	0	0
Diet Red Pop	1 can (12 oz)	0	0	0
Diet Root Beer	1 can (12 oz)	0	0	0
Diet Strawberry	1 can (12 oz)	0	0	0
Diet Strawberry-Peach	1 can (12 oz)	0	0	0
Doc Shasta	1 can (12 oz)	160	0	0
Fruit Punch	1 can (12 oz)	200	0	0
Ginger Ale	1 can (12 oz)	130	0	0
Grape	1 can (12 oz)	190	0	0
Kiwi-Strawberry	1 can (12 oz)	170	0	0
Lemon-Lime Twist	1 can (12 oz)	150	0	0
Moon Mist	1 can (12 oz)	180	0	0
Orange	1 can (12 oz)	200	0	0
Peach	1 can (12 oz)	170	0	0
Pineapple	1 can (12 oz)	200	0	0
Pineapple-Orange	1 can (12 oz)	180	0	0
Quinine/Tonic	1 can (12 oz)	130	0	0
Raspberry Creme	1 can (12 oz)	170	0	0
Red Pop	1 can (12 oz)	170	0	0
Root Beer	1 can (12 oz)	170	0	0

FOOD	PORTION	CALS.	SAT. FAT	FAT
Shasta (CONT.)				
Strawberry	1 can (12 oz)	190	0	0
Strawberry-Peach	1 can (12 oz)	170	0	0
Slice				
Diet Lemon Lime	8 fl oz	5	0	0
Diet Mandarin	8 fl oz	5	0	0
Lemon Lime	8 fl oz	100	0	0
Mandarin Orange	8 fl oz	128	0	0
Red	8 fl oz	128	0	0
Snapple				
Amazin' Grape	8 fl oz	120	0	0
Cherry Lime Ricky	8 fl oz	110	0	0
Creme D'Vanilla	8 fl oz	130	0	0
French Cherry	8 fl oz	120	0	0
Kiwi Peach	8 fl oz	120	0	0
Kiwi Strawberry	8 fl oz	130	0	0
Mango Madness	8 fl oz	130	0	0
Passion Supreme	8 fl oz	120	0	0
Peach Melba	8 fl oz	120	0	0
Raspberry	8 fl oz	120	0	0
Seltzer Black Cherry	8 fl oz	0	0	0
Seltzer Lemon Lime	8 fl oz	0	0	0
Seltzer Original	8 fl oz	0	0	0
Seltzer Tangerine	8 fl oz	0	0	0
Tru Root Beer	8 fl oz	110	0	0
Sprite				
Diet	8 fl oz	3	0	0
Soda	8 fl oz	100	0	0
Sundrop				
Cherry	8 fl oz	130	0	0
Diet	8 fl oz	5	0	0
Soda	8 fl oz	140	0	0
Sunkist				
Cactus Cooler	8 fl oz	110	0	0
Cherry	8 fl oz	140	0	0
Diet Citrus	8 fl oz	0	0	0
Diet Orange	8 fl oz	5	0	0
Fruit Punch	8 fl oz	130	0	0
Orange	8 fl oz	140	0	0
Peach	8 fl oz	120	0	0
Pineapple	8 fl oz	140	0	0
Strawberry	8 fl oz	140	0	0
TAB				
Soda	8 fl oz	1	0	0

FOOD	PORTION	CALS.	SAT. FAT	FAT
Tropical Chill				
Cola	8 fl oz	117	0	0
Diet	8 fl oz	1	0	0
Upper 10				
Diet	8 fl oz	3	0	0
Diet Salt/Sodium Free	8 fl oz	3	0	0
Salt Free	8 fl oz	100	0	0
Soda	8 fl oz	100	0	0
Welch's				
Sparkling Apple	12 oz	180	—	0
Sparkling Grape	12 oz	180	—	0
Sparkling Orange	12 oz	180	—	0
Sparkling Strawberry	12 oz	180	—	0
Wink				
Diet	8 fl oz	5	0	0
Soda	8 fl oz	130	0	0
Yoo-Hoo				
Original	9 fl oz	150	tr	tr
SOLDIER BEANS				
Bean Cuisine				
Dried	½ cup	115	—	1
SOLE				
FRESH				
cooked	3 oz	99	tr	1
cooked	1 fillet (4.5 oz)	148	tr	2
FROZEN				
Gorton's				
Fishmarket Fresh	5 oz	110	—	1
Microwave Entree In Lemon Butter	1 pkg	380	11	24
Microwave Entree In Wine Sauce	1 pkg	180	3	8
Mrs. Paul's				
Light Fillets	1 fillet	240	—	10
Van De Kamp's				
Lightly Breaded Fillets	1 (4 oz)	220	2	11
Natural Fillets	1 (4 oz)	110	0	2
TAKE-OUT				
battered & fried	3.2 oz	211	3	11
breaded & fried	3.2 oz	211	3	11

SORBET
(see ICES AND ICE POPS)

FOOD	PORTION	CALS.	SAT. FAT	FAT

SORGHUM

FOOD	PORTION	CALS.	SAT. FAT	FAT
sorghum	1 cup (6.7 oz)	651	1	6

SOUFFLE

FOOD	PORTION	CALS.	SAT. FAT	FAT
lemon chilled	1 cup	176	—	tr
raspberry chilled	1 cup	173	—	tr
spinach	1 cup	218	7	18

SOUP
CANNED

FOOD	PORTION	CALS.	SAT. FAT	FAT
asparagus cream of as prep w/ milk	1 cup	161	3	8
asparagus cream of as prep w/ water	1 cup	87	1	4
beef broth ready-to-serve	1 can (14 oz)	27	tr	1
beef broth ready-to-serve	1 cup	16	tr	1
beef noodle as prep w/water	1 cup	84	1	3
black bean turtle soup	1 cup	218	tr	1
black bean as prep w/water	1 cup	116	tr	2
celery cream of as prep w/ milk	1 cup	165	4	10
celery cream of as prep w/ water	1 cup	90	1	6
celery cream of not prep	1 can (10.75 oz)	219	3	14
cheese as prep w/ milk	1 cup	230	9	15
cheese as prep w/ water	1 cup	155	7	10
cheese not prep	1 can (11 oz)	377	16	25
chicken broth as prep w/ water	1 cup	39	tr	1
chicken cream of as prep w/ milk	1 cup	191	5	11
chicken cream of as prep w/ water	1 cup	116	2	7
chicken gumbo as prep w/ water	1 cup	56	tr	1
chicken noodle as prep w/ water	1 cup	75	1	2
chicken rice as prep w/ water	1 cup	251	tr	2
clam chowder new england as prep w/ water	1 cup	95	tr	3
clam chowder new england as prep w/ milk	1 cup	163	3	7
consomme w/ gelatin not prep	1 can (10.5 oz)	71	0	0
consomme w/ gelatin as prep w/ water	1 cup	29	0	0
escarole ready-to-serve	1 cup	27	1	2
french onion as prep w/ water	1 cup	57	tr	2
gazpacho ready-to-serve	1 cup	57	tr	2
minestrone as prep w/water	1 cup	83	1	3

FOOD	PORTION	CALS.	SAT. FAT	FAT
mushroom cream of as prep w/ milk	1 cup	203	5	14
mushroom cream of as prep w/ water	1 cup	129	2	9
oyster stew as prep w/ milk	1 cup	134	5	8
oyster stew as prep w/ water	1 cup	59	3	4
pepperpot as prep w/ water	1 cup	103	2	5
potato cream of as prep w/ milk	1 cup	148	4	6
potato cream of as prep w/ water	1 cup	73	1	2
scotch broth as prep w/ water	1 cup	80	1	3
split pea w/ ham as prep w/ water	1 cup	189	2	4
tomato as prep w/ milk	1 cup	160	3	6
tomato as prep w/water	1 cup	86	tr	2
vegetarian vegetable as prep w/ water	1 cup	72	tr	2
vichyssoise	1 cup	148	4	6
Campbell				
Chicken & Pasta With Garden Vegetables	1 cup (8.4 oz)	90	0	1
Home Cookin' Chicken With Egg Noodles	1 cup (8.4 oz)	90	1	2
Home Cookin' Oriental Noodles w/ Vegetables	1 cup (8.4 oz)	100	1	1
College Inn				
Beef Broth	½ can (7 oz)	16	0	0
Chicken Broth	½ can (7 oz)	35	1	3
Chicken Broth Lower Salt	½ can (7 oz)	20	1	2
Gold's				
Russian Borscht	8 oz	70	0	0
Gorton's				
New England Clam Chowder as prep w/ whole milk	¼ can	140	—	5
Goya				
Black Bean	7.5 oz	160	—	4
Hain				
Chicken Broth	8.75 fl oz	70	—	6
Chicken Broth No Salt Added	8.75 fl oz	60	—	5
Chicken Noodle	9.5 fl oz	120	—	4
Chicken Noodle No Salt Added	9.5 fl oz	120	—	4
Creamy Mushroom	9.25 fl oz	110	—	4
Italian Vegetable Pasta	9.5 fl oz	160	—	5
Italian Vegetable Pasta Low Sodium	9.5 fl oz	140	—	6
Minestrone	9.5 fl oz	170	—	2

FOOD	PORTION	CALS.	SAT. FAT	FAT
Hain (CONT.)				
Minestrone No Salt Added	9.5 fl oz	160	—	4
Mushroom Barley	9.5 fl oz	100	—	2
New England Clam Chowder	9.5 fl oz	180	—	4
Split Pea	9.5 fl oz	170	—	1
Split Pea No Salt Added	9.5 fl oz	170	—	1
Turkey Rice	9.5 fl oz	100	—	3
Turkey Rice No Salt Added	9.5 fl oz	120	—	4
Vegetable Chicken	9.5 fl oz	120	—	4
Vegetable Chicken No Salt Added	9.5 fl oz	130	—	4
Vegetable Broth	9.5 fl oz	45	—	0
Vegetable Broth Low Sodium	9.5 fl oz	40	—	tr
Vegetable Split Pea	9.5 fl oz	170	—	1
Vegetable Split Pea No Salt Added	9.5 fl oz	170	—	1
Vegetarian Lentil	9.5 fl oz	160	—	3
Vegetarian Lentil No Salt Added	9.5 fl oz	160	—	3
Vegetarian Vegetable	9.5 fl oz	140	—	4
Vegetarian Vegetable No Salt Added	9.5 fl oz	150	—	5
Health Valley				
5 Bean Vegetable	1 cup	250	0	0
Beef Broth Fat Free	1 cup	20	0	0
Beef Broth Fat Free No Salt	1 cup	20	0	0
Black Bean & Vegetable	1 cup	110	0	0
Chicken Broth	1 cup	45	—	2
Chicken Broth Fat Free	1 cup	30	0	0
Chicken Broth No Salt	1 cup	45	—	2
Country Corn & Vegetable	1 cup	70	0	0
Garden Vegetable	1 cup	80	0	0
Italian Plus Carotene	1 cup	80	0	0
Lentil & Carrot	1 cup	100	0	0
Organic Black Bean	1 cup	110	0	0
Organic Lentil No Salt	1 cup	90	0	0
Organic Minestrone	1 cup	100	0	0
Organic Mushroom Barley No Salt	1 cup	60	0	0
Organic Potato Leek	1 cup	70	0	0
Organic Potato Leek No Salt	1 cup	70	0	0
Organic Split Pea	1 cup	110	0	0
Organic Split Pea No Salt	1 cup	110	0	0
Organic Tomato	1 cup	90	0	0

FOOD	PORTION	CALS.	SAT. FAT	FAT
Health Valley (CONT.)				
Organic Vegetable No Salt	1 cup	80	0	0
Pasta Bolognese	1 cup	100	0	0
Pasta Cacciatore	1 cup	100	0	0
Pasta Romano	1 cup	100	0	0
Real Italian Minestrone	1 cup	90	0	0
Rotini & Vegetable	1 cup	100	0	0
Split Pea & Carrots	1 cup	110	0	0
Super Broccoli Carotene	1 cup	70	0	0
Tomato Vegetable	1 cup	80	0	0
Vegetable Barley	1 cup	90	0	0
Vegetable Power Carotene	1 cup	70	0	0
Healthy Choice				
Beef & Potato	1 cup (8.5 oz)	119	1	2
Chicken Corn Chowder	1 cup (8.8 oz)	176	1	3
Chicken Pasta	1 cup (8.6 oz)	118	1	3
Chicken With Rice	1 cup (8.4 oz)	108	1	3
Chili Beef	1 cup (9.1 oz)	166	1	1
Clam Chowder	1 cup (8.8 oz)	123	1	1
Country Vegetable	1 cup (8.6 oz)	104	tr	1
Cream Of Mushroom	1 cup (8.8 oz)	77	tr	1
Cream Of Chicken With Mushrooms	1 cup (8.9 oz)	127	1	2
Cream Of Chicken With Vegetables	1 cup (8.9 oz)	127	1	2
Garden Vegetable	1 cup (8.6 oz)	118	tr	1
Hearty Chicken	1 cup (8.7 oz)	132	1	3
Lentil	1 cup (8.7 oz)	146	tr	1
Minestrone	1 cup (8.6 oz)	112	tr	1
Old Fashion Chicken Noodle	1 cup (8.8 oz)	137	1	3
Split Pea & Ham	1 cup (8.8 oz)	155	1	2
Tomato Garden	1 cup (8.6 oz)	106	1	2
Turkey With Wild Rice	1 cup (8.4 oz)	92	tr	2
Vegetable Beef	1 cup (8.8 oz)	130	tr	1
Herb-Ox				
Beef Liquid	2 tsp (0.4 oz)	20	0	0
Chicken Liquid	2 tsp (0.4 oz)	15	0	0
Natural Choice				
Orangic Vegan Classic Tomato	1 cup	100	0	1
Organic Vegan Classic Mushroom	1 cup	50	0	2
Organic Vegan Country Corn	1 cup	100	0	1
Organic Vegan Kabocha Squash	1 cup	60	0	1

FOOD	PORTION	CALS.	SAT. FAT	FAT
Natural Choice (CONT.)				
Organic Vegan Southern Greens	1 cup	80	0	3
Organic Vegan Split Pea	1 cup	120	0	1
Organic Vegan Vegetable Curry	1 cup	110	1	4
Old El Paso				
Black Bean With Bacon	1 cup (8.6 oz)	160	1	2
Chicken Vegetable	1 cup (8.4 oz)	110	1	3
Chicken With Rice	1 cup (8.4 oz)	90	1	3
Garden Vegetable	1 cup (8.4 oz)	110	1	3
Hearty Beef	1 cup (8.4 oz)	120	2	3
Hearty Chicken Noodle	1 cup (8.4 oz)	110	1	3
Pritikin				
Chicken & Rice	1 cup (8.8 oz)	80	0	1
Chicken Broth	1 cup (8.5 oz)	15	0	0
Chicken Pasta	1 cup (8.6 oz)	100	0	1
Hearty Vegetable	1 cup (8.8 oz)	90	0	1
Lentil	1 cup (8.4 oz)	130	0	1
Minestrone	1 cup (8.8 oz)	90	0	1
Split Pea	1 cup (9.2 oz)	140	0	1
Three Bean Chili	½ cup (4.5 oz)	90	0	1
Vegetable Broth	1 cup (8.3 oz)	20	0	0
Vegetarian Vegetables	1 cup (9 oz)	100	0	0
Progresso				
Bean And Ham	1 cup (8.4 oz)	160	1	2
Beef	1 can (10.5 fl oz)	180	—	6
Beef Barley	1 cup (8.5 oz)	130	2	4
Beef Minestrone	1 cup (8.5 oz)	140	2	4
Beef Noodle	1 cup (8.5 oz)	140	2	4
Beef Vegetable & Rotini	1 cup (8 oz)	120	2	4
Broccoli & Shells	1 cup (8.5 oz)	70	0	1
Chickarina	1 cup (8.3 oz)	120	2	5
Chicken Minestrone	1 cup (8.4 oz)	120	1	4
Chicken Vegetables & Penne	1 cup (8.4 oz)	100	1	3
Chicken & Wild Rice	1 cup (8.4 oz)	100	1	2
Chicken Barley	1 cup (8.5 oz)	110	1	3
Chicken Broth	1 cup ((8.2 oz)	20	—	1
Chicken Noodle	1 cup (8.4 oz)	80	1	2
Chicken Noodle	1 can (10.5 oz)	110	1	3
Chicken Rice Vegetable	1 cup (8.4 oz)	110	1	3
Chicken Rice Vegetable	1 can (10.5 oz)	130	1	4
Clam & Rotini Chowder	1 cup (8.8 oz)	200	2	9
Corn Chowder	1 cup (8.6 oz)	180	4	10

FOOD	PORTION	CALS.	SAT. FAT	FAT
Progresso (CONT.)				
Cream Of Chicken	1 cup (8.4 oz)	170	4	10
Cream Of Mushroom	1 cup (8.4 oz)	140	4	8
Creamy Tortellini	1 cup (8.4 oz)	210	8	15
Escarole In Chicken Broth	1 cup (8.1 oz)	25	0	1
Green Split Pea	1 cup (8.6 oz)	170	1	3
Healthy Classics Beef Barley	1 cup (8.5 oz)	140	1	2
Healthy Classics Beef Vegetable	1 cup (8.5 oz)	150	1	2
Healthy Classics Chicken Noodle	1 cup (8.3 oz)	80	1	2
Healthy Classics Chicken Rice With Vegetables	1 cup (8.4 oz)	90	0	2
Healthy Classics Cream Of Broccoli	1 cup (8.6 oz)	90	1	3
Healthy Classics Garlic & Pasta	1 cup (8.5 oz)	100	0	2
Healthy Classics Lentil	1 cup (8.5 oz)	120	0	3
Healthy Classics Minestrone	1 cup (8.5 oz)	120	0	3
Healthy Classics New England Clam Chowder	1 cup (8.6 oz)	120	1	2
Healthy Classics Split Pea	1 cup (8.9 oz)	180	1	3
Healthy Classics Tomato Garden Vegetable	1 cup (8.6 oz)	100	0	1
Healthy Classics Vegetable	1 cup (8.4 oz)	80	0	2
Hearty Minestrone With Shells	1 cup (8.4 oz)	120	0	2
Hearty Black Bean	1 cup (8.5 oz)	170	0	2
Hearty Chicken	1 can (10.5 fl oz)	120	1	3
Hearty Chicken & Rotini	1 cup (8.4 oz)	90	1	2
Hearty Penne In Chicken Broth	1 cup (8.4 oz)	70	0	1
Hearty Tomato & Rotini	1 cup (8.4 oz)	90	0	1
Hearty Vegetable With Rotini	1 cup (8.4 oz)	110	0	1
Homestyle Chicken Vegetable	1 cup (8.4 oz)	100	1	3
Lentil	1 can (10.5 fl oz)	170	0	3
Lentil	1 cup (8.5 oz)	140	0	2
Lentil & Shells	1 cup (8.5 oz)	130	0	2
Lentil With Sausage	1 cup (8.5 oz)	170	2	7
Macaroni & Bean	1 cup (8.6 oz)	160	1	4
Manhattan Clam Chowder	1 cup (8.4 oz)	110	0	2
Meatballs & Pasta Pearls	1 cup (8.3 oz)	140	3	7
Minestrone	1 cup (8.4 oz)	130	1	3
Minestrone	1 can (10.5 fl oz)	170	1	4
New England Clam Chowder	1 can (10.5 oz)	220	4	12
New England Clam Chowder	1 cup (8.4 oz)	180	3	10
Spicy Chicken & Penne	1 cup (8.5 oz)	120	1	4

FOOD	PORTION	CALS.	SAT. FAT	FAT
Progresso (CONT.)				
Split Pea With Ham	1 cup (8.5 oz)	160	2	4
Tomato	1 cup (8.5 oz)	90	0	2
Tomato Tortellini	1 cup (8.4 oz)	120	2	5
Tomato Beef & Rotini	1 cup (8.5 oz)	140	2	5
Tortellini In Chicken Broth	1 cup (8.3 oz)	80	1	2
Vegetable	1 cup (8.4 oz)	90	1	2
Zesty Minestrone	1 cup (8.3 oz)	150	3	6
Snow's				
Manhattan Clam Chowder as prep w/ water	7.5 fl oz	70	—	2
New England Clam Chowder as prep w/ milk	7.5 fl oz	140	—	6
New England Corn Chowder as prep w/ milk	7.5 fl oz	150	—	6
New England Fish Chowder as prep w/ milk	7.5 fl oz	130	—	6
New England Seafood Chowder as prep w/ milk	7.5 fl oz	130	—	6
Swanson				
Beef Broth	7.25 oz	18	—	1
Chicken Broth	7.25 oz	30	—	2
Chicken Broth Seasoned w/ Italian Herbs	1 cup (8 oz)	25	0	1
Chicken Broth Seasoned w/ Italian Herbs	1 cup (8 oz)	25	0	1
Natural Goodness Clear Chicken Broth	7.25 oz	20	—	1
Vegetable Broth	7.25 fl oz	20	—	1
Weight Watchers				
Chicken & Rice	1 can (10.5 oz)	110	0	2
Chicken Noodle	1 can (10.5 oz)	150	1	2
Minestrone	1 can (10.5 oz)	130	1	2
Vegetable	1 can (10.5 oz)	130	0	1
FROZEN				
Tabatchnick				
Barley Mushroom	1 serv (7.5 oz)	70	0	0
Barley Mushroom No Salt Added	1 serv (7.5 oz)	70	0	0
Broccoli Cream Of	1 serv (7.5 oz)	90	2	4
Cabbage	1 serv (7.5 oz)	60	0	0
Chicken With Dumplings	1 serv (7.5 oz)	70	0	2
Corn Chowder	1 serv (7.5 oz)	150	2	6
Minestrone	1 serv (7.5 oz)	150	0	1

FOOD	PORTION	CALS.	SAT. FAT	FAT
Tabatchnick (CONT.)				
New England Potato	1 serv (7.5 oz)	150	3	6
New York Chicken	1 serv (7.5 oz)	35	0	0
Old Fashion Potato	1 serv (7.5 oz)	70	0	0
Pea	1 serv (7.5 oz)	180	0	2
Pea No Salt Added	1 serv (7.5 oz)	180	0	2
Spinach Cream Of	1 serv (7.5 oz)	90	2	4
Vegetable	1 serv (7.5 oz)	110	0	1
Vegetable No Salt Added	1 serv (7.5 oz)	110	0	1
Wisconsin Cheddar Vegetable	1 serv (7.5 oz)	140	3	9
Yankee Bean	1 serv (7.5 oz)	160	0	2
MIX				
asparagus cream of as prep w/ water	1 cup	59	tr	2
beef broth	1 pkg (0.2 oz)	14	tr	1
beef broth cube	1 cube (3.6 g)	6	tr	tr
beef broth cube as prep w/water	1 cup	8	tr	tr
celery cream of as prep w/ water	1 cup	63	tr	2
chicken broth	1 pkg (0.2 oz)	16	tr	1
chicken broth as prep w/water	1 cup	21	tr	1
chicken broth cube	1 cube (4.8 g)	9	tr	tr
chicken broth cube, as prep w/ water	1 cup	13	tr	tr
chicken cream of as prep w/ water	1 cup	107	3	5
chicken noodle as prep w/ water	1 cup	53	tr	1
french onion not prep	1 pkg (1.4 oz)	115	1	2
leek as prep w/ water	1 cup	71	1	2
onion as prep w/ water	1 cup	28	tr	1
tomato as prep w/ water	1 cup	102	1	2
Armour				
Bouillon Cubes Beef	1 (4 g)	5	0	0
Bouillon Cubes Chicken	1 (4 g)	5	0	0
Arrowhead				
Bean & Barley	¼ cup (1.9 oz)	170	0	0
Bean Cuisine				
Bean Bouillabisse	1 cup (7.5 fl oz)	174	tr	tr
Island Black Bean	1 cup (8.7 fl oz)	210	1	4
Lots of Lentil	1 cup (7.7 oz)	166	tr	tr
Mesa Maize	1 cup (9.2 fl oz)	179	tr	tr
Rocky Mountain Red Bean	1 cup (8.6 oz)	202	tr	tr
Sante Fe Corn Chowder	1 cup (9.2 oz)	179	tr	tr

FOOD	PORTION	CALS.	SAT. FAT	FAT
Bean Cuisine (CONT.)				
Thick As Fog Split Pea	1 cup (8.6 fl oz)	189	tr	tr
Ultima Pasta E Fagioli	1 cup (8.6 fl oz)	179	0	tr
White Bean Provencal	1 cup (7.7 fl oz)	166	tr	tr
Casbah				
Black Bean	1 pkg (1.7 oz)	170	0	2
Split Pea	1 pkg (2.3 oz)	230	0	1
Sweet Corn Chowder	1 pkg (1.2 oz)	125	0	1
Vegetarian Chili	1 pkg (1.8 oz)	170	0	2
Cup-A-Ramen				
Beef With Vegetables Low Fat as prep	8 oz	220	—	2
Beef With Vegetables as prep	8 oz	270	—	10
Chicken With Vegetables Low Fat as prep	8 oz	220	—	2
Chicken With Vegetables as prep	8 oz	270	—	10
Oriental With Vegetables Low Fat as prep	8 oz	220	—	2
Oriental With Vegetables as prep	8 oz	270	—	10
Shrimp With Vegetables Low Fat as prep	8 oz	230	—	2
Shrimp With Vegetables as prep	8 oz	280	—	10
Cup-a-Soup				
Broccoli & Cheese as prep	1 serv (6 oz)	70	1	3
Chicken Vegetable as prep	1 serv (6 oz)	50	0	1
Chicken Broth as prep	1 serv (6 oz)	20	0	0
Chicken Broth w/ Pasta Fat Free as prep	1 serv (6 oz)	45	0	0
Chicken Noodle as prep	1 serv (6 oz)	50	0	1
Cream Of Chicken as prep	1 serv (6 oz)	70	0	2
Creamy Chicken Vegetable as prep	1 serv (6 oz)	80	2	5
Creamy Mushroom as prep	1 serv (6 oz)	60	0	2
Green Pea as prep	1 serv (6 oz)	80	0	1
Hearty Chicken Noodle as prep	1 serv (6 oz)	60	0	1
Ring Noodle as prep	1 serv (6 oz)	50	0	1
Spring Vegetable as prep	1 serv (6 oz)	45	0	1
Tomato as prep	1 serv (6 oz)	100	0	1
Emes				
Beef Base	1 tsp	18	0	tr
Chicken Base	1 tsp	18	0	tr

FOOD	PORTION	CALS.	SAT. FAT	FAT
Fantastic				
Cha-Cha Chili Low Fat	1 pkg	220	0	1
George Washington				
Broth & Brown Seasoning	1 serv	6	—	0
Broth & Golden Seasoning	1 serv	6	—	0
Broth & Onion Seasoning	1 serv	12	—	0
Broth & Vegetable Seasoning	1 serv	12	—	0
Goodman's				
Cup Of Soup Beef	1 pkg (1½ cups)	180	1	3
Cup Of Soup Chicken Noodle	1 pkg (1½ cups)	180	1	3
Cup Of Soup Vegetable	1 pkg (1½ cups)	180	1	3
Matzo Ball & Soup	1 cup	40	0	1
Matzo Ball & Soup 50% Less Salt	1 serv	50	0	1
Noodleman	1 cup	45	0	1
Noodleman Low Sodium	1 cup	50	0	1
Onion	1 cup	30	1	1
Onion Low Sodium	1 cup	30	0	1
Hain				
Cheese & Broccoli	¾ cup	310	—	22
Cheese Savory	¾ cup	250	—	16
Savory Lentil	¾ cup	130	—	2
Savory Minestrone	¾ cup	110	—	1
Savory Mushroom	¾ cup	210	—	15
Savory Mushroom No Salt Added	¾ cup	250	—	20
Savory Onion	¾ cup	50	—	2
Savory Onion No Salt Added	¾ cup	50	—	1
Savory Potato Leek	¾ cup	260	—	18
Savory Split Pea	¾ cup	310	—	10
Savory Tomato	¾ cup	220	—	14
Savory Vegetable	¾ cup	80	—	1
Savory Vegetable No Salt Added	¾ cup	80	—	1
Health Valley				
Chicken Noodles w/ Vegetables	1 serv	110	0	0
Corn Chowder w/ Tomatoes	1 serv	100	0	0
Creamy Potatoe w/ Broccoli	1 serv	70	0	0
Garden Split Pea w/ Carrots	1 serv	130	0	0
Lentil w/ Couscous	1 serv	130	0	0
Pasta Italiano	1 serv	140	0	0
Pasta Marinara	1 serv	100	0	0
Pasta Parmesan	1 serv	100	0	0

FOOD	PORTION	CALS.	SAT. FAT	FAT
Health Valley (CONT.)				
Spicy Black Bean w/ Couscous	1 serv	130	0	0
Zesty Black Bean w/ Rice	1 serv	100	0	0
Herb-Ox				
Beef Bouillon	1 cube (3.5 g)	5	0	0
Beef Instant Bouillon Powder	1 tsp (4 g)	5	0	0
Beef Instant Broth & Seasoning Pack	1 pkg (4.5 g)	5	0	0
Beef Instant Broth & Seasoning Pack Low Sodium	1 pkg (4 g)	10	0	0
Chicken Bouillon	1 cube (4 g)	5	0	0
Chicken Instant Bouillon Powder	1 tsp (4 g)	5	0	0
Chicken Instant Broth & Seasoning Pack	1 pkg (4 g)	5	0	0
Chicken Instant Broth & Seasoning Pack Low Sodium	1 pkg (4 g)	10	0	0
Vegetable Bouillon	1 cube (4 g)	5	0	0
Hodgson Mill				
13 Bean not prep	1.5 oz	100	0	1
Hurst				
15 Bean Soup Beef	1 serv (6 oz)	120	0	1
15 Bean Soup Cajun	1 serv	120	0	1
15 Bean Soup Chicken	1 serv (6 oz)	120	0	1
15 Bean Soup Chili	1 serv (6 oz)	120	0	1
15 Bean Soup Ham	1 serv	120	0	1
HamBeens Great Northern Bean	1 serv	120	0	1
HamBeens Navy Bean	1 serv	120	0	1
Pasta Fagioli	1 serv	120	0	1
Spanish American Pinto Bean	1 serv	120	0	1
Spanish-American Black Bean	1 serv	120	0	1
Knorr				
Black Bean Cup-A-Soup as prep	1 pkg	200	0	1
Broccoli as prep	8 fl oz	160	—	8
Cauliflower as prep	8 fl oz	100	—	3
Chef's Series Wild Mushroom as prep	8 fl oz	100	—	3
Chick 'N Pasta as prep	8 fl oz	90	—	2
Chicken Bouillon as prep	8 fl oz	16	—	1
Chicken Flavored Noodle as prep	8 fl oz	100	—	2

FOOD	PORTION	CALS.	SAT. FAT	FAT
Knorr (CONT.)				
Chicken Noodle Instant as prep	6 fl oz	25	—	tr
Fine Herb as prep	8 fl oz	130	—	6
Fish Bouillon as prep	8 fl oz	10	—	tr
French Onion as prep	8 fl oz	50	—	1
Hearty Minestrone Cup-A-Soup as prep	1 pkg	150	1	1
Lentil Cup-A-Soup as prep	1 pkg	220	0	0
Mushroom as prep	8 fl oz	100	—	4
Navy Bean Cup-A-Soup as prep	1 pkg	140	0	0
Oriental Hot And Sour as prep	8 fl oz	50	—	1
Oxtail Hearty Beef as prep	8 fl oz	70	—	2
Potato Leek Cup-A-Soup as prep	1 pkg	120	0	0
Spinach as prep	8 fl oz	100	—	5
Spring Vegetable With Herbs as prep	8 fl oz	30	—	tr
Tomato Basil as prep	8 fl oz	90	—	3
Tortellini In Brodo as prep	8 fl oz	60	—	1
Vegetable Cup-A-Soup as prep	1 pkg	100	0	0
Vegetable as prep	8 fl oz	35	—	1
Vegetarian Vegetable Bouillon as prep	8 fl oz	16	—	1
Kojel				
Hearty Potato With Vegetables Instant	1 serv (6 fl oz)	60	0	0
Noodle Soup Chicken Flavor Instant	1 serv (6 fl oz)	70	0	1
Split Pea Instant	1 serv (6 fl oz)	60	0	tr
Tomato Instant	1 serv (6 fl oz)	50	0	0
Vegetable Chicken Couscous Instant	1 serv (6 fl oz)	80	tr	1
Lipton				
Chicken Noodle w/ White Chicken Meat as prep	1 cup	80	1	2
Extra Noodle w/ Chicken Broth as prep	1 cup	90	1	2
Giggle Noodle w/ Chicken Broth as prep	1 cup	70	1	2
Recipe Secrets Beefy Mushroom	1½ tbsp (0.4 oz)	35	0	0
Recipe Secrets Beefy Onion	1 tbsp (0.3 oz)	25	0	1

FOOD	PORTION	CALS.	SAT. FAT	FAT
Lipton (CONT.)				
Recipe Secrets Fiesta Herb w/ Red Pepper as prep	1 cup	30	0	0
Recipe Secrets Golden Herb w/ Lemon as prep	1 cup	35	0	1
Recipe Secrets Golden Onion	1⅔ tbsp (0.5 oz)	50	0	1
Recipe Secrets Italian Herb w/ Tomato as prep	1 cup	40	0	1
Recipe Secrets Onion as prep	1 cup	20	0	0
Recipe Secrets Onion Mushroom as prep	1 cup	30	0	1
Recipe Secrets Savory Herb With Garlic as prep	1 cup	30	0	0
Recipe Secrets Vegetable as prep	1 cup	30	0	0
Ring-O-Noodle w/ Chicken Broth as prep	1 cup	70	1	2
Soup Secrets Chicken 'N Onion as prep	1 cup	120	0	2
Soup Secrets Chicken w/ Pasta & Beans as prep	1 cup	110	0	2
Soup Secrets Country Chicken w/ Pasta & Herbs as prep	1 cup	100	0	2
Soup Secrets Homestyle Lentil w/ Bow Tie Pasta as prep	1 cup	130	0	1
Soup Secrets Minestrone as prep	1 cup	110	0	1
Sprial Pasta w/ Chicken Broth as prep	1 cup	60	0	1
Lite Line				
Beef Bouillon Instant Low Sodium	1 tsp	12	—	tr
Chicken Bouillon Instant Low Sodium	1 tsp	12	—	tr
Maruchan				
Instant Lunch Oriental Noodles Beef	1 pkg (2.25 oz)	290	—	13
Instant Lunch Oriental Noodles Chicken	1 pkg (2.25 oz)	290	7	13
Instant Lunch Oriental Noodles Chicken Mushroom	1 pkg (2.25 oz)	280	—	13
Instant Lunch Oriental Noodles Mushroom	1 pkg (2.25 oz)	290	—	13
Instant Lunch Oriental Noodles Pork	1 pkg (2.25 oz)	290	—	13

FOOD	PORTION	CALS.	SAT. FAT	FAT
Maruchan (CONT.)				
Instant Lunch Oriental Noodles Shrimp	1 pkg (2.25 oz)	290	—	13
Instant Lunch Oriental Noodles Toast Onion	1 pkg (2.25 oz)	270	—	12
Instant Lunch Oriental Noodles Vegetable Beef	1 pkg (2.25 oz)	290	—	12
Instant Wonton Chicken	1 pkg (1.49 oz)	200	—	12
Instant Wonton Hot & Sour	1 pkg (1.49 oz)	200	—	11
Instant Wonton Oriental	1 pkg (1.49 oz)	190	—	12
Instant Wonton Pork	1 pkg (1.49 oz)	200	—	12
Instant Wonton Shrimp	1 pkg (1.49 oz)	200	—	12
Oriental Noodle Picante Style Beef	1 pkg (2.25 oz)	290	—	15
Oriental Noodle Picante Style Chicken	1 pkg (2.25 oz)	290	—	15
Oriental Noodle Picante Style Shrimp	1 pkg (2.25 oz)	300	—	16
Ramen Beef	½ pkg (1.5 oz)	190	—	9
Ramen Chicken	½ pkg (1.5 oz)	190	—	8
Ramen Chicken Mushroom	½ pkg (1.5 oz)	190	—	8
Ramen Chili	½ pkg (1.5 oz)	190	—	9
Ramen Mushroom	½ pkg (1.5 oz)	190	—	9
Ramen Oriental	½ pkg (1.5 oz)	190	—	9
Ramen Pork	½ pkg (1.5 oz)	190	—	9
Ramen Shrimp	½ pkg (1.5 oz)	190	—	9
Wonton Beef	⅓ pkg (0.68 oz)	90	—	5
Wonton Chicken	⅓ pkg (0.67 oz)	90	—	5
Wonton Pork	⅓ pkg (0.68 oz)	90	—	5
Wonton Vegetable	⅓ pkg (0.7 oz)	90	—	6
Morga				
Vegetable Bouillon No Salt Added	½ cube (5 g)	25	1	2
Vegetable Broth Fat Free	1 tsp (4 g)	10	0	0
Nile Spice				
Couscous Almondine	1 pkg	200	0	3
Couscous Garbanzo	1 pkg	220	0	3
Couscous Lentil Curry	1 pkg	200	0	2
Couscous Minestrone	1 pkg	180	0	2
Couscous Parmesan	1 pkg	200	2	3
Homestyle Black Bean	1 pkg	190	0	2
Homestyle Chicken Flavored Vegetable	1 pkg	120	1	2
Homestyle Lentil	1 pkg	180	0	2
Homestyle Minestrone	1 pkg	160	0	2

FOOD	PORTION	CALS.	SAT. FAT	FAT
Nile Spice (CONT.)				
Homestyle Red Beans & Rice	1 pkg	190	0	2
Homestyle Split Pea	1 pkg	200	0	2
Homestyle Sweet Corn Chowder	1 pkg	120	1	3
Italian Tomato	1 pkg	140	3	4
Potato Leek	1 pkg	150	4	6
Potato Romano	1 pkg	140	4	5
Ramen Noodle				
Beef Low Fat as prep	8 oz	160	—	1
Beef as prep	8 oz	190	—	8
Chicken Low Fat as prep	8 oz	160	—	1
Chicken as prep	8 oz	190	—	8
Oriental Low Fat as prep	8 oz	150	—	1
Oriental as prep	8 oz	190	—	8
Pork Low Fat as prep	8 oz	150	—	1
Pork as prep	8 oz	200	—	8
Ultra Slim-Fast				
Beef Noodle	6 oz	45	—	tr
Chicken Leek	6 oz	50	—	tr
Chicken Noodle	6 oz	45	—	tr
Creamy Broccoli	6 oz	75	—	tr
Creamy Tomato	6 oz	60	—	tr
Hearty Vegetable	6 oz	50	—	tr
Onion	6 oz	45	—	tr
Potato Leek	6 oz	80	—	tr
Weight Watchers				
Instant Beef Broth	1 pkg (0.16 oz)	10	0	0
Instant Chicken Broth	1 pkg (0.16 oz)	10	0	0
Wyler's				
Beef Bouillon Instant	1 tsp	6	—	tr
Beef Bouillon Instant Cube	1	6	—	tr
Chicken Bouillon Instant	1 tsp	8	—	tr
Chicken Bouillon Instant Cube	1	8	—	tr
Onion Bouillon Instant	1 tsp	10	—	tr
Vegetable Bouillon Instant	1 tsp	6	—	tr
SHELF-STABLE				
Hormel				
Micro Cup Bean & Ham	1 cup (7.5 oz)	190	1	4
Micro Cup Beef Vegetable	1 cup (7.5 oz)	90	0	1
Micro Cup Broccoli Cheese w/ Ham	1 cup (7.5 oz)	170	5	13
Micro Cup Chicken & Rice	1 cup (7.5 oz)	110	1	3
Micro Cup Chicken Noodle	1 cup (7.5 oz)	110	2	3

FOOD	PORTION	CALS.	SAT. FAT	FAT
Hormel (CONT.)				
Micro Cup New England Clam Chowder	1 cup (7.5 oz)	130	3	5
Micro Cup Potato Cheese w/ Ham	1 cup (7.5 oz)	190	5	13
Lunch Bucket				
Chicken Noodle	1 pkg (7.25 oz)	80	1	2
Country Vegetable	1 pkg (7.25 oz)	60	0	1
TAKE-OUT				
beef stew soup	1 cup (8.8 oz)	221	2	5
black bean turtle soup	1 cup	241	tr	1
brunswick stew soup	1 cup (8.5 oz)	232	2	6
gazpacho	1 cup	46	—	tr
hot & sour	1 serv (14 oz)	173	2	8
onion soup gratinee	1 serv	492	16	27
pasta e fagioll	1 cup (8.8 oz)	194	1	5
ratatouille	1 cup (7.5 oz)	266	3	25

SOUR CREAM
(see also SOUR CREAM SUBSTITUTES)

FOOD	PORTION	CALS.	SAT. FAT	FAT
sour cream	1 cup (8 oz)	493	30	48
sour cream	1 tbsp (0.4 oz)	26	2	3
Breakstone's				
Free	2 tbsp (1.1 oz)	35	0	0
Reduced Fat	2 tbsp (1.1 oz)	45	3	4
Sour Cream	2 tbsp (1 oz)	60	4	5
Cabot				
Light	1 oz	33	—	2
Sour Cream	1 oz	60	4	6
Friendship				
Light	2 tbsp (1 oz)	35	2	3
Sour Cream	2 tbsp (1 oz)	60	4	5
Heluva Good Cheese				
Fat-Free	2 tbsp (1.1 oz)	20	0	0
Light	2 tbsp (1.1 oz)	40	2	3
Sour Cream	2 tbsp (1.1 oz)	60	4	5
Hood				
Fat Free	2 tbsp (1 oz)	20	0	0
Light	2 tbsp (1 oz)	40	2	3
Sour Cream	2 tbsp (1 oz)	60	4	5
Knudsen				
Free	2 tbsp (1.1 oz)	35	0	0
Hampshire	2 tbsp (1 oz)	60	4	6
Light	2 tbsp (1.1 oz)	50	2	3

FOOD	PORTION	CALS.	SAT. FAT	FAT
Naturally Yours				
No Fat	2 tbsp (1 fl oz)	15	0	0
SOUR CREAM SUBSTITUTES				
nondairy	1 oz	59	5	6
nondairy	1 cup	479	41	45
Pet				
Imitation	1 tbsp	25	—	2
Tofutti				
Better Than Sour Cream Sour Supreme	1 oz	50	2	5
SOURSOP				
fresh	1	416	—	2
fresh cut up	1 cup	150	—	1
SOY				

(see also CHEESE SUBSTITUTES, ICE CREAM AND FROZEN DESSERTS, MILK SUBSTITUTES, MISO, SOYBEANS, SOY SAUCE, TEMPH, TOFU, YOGURT FROZEN)

FOOD	PORTION	CALS.	SAT. FAT	FAT
lecithin	1 tbsp	104	2	14
soy milk	1 cup	79	1	5
Loma Linda				
Soyagen All Purpose	¼ cup (1 oz)	130	1	6
Soyagen Carob	¼ cup (1 oz)	130	1	6
Soyagen No Sucrose	¼ cup (1 oz)	130	1	6
SOYBEANS				

(see also MILK SUBSTITUTES, MISO, SOY, SOY SAUCE, TEMPH, TOFU)

FOOD	PORTION	CALS.	SAT. FAT	FAT
dried cooked	1 cup	298	2	15
dry-roasted	½ cup	387	3	19
green cooked	½ cup	127	1	6
honey toasted	¼ cup (1 oz)	130	1	4
roasted	½ cup	405	3	22
roasted & toasted	1 oz	129	1	7
roasted & toasted	1 cup	490	3	26
roasted & toasted salted	1 oz	129	1	7
roasted & toasted salted	1 cup	490	3	26
sprouts raw	½ cup	43	tr	2
sprouts steamed	½ cup	38	tr	2
sprouts stir fried	1 cup	125	1	7
Dakota Gourmet				
Soy Nuts	1 oz	129	1	7
SOY SAUCE				
shoyu	1 tbsp	9	tr	tr
soy sauce	1 tbsp	7	tr	tr
tamari	1 tbsp	11	tr	tr

FOOD	PORTION	CALS.	SAT. FAT	FAT
Eden				
Shoyu Organic	1 tbsp (0.5 oz)	15	0	0
Shoyu Traditional	1 tbsp (0.5 oz)	15	0	0
Tamari Organic Domestic	1 tbsp (0.5 oz)	15	0	0
Tamari Organic Imported	1 tbsp (0.5 oz)	15	0	0
House Of Tsang				
Dark	1 tbsp (0.6 oz)	10	0	0
Ginger Flavored	1 tbsp (0.6 oz)	20	0	0
Light	1 tbsp (0.6 oz)	5	0	0
Low Sodium	1 tbsp (0.6 oz)	5	0	0
Low Sodium Ginger	1 tbsp (0.6 oz)	10	0	0
Low Sodium Mushroom	1 tbsp (0.6 oz)	10	0	0
Ka-Me				
Chinese Light	1 tbsp (0.5 fl oz)	5	0	0
Trappey				
Chef Magic	1 tbsp (0.5 oz)	23	tr	tr
Tree Of Life				
Shoyu	1 tbsp (0.5 oz)	15	0	0
Tamari Reduced Sodium	1 tbsp (0.5 oz)	20	0	0
Tamari Wheat Free	1 tbsp (0.5 oz)	15	0	0

SPAGHETTI

(see PASTA, PASTA DINNERS, PASTA SALAD, SPAGHETTI SAUCE)

SPAGHETTI SAUCE

(see also PIZZA SAUCE, TOMATO)

JARRED				
marinara sauce	1 cup	171	tr	8
spaghetti sauce	1 cup	272	2	12
Classico				
Beef & Pork	4 fl oz	80	—	4
Four Cheese	4 fl oz	70	—	4
Ripe Olives & Mushrooms	4 fl oz	50	—	2
Spicy Red Pepper	4 fl oz	50	—	2
Sweet Peppers & Onions	4 fl oz	50	—	4
Tomato & Basil	4 fl oz	60	—	3
Contadina				
Italian	¼ cup	15	0	0
Sauce	¼ cup	20	0	0
Thick & Zesty	¼ cup	15	0	0
Del Monte				
Traditional	½ cup (4.4 oz)	80	0	1
Traditional No Sugar Added	½ cup (4.4 oz)	60	0	1
With Garlic & Onion	½ cup (4.4 oz)	70	0	1
With Green Peppers & Mushrooms	½ cup (4.4 oz)	70	0	1

FOOD	PORTION	CALS.	SAT. FAT	FAT
Del Monte (CONT.)				
With Meat	½ cup (4.4 oz)	40	0	2
With Mushrooms	½ cup (4.4 oz)	80	0	2
Eden				
Organic No Salt Added	½ cup (4.4 oz)	80	0	3
Enrico's				
Fat Free Organic Basil	½ cup (4 oz)	50	0	0
Fat Free Organic Garlic	½ cup (4 oz)	50	0	0
Fat Free Organic Hot Pepper	½ cup (4 oz)	50	0	0
Fat Free Organic Mushroom	½ cup (4 oz)	60	0	0
Fat Free Organic Traditional	½ cup (4 oz)	45	0	0
Healthy Choice				
Extra Chunky Garlic & Onion	½ cup (4.4 oz)	43	0	tr
Extra Chunky Italian Vegetable	½ cup (4.4 oz)	39	0	tr
Extra Chunky Mushroom	½ cup (4.4 oz)	41	0	tr
Garlic & Herbs	½ cup (4.4 oz)	47	—	1
Super Chunky Mushroom & Sweet Peppers	½ cup (4.4 oz)	44	0	tr
Super Chunky Tomato, Mushroom & Garlic	½ cup (4.4 oz)	46	0	tr
Super Chunky Vegetable Primavera	½ cup (4.4 oz)	46	0	tr
Traditional	½ cup (4.4 oz)	47	0	1
With Meat	½ cup (4.4 oz)	47	tr	1
With Mushrooms	½ cup (4.4 oz)	47	—	1
Hunt's				
Chunky Marinara	½ cup (4.4 oz)	60	tr	2
Chunky Tomato Garlic & Onion	½ cup (4.4 oz)	61	tr	1
Chunky Vegetable	½ cup (4.4 oz)	63	tr	1
Classic Garlic & Onion	½ cup (4.4 oz)	58	tr	2
Classic Tomato & Basil	½ cup (4.4 oz)	48	tr	2
Classic Italian With Parmesan	½ cup (4.4 oz)	50	tr	2
Home Style With Meat	½ cup (4.4 oz)	56	1	2
Home Style With Mushrooms	½ cup (4.4 oz)	56	tr	2
Homestyle Traditional	½ cup (4.4 oz)	56	tr	3
Italian Cheese & Garlic	½ cup (4.5 oz)	65	1	2
Italian Sausage	½ cup (4.5 oz)	77	1	3
Old Country Garlic & Herbs	½ cup (4.4 oz)	63	tr	3
Old Country Italian Style Vegetables	½ cup (4.4 oz)	64	tr	3
Old Country Traditional	½ cup (4.4 oz)	53	tr	3
Old Country With Meat	½ cup (4.4 oz)	56	1	3

FOOD	PORTION	CALS.	SAT. FAT	FAT
Hunt's (CONT.)				
Old Country With Mushrooms	½ cup (4.4 oz)	53	tr	3
Original Traditional	½ cup (4.4 oz)	65	tr	2
Original With Meat	½ cup (4.4 oz)	65	1	2
Original With Mushrooms	½ cup (4.4 oz)	65	tr	2
Mama Rizzo's				
Mushroom Onion	½ cup (4.3 oz)	60	0	2
Pepper Mushroom Onion	½ cup (4.3 oz)	60	0	2
Pepper Primavera Vegetable	½ cup (4.2 oz)	50	0	2
Pepper Tomato Basil Garlic	½ cup (4.7 oz)	60	0	2
Primavera Vegetable	½ cup (4.2 oz)	50	0	2
Tomato Basil Garlic	½ cup (4.6 oz)	60	0	2
Muir Glen				
Organic Cabernet Marinara	½ cup (4.4 oz)	45	—	0
Organic Chunky Style	½ cup (4.5 oz)	80	—	2
Organic Fat Free Tomato Basil	½ cup (4.3 oz)	50	0	0
Organic Garlic Onion	½ cup (4.3 oz)	50	—	0
Organic Garlic Roasted Garlic	½ cup (4.4 oz)	45	—	0
Organic Green Pepper & Mushroom	½ cup (4.5 oz)	70	—	2
Organic Italian Herb	½ cup (4.5 oz)	60	—	0
Organic Romano Cheese	½ cup (4.5 oz)	90	—	3
Organic Sun Dried Tomato	½ cup (4.4 oz)	40	—	0
Organic Sweet Pepper Onion	½ cup (4.4 oz)	40	—	0
Organic Tomato Basil	½ cup (4.3 oz)	50	—	0
Newman's Own				
Marinara Ventian	½ cup (4.4 oz)	60	0	2
Marinara Ventian w/ Mushrooms	½ cup (4.4 oz)	60	0	2
Pasta Sauce Bambolina	½ cup (4.5 oz)	100	1	5
Pasta Sauce Roasted Garlic & Red & Green Peppers	½ cup (4.7 oz)	70	0	3
Pasta Sauce Say Cheese	½ cup (4.4 oz)	90	2	3
Sockarooni	½ cup (4.4 oz)	60	0	2
Prego				
Chunky Sausage & Green Peppers	4 oz	160	—	8
Extra Chunky Garden Combination	4 oz	80	—	2
Extra Chunky Mushroom & Tomato	4 oz	110	—	5
Extra Chunky Mushroom & Green Pepper	4 oz	100	—	4

FOOD	PORTION	CALS.	SAT. FAT	FAT
Prego (CONT.)				
Extra Chunky Mushroom & Onion	4 oz	100	—	4
Extra Chunky Mushroom With Extra Spice	4 oz	100	—	3
Extra Chunky Tomato & Onion	4 oz	110	—	5
Marinara	4 oz	100	—	6
Meat Flavored	4 oz	140	—	6
Mushroom	4 oz	130	—	5
Onion & Garlic	4 oz	110	—	4
Regular	4 oz	130	—	5
Three Cheese	4 oz	100	—	2
Tomato & Basil	4 oz	100	—	2
Pritikin				
Chunky Garden	½ cup (4 oz)	50	0	1
Marinara	½ cup (4 oz)	60	0	0
Original	½ cup (4 oz)	60	0	1
Progresso				
Marinara	½ cup (4.3 oz)	90	1	5
Meat Flavored	½ cup (4.4 oz)	100	1	5
Mushroom	½ cup (4.4 oz)	100	1	5
Sauce	½ cup (4.4 oz)	100	1	5
Ragu				
Fino Italian Garden Medley	½ cup (4.5 oz)	90	0	3
Fino Italian Garlic & Basil	½ cup (4.5 oz)	90	0	3
Fino Italian Parmesan	½ cup (4.5 oz)	100	1	3
Fino Italian Sliced Mushroom	½ cup (4.5 oz)	90	0	3
Fino Italian Tomato & Herb	½ cup (4.5 oz)	90	0	3
Fino Italian Zesty Tomato	½ cup (4.5 oz)	90	0	3
Gardenstyle Chunky Garden Combination	½ cup (4.5 oz)	120	1	4
Gardenstyle Chunky Green & Red Pepper	½ cup (4.5 oz)	120	1	4
Gardenstyle Chunky Mushroom & Green Pepper	½ cup (4.5 oz)	120	1	4
Gardenstyle Chunky Mushroom & Onion	½ cup (4.5 oz)	120	1	4
Gardenstyle Chunky Tomato Garlic & Onion	½ cup (4.5 oz)	120	1	4
Gardenstyle Super Mushroom	½ cup (4.5 oz)	120	1	4
Gardenstyle Super Vegetable Primavera	½ cup (4.5 oz)	110	1	4
Homestyle Mushroom	½ cup (4.5 oz)	120	1	4
Homestyle Tomato & Herb	½ cup (4.5 oz)	120	1	4

FOOD	PORTION	CALS.	SAT. FAT	FAT
Ragu (CONT.)				
Homestyle With Meat	½ cup (4.5 oz)	130	1	4
Light Chunky Mushroom	½ cup (4.4 oz)	50	0	0
Light Garden Harvest	½ cup (4.4 oz)	50	0	0
Light No Sugar Added	½ cup (4.4 oz)	60	0	0
Light Tomato & Herb	½ cup (4.4 oz)	50	0	0
Old World Style Marinara	½ cup (4.4 oz)	90	1	5
Old World Style Mushrooms	½ cup (4.4 oz)	80	1	3
Old World Style Traditional	½ cup (4.4 oz)	80	1	3
Old World Style With Meat	½ cup (4.4 oz)	90	1	5
Sauce	4 fl oz	80	—	4
Thick & Hearty Mushroom	½ cup (4.5 oz)	120	1	3
Thick & Hearty Spaghetti Sauce	4 oz	100	—	3
Thick & Hearty Tomato & Herb	½ cup (4.5 oz)	120	1	3
Thick & Hearty With Meat	1.2 cup (4.5 oz)	130	1	5
Tree Of Life				
Pasta Sauce	½ cup (4 oz)	50	—	2
Pasta Sauce Calabrese	½ cup (3.9 oz)	60	—	3
Pasta Sauce Fat Free Classic	½ cup (3.9 oz)	40	0	0
Pasta Sauce Fat Free Mushroom & Basil	½ cup (3.9 oz)	30	0	0
Pasta Sauce Fat Free Onion & Garlic	½ cup (3.9 oz)	30	0	0
Pasta Sauce Fat Free Sweet Pepper	½ cup (3.9 oz)	30	0	0
Pasta Sauce No Salt	½ cup (3.9 oz)	50	—	2
MIX				
Durkee				
Spaghetti Sauce as prep	½ cup	15	0	0
With Mushrooms as prep	½ cup	15	0	0
French's				
Italian as prep	½ cup	16	0	0
Mushroom as prep	½ cup	20	0	1
Thick as prep	½ cup	10	0	0
REFRIGERATED				
Contadina				
Alfredo	½ cup (4.2 fl oz)	400	21	38
Four Cheese Sauce With White Wine & Shallots	½ cup (4.2 fl oz)	320	14	25
Light Alfredo	½ cup (4.2 fl oz)	190	7	13
Light Chunky Tomato	½ cup (4.4 fl oz)	45	0	0
Light Garden Vegetable	½ cup (4.4 fl oz)	45	0	1

FOOD	PORTION	CALS.	SAT. FAT	FAT
Contadina (CONT.)				
Marinara	½ cup (4.4 fl oz)	80	1	4
Pesto With Basil	¼ cup (2 oz)	310	5	30
Pesto With Sun Dried Tomatoes	¼ cup (2 oz)	250	4	24
Plum Tomato With Basil	½ cup (4.4 fl oz)	70	1	3
Spicy Italian Sausage & Bell Pepper	½ cup (4.4 fl oz)	100	1	5
Di Giorno				
Alfredo	¼ cup (2.2 oz)	180	7	18
Basil Pesto	¼ cup (2.2 oz)	320	6	31
Four Cheese	¼ cup (2.2 oz)	160	7	15
Garlic Pesto	¼ cup (2.1 oz)	340	7	33
Light Alfredo Sauce	¼ cup (2.4 oz)	140	6	9
Marinara	½ cup (4.5 oz)	70	0	0
Plum Tomato Cream Sauce	½ cup (4.4 oz)	160	7	13
Plum Tomato & Mushroom	½ cup (4.4 oz)	60	0	0
Roasted Red Bell Pepper Cream Sauce	¼ cup (2.3 oz)	140	6	10

SPANISH FOOD

(see also BEANS, CHIPS, CHILI, DINNER, PEPPERS, SALSA, SNACKS, SAUCE, TORTILLA)

CANNED

FOOD	PORTION	CALS.	SAT. FAT	FAT
Chi-Chi's				
Pico De Gallo	2 tbsp (1.2 oz)	10	0	0
Derby				
Tamales	2	160	3	7
El Molino				
Enchilada Sauce Hot	2 tbsp	16	—	1
Green Chili Sauce Mild	2 tbsp	10	0	0
Gebhardt				
Enchiladas	2	310	9	24
Tamales	2	290	8	22
Tamales Jumbo	2	400	11	30
Hormel				
Tamales Beef	3 (7.5 oz)	280	8	21
Tamales Chicken	3 (7.5 oz)	210	4	11
Tamales Hot Spicy Beef	3 (7.5 oz)	280	8	21
Tamales Jumbo Beef	2 (6.9 oz)	270	8	20
Old El Paso				
Tamales	3 (7.2 oz)	330	7	19
Rosarita				
Enchilada Sauce Mild	2.5 oz	25	tr	1
Picante Chunky Hot	3 tbsp (2 fl oz)	18	—	tr

FOOD	PORTION	CALS.	SAT. FAT	FAT
Rosarita (CONT.)				
Picante Chunky Medium	3 tbsp (2 fl oz)	16	—	tr
Picante Chunky Mild	3 tbsp (2 oz)	25	—	tr
Van Camp's				
Tamales	2 (5.1 oz)	210	5	13
FROZEN				
Amy's Organic				
Black Bean Vegetable Enchilada	1 (4.75 oz)	130	0	4
Burritos Bean & Cheese	1 (6 oz)	280	3	8
Burritos Bean & Rice Non-Dairy	1 (6 oz)	250	tr	5
Burritos Black Bean Vegetable	1 (6 oz)	320	1	8
Burritos Breakfast	1 (6 oz)	230	tr	5
Cheese Enchilada	1 (4.7 oz)	210	3	9
Mexican Tamale Pie	1 (8 oz)	220	0	3
Pocket Sandwich Tamale	1 (4.5 oz)	250	3	7
Whole Meals Cheese Enchilada	1 pkg (9 oz)	330	7	14
Whole Meals Enchilada	1 pkg (10 oz)	250	1	8
Banquet				
Beef Enchilada	1 pkg (11 oz)	320	5	12
Chimichanga Meal	1 pkg (9.5 oz)	470	7	23
Enchilada Cheese	1 pkg (11 oz)	350	3	6
Enchilada Chicken	1 pkg (11 oz)	360	3	10
Family Entree Beef Enchilada w/ Cheese	1 serv (4.67 oz)	130	2	4
Chi-Chi's				
Burro Beef	1 pkg (15.9 oz)	590	8	19
Burro Chicken	1 pkg (15.9 oz)	540	5	14
Chimichanga Beef	1 pkg (15.9 oz)	630	9	24
Chimichanga Chicken	1 pkg (15.9 oz)	580	6	19
Enchilada Chicken Suprema	1 pkg (15.9 oz)	600	9	20
Enchilida Baja	1 pkg (15.9 oz)	590	9	20
Healthy Choice				
Beef Burrito Ranchero Medium	1 (5.4 oz)	290	3	7
Beef Burrito Ranchero Mild	1 (5.4 oz)	300	3	7
Beef Enchilada Rio Grande	1 meal (13.4 oz)	410	3	8
Burrito Chicken Con Queso	1 (5.4 oz)	280	2	6
Chicken Enchilada Supreme	1 meal (13.4 oz)	390	5	9
Enchiladas Suiza Chicken	1 meal (10 oz)	270	2	4
Fiesta Chicken Fajitas	1 meal (7 oz)	260	1	4

FOOD	PORTION	CALS.	SAT. FAT	FAT
Jimmy Dean				
Burrito Breakfast Bacon	1 (4 oz)	260	3	8
Burrito Breakfast Sausage	1 (4 oz)	250	3	8
Le Menu				
Entree LightStyle Enchiladas Chicken	8 oz	280	—	8
Lean Cuisine				
Chicken Enchilada Suiza w/ Mexican Style Rice	1 pkg (9 oz)	280	2	5
Life Choice				
Burrito Black Bean	1 meal (13.2 oz)	410	0	2
Vegetable Enchilada Sonora	1 meal (14 oz)	420	0	2
Old El Paso				
Burrito Bean & Cheese	1 (4.9 oz)	290	5	9
Burrito Beef & Bean Hot	1 (5 oz)	320	4	10
Burrito Beef & Bean Medium	1 (5 oz)	320	4	10
Burrito Beef & Bean Mild	1 (5 oz)	330	3	9
Chimichanga Beef	1 (4.5 oz)	370	5	20
Chimichanga Chicken	1 (4.5 oz)	350	4	16
Patio				
Burrito Bean & Cheese	1 (5 oz)	270	2	5
Burrito Chicken	1 (5 oz)	260	2	4
Burrito Red Chili	1 (5 oz)	270	2	6
Burritos Beef & Bean	1 (5 oz)	280	3	7
Burritos Beef & Bean Green Chili	1 (5 oz)	260	2	5
Burritos Beef & Bean Red Chili	1 (5 oz)	260	2	5
Enchilada Beef Dinner	1 meal (12 oz)	320	3	8
Enchilada Cheese Dinner	1 meal (12 oz)	330	3	8
Enchilada Chicken	1 pkg (12 oz)	380	3	9
Family Entree Beef Enchilada	2 (5.7 oz)	170	2	4
Family Entree Enchilada Beef	2 (5.3 oz)	250	3	7
Family Entree Enchilada Cheese	2 (5.7 oz)	170	2	4
Fiesta Dinner	1 meal (12 oz)	340	4	9
Mexican Dinner	1 meal (13.25 oz)	440	6	15
Salis Con Queso	1 pkg (11 oz)	390	11	20
Patio Britos				
Beef & Bean	10 (6 oz)	420	7	19
Nacho Beef	10 (6 oz)	410	5	18
Nacho Cheese	10 (6 oz)	360	4	13
Spicy Chicken	10 (6 oz)	400	4	16

FOOD	PORTION	CALS.	SAT. FAT	FAT
Rudy's Farm				
Burrito Beef/Bean	1 (5 oz)	326	4	12
Burrito Hot Beef/Bean	1 (5 oz)	305	3	9
Senor Felix's				
Burrito Black Bean	1 (10 oz)	540	9	18
Burrito Black Bean Soy	1 (5 oz)	240	1	7
Burrito Chicken	1 (10 oz)	520	4	20
Burrito Hot Potato	1 (10 oz)	560	9	24
Burrito Soy Hot	1 (10 oz)	520	3	20
Burritos Charbroiled Chicken	1 + 4 tsp sauce (6.7 oz)	320	3	11
Burritos Sonora Style	1 + 4 tsp sauce (6.7 oz)	280	2	8
Burritos Yucatan Style	1 + 4 tsp sauce (6.7 oz)	310	2	9
Empanadas Chicken	1 (4.7 oz)	340	30	15
Empanadas Corn & Rice	1 (4.7 oz)	280	4	13
Empanadas Pumpkin & Mushroom	1 (4.7 oz)	260	4	11
Empanadas Spinach & Ricotta	1 (4.7 oz)	260	4	12
Enchilada Red Pepper	1 (10 oz)	420	5	19
Enchilada Soy Verda	1 (10 oz)	430	3	24
Enchilada Supreme Soy Cheese	1 (10 oz)	460	4	23
Enchilada Verde	1 (5 oz)	423	5	23
Tamales Blue Corn & Soy Cheese	2 + 4 tsp sauce (5.7 oz)	240	3	10
Tamales Chicken	2 + 4 tsp sauce (5.7 oz)	240	2	9
Tamales Gourmet Vegetarian	2 + 4 tsp sauce	240	2	9
Taquitos Blue Corn Soy	3 + 4 tsp sauce (5.2 oz)	230	2	11
Taquitos Chicken	2 + 4 tsp sauce (5.7 oz)	240	3	10
Stouffer's				
Chicken Enchilada	1 serv (4.8 oz)	230	5	11
Swanson				
Enchiladas Beef	13¾ oz	480	—	21
Mexican Style Combination	14¼ oz	490	—	18
Mexican Style Hungry Man	20¼ oz	820	—	41
Today's Tamales				
Cheese & Chili	1 pkg (7 oz)	390	10	21
Del Sol	1 pkg (6.5 oz)	310	2	15

FOOD	PORTION	CALS.	SAT. FAT	FAT
Today's Tamales (CONT.)				
Original Bean	1 pkg (7 oz)	330	1	11
Spicy Taco	1 pkg (7 oz)	310	1	15
Tyson				
Beef Fajita	3½ pieces (12.5 oz)	550	4	16
Chicken Fajita	3½ pieces (13.1 oz)	460	3	11
Weight Watchers				
Smart Ones Chicken Enchiladas Suiza	1 pkg (9 oz)	270	5	9
Smart Ones Santa Fe Style Rice & Beans	1 pkg (10 oz)	290	4	8
MIX				
Gebhardt				
Menudo Mix	1 tsp	5	—	tr
Hain				
Taco Seasoning Mix	⅒ pkg	10	0	0
Old El Paso				
Burrito Seasoning Mix	2 tsp (6 g)	20	0	0
Dinner Kit Burrito as prep	1	280	3	7
Dinner Kit Soft Taco as prep	2	380	4	10
Dinner Kit Taco as prep	2	270	5	13
Enchilada Sauce Mix	2 tsp (4 g)	10	0	0
Taco Mix 40% Less Sodium	2 tsp (6 g)	20	0	0
Taco Seasoning Mix	2 tsp (6 g)	20	0	0
Ortega				
Taco Meat Seasoning Mix Mild	1 filled taco	90	0	1
Taco Bell				
Home Originals Chicken Fajita Dinner as prep	2 (6.9 oz)	340	2	9
Home Originals Chicken Fajita Seasoning Mix	1 tbsp (8 g)	25	0	0
Home Originals Soft Taco Dinner as prep	2 (6.3 oz)	410	4	18
Home Originals Taco Dinner as prep	2 (4.4 oz)	280	5	15
Home Originals Taco Seasoning Mix	2 tsp (6 g)	20	0	0
Home Originals Ultimate Bean Burrito Dinner as prep	1 (4.4 oz)	200	2	5
Home Originals Ultimate Nachos as prep	12 pieces (4.6 oz)	240	3	11
READY-TO-EAT				
taco shell baked	1 med (0.5 oz)	61	tr	3
taco shell baked w/o salt	1 med (½ oz)	61	tr	3

FOOD	PORTION	CALS.	SAT. FAT	FAT
Casa Fiesta				
Taco Shells	3.5 oz	480	—	23
Chi-Chi's				
Taco Shells White Corn	2 (1.2 oz)	170	2	8
Taco Shells Yellow Corn	2 shells (1.2 oz)	170	0	8
Gebhardt				
Taco Shells	1	50	2	2
La Mexicana				
Flour Burritos	1 (1.6 oz)	160	1	5
Old El Paso				
Taco Shells Mini	7 (1.1 oz)	160	2	10
Taco Shells Regular	3 (1.1 oz)	170	2	10
Taco Shells Super	2 (1.3 oz)	190	2	12
Taco Shells White Corn	3 (1.1 oz)	170	2	10
Tostaco Shells	1 (0.8 oz)	130	1	7
Tostada Shells	3 (1.1 oz)	160	2	10
Rosarita				
Taco Shells	1 shell (11 g)	50	2	2
Tostada Shells	1 shell (14 g)	60	2	3
Taco Bell				
Home Originals Taco Shells	3 (1.1 oz)	150	1	6
TAKE-OUT				
burrito w/ apple	1 sm (2.6 oz)	231	5	10
burrito w/ apple	1 lg (5.4 oz)	484	7	20
burrito w/ beans	2 (7.6 oz)	448	7	14
burrito w/ beans & cheese	2 (6.5 oz)	377	7	12
burrito w/ beans & chili peppers	2 (7.2 oz)	413	8	15
burrito w/ beans & meat	2 (8.1 oz)	508	8	18
burrito w/ beans cheese & beef	2 (7.1 oz)	331	7	13
burrito w/ beans cheese & chili peppers	2 (11.8 oz)	663	11	23
burrito w/ beef	2 (7.7 oz)	523	10	21
burrito w/ beef & chili peppers	2 (7.1 oz)	426	8	17
burrito w/ beef cheese & chili peppers	2 (10.7 oz)	634	10	25
burrito w/ cherry	1 sm (2.6 oz)	231	5	10
burrito w/ cherry	1 lg (5.4 oz)	484	7	20
chimichanga w/ beef	1 (6.1 oz)	425	9	20
chimichanga w/ beef & cheese	1 (6.4 oz)	443	11	23
chimichanga w/ beef & red chili peppers	1 (6.7 oz)	424	8	19
chimichanga w/ beef cheese & red chili peppers	1 (6.3 oz)	364	8	18
enchilada eggplant	1	142	—	5

FOOD	PORTION	CALS.	SAT. FAT	FAT
enchilada w/ cheese	1 (5.7 oz)	320	11	19
enchilada w/ cheese & beef	1 (6.7 oz)	324	9	18
enchirito w/ cheese beef & beans	1 (6.8 oz)	344	8	16
frijoles w/ cheese	1 cup (5.9 oz)	226	4	8
nachos w/ cheese	6 to 8 (4 oz)	345	8	19
nachos w/ cheese & jalapeno peppers	6 to 8 (7.2 oz)	607	14	34
nachos w/ cheese beans ground beef & peppers	6 to 8 (8.9 oz)	568	12	31
nachos w/ cinnamon & sugar	6 to 8 (3.8 oz)	592	18	36
taco	1 sm (6 oz)	370	11	21
taco salad	1½ cups	279	7	15
taco salad w/ chili con carne	1½ cups	288	6	13
tostada w/ beans & cheese	1 (5.1 oz)	223	5	10
tostada w/ beans beef & cheese	1 (7.9 oz)	334	11	17
tostada w/ beef & cheese	1 (5.7 oz)	315	10	16
tostada w/ guacamole	2 (9.2 oz)	360	10	23

SPARE RIBS
(see PORK)

SPELT
Arrowhead
Spelt	1 oz	83	tr	1

SPICES
(see INDIVIDUAL NAMES, HERBS/SPICES)

SPINACH
CANNED
spinach	½ cup	25	tr	1
Del Monte				
50% Less Salt	½ cup (4 oz)	30	0	0
Chopped	½ cup (4 oz)	30	0	0
No Salt Added	½ cup (4 oz)	30	0	0
Whole Leaf	½ cup (4 oz)	30	0	0
Popeye				
Chopped	½ cup (4.1 oz)	40	0	1
Leaf	½ cup (4.2 oz)	45	0	1
Low Sodium	½ cup (4.2 oz)	35	0	1
Sunshine				
Chopped	½ cup (4.1 oz)	40	0	1
FRESH				
cooked	½ cup	21	tr	tr
malabar cooked	1 cup (1.5 oz)	10	—	tr
mustard chopped cooked	½ cup	14	—	tr
mustard raw chopped	½ cup	17	—	tr

FOOD	PORTION	CALS.	SAT. FAT	FAT
new zealand chopped cooked	½ cup	11	tr	tr
new zealand raw	½ cup	4	tr	tr
raw chopped	½ cup	6	tr	tr
raw chopped	1 pkg (10 oz)	46	tr	1
Dole				
Baby Spinach	3½ cups (3 oz)	35	0	0
Fresh Express				
Spinach	1½ cups (3 oz)	40	0	0
FROZEN				
cooked	½ cup	27	tr	tr
Amy's Organic				
Pocket Sandwich Spinach Feta	1 (4.5 oz)	200	3	7
Birds Eye				
Creamed	½ cup (4.3 oz)	100	3	7
Whole Leaf	1 cup (2.8 oz)	20	0	0
Budget Gourmet				
Au Gratin	1 pkg (5.5 oz)	160	—	11
Fresh Like				
Cut Leaf	3.5 oz	21	—	tr
Green Giant				
Butter Sauce	½ cup (3.4 oz)	40	1	2
Creamed	½ cup (3.8 oz)	80	2	3
Cut Leaf	¾ cup (2.6 oz)	25	0	0
Harvest Fresh	½ cup (3.5 oz)	25	0	0
Stouffer's				
Creamed	1 serv (4.5 oz)	160	4	12
Souffle	1 serv (4 oz)	150	2	10
Tabatchnick				
Creamed	7.5 oz	60	1	2
TAKE-OUT				
indian saag	1 serv	28	tr	2
spanakopita spinach pie	1 cup (6 oz)	196	2	3

SPORTS DRINKS

(see also NUTRITION SUPPLEMENTS)

FOOD	PORTION	CALS.	SAT. FAT	FAT
Gatorade				
Citrus Cooler	1 cup (8 oz)	50	0	0
Fruit Punch	1 cup (8 oz)	50	0	0
Grape	1 cup (8 oz)	50	0	0
Iced Tea Cooler	1 cup (8 oz)	50	0	0
Lemon-Lime	1 cup (8 oz)	50	0	0
Lemonade	1 cup (8 oz)	50	0	0
Orange	1 cup (8 fl oz)	50	0	0
Tropical Fruit	1 cup (8 oz)	50	0	0

FOOD	PORTION	CALS.	SAT. FAT	FAT
Powerade				
Fruit Punch	8 fl oz	72	0	0
Grape	8 fl oz	73	0	0
Lemon-Lime	8 fl oz	70	0	0
Orange	8 fl oz	72	0	0
Slice				
All Sport Diet Lemon Lime	8 fl oz	1	0	0
All Sport Lemon Lime	8 fl oz	72	0	0
All Sport Orange	8 fl oz	74	0	0
All Sport Punch	8 fl oz	81	0	0
Snapple				
Sport Fruit	1 bottle	80	0	0
Sport Lemon	1 bottle	80	0	0
Sport Lemon Lime	1 bottle	80	0	0
Sport Orange	1 bottle	80	0	0
Ultra Fuel				
Lemon Lime	16 fl oz	400	0	0
SPOT				
baked	3 oz	134	2	5
SPROUTS				
(see also ALFALFA)				
kidney bean	½ cup	27	tr	tr
kidney bean cooked	1 lb	152	tr	3
lentil sprouts	½ cup	40	tr	tr
mung bean	½ cup	16	tr	tr
mung bean canned	½ cup	8	tr	tr
mung bean cooked	½ cup	13	tr	tr
navy bean	½ cup	35	—	tr
navy bean cooked	3½ oz	78	—	1
pea	½ cup	77	—	tr
pinto bean	3½ oz	62	—	1
pinto bean cooked	3½ oz	22	—	tr
radish	½ cup	8	tr	tr
Fresh Alternatives				
BroccoSprouts	½ cup (1 oz)	10	0	0
Deli Blend	½ cup (1 oz)	10	0	0
Salad Blend	½ cup (1 oz)	10	0	0
Sandwich Blend	½ cup (1 oz)	5	0	0
TAKE-OUT				
mung bean stir fried	½ cup	31	tr	tr
SQUAB				
boneless baked	3.5 oz	175	1	3
breast w/o skin raw	1 (3.5 oz)	135	1	5
w/o skin raw	1 squab (5.9 oz)	239	3	13

FOOD	PORTION	CALS.	SAT. FAT	FAT
SQUASH				
(see also ZUCCHINI)				
CANNED				
crookneck sliced	½ cup	14	tr	tr
Allen				
Yellow	½ cup (4.2 oz)	25	0	0
Sunshine				
Yellow	½ cup (4.2 oz)	25	0	0
FRESH				
acorn cooked mashed	½ cup	41	tr	tr
acorn cubed baked	½ cup	57	tr	tr
butternut baked	½ cup	41	tr	tr
crookneck raw sliced	½ cup	12	tr	tr
crookneck sliced cooked	½ cup	18	tr	tr
hubbard baked	½ cup	51	tr	tr
hubbard cooked mashed	½ cup	35	tr	tr
scallop sliced cooked	½ cup	14	tr	tr
spaghetti cooked	½ cup	23	tr	tr
Nature's Pasta				
Spaghetti Squash	1 cup (5.5 oz)	20	0	0
FROZEN				
butternut cooked mashed	½ cup	47	tr	tr
crookneck sliced cooked	½ cup	24	tr	tr
Southland				
Butternut	4 oz	45	—	0
Prepared Squash	3.6 oz	80	—	2
SEEDS				
dried	1 oz	154	2	13
dried	1 cup	747	12	63
roasted	1 cup	1184	18	96
roasted	1 oz	148	2	12
salted & roasted	1 oz	148	2	12
salted & roasted	1 cup	1184	18	96
whole roasted	1 oz	127	1	6
whole roasted	1 cup	285	2	12
whole salted roasted	1 cup	285	2	12
whole salted roasted	1 oz	127	1	6
SQUID				
fried	3 oz	149	2	6
raw	3 oz	78	tr	1
SQUIRREL				
roasted	3 oz	147	tr	4
STAR FRUIT				
fresh	1	42	—	tr

FOOD	PORTION	CALS.	SAT. FAT	FAT
Sonoma				
Dried	7-9 pieces (1.4 oz)	140	0	0

STRAWBERRIES
CANNED
in heavy syrup	½ cup	117	tr	tr

FRESH
strawberries	1 cup	45	tr	1
strawberries	1 pint	97	tr	1
Dole				
Strawberries	8	50	—	0

FROZEN
sweetened sliced	1 cup	245	tr	tr
sweetened sliced	1 pkg (10 oz)	273	tr	tr
unsweetened	1 cup	52	tr	tr
whole sweetened	1 cup	200	tr	tr
whole sweetened	1 pkg (10 oz)	223	tr	tr
Big Valley				
Strawberries	⅔ cup (4.9 oz)	50	0	0
Birds Eye				
Halves	½ cup (4.7 oz)	120	0	0
Halves In Lite Syrup	½ cup (4.6 oz)	70	0	0
Whole	½ cup (4.5 oz)	100	0	0

STRAWBERRY JUICE
Capri Sun				
Strawberry Cooler Drink	1 pkg (7 oz)	90	0	0
Kern's				
Nectar	6 fl oz	110	0	0
Kool-Aid				
Drink as prep w/ sugar	1 serv (8 oz)	100	0	0
Drink Mix as prep	1 serv (8 oz)	60	0	0
Libby				
Nectar	1 can (11.5 fl oz)	210	0	0
Veryfine				
Juice-Ups	8 fl oz	140	0	0

STUFFING/DRESSING
bread dry as prep	½ cup	178	2	9
combread as prep	½ cup	179	2	9
Arnold				
All Purpose Seasoned	½ oz	50	0	0
Corn	½ oz	50	0	1
Herb Seasoned	½ oz	50	—	tr
Sage & Onion	½ oz	50	0	tr

FOOD	PORTION	CALS.	SAT. FAT	FAT
Kellogg's				
Croutettes Mix	1 cup (1.2 oz)	120	0	0
Pepperidge Farm				
Corn Bread	¾ cup (1.5 oz)	170	0	2
Herb Seasoned	¾ cup (1.5 oz)	170	0	2
Herb Seasoned Cubed	¾ cup (1.3 oz)	140	0	2
One Step Chicken	½ cup (1.2 oz)	140	1	4
One Step Southwestern Corn Bread	½ cup (1.2 oz)	150	1	5
One Step Turkey	½ cup (1.2 oz)	150	1	5
Stove Top				
Chicken as prep w/ margarine	½ cup (3.6 oz)	170	2	9
Cornbread as prep w/ margarine	½ cup (3.6 oz)	170	2	8
Flexible Serve Chicken as prep w/ margarine	½ cup (3.3 oz)	170	2	8
Flexible Serve Cornbread as prep w/ margarine	½ cup (3.3 oz)	160	2	8
Flexible Serve Homestyle Herb as prep w/ margarine	½ cup (3.3 oz)	170	2	8
For Beef as prep w/ margarine	½ cup (3.7 oz)	180	2	9
For Pork as prep w/ margarine	½ cup (3.6 oz)	170	2	9
For Turkey as prep w/ margarine	½ cup (3.6 oz)	170	2	9
Long Grain & Wild Rice as prep w/ margarine	½ cup (3.7 oz)	180	2	9
Lower Sodium Chicken as prep w/ margarine	½ cup (3.6 oz)	180	2	9
Microwave Chicken as prep w/ margarine	½ cup (3.5 oz)	160	2	7
Microwave Homestyle Cornbread as prep w/ margarine	½ cup (3 oz)	160	2	7
Mushroom & Onion as prep w/ margarine	½ cup (3.6 oz)	180	2	9
San Francisco Style as prep w/ margarine	½ cup (3.6 oz)	170	2	9
Savory Herb as prep w/ margarine	½ cup (3.6 oz)	170	2	9
Traditional Sage as prep w/ margarine	½ cup (3.6 oz)	180	2	9

FOOD	PORTION	CALS.	SAT. FAT	FAT
TAKE-OUT				
bread	½ cup (3½ oz)	195	2	8
STURGEON				
cooked	3 oz	115	1	4
raw	3 oz	90	1	3
roe raw	3.5 oz	207	—	10
smoked	1 oz	48	tr	1
smoked	3 oz	147	1	4
SUCKER				
white baked	3 oz	101	tr	3
SUGAR				
(see also FRUCTOSE, SUGAR SUBSTITUTES, SYRUP)				
brown packed	1 cup (7.7 oz)	828	0	0
brown unpacked	1 cup (5.1 oz)	546	0	0
maple	1 piece (1 oz)	100	—	tr
powdered	1 tbsp (0.3 oz)	31	0	0
powdered unsifted	1 cup (4.2 oz)	467	—	tr
white	1 cup (7 oz)	773	0	0
white	1 packet (6 g)	25	0	0
white	1 tbsp	45	0	0
white	1 tsp (4 g)	15	0	0
C&H				
White	1 tsp	16	0	0
Domino				
White	1 tsp	16	0	0
Hain				
Turbinado	1 tbsp	50	0	0
Hollywood				
Turbinado	1 tbsp	50	0	0
SUGAR SUBSTITUTES				
(see also FRUCTOSE)				
Mrs. Bateman's				
Sugarlike	1 tsp (4 g)	4	0	0
NatraTaste				
Packet	1 pkg (1 g)	0	0	0
Sweet One				
Packet	1 pkg (1 g)	4	0	0
Sweet'N Low				
Granulated	1 pkg (1g)	4	0	0
Weight Watchers				
Sweetener	1 serv (1 g)	5	0	0

FOOD	PORTION	CALS.	SAT. FAT	FAT
SUGAR-APPLE				
fresh	1	146	—	tr
fresh cut up	1 cup	236	—	1
SUNCHOKE				
fresh raw sliced	½ cup	57	0	tr
SUNDAE TOPPINGS				
(see ICE CREAM TOPPINGS)				
SUNFISH				
pumpkinseed baked	3 oz	97	tr	1
SUNFLOWER				
seeds dried	1 oz	162	7	14
seeds dried	1 cup	821	7	71
seeds dry roasted	1 oz	165	1	14
seeds dry roasted	1 cup	745	7	64
seeds dry roasted salted	1 cup	745	7	64
seeds dry roasted salted	1 oz	165	1	14
seeds oil roasted	1 cup	830	8	78
seeds oil roasted salted	1 oz	175	2	16
seeds oil roasted salted	1 cup	830	8	78
seeds toasted	1 oz	176	2	16
seeds toasted	1 cup	826	8	76
seeds toasted salted	1 oz	176	2	16
seeds toasted salted	1 cup	826	8	76
sunflower butter	1 tbsp	93	1	8
sunflower butter w/o salt	1 tbsp	93	1	8
Dakota Gourmet				
Honey Roasted Kernels	1 pkg (1 oz)	158	1	12
Lightly Salted Kernels	1 pkg (1 oz)	168	1	14
Fisher				
Seeds Oil Roasted	1 oz	170	2	15
Seeds Salted In Shell shelled	1 oz	160	1	14
Seeds Salted In Shell unshelled	1 oz	170	2	15
Frito Lay				
Seeds	1 oz	180	2	15
Lance				
Seeds In Shell	⅔ cup (1.8 oz)	160	3	13
Seeds Roasted & Shelled	1 pkg (1⅛ oz)	190	3	16
Planters				
Kernels	1 pkg (1.7 oz)	290	3	25
Kernels	1 pkg (2 oz)	340	3	29
Kernels Barbecue	1 pkg (1.7 oz)	290	3	25

FOOD	PORTION	CALS.	SAT. FAT	FAT
Planters (CONT.)				
Kernels Honey Roasted	1 pkg (1.7 oz)	280	3	22
Kernels Salted	1 oz	170	2	14
Munch'N Go Singles Dry Roasted	1 pkg	120	1	11
Nuts Dry Roasted	¼ cup (1.1 oz)	190	2	17
Original With Shell Dry Roasted	¾ cup	160	2	15
Stone-Buhr				
Seeds Raw	4 tsp (1 oz)	170	2	14

SUSHI
TAKE-OUT

FOOD	PORTION	CALS.	SAT. FAT	FAT
california roll	1 piece (0.8 oz)	28	tr	1
kim chi	½ cup (5.8 oz)	18	tr	tr
sashimi	1 serv (6 oz)	198	1	7
tuna roll	1 piece (0.7 oz)	23	tr	tr
vegetable roll	1 piece (1.2 oz)	27	tr	1
vinegared ginger	⅓ cup (1.6 oz)	48	tr	tr
wasabi	2 tsp (0.3 oz)	5	0	tr
yellowtail roll	1 piece (0.6 oz)	25	tr	1

SWAMP CABBAGE

FOOD	PORTION	CALS.	SAT. FAT	FAT
chopped cooked	½ cup	10	—	tr
raw chopped	1 cup	11	—	tr

SWEET POTATO
(see also YAM)
CANNED

FOOD	PORTION	CALS.	SAT. FAT	FAT
in syrup	½ cup	106	tr	tr
pieces	1 cup	183	tr	tr
Princella				
Mashed	⅔ cup (5.1 oz)	120	0	1
Royal Prince				
Candied	½ cup (4.9 oz)	210	0	1
Halves	3 pieces (5.7 oz)	190	0	1
Orange Pineapple	½ cup (4.8 oz)	210	0	1
Sugary Sam				
Mashed	⅔ cup (5.1 oz)	120	0	1

FRESH

FOOD	PORTION	CALS.	SAT. FAT	FAT
baked w/ skin	1 (3½ oz)	118	tr	tr
leaves cooked	½ cup	11	tr	tr
mashed	½ cup	172	tr	tr

FROZEN

FOOD	PORTION	CALS.	SAT. FAT	FAT
cooked	½ cup	88	tr	tr

FOOD	PORTION	CALS.	SAT. FAT	FAT
Mrs. Paul's				
Candied Sweet Potatoes	4 oz	170	—	0
Candied Sweets 'N Apples	4 oz	160	—	0
TAKE-OUT				
candied	3½ oz	144	1	3

SWEETBREADS

FOOD	PORTION	CALS.	SAT. FAT	FAT
beef braised	3 oz	230	—	15
lamb braised	3 oz	199	6	13
veal braised	3 oz	218	—	12

SWISS CHARD

FOOD	PORTION	CALS.	SAT. FAT	FAT
cooked	½ cup	18	—	tr
raw chopped	½ cup	3	—	tr

SWORDFISH

FOOD	PORTION	CALS.	SAT. FAT	FAT
cooked	3 oz	132	1	4
raw	3 oz	103	1	3

SYRUP
(see also ICE CREAM TOPPINGS, PANCAKE/WAFFLE SYRUP)

FOOD	PORTION	CALS.	SAT. FAT	FAT
corn	2 tbsp	122	0	0
corn dark	1 tbsp (0.7 oz)	56	—	0
corn dark	1 cup (11.5 oz)	925	—	tr
corn light	1 cup (11.5 oz)	925	—	tr
corn light	1 tbsp (0.7 oz)	56	—	0
malt	1 tbsp (0.8 oz)	76	—	0
malt	1 cup (13 oz)	1222	—	tr
maple	1 tbsp (0.8 oz)	52	—	0
maple	1 cup (11.1 oz)	824	—	1
rose hip	3.5 oz	33	0	0
sorghum	1 cup (11.6 oz)	957	0	0
sorghum	1 tbsp (0.7 oz)	61	0	0
Estee				
Blueberry	¼ cup	80	0	0
Hershey				
Strawberry	2 tbsp (1.4 oz)	100	0	0
McIlhenny				
Cane	2 tbsp (1.4 oz)	130	0	0
Quik				
Strawberry	2 tbsp (1.5 oz)	110	0	0
Red Wing				
Strawberry	2 tbsp (1.4 oz)	110	0	0
Tree Of Life				
Maple	¼ cup (2.1 oz)	200	0	0
Rice Syrup	2 tbsp (1 oz)	120	—	1

FOOD	PORTION	CALS.	SAT. FAT	FAT
Whistling Wings				
Blueberry	1 oz	45	—	tr
Raspberry	1 oz	60	—	tr
TACO				
(see SPANISH FOOD)				
TAHINI				
(see SESAME)				
TAMARIND				
fresh	1	5	tr	tr
fresh cut up	1 cup	287	tr	1
TANGERINE				
CANNED				
in light syrup	½ cup	76	tr	tr
juice pack	½ cup	46	tr	tr
FRESH				
sections	1 cup	86	tr	tr
tangerine	1	37	tr	tr
Dole				
Tangerine	2	70	—	1
TANGERINE JUICE				
canned sweetened	1 cup	125	tr	1
fresh	1 cup	106	tr	tr
frzn sweetened as prep	1 cup	110	tr	tr
frzn sweetened not prep	6 oz	344	tr	1
After The Fall				
Juice	1 can (12 oz)	170	0	0
Fresh Samantha				
Fresh Juice	1 cup (8 oz)	106	0	1
Minute Maid				
Frozen	8 fl oz	120	0	0
TAPIOCA				
pearl dry	½ cup (2.7 oz)	272	tr	tr
Minute				
Minute Tapioca	1½ tsp (6 g)	20	0	0
TARO				
chips	10 (0.8 oz)	115	1	6
chips	1 oz	141	2	7
leaves cooked	½ cup	18	tr	tr
raw sliced	½ cup	56	tr	tr
shoots sliced cooked	½ cup	10	tr	tr
sliced cooked	½ cup (2.3 oz)	94	tr	tr
tahitian sliced cooked	½ cup	30	tr	tr

FOOD	PORTION	CALS.	SAT. FAT	FAT
TARRAGON				
ground	1 tsp	5	—	tr
TEA/HERBAL TEA				
(see also ICED TEA)				
HERBAL				
Bigelow				
Almond Orange	5 fl oz	tr	—	tr
Apple Orchard	5 fl oz	5	—	tr
Apple Spice	5 fl oz	tr	—	tr
Chamomile	5 fl oz	tr	—	tr
Chamomile Mint	5 fl oz	tr	—	tr
Cinnamon Orange	5 fl oz	tr	—	tr
Early Riser	5 fl oz	3	—	tr
Feeling Free	5 fl oz	1	—	tr
Fruit & Almond	5 fl oz	1	—	tr
Hibiscus & Rose Hips	5 fl oz	1	—	tr
I Love Lemon	5 fl oz	1	—	tr
Lemon & C	5 fl oz	tr	—	tr
Looking Good	5 fl oz	1	—	tr
Mint Blend	5 fl oz	tr	—	tr
Mint Medley	5 fl oz	1	—	tr
Orange & C	5 fl oz	tr	—	tr
Orange & Spice	5 fl oz	1	—	tr
Peppermint	5 fl oz	tr	—	tr
Roasted Grains & Carob	5 fl oz	3	—	tr
Spearmint	5 fl oz	tr	—	tr
Sweet Dreams	5 fl oz	1	—	tr
Take-A-Break	5 fl oz	3	—	tr
Celestial Seasonings				
Almond Sunset	8 fl oz	3	—	tr
Bengal Spice	8 fl oz	5	—	tr
Caffeine Free	8 fl oz	2	—	tr
Chamomile	8 fl oz	2	—	tr
Cinnamon Apple Spice	8 fl oz	<3	—	tr
Cinnamon Rose	8 fl oz	<4	—	tr
Country Peach Spice	8 fl oz	3	—	tr
Cranberry Cove	8 fl oz	2	—	tr
Emperor's Choice	8 fl oz	4	—	tr
Ginseng Plus	8 fl oz	3	—	tr
Grandma's Tummy Mint	8 fl oz	2	—	tr
Lemon Mist	8 fl oz	3	—	tr
Lemon Zinger	8 fl oz	4	—	tr
Mama Bear's Cold Care	8 fl oz	6	—	tr
Mandarin Orange Spice	8 fl oz	5	—	tr

FOOD	PORTION	CALS.	SAT. FAT	FAT
Celestial Seasonings (CONT.)				
Mellow Mint	8 fl oz	2	—	tr
Mint Magic	8 fl oz	1	—	tr
Orange Zinger	8 fl oz	6	—	tr
Peppermint	8 fl oz	2	—	tr
Raspberry Patch	8 fl oz	4	—	tr
Red Zinger	8 fl oz	4	—	tr
Roastaroma	8 fl oz	10	—	tr
Sleepytime	8 fl oz	4	—	tr
Spearmint	8 fl oz	5	—	1
Strawberry Fields	8 fl oz	4	—	tr
Sunburst C	8 fl oz	3	—	tr
Tropical Escape	8 fl oz	1	—	tr
Wild Forest Blackberry	8 fl oz	2	—	tr
Lipton				
Bedtime Story	1 tea bag	0	0	0
Cinnamon Apple	1 tea bag	0	0	0
Country Cranberry	1 tea bag	0	0	0
Gentle Orange	1 tea bag	0	0	0
Ginger Twist	1 tea bag	0	0	0
Golden Lemon Honey	1 tea bag	0	0	0
Lemon Soother	1 tea bag	0	0	0
Peppermint Breeze	1 tea bag	0	0	0
REGULAR				
brewed tea	6 oz	2	0	0
instant unsweetened as prep w/ water	8 oz	2	0	0
Bigelow				
Chinese Fortune	5 fl oz	1	—	tr
Cinnamon Stick	5 fl oz	1	—	tr
Constant Comment	5 fl oz	1	—	tr
Darjeeling Blend	5 fl oz	1	—	tr
Earl Gray	5 fl oz	1	—	tr
English Teatime	5 fl oz	1	—	tr
Lemon Lift	5 fl oz	1	—	tr
Orange Pekoe	5 fl oz	1	—	tr
Peppermint Stick	5 fl oz	1	—	tr
Plantation Mint	5 fl oz	1	—	tr
Raspberry Royale	5 fl oz	1	—	tr
Celestial Seasonings				
Cinnamon Vienna	8 fl oz	2	—	tr
Earl Grey Extraordinary	8 fl oz	3	—	tr
English Breakfast Classic	8 fl oz	3	—	tr
Lemon	8 fl oz	7	—	tr

FOOD	PORTION	CALS.	SAT. FAT	FAT
Celestial Seasonings (CONT.)				
Mint	8 fl oz	4	—	tr
Morning Thunder	8 fl oz	3	—	tr
Naturally Decaffeinated	8 fl oz	10	—	1
Orange Spice	8 fl oz	7	—	tr
Orange Spice Decaff	8 fl oz	7	—	tr
Organically Grown	8 fl oz	12	—	tr
Raspberry	8 fl oz	7	—	tr
General Foods				
International Instant Tea Decaffeinated English Breakfast Creme	1 serv (8 oz)	70	1	2
International Instant Tea Decaffeinated Viennese Cinnamon Creme	1 serv (8 oz)	70	1	2
International Instant Tea English Breakfast Creme as prep	1 serv (8 oz)	70	1	2
International Instant Tea English Raspberry Creme as prep	1 serv (8 oz)	70	1	2
International Instant Tea Island Orange Creme as prep	1 serv (8 oz)	70	1	2
International Instant Tea Viennese Cinnamon Creme as prep	1 serv (8 oz)	70	1	2
Lipton				
Brisk Tea as prep	1 serv	0	0	0
Decaffeinated Brisk Tea as prep	1 serv	0	0	0
English Blend as prep	1 cup	0	0	0
Flavored Blackberry	1 tea bag	0	0	0
Flavored Decaffeinated Orange & Spice	1 tea bag	0	0	0
Flavored Honey & Lemon	1 tea bag	0	0	0
Flavored Mint	1 tea bag	0	0	0
Flavored Orange & Spice	1 tea bag	0	0	0
Flavored Raspberry	1 tea bag	0	0	0
Green Tea	1 tea bag	0	0	0
Green Tea Orange, Passionfruit & Jasmine	1 tea bag	0	0	0
Loose Tea	1 tsp (2 g)	0	0	0
Paradise				
Tropical Tea	8 fl oz	1	0	0
Tropical Tea Decafe	8 fl oz	1	0	0
Tropical Tea Passion Fruit	8 fl oz	1	0	0

FOOD	PORTION	CALS.	SAT. FAT	FAT
Tetley				
Tea Bag as prep	1	0	0	0
TEFF				
Arrowhead				
Whole Grain	¼ cup (1.6 oz)	160	0	1
TEMPEH				
tempeh	½ cup	165	1	6
Lightlife				
Garden Vege	4 oz	142	1	4
Quinoa Sesame	4 oz	190	1	3
Smokey Strips	3 slices	80	1	3
Soy	4 oz	182	2	6
Three Grain	4 oz	190	2	4
Wild Rice	4 oz	190	1	4
White Wave				
Burger	1 patty (3 oz)	110	0	3
Lemon Broil	1 patty (2 oz)	130	1	6
Organic Wild Rice	½ block (2.7 oz)	140	1	4
Teriyaki Burger	1 patty (3 oz)	110	0	2
THYME				
ground	1 tsp	4	tr	tr
Watkins				
Thyme	¼ tsp (0.5 oz)	0	0	0
TILEFISH				
cooked	3 oz	125	1	4
cooked	½ fillet (5.3 oz)	220	1	7
raw	3 oz	81	tr	2
TOFU				
firm	¼ block (3 oz)	118	1	7
fresh fried	1 piece (0.5 oz)	35	tr	3
Casbah				
Gyro as prep w/ tofu	1 patty (2 oz)	105	0	3
Galaxy				
Slices Hickory Smoked	1 slice (1 oz)	50	0	2
Slices Italian Garlic Herb	1 slice (1 oz)	50	0	2
Slices Original	1 slice (1 oz)	50	0	2
Slices Savory	1 slice (1 oz)	50	0	2
Hinoichi				
Firm	1 inch slice (3 oz)	60	0	3
Long Life				
Tofu	3 oz	60	0	3

FOOD	PORTION	CALS.	SAT. FAT	FAT
Mori-Nu				
Extra Firm	1 in slice (3 oz)	55	0	2
Firm	1 in slice (3 oz)	50	0	3
Lite Extra Firm	1 in slice (3 oz)	35	0	1
Lite Firm	1 in slice (3 oz)	35	0	1
Soft	1 in slice (3 oz)	45	0	3
Nasoya				
Chinise 5 Spice	¼ block (3 oz)	68	1	4
Extra Firm	⅕ block (3.2 oz)	92	1	5
Firm	⅕ block (3.2 oz)	76	1	4
French Country	⅕ block (3 oz)	68	1	4
Silken	⅕ block (3.2 oz)	48	tr	2
Soft	⅕ block (3.2 oz)	63	tr	3
Tree Of Life				
Baked	⅕ block (3.2 oz)	150	1	8
Firm	⅕ block (3.2 oz)	100	—	5
Raw Firm	⅕ block (3.2 oz)	100	—	5
Ready Ground Hot & Spicy	⅓ pkg (3 oz)	60	1	4
Ready Ground Original	⅓ pkg (3 oz)	60	1	4
Ready Ground Savory Garlic	⅓ pkg (3 oz)	60	1	4
Reduced Fat	⅕ block (3.2 oz)	90	—	4
Savory Baked	⅕ block (3.2 oz)	140	1	8
Smoked Hot'N Spicy	½ block (3 oz)	120	1	5
Smoked Original	½ block (3 oz)	120	1	5
White Wave				
Baked Tofu Teriyaki Oriental Style	¼ block (2 oz)	120	1	6
Hard	4 oz	120	—	7
International Baked Italian Garlic Herb	¼ pkg (2 oz)	120	1	6
International Baked Mexican Jalapeno	¼ pkg (2 oz)	120	1	6
International Baked Oriental Teriyaki	¼ pkg (2 oz)	120	1	6
International Baked Thai Sesame Peanut	¼ pkg (2 oz)	120	1	6
Soft	4 oz	120	—	7
YOGURT				
Stir Fruity				
Black Cherry	6 oz	141	—	2
Blueberry	6 oz	140	—	1
Lemon Chiffon	6 oz	152	—	3
Mixed Berry	6 oz	149	—	2
Orange	6 oz	143	—	2

FOOD	PORTION	CALS.	SAT. FAT	FAT
Stir Fruity (CONT.)				
Peach	6 oz	160	—	3
Pina Colada	6 oz	162	—	3
Raspberry	6 oz	155	—	2
Spiced Apple	6 oz	167	—	2
Strawberry	6 oz	140	—	2
Tropical Fruit	6 oz	170	—	2
TOMATILLO				
fresh	1 (1.2 oz)	11	—	tr
TOMATO				
(see also PIZZA, SPAGHETTI SAUCE)				
CANNED				
red whole	½ cup	24	tr	tr
sauce w/ mushrooms	½ cup	42	tr	tr
sauce w/ onion	½ cup	52	tr	tr
stewed	½ cup	34	tr	tr
w/ green chiles	½ cup	18	tr	tr
wedges in tomato juice	½ cup	34	tr	tr
Amore				
Sun-Dried Tomato Paste	1 tsp (6 g)	15	0	1
Big R				
Cajun Stewed	½ cup (4.2 oz)	25	0	0
Diced w/ Chilies	½ cup (4.2 oz)	25	0	0
Mexican Stewed	½ cups (4.2 oz)	25	0	0
Stewed	½ cup (4.2 oz)	25	0	0
Whole	½ cup (4.2 oz)	25	0	0
Claussen				
Kosher	1	9	—	tr
Contadina				
California Sliced	½ cup	40	—	tr
Crushed	¼ cup	20	0	0
Italian Paste	2 tbsp	40	—	1
Italian Style Pear	½ cup	25	0	0
Italian Style Stewed	½ cup	40	0	0
Mexican Style Stewed	½ cup	40	0	0
Pasta Ready Primavera	½ cup	50	1	2
Pasta Ready Tomatoes	½ cup	50	0	2
Pasta Ready With Crushed Red Pepper	½ cup	60	1	3
Pasta Ready With Mushrooms	½ cup	50	1	2
Pasta Ready With Olives	½ cup	60	1	3
Pasta Ready With Three Cheeses	½ cup	70	0	4

FOOD	PORTION	CALS.	SAT. FAT	FAT
Contadina (CONT.)				
Paste	2 tbsp	30	0	0
Peeled Whole	½ cup	25	0	0
Puree	¼ cup	20	0	0
Recipe Ready	½ cup	25	0	0
Stewed	½ cup	40	0	0
Del Monte				
Paste	2 tbsp (1.2 oz)	30	0	0
Peeled Diced	½ cup (4.4 oz)	25	0	0
Puree	¼ cup (2.2 oz)	30	0	0
Sauce	¼ cup (2.1 oz)	20	0	0
Sauce No Salt Added	¼ cup (2.1 oz)	20	0	0
Stewed Cajun Style	½ cup (4.4 oz)	35	0	0
Stewed Chunky Chili	½ cup (4.5 oz)	30	0	0
Stewed Chunky Pasta	½ cup (4.5 oz)	45	0	0
Stewed Chunky Pizza	½ cup (4.5 oz)	35	0	0
Stewed Chunky Salsa	½ cup (4.5 oz)	35	0	0
Stewed Italian Style	½ cup (4.4 oz)	30	0	0
Stewed Mexican Style	½ cup (4.4 oz)	35	0	0
Stewed Original	½ cup (4.4 oz)	35	0	0
Stewed Original No Salt Added	½ cup (4.4 oz)	35	0	0
Wedges	½ cup (4.4 oz)	35	0	0
Whole Peeled	½ cup (4.4 oz)	25	0	0
Eden				
Crushed Organic	¼ cup (2.1 oz)	20	0	0
Sauce Lightly Seasoned	¼ cup (2.1 oz)	25	0	0
Hebrew National				
Pickled	⅓ tomato (1 oz)	4	0	0
Hunt's				
Choice Cut	½ cup (4.2 oz)	22	0	tr
Choice Cut Diced Tomatoes & Green Chiles	2 tbsp (0.4 oz)	1	0	0
Choice Cut Diced Tomatoes & Roasted Garlic	½ cup (4.2 oz)	24	0	0
Crushed	½ cup (4.2 oz)	29	0	tr
Crushed Angela Mia	½ cup (4.2 oz)	27	0	tr
Paste	2 tbsp (1.2 oz)	30	0	tr
Paste Italian	2 tbsp (1.2 oz)	27	0	tr
Paste No Salt Added	2 tbsp (1.2 oz)	30	0	tr
Paste With Garlic	2 tbsp (1.2 oz)	28	0	tr
Pear Shaped	½ cup (4.6 oz)	20	0	tr
Puree	¼ cup (2.2 oz)	24	0	tr
Ready Sauce Chunky Chili	¼ cup (2.2 oz)	22	0	tr

FOOD	PORTION	CALS.	SAT. FAT	FAT
Hunt's (CONT.)				
Ready Sauce Chunky Italian	¼ cup (2.2 oz)	26	0	tr
Ready Sauce Chunky Mexican	¼ cup (2.2 oz)	21	0	tr
Ready Sauce Chunky Special	¼ cup (2.2 oz)	21	0	tr
Ready Sauce Chunky Tomato	¼ cup (2.2 oz)	15	0	0
Ready Sauce Country Herb	¼ cup (2.2 oz)	33	tr	1
Ready Sauce Garlic	¼ cup (2.2 oz)	29	tr	1
Ready Sauce Garlic & Herb	¼ cup (2.2 oz)	26	0	tr
Ready Sauce Meatloaf Fixins	¼ cup (2.2 oz)	23	0	tr
Ready Sauce Original	¼ cup (2.2 oz)	30	0	1
Ready Sauce Salsa	¼ cup (2.2 oz)	18	0	tr
Sauce	¼ cup (2.2 oz)	16	0	tr
Sauce Italian	¼ cup (2.2 oz)	32	0	1
Sauce No Salt Added	¼ cup (2.2 oz)	16	0	tr
Sauce With Herb	¼ cup (2.2 oz)	32	0	1
Stewed	½ cup (4.2 oz)	33	0	tr
Stewed Italian	4 oz	40	—	tr
Tomatoes	½ cup (4.2 oz)	33	0	tr
Whole	2 (5.2 oz)	22	0	tr
Muir Glen				
Organic Chunky Sauce	¼ cup (2.3 oz)	20	0	0
Organic Crushed With Basil	¼ cup (2.3 oz)	25	0	0
Organic Diced	½ cup (4.5 oz)	25	—	0
Organic Diced No Salt Added	½ cup (4.5 oz)	25	0	0
Organic Ground Peeled	¼ cup (2.3 oz)	10	0	0
Organic Italian Style Diced	½ cup (4.4 oz)	25	—	0
Organic Paste	2 tbsp (1.2 oz)	30	0	0
Organic Puree	¼ cup (2.2 oz)	20	0	0
Organic Sauce	¼ cup (2.2 oz)	20	0	0
Organic Sauce No Salt Added	¼ cup (2.2 oz)	20	0	0
Organic Stewed	½ cup (4.5 oz)	30	0	0
Organic Stewed Italian Style	½ cup (4.4 oz)	30	0	0
Organic Stewed Mexican Style	½ cup (4.4 oz)	30	0	0
Organic Whole Peeled	½ cup (4.6 oz)	30	0	0
Old El Paso				
Tomatoes & Jalapenos	¼ cup (2 oz)	15	0	0
Tomatoes & Green Chilies	¼ cup (2 oz)	10	—	0
Progresso				
Crushed	¼ cup (2.1 oz)	20	0	0
Paste	2 tbsp (1.2 oz)	30	0	0
Peeled Whole	½ cup (4.2 oz)	25	0	0
Peeled w/ Basil	½ cup (4.2 oz)	25	0	0
Puree	¼ cup (2.2 oz)	25	0	0
Puree Thick Style	¼ cup (2.2 oz)	30	0	0
Sauce	¼ cup (2.1 oz)	20	0	0

FOOD	PORTION	CALS.	SAT. FAT	FAT
Ro-Tel				
Diced Tomatoes & Green Chilies	½ cup (4.4 oz)	20	0	0
Rosoff's				
Pickled	⅓ tomato (1 oz)	5	0	0
Schorr's				
Pickled	⅓ tomato (1 oz)	4	0	0
Sonoma				
Dried Spice Medley oil drained	1 tbsp (0.5 oz)	50	0	4
Pesto	¼ cup (2 oz)	110	2	9
Tapenade	1 tbsp (0.7 oz)	70	1	6
Tree Of Life				
Sauce	¼ cup (2 oz)	20	0	0
DRIED				
sun dried	1 piece	5	tr	tr
sun dried in oil	1 piece (3 g)	6	tr	tr
Sonoma				
Bits	2-3 tsp (5 g)	15	0	0
Dried	2-3 halves (5 g)	15	0	0
Halves	2-3 halves (5 g)	15	0	0
Julienne	7-9 pieces (5 g)	15	0	0
Pasta Toss	½ cup (0.7 oz)	70	0	0
Season It	2-3 tsp (5 g)	20	0	0
FRESH				
green	1	30	tr	tr
red	1 (4.5 oz)	26	tr	tr
TAKE-OUT				
stewed	1 cup	80	1	3
TOMATO JUICE				
beef broth & tomato	5½ oz	61	tr	tr
clam & tomato	1 can (5½ oz)	77	tr	tr
tomato juice	6 oz	32	tr	tr
tomato juice	½ cup	21	tr	tr
Campbell				
Juice	6 oz	40	—	0
Del Monte				
Snap-E-Tom	6 fl oz	40	0	0
Snap-E-Tom	8 fl oz	50	0	0
Snap-E-Tom	10 fl oz	60	0	0
Dole				
Juice	1 bottle (12 oz)	85	0	0
Hunt's				
Juice	8 fl oz	22	0	tr
No Salt Added	8 fl oz	34	0	tr

FOOD	PORTION	CALS.	SAT. FAT	FAT
Mott's				
Beefamato	8 fl oz	80	0	0
Clamato	8 fl oz	100	0	0
Clamato Caesar	8 fl oz	100	0	0
Muir Glen				
Organic	8 oz	40	—	0
TONGUE				
beef simmered	3 oz	241	8	18
lamb braised	3 oz	234	7	17
pork braised	3 oz	230	5	16
TOPPINGS				
(see ICE CREAM TOPPINGS)				
TORTILLA				
(see also CHIPS, SPANISH FOOD)				
corn	1 (6 in diam)	56	tr	1
corn w/o salt	1-6 in diam (.9 oz)	56	tr	1
flour w/o salt	1-8 in diam (1.2 oz)	114	tr	3
Alvarado St. Bakery				
Burrito Size	1 (2.2 oz)	170	0	4
Fajita Size	1 (1.6 oz)	130	0	3
La Mexicana				
Corn	1 (0.8 oz)	50	0	1
Flour	1 (0.8 oz)	80	1	3
Tortillas de Trigo	1 (1 oz)	140	1	7
Mariachi				
Tortilla	1	112	—	3
Old El Paso				
Flour	1 (1.4 oz)	150	1	3
Soft Taco Tortilla	2 (1.8 oz)	180	1	4
Tyson				
Flour	1 (1.7 oz)	150	1	4
Flour Heat Pressed	2 (2 oz)	170	1	4
White Corn	2 (1.8 oz)	100	0	1
Whole Wheat Heat				
Pressed	1 (1.4 oz)	120	1	3
Yellow Corn	3 (1.9 oz)	140	0	2
Zapata				
Tortilla	1 (1.2 oz)	100	0	2
TORTILLA CHIPS				
(see CHIPS)				
TREE FERN				
chopped cooked	½ cup	28	—	tr

FOOD	PORTION	CALS.	SAT. FAT	FAT
TRITICALE				
dry	1 cup (6.7 oz)	645	1	4
triticale not prep	3.5 oz	329	—	2
TROUT				
baked	3 oz	162	1	7
rainbow cooked	3 oz	129	1	4
Clear Springs				
Rainbow	3.5 oz	140	—	7
TUMERIC				
ground	1 tsp	8	—	tr
TUNA				
(see also TUNA DISHES)				
CANNED				
light in oil	3 oz	169	1	7
light in oil	1 can (6 oz)	399	3	14
white in oil	3 oz	158	—	7
white in oil	1 can (6.2 oz)	331	—	14
Bumble Bee				
Chunk Light In Oil	2 oz	160	3	12
Chunk Light In Water	2 oz	60	1	1
Chunk White In Oil	2 oz	160	3	12
Chunk White In Water	2 oz	70	1	2
Chunk White In Water Diet	2 oz	60	—	1
Solid White In Oil	2 oz	130	2	8
Solid White In Water	2 oz	70	1	2
Progresso				
In Olive Oil	¼ cup (2 oz)	160	2	12
Tree Of Life				
Tongol In Spring Water	2 oz	60	0	0
Tongol In Spring Water No Salt Water	2 oz	70	0	0
FRESH				
bluefin cooked	3 oz	157	1	5
bluefin raw	3 oz	122	1	4
yellowfin baked	3 oz	118	tr	1
TUNA DISHES				
FROZEN				
Mrs. Paul's				
Microwave Tuna Sandwich	1	200	—	6
MIX				
Bumble Bee				
Tuna Mix-ins Classic Italian	⅓ pkg (0.17 oz)	25	0	0
Tuna Mix-ins Garden & Herb	⅓ pkg (0.17 oz)	25	—	0

FOOD	PORTION	CALS.	SAT. FAT	FAT
Bumble Bee (CONT.)				
Tuna Mix-ins Lemon Herb	⅓ pkg (0.17 oz)	25	0	0
Tuna Mix-ins Zesty Tomato	⅓ pkg (0.17 oz)	25	0	0
Tuna Helper				
AuGratin 50% Less Fat Recipe as prep	1 cup	240	2	6
AuGratin as prep	1 cup	300	3	11
Cheesy Broccoli 50% Less Fat Recipe as prep	1 cup	240	2	5
Cheesy Broccoli as prep	1 cup	290	3	9
Cheesy Pasta 50% Less Fat Recipe as prep	1 cup	230	2	5
Cheesy Pasta as prep	1 cup	280	3	11
Creamy Broccoli 50% Less Fat Recipe as prep	1 cup	240	2	5
Creamy Broccoli as prep	1 cup	310	3	12
Creamy Pasta 50% Less Fat Recipe as prep	1 cup	230	2	6
Creamy Pasta as prep	1 cup	300	4	13
Fettuccine Alfredo 50% Less Fat Recipe as prep	1 cup	240	2	6
Fettuccine Alfredo as prep	1 cup	310	4	14
Garden Cheddar 50% Less Fat Recipe as prep	1 cup	240	2	5
Garden Cheddar as prep	1 cup	290	3	11
Pasta Salad Low Fat Recipe as prep	⅔ cup	230	0	2
Pasta Salad as prep	⅔ cup	380	3	27
Tetrazzini 50% Less Fat Recipe as prep	1 cup	230	2	5
Tetrazzini as prep	1 cup	300	4	12
Tuna Melt Reduced Fat Recipe as prep	1 cup	240	2	6
Tuna Melt as prep	1 cup	300	4	12
Tuna Pot Pie as prep	1 cup	440	7	24
Tuna Romanoff 50% Less Fat Recipe as prep	1 cup	240	1	3
Tuna Romanoff as prep	1 cup	280	2	8
READY-TO-EAT				
The Spreadables				
Tuna Salad	¼ can	90	—	6
Wampler				
Salad	⅓ cup	180	—	12
Salad Chunky	⅓ cup	180	—	13

FOOD	PORTION	CALS.	SAT. FAT	FAT
TAKE-OUT				
tuna salad	3 oz	159	1	8
tuna salad	1 cup	383	3	19
TURBOT				
european baked	3 oz	104	—	3
TURKEY				
(see also DINNER, HOT DOG, TURKEY DISHES, TURKEY SUBSTITUTES)				
CANNED				
w/ broth	1 can (5 oz)	231	3	10
w/ broth	½ can (2.5 oz)	116	1	5
Hormel				
Chunk Turkey Ham	2 oz	70	2	4
Swanson				
White	2½ oz	80	—	1
Underwood				
Chunky Light	2.08 oz	75	tr	2
FRESH				
back w/ skin roasted	½ back (9 oz)	637	11	38
breast w/ skin roasted	4 oz	212	2	8
dark meat w/ skin roasted	3.6 oz	230	4	12
dark meat w/o skin roasted	1 cup (5 oz)	262	3	10
dark meat w/o skin roasted	3 oz	170	2	7
ground cooked	3 oz	188	3	11
leg w/ skin roasted	1 (1.2 lbs)	1133	17	54
leg w/ skin roasted	2.5 oz	147	2	7
light meat w/ skin roasted	4.7 oz	268	3	11
light meat w/ skin roasted	from ½ turkey (2.3 lbs)	2069	25	87
light meat w/o skin roasted	4 oz	183	1	4
neck simmered	1 (5.3 oz)	274	4	11
skin roasted	from ½ turkey (9 oz)	1096	26	98
skin roasted	1 oz	141	3	13
w/ skin roasted	½ turkey (4 lbs)	3857	53	181
w/ skin roasted	8.4 oz	498	7	23
w/ skin neck & giblets roasted	½ turkey (8.8 lbs)	4123	56	190
w/o skin roasted	1 cup (5 oz)	238	2	7
w/o skin roasted	7.3 oz	354	3	10
wing w/ skin roasted	1 (6.5 oz)	426	6	23
Butterball				
Ground All White Meat	3 oz	100	—	3
Louis Rich				
Ground	4 oz	190	4	12
Patties White	1 (4 oz)	170	3	10

FOOD	PORTION	CALS.	SAT. FAT	FAT
Mr. Turkey				
Ground 85% Fat Free	3.5 oz	210	—	16
Ground 91% Fat Free	3.5 oz	170	—	10
Perdue				
Breast Tenderloins Cooked	3 oz	110	1	1
Breast Boneless Cooked	3 oz	110	0	1
Breast Cutlets Thin Sliced Cooked	1 (2.5 oz)	90	1	1
Breast Fillets Cooked	3 oz	110	1	1
Burger Cooked	1 (3 oz)	170	3	9
Cubed Steak Cooked	3 oz	120	1	3
Dark Cooked	3 oz	200	5	14
Drumsticks Roasted	3 oz	150	2	7
Drumsticks Cooked	3 oz	150	2	7
Ground Cooked	3 oz	170	3	9
Ground Breast Cooked	3 oz	110	1	2
Half Breast Cooked	3 oz	170	3	8
Thighs Cooked	3 oz	180	4	11
Tom Wings Cooked	3 oz	160	3	8
White Cooked	3 oz	170	3	9
Whole Breast Cooked	3 oz	170	3	8
Wings Roasted	1 (3 oz)	180	3	10
Wings Drummettes Roasted	1 (3.5 oz)	180	3	9
Shady Brook				
Cutlets	4 oz	130	0	1
Drumstick	4 oz	170	3	9
Ground Breast	4 oz	120	0	1
Ground Lean	4 oz	170	3	9
Ground Turkey 85%	4 oz	220	5	15
Mesquite Seasoned Tenderloin	4 oz	110	0	1
OnlyOne Boneless Breast Roast	4 oz	130	0	1
Split Breast	4 oz	190	3	9
Tenderloin	4 oz	130	0	1
Teriyaki Seasoned Tenderloin	4 oz	120	0	1
Thigh	4 oz	220	5	15
Turkey Burgers	4 oz	170	3	9
Turkey Meatloaf Lean	4 oz	150	2	7
Whole Breast	4 oz	190	3	9
Whole Turkey	4 oz	180	3	9
Wing	4 oz	220	4	14
Zesty Lemon Seasoned Tenderlion	4 oz	120	0	1
Swift-Eckrich				
Ground All White	3 oz	100	—	3

FOOD	PORTION	CALS.	SAT. FAT	FAT
The Turkey Store				
Breakfast Sausage Patties Mild	2 patties (2.3 oz)	160	4	13
Seasoned Cuts Turkey Breast Roast	4 oz	110	0	1
Wampler				
Boneless Breast Roast	4 oz	160	1	6
Breast Half	4 oz	160	1	6
Breast Steaks	4 oz	120	—	1
Burger	1 (4 oz)	160	2	9
Drumsticks	4 oz	180	3	10
Ground	4 oz	210	3	15
Ground Breast	4 oz	130	0	1
Ground Lean	4 oz	160	2	8
Thighs	4 oz	170	2	10
Wings	4 oz	220	4	14
FROZEN				
roast boneless seasoned light & dark meat roasted	1 pkg (1.7 lbs)	1213	—	45
Empire				
Patties	1 (3.1 oz)	200	2	10
Wampler				
Burger BBQ	1 (4 oz)	240	—	17
Burger Seasoned	1 (4 oz)	180	—	11
READY-TO-EAT				
bologna	1 oz	57	—	4
breast	1 slice (0.75 oz)	23	tr	tr
diced light & dark seasoned	½ lb	313	4	14
diced light & dark seasoned	1 oz	39	1	2
ham thigh meat	2 oz	73	1	3
ham thigh meat	1 pkg (8 oz)	291	4	12
pastrami	2 oz	80	1	4
pastrami	1 pkg (8 oz)	320	4	14
patties battered & fried	1 (3.3 oz)	266	—	17
patties battered & fried	1 (2.3 oz)	181	—	12
patties breaded & fried	1 (3.3 oz)	266	—	17
patties breaded & fried	1 (2.3 oz)	181	—	12
poultry salad sandwich spread	1 tbsp	109	tr	2
poultry salad sandwich spread	1 oz	238	1	4
prebasted breast w/ skin roasted	1 breast (3.8 lbs)	2175	17	60
prebasted breast w/ skin roasted	½ breast (1.9 lbs)	1087	8	30
prebasted thigh w/ skin roasted	1 thigh (11 oz)	494	8	27

FOOD	PORTION	CALS.	SAT. FAT	FAT
roll light & dark meat	1 oz	42	1	2
roll light meat	1 oz	42	1	2
salami cooked	2 oz	111	—	8
salami cooked	1 pkg (8 oz)	446	—	31
turkey loaf breast meat	1 pkg (6 oz)	187	1	3
turkey loaf breast meat	2 slices (1.5 oz)	47	tr	1
turkey sticks battered & fried	1 stick (2.3 oz)	178	—	11
turkey sticks breaded & fried	1 stick (2.3 oz)	178	—	11
Alpine Lace				
Breast Fat Free	2 oz	50	25	0
Boar's Head				
Breast Cracked Pepper Smoked	2 oz	60	0	1
Breast Golden Skin On	2 oz	60	1	2
Breast Golden Skinless	2 oz	60	0	1
Breast Hickory Smoked	2 oz	70	1	2
Breast Low Sodium Skinless	2 oz	60	0	1
Breast Lower Sodium Skin On	2 oz	60	1	2
Breast Maple Glazed Honey Coat	2 oz	70	0	1
Breast Ovengold Skin On	2 oz	60	0	2
Breast Ovengold Skinless	2 oz	60	0	1
Breast Roasted Mesquite Smoked Skin On	2 oz	60	0	1
Breast Roasted Mesquite Smoked Skinless	2 oz	60	0	1
Breast Roasted Salsalito	2 oz	60	0	1
Pastrami Seasoned	2 oz	60	0	1
Carl Buddig				
Honey Roasted Turkey Breast	1 pkg (2.5 oz)	120	3	7
Lean Slices Honey Roasted Breast	1 pkg (2.5 oz)	70	1	1
Lean Slices Oven Roasted Breast	1 pkg (2.5 oz)	70	1	1
Lean Slices Smoked Breast	1 pkg (2.5 oz)	70	1	1
Oven Roasted Breast	1 pkg (2.5 oz)	110	3	7
Smoked Breast	1 pkg (2.5 oz)	110	3	7
Turkey Ham	1 pkg (2.5 oz)	100	2	5
Empire				
Barbecue Whole	5 oz	250	4	12
Bologna	3 slices (1.8 oz)	90	2	6
Oven Prepared Breast Slices	3 slices (1.8 oz)	50	0	1
Pastrami	3 slices (1.8 oz)	60	5	2
Salami	3 slices (1.8 oz)	70	1	4
Smoked Breast Slices	3 slices (1.8 oz)	40	0	0

FOOD	PORTION	CALS.	SAT. FAT	FAT
Falls				
BBQ	3 oz	140	—	8
Gourmet Breast	3 oz	80	—	1
Premium Cooked Breast	3 oz	100	—	2
Hansel n'Gretel				
Breast Gourmet	1 oz	28	—	1
Breast Gourmet Smoked	1 oz	31	—	1
Breast Honey	1 oz	28	—	1
Breast Lessalt Cooked	1 oz	25	—	1
Breast Oven Cooked	1 oz	26	—	tr
Doubledecker Turkey Corned Beef	1 oz	30	—	1
Doubledecker Turkey Ham	1 oz	30	—	1
Healthy Choice				
Deli-Thin Honey Roast & Smoked	6 slices (2 oz)	70	1	2
Deli-Thin Roasted Breast	6 slices (2 oz)	60	1	2
Deli-Thin Smoked Breast	6 slices (2 oz)	60	1	2
Deli-Thin Turkey Ham	6 slices (2 oz)	60	1	2
Fresh-Trak Honey Roast & Smoked Breast	1 slice (1 oz)	35	0	1
Fresh-Trak Oven Roasted Breast	1 slice (1 oz)	35	0	1
Honey Roasted & Smoked	1 slice (1 oz)	35	0	1
Oven Roasted Breast	1 slice (1 oz)	35	0	1
Smoked Breast	1 slice (1 oz)	30	0	1
Variety Pack Regular	3 slices (2.2 oz)	70	1	2
Hebrew National				
Deli Thin Hickory Smoked	1.8 oz	55	—	1
Deli Thin Lemon Garlic	1.8 oz	50	—	1
Deli Thin Oven Roasted	1.8 oz	80	—	1
Hillshire				
Deli Select Honey Roasted Breast	1 slice	10	—	tr
Deli Select Oven Roasted Breast	1 slice	10	—	tr
Deli Select Smoked Breast	1 slice	10	—	tr
Deli Select Turkey Ham	1 slice	10	—	tr
Flavor Pack 90-99% Fat Free Honey Roasted Breast	1 slice (0.75 oz)	20	—	tr
Flavor Pack 90-99% Fat Free Oven Roasted Breast	1 slice (0.75 oz)	20	—	tr
Flavor Pack 90-99% Fat Free Smoked Breast	1 slice (0.75 oz)	20	—	tr
Honey Cured Breast	1 oz	35	—	1

FOOD	PORTION	CALS.	SAT. FAT	FAT
Hillshire (CONT.)				
Lunch 'N Munch Smoked Turkey/Cheddar	1 pkg (4.5 oz)	350	—	21
Lunch 'N Munch Smoked Turkey/Cheddar/ Brownie	1 pkg (4.5 oz)	400	—	22
Lunch 'N Munch Turkey/ Cheddar/Brownie/Hi-C	1 pkg (4.5 oz + 6 fl oz)	500	—	22
Smoked Breast	1 oz	35	—	1
Hormel				
Light & Lean 97 Breast Sliced	1 slice (1 oz)	30	0	1
Light & Lean 97 Mesquite Smoked Breast	1 slice (1 oz)	30	0	1
turkey pepperoni	17 slices (1 oz)	80	2	4
Jordan's				
Healthy Trim Fat Free Oven Roasted Breast	1 slice (1 oz)	20	0	0
Healthy Trim Fat Free Oven Roasted Smoked Breast	1 slice (1 oz)	20	0	0
Louis Rich				
Bologna	1 slice (28 g)	50	1	4
Breaded Nuggets	4 (3.2 oz)	260	3	16
Breaded Patties	1 (3 oz)	220	3	13
Breaded Sticks	3 (3 oz)	230	3	15
Breast Skinless Hickory Smoked	2 oz	50	0	0
Breast Skinless Honey Roasted	2 oz	60	0	0
Breast Skinless Oven Roasted	2 oz	50	0	0
Breast Skinless Rotisserie	2 oz	50	0	0
Breast Slices Hickory Smoked	1 slice (2 oz)	50	0	0
Breast Slices Honey Roasted	1 slice (2 oz)	60	0	0
Breast Slices Oven Roasted	1 slice (2 oz)	50	0	0
Breast Slices Rotisserie	1 slice (2 oz)	50	0	0
Carving Board Hickory Smoked	2 slices (1.6 oz)	40	0	1
Carving Board Oven Roasted Thin	6 slices (2.1 oz)	60	0	1
Carving Board Oven Roasted Traditional	2 slices (1.6 oz)	40	0	1
Carving Board Rotisserie	2 slices (1.6 oz)	40	0	1
Cotto Salami	1 slice (28 g)	40	1	3
Deli-Thin Oven Roasted	4 slices (1.8 oz)	50	0	1
Deli-Thin Smoked	4 slices (1.8 oz)	50	1	2
Fat Free Hickory Smoked Breast	1 slice (1 oz)	25	0	0

FOOD	PORTION	CALS.	SAT. FAT	FAT
Louis Rich (CONT.)				
Fat Free Oven Roasted Breast	1 slice (1 oz)	25	0	0
Fat Free Oven Roasted Deli-Thin Breast	4 slices (1.8 oz)	45	0	0
Fat Free Turkey Ham Honey	2 slices (1.7 oz)	35	0	0
Fat Free Turkey Ham Smoked	2 slices (1.7 oz)	35	0	0
Hickory Smoked	1 slice (1 oz)	30	0	1
Oven Roasted	1 slice (1 oz)	30	0	1
Pastrami	1 slice (1 oz)	30	0	1
Salami	1 slice (28 g)	40	1	3
Smoked	1 slice (1 oz)	30	0	1
Turkey Ham	1 slice (1 oz)	30	0	1
Turkey Ham Chopped	1 slice (1 oz)	45	1	3
Turkey Ham Honey Cured	1 slice (1 oz)	30	0	1
Mr. Turkey				
Deli Cuts Hardwood Smoked Breast	3 slices	30	—	1
Deli Cuts Honey Roasted Breast	3 slices	30	—	1
Deli Cuts Oven Roasted Breast	3 slices	30	—	1
Deli Cuts Turkey Ham	3 slices	35	—	2
Deli Cuts Turkey Pastrami	3 slices	35	—	1
Hardwood Smoked Breast	1 slice	30	—	1
Hardwood Smoked Turkey Ham	1 slice	35	—	2
Honey Cured Turkey Ham	1 slice	30	—	1
Oven Roasted Breast	1 slice	30	—	1
Smoked Breakfast Turkey Ham	1 oz	30	—	1
Turkey Bologna	1 slice	70	—	5
Turkey Cotto Salami	1 slice	50	—	4
Turkey Ham	1 slice	35	—	2
Turkey Pastrami	1 slice	30	—	1
Oscar Mayer				
Free Oven Roasted Breast	4 slices (1.8 oz)	40	0	0
Free Smoked Breast	4 slices (1.8 oz)	40	0	0
Lunchables Fun Pack Turkey/ Pacific Cooler	1 pkg (11.2 oz)	460	10	21
Lunchables Fun Pack Turkey/ Surger Cooler	1 pkg (11.2 oz)	440	8	16
Lunchables Turkey/Cheddar	1 pkg (4.5 oz)	360	11	22
Oven Roasted White	1 slice (1 oz)	30	0	1
Smoked White	1 slice (1 oz)	30	0	1
Perdue				
Nuggets Dinosaur	3 (3 oz)	200	3	12

FOOD	PORTION	CALS.	SAT. FAT	FAT
Sara Lee				
Hardwood Smoked Breast Of Turkey	2 oz	60	0	1
Hardwood Smoked Turkey Ham	2 oz	60	1	2
Honey Roasted Breast Of Turkey	2 oz	60	0	0
Honey Roasted Turkey Ham	2 oz	70	1	3
Mesquite Smoked Breast Of Turkey	2 oz	60	1	2
Oven Roasted Breast Of Turkey	2 oz	60	1	2
Peppered Breast Of Turkey	2 oz	50	0	0
Seasoned Breast Of Turkey Pastrami	2 oz	60	0	1
Shady Brook				
Black Forest Turkey Ham	2 oz	70	1	3
Browned Homestyle Oven Roasted Breast	2 oz	60	0	1
Browned Slow Roasted Breast	2 oz	60	0	0
Carved Breast Italian Seasoned	2 oz	60	0	0
Carved Breast Natural Roast	2 oz	60	0	0
Carved Breast Peppered	2 oz	60	0	0
Hickory Smoked Breast	2 oz	50	0	0
Honey Roasted Breast	2 oz	60	0	1
Honey Roasted Breast Covered w/ Cracked Pepper	2 oz	60	0	0
Meatballs Italian Style	3 oz	130	3	7
Smoked Drumstick	3 oz	180	3	8
Smoked Neck	3 oz	150	2	6
Smoked Whole Turkey	3 oz	150	2	4
Smoked Wing	3 oz	200	3	10
Wampler				
Bologna	2 oz	130	—	11
Dark Cured	2 oz	80	—	5
Deli Roast Breast	2 oz	50	—	1
Deli Roast Classic Spiced Breast	2 oz	70	—	1
Deli Roast Pan Roasted Breast	2 oz	70	—	2
Deli Roast Pan Roasted Skinless Breast	2 oz	50	—	0
Deli Roast Peppered Breast	2 oz	40	—	0
Deli Roast Rotisserie Breast	2 oz	50	—	2

FOOD	PORTION	CALS.	SAT. FAT	FAT
Wampler (CONT.)				
Pastrami	2 oz	90	—	5
Salami	2 oz	90	—	6
Turkey Ham	2 oz	60	—	3

TURKEY DISHES

(see also DINNER, TURKEY SUBSTITUTES)

CANNED

Dinty Moore

Stew	1 cup (8.5 oz)	140	1	3

FROZEN

gravy & turkey	1 cup (8.4 oz)	160	2	6
gravy & turkey	1 pkg (5 oz)	95	1	4

Hot Pocket

Stuffed Sandwich Turkey & Ham With Cheese	1 (4.5 oz)	320	6	13

Lean Pockets

Stuffed Sandwich Turkey & Ham With Cheddar	1 (4.5 oz)	260	3	7
Stuffed Sandwich Turkey Broccoli & Cheese	1 (4.5 oz)	260	3	8

Luigino's

Gravy Dressing & Turkey	1 pkg (8 oz)	340	4	15

READY-TO-EAT

Shady Brook

Meatloaf	1 serv (16 oz)	470	10	17

Spreadables

Turkey Salad	¼ can	100	—	6

Wampler

Turkey Ham Salad	⅓ cup	150	—	10

SHELF-STABLE

Dinty Moore

Microwave Cup Stew	1 pkg (7.5 oz)	130	1	3

TURKEY SUBSTITUTES

Harvest Direct

TVP Poultry Chunks	3.5 oz	280	tr	1
TVP Poultry Ground	3.5 oz	280	tr	1

Soy Is Us

Turkey Not!	½ cup (1.75 oz)	140	1	2

White Wave

Meatless Sandwich Slices	2 slices (1.6 oz)	80	0	0

Worthington

Smoked Turkey Meatless	3 slices (2 oz)	140	2	10
Turkee Slices	3 slices (3.3 oz)	130	3	14

FOOD	PORTION	CALS.	SAT. FAT	FAT
TURNIPS				
CANNED				
greens	½ cup	17	tr	tr
Allen				
Chopped Greens And Diced Turnip	½ cup (4.2 oz)	30	0	1
Greens	½ cup (4.2 oz)	25	0	1
Sunshine				
Chopped Greens And Diced Turnip	½ cup (4.2 oz)	30	0	1
Greens	½ cup (4.2 oz)	25	0	1
FRESH				
cooked mashed	½ cup (4.2 oz)	47	tr	tr
cubed cooked	½ cup (3 oz)	33	tr	tr
greens chopped cooked	½ cup	15	tr	tr
raw cubed	½ cup (2.4 oz)	25	tr	tr
FROZEN				
Birds Eye				
Chopped Greens	1 cup (3.1 oz)	30	0	0
Greens w/ Diced Root	1 cup (3 oz)	25	0	0
Southland				
Mashed	3.6 oz	90	—	6
Rutabaga Yellow Turnips	4 oz	50	—	0
VANILLA				
Virginia Dare				
Vanilla Extract	1 tsp	10	—	0
VEAL				
(see also DINNER, VEAL DISHES)				
cutlet lean only braised	3 oz	172	2	4
cutlet lean only fried	3 oz	156	1	4
ground broiled	3 oz	146	3	6
loin chop w/ bone lean & fat braised	1 chop (2.8 oz)	227	5	14
loin chop w/ bone lean only braised	1 chop (2.4 oz)	155	2	6
shoulder w/ bone lean only braised	3 oz	169	1	5
sirloin w/ bone lean & fat roasted	3 oz	171	4	9
sirloin w/ bone lean only roasted	3 oz	143	2	5
VEGETABLE JUICE				
vegetable juice cocktail	6 fl oz	34	tr	tr
vegetable juice cocktail	½ cup	22	tr	tr

FOOD	PORTION	CALS.	SAT. FAT	FAT
Dole				
Vegetable Blend	1 bottle (12 oz)	90	0	0
Mott's				
Vegetable Juice as prep	8 fl oz	60	0	0
Muir Glen				
Organic	8 oz	70	—	0
Organic Reduced Sodium	8 oz	70	—	0
Odwalla				
Vegetable Cocktail	8 fl oz	70	0	0
V8				
No Salt Added	6 fl oz	35	—	0
Original	6 fl oz	35	—	0
Spicy Hot	6 fl oz	35	—	0
Splash Tropical Blend	8 fl oz	120	0	0

VEGETABLES MIXED
(see also VEGETABLE JUICE)

CANNED

FOOD	PORTION	CALS.	SAT. FAT	FAT
mixed vegetables	½ cup	39	tr	tr
peas & carrots	½ cup	48	tr	tr
peas & onions	½ cup	30	tr	tr
succotash	½ cup	102	tr	1
Allen				
Green Beans And Potatoes	½ cup (4.2 oz)	35	0	0
Okra & Tomatoes	½ cup (4 oz)	25	0	0
Okra Tomatoes & Corn	½ cup (4.1 oz)	30	0	0
Chi-Chi's				
Diced Tomatoes & Green Chilies	¼ cup (2.5 oz)	20	0	0
Del Monte				
Mixed	½ cup (4.4 oz)	40	0	0
Peas And Carrots	½ cup (4.5 oz)	60	0	0
Green Giant				
Garden Medley	½ cup (4.2 oz)	40	0	0
Mixed	½ cup (4.3 oz)	60	0	0
Sweet Peas & Carrots	½ cup (4.3 oz)	50	0	0
Sweet Peas & Tiny Pearl Onion	½ cup (4.4 oz)	60	0	0
Hanover				
Mixed	½ cup	110	—	0
Vegetable Salad	½ cup	90	—	0
House Of Tsang				
Vegetables & Sauce Cantonese Classic	½ cup (4.2 oz)	70	0	1
Vegetables & Sauce Hong Kong Sweet & Sour	½ cup (4.5 oz)	160	0	0

FOOD	PORTION	CALS.	SAT. FAT	FAT
House Of Tsang (CONT.)				
Vegetables & Sauce Szechuan Hot & Spicy	½ cup (4.2 oz)	70	0	1
Vegetables & Sauce Tokyo Teriyaki	½ cup (4.4 oz)	100	0	0
LeSueur				
Early Peas w/ Mushrooms & Pearl Onions	½ cup (4.3 oz)	60	0	0
Seneca				
Peas & Carrots	½ cup	60	0	0
Succotash	½ cup	90	0	0
Sunshine				
Green Beans And Potatoes	½ cup (4.2 oz)	35	0	0
Trappey				
Okra & Tomatoes	½ cup (4 oz)	25	0	0
Okra Tomatoes & Corn	½ cup (4.1 oz)	30	0	0
FROZEN				
peas & carrots cooked	½ cup	38	tr	tr
peas & onions cooked	½ cup	40	tr	tr
succotash cooked	½ cup	79	tr	1
Amy's Organic				
Pocket Sandwich Mediterranean Vegetables	1 (4.5 oz)	220	4	7
Pocket Sandwich Roasted Vegetables	1 (4.5 oz)	220	2	8
Pocket Sandwich Vegetable Pie	1 (5 oz)	230	1	6
Big Valley				
California Blend	¾ cup (3 oz)	25	0	0
Italian Blend	¾ cup (3 oz)	30	0	0
Oriental Blend	¾ cup (3 oz)	25	0	0
Stew Vegetables	⅔ cup (3 oz)	40	0	0
Winter Blend	¾ cup (3 oz)	25	0	0
Birds Eye				
Baby Bean & Carrot Blend	1 cup (2.9 oz)	30	0	0
Broccoli Cauliflower Carrots w/ Cheese	½ cup (3.9 oz)	70	1	4
Brussels Sprouts Cauliflower Carrots	½ cup (3.1 oz)	30	0	0
Chicken Viola Garlic	2 cups (6.2 oz)	260	3	11
Chicken Viola Pesto	2¼ cups (6.6 oz)	250	3	9
Chicken Viola Three Cheese	1¾ cups (6.2 oz)	240	3	9
Chicken Voila Teriyaki	2⅓ cups (6.1 oz)	230	2	6
Farm Fresh Broccoli Carrots Water Chestnuts	½ cup (3.3 oz)	30	0	0

FOOD	PORTION	CALS.	SAT. FAT	FAT
Birds Eye (CONT.)				
Farm Fresh Broccoli Cauliflower	½ cup (3.2 oz)	20	0	0
Farm Fresh Broccoli Cauliflower Carrots	½ cup (3.2 oz)	25	0	0
Farm Fresh Broccoli Cauliflower Red Peppers	½ cup (3.3 oz)	20	0	0
Farm Fresh Broccoli Corn Red Peppers	½ cup (3.6 oz)	50	0	0
Farm Fresh Broccoli Red Peppers Onions Mushrooms	½ cup (3.5 oz)	25	0	0
Farm Fresh Brussels Sprouts Cauliflower Carrots	½ cup (3.1 oz)	30	0	0
Farm Fresh Cauliflower Carrots Snow Peas Pods	½ cup (3.2 oz)	30	0	0
For Soup	⅔ cup (3 oz)	45	0	0
For Stew	¾ cup (2.9 oz)	40	0	0
Gumbo Blend	¾ cup (3 oz)	40	0	0
International French Country Style	⅔ cup (4.4 oz)	110	3	6
International New England Style	1 pkg (9 oz)	260	5	14
International Oriental Style	½ cup (3 oz)	60	2	4
International Stir Fry Style	½ cup 3.6 oz)	60	2	4
Internationals Bavarian Style	1 cup (5.5 oz)	150	4	8
Internationals California Style	½ cup (3 oz)	100	2	5
Internationals Italian Style	1 cup (5.8 oz)	150	3	10
Peas & Carrots	⅔ cup (3 oz)	50	0	0
Peas & Pearl Onions	⅔ cup (4.2 oz)	90	0	1
Peas & Potatoes In Cream Sauce	½ cup (4.4 oz)	90	1	3
Seasoning Blend	¾ cup (2.9 oz)	20	0	0
Stir Fry Asparagus	2 cups (5.8 oz)	90	0	1
Stir Fry Broccoli	1 cup (3.3 oz)	30	0	0
Stir Fry Pepper	1 cup (2.9 oz)	25	0	0
Stir Fry Sugar Snap	¾ cup (2.6 oz)	35	0	0
Stir Fry Whole Green Bean	1¾ cup (5.3 oz)	100	0	1
Budget Gourmet				
Mandarin Vegetables	1 pkg (5.25 oz)	160	—	11
New England Recipe Vegetables	1 pkg (5.5 oz)	230	—	13
Spring Vegetables In Cheese Sauce	1 pkg (5 oz)	130	—	8
Fresh Like				
California Blend	3.5 oz	31	—	tr

FOOD	PORTION	CALS.	SAT. FAT	FAT
Fresh Like (CONT.)				
Chuckwagon Blend	3.5 oz	71	—	1
Italian Blend	3.5 oz	33	—	tr
Midwestern Blend	3.5 oz	42	—	tr
Mixed	3.5 oz	69	—	tr
Oriental Blend	3.5 oz	26	—	tr
Peas & Carrots	3.5 oz	63	—	tr
Winter Blend	3.5 oz	26	—	tr
Green Giant				
American Mixtures Broccoli Carrots Cauliflower	¾ cup (2.6 oz)	25	0	0
American Mixtures Broccoli Carrots Waterchestnuts	¾ cup (3 oz)	30	0	0
American Mixtures Carrots Green Bean Cauliflower	¾ cup (2.7 oz)	25	0	0
American Mixtures Cauliflower Broccoli Sugar Snap & Sweet Pea	¾ cup (2.8 oz)	35	0	0
American Mixtures Corn Broccoli Red Pepper	¾ cup (3.1 oz)	60	0	0
American Mixtures Green Beans Potatoes Onions Red Peppers	¾ cup (2.8 oz)	45	0	1
American Mixtures Sweet Peas Potatoes Carrots	⅔ cup (3 oz)	70	0	2
Butter Sauce Broccoli Cauliflower Carrots Corn Sweet Peas	¾ cup (3.6 oz)	60	2	2
Butter Sauce Broccoli Pasta Sweet Peas Corn Red Peppers	¾ cup (3.5 oz)	70	2	2
Butter Sauce Mixed	¾ cup (3.6 oz)	70	1	2
Cheese Sauce Broccoli Cauliflower Carrots	⅔ cup (4.3 oz)	80	2	3
Harvest Fresh Broccoli Cauliflower Carrots	1 cup (3.4 oz)	30	0	0
Harvest Fresh Mixed Vegetables	⅔ cup (3.1 oz)	50	0	0
Harvest Fresh Sweet Peas & Pearl Onions	½ cup (2.7 oz)	55	0	0
Mixed	¾ cup (2.9 oz)	50	0	0
Select Sweet Peas & Pearl Onions	⅔ cup (3.1 oz)	60	0	0
Hanover				
Broccoli Cut & Cauliflower Cut	½ cup	20	—	0

FOOD	PORTION	CALS.	SAT. FAT	FAT
Hanover (CONT.)				
Caribbean Blend	½ cup	20	—	0
Garden Medley	½ cup	20	—	0
Mixed	½ cup	50	—	0
Oriental Blend	½ cup	25	—	0
Succotash	½ cup	80	—	0
Summer Vegetables	½ cup	35	—	0
Vegetables For Soup	½ cup	60	—	0
Ore Ida				
Stew Vegetables	⅔ cup (3 oz)	50	0	0
Soglowek				
Golden Vegetarian Nuggets	4 pieces (2.5 oz)	190	2	11
Southland				
Peppers & Onions	2 oz	15	—	0
Soup Mix Vegetables	3.2 oz	50	—	0
Stew Vegetables	4 oz	60	—	0
Tree Of Life				
Mixed	½ cup (3 oz)	65	0	0
Veg-All				
Country Wisconsin Blend	3.5 oz	52	—	tr
Scandinavian Blend	3.5 oz	48	—	tr
Vegetables For Soup (Eight)	3.5 oz	34	—	tr
Vegetables For Soup (Potatoes)	3.5 oz	53	—	tr
Vegetables For Stew 4-Way	3.5 oz	51	—	tr
Vegetables For Stew 5-Way	3.5 oz	54	—	tr
TAKE-OUT				
caponata	¼ cup	28	—	1
gyoza potstickers vegetable	8 (4.9 oz)	210	1	4
ratatouille	1 serv (3.5 oz)	96	1	7
succotash	½ cup	111	tr	1
VENISON				
roasted	3 oz	134	1	3
Broken Arrow Ranch				
Antelope Chili Meat	3.5 oz	115	1	2
Antelope Ground Venison	3.5 oz	110	1	2
Antelope Stew Meat	3.5 oz	110	1	2
Nilgai Chili Meat	3.5 oz	115	1	2
Nilgai Leg	3.5 oz	100	tr	1
Nilgai Stew Meat	3.5 oz	110	1	2
Venison & Beef Smoked Sausage	6 oz	432	—	30
Venison Meat Chunks	6 oz	175	—	2
Venison Salami	6 oz	252	—	8

FOOD	PORTION	CALS.	SAT. FAT	FAT
VINEGAR				
balsamic	1 tbsp (0.5 oz)	5	0	0
cider	1 tbsp	tr	0	0
Hain				
Cider	1 tbsp	2	0	0
Nakano				
Rice	1 tbsp	0	0	0
Regina				
Red Wine	1 oz	4	0	0
Tree Of Life				
Apple Cider Organic	1 tbsp (0.5 oz)	0	0	0
Brown Rice	1 tbsp (0.5 oz)	2	0	0
Victoria				
Balsamic	1 tbsp (0.5 oz)	5	0	0
White House				
Apple Cider	1 tbsp (0.5 oz)	0	0	0
White	1 tbsp (0.5 oz)	0	0	0
WAFFLES				
FROZEN				
buttermilk	1 4 in sq (1.2 oz)	88	tr	3
plain	1 4 in sq (1.2 oz)	88	tr	3
Aunt Jemima				
Blueberry	2 (2.5 oz)	190	2	7
Buttermilk	2 (2.5 oz)	170	2	6
Cinnamon	2 (2.5 oz)	180	2	6
Oatmeal	2 (2.5 oz)	170	1	7
Whole Grain	2 (2.5 oz)	170	1	7
Belgian Chef				
Belgian	2 (2.5 oz)	140	1	3
Downyflake				
Blueberry	2	180	—	4
Buttermilk	2	190	—	5
Multi-Grain	2	250	—	14
Oat Bran	2	260	—	13
Regular	2	120	—	3
Regular Jumbo	2	170	—	4
Rice Bran	2	210	—	11
Roman Meal	2	280	—	14
Waffles	2	180	—	6
Eggo				
Apple Cinnamon	2 (2.7 oz)	220	2	8
Banana Bread	2 (2.7 oz)	200	1	7
Blueberry	2 (2.7 oz)	220	2	9
Buttermilk	2 (2.7 oz)	220	2	8
Golden Oat	2 (2.7 oz)	150	1	3

FOOD	PORTION	CALS.	SAT. FAT	FAT
Eggo (CONT.)				
Homestyle	2 (2.7 oz)	220	2	8
Minis Cinnamon Toast	12 (3.2 oz)	290	2	10
Minis Cinnamon Toast	12 (3.2 oz)	280	2	9
Minis Homestyle	12 (3.3 oz)	260	2	9
Nut & Honey	2 (2.7 oz)	240	2	10
Nutri-Grain	2 (2.7 oz)	190	1	6
Nutri-Grain Multi-Bran	2 (2.7 oz)	180	1	6
Nutri-Grain Raisin & Bran	2 (2.9 oz)	210	1	6
Special K	2 (2 oz)	120	0	0
Strawberry	2 (2.7 oz)	220	2	8
Kellogg's				
Homestyle Low Fat	2 (2.7 oz)	180	1	3
Nutri-Grain Low Fat	2 (2.7 oz)	160	0	3
Nutri-Grain Low Fat Blueberry	2 (2.7 oz)	160	0	2
Van's				
7 Grain Belgain	2	152	0	4
Belgian Original	2	145	0	4
Belgian Original Toaster	2	145	0	4
Blueberry Toaster	2	157	0	4
Blueberry Wheat Free Toaster	2	225	1	5
Fat Free	2	155	0	2
Mini	4	107	0	4
Multigrain Toaster	2	160	0	4
Organic Whole Wheat	2	190	0	5
Organic Whole Wheat Blueberry	2	190	0	5
Wheat Free Cinnamon Apple Toaster	2	220	1	5
Wheat Free Toaster	2	220	1	5
HOME RECIPE				
plain	1 (7 in diam)	218	2	11
MIX				
plain as prep	1 7 in diam (2.6 oz)	218	2	10

WALNUTS

FOOD	PORTION	CALS.	SAT. FAT	FAT
black dried chopped	1 cup	759	5	71
Planters				
Black	1 pkg (2 oz)	340	2	31
Gold Measure Halves	1 pkg (2 oz)	380	4	38
Halves	⅓ cup (1.2 oz)	220	3	22
Pieces	¼ cup (1 oz)	190	2	20

WASABI

FOOD	PORTION	CALS.	SAT. FAT	FAT
root raw	1 (5.9 oz)	184	—	1
root raw sliced	1 cup (4.6 oz)	142	—	1

FOOD	PORTION	CALS.	SAT. FAT	FAT
WATER				
Canada Dry				
Sparkling Water	8 fl oz	0	0	0
Crystal Geyser				
Sparkling Lemon	1 bottle (12 fl oz)	0	0	0
Sparkling Mineral	1 bottle (12 fl oz)	0	0	0
Sparkling Natural Cola Berry	1 bottle (12 fl oz)	0	0	0
Sparkling Natural Wild Cherry	1 bottle (12 fl oz)	0	0	0
Sparkling Orange	1 bottle (12 fl oz)	0	0	0
Diamond Spring				
Water	1 qt	0	0	0
Evian				
Water	1 liter	0	0	0
Glacier Springs				
Drinking Water	8 fl oz	0	0	0
Glennpatrick				
Irish Spring Pure	8 oz	0	—	0
LaCroix				
Sparkling Berry	12 fl oz	0	0	0
Sparkling Lemon	12 fl oz	0	0	0
Sparkling Lime	12 fl oz	0	0	0
Sparkling Orange	12 fl oz	0	0	0
Sparkling Regular	12 fl oz	0	0	0
Spring	1 bottle (12 oz)	0	0	0
Meridian				
Clear All Flavors	8 oz	100	0	0
Mountain Valley				
Mineral Water	1 qt	0	0	0
Mt Shasta				
Natural Spring	1 bottle (20 oz)	0	0	0
San Pellegrino				
Acqua Panna	8 fl oz	0	0	0
Mineral Water	1 liter (33.8 oz)	0	0	0
Saratoga				
Sparkling	1 liter	0	0	0
Snapple				
Natural Spring	8 fl oz	0	0	0
Veryfine				
Fruit 2 0 Lemon	8 oz	0	0	0
Water Joe				
Caffeine Enhanced	8 fl oz	0	0	0
WATER CHESTNUTS				
CANNED				
chinese sliced	½ cup	35	—	tr

FOOD	PORTION	CALS.	SAT. FAT	FAT
FRESH				
sliced	½ cup	66	—	tr
WATERCRESS				
(see also CRESS)				
raw chopped	½ cup	2	tr	tr
WATERMELON				
cut up	1 cup	50		1
seeds dried	1 oz	158	3	13
seeds dried	1 cup	602	3	51
wedge	⅛	152	—	2
WATERMELON JUICE				
Kool-Aid				
Splash Drink	1 serv (8 oz)	110	0	0
WAX BEANS				
CANNED				
Del Monte				
Cut Golden	½ cup (4.3 oz)	20	0	0
Owatonna				
Cut	½ cup	20		0
Seneca				
Cuts Natural Pack	½ cup	25	0	0
Wax Beans	½ cup	25	0	0
WHALE				
raw	3.5 oz	134	—	3
WHEAT				
(see also BULGUR, BRAN, CEREAL, COUSCOUS, FLOUR, WHEAT GERM)				
sprouted	1 cup (3.8 oz)	214	tr	1
Arrowhead				
Kamut Grain	¼ cup (1.7 oz)	140	0	1
Seitan Quick Mix	⅓ cup (1.4 oz)	150	0	1
Hodgson Mill				
Vital Wheat Gluten Plus Ascorbic Acid	1 tbsp (0.3 oz)	30	0	0
Near East				
Taboule Salad Mix as prep	⅔ cup	120	1	3
Wheat Pilaf as prep	1 cup	220	1	5
Sonoma				
Wheat Nuts Salted	2 tbsp (0.5 oz)	60	0	3
White Wave				
Seitan	½ pkg (4 oz)	140	0	0
Seitan Fajita Strips	⅓ cup (1.8 oz)	60	0	0
Seitan Marinated Slices	3 slices (1.8 oz)	60	0	0

FOOD	PORTION	CALS.	SAT. FAT	FAT
WHEAT GERM				
plain toasted	¼ cup (1 oz)	108	1	3
Arrowhead				
Wheat Germ	3 tbsp (0.5 oz)	50	0	1
Hodgson Mill				
Wheat Germ	2 tbsp (0.5 oz)	55	0	1
Stone-Buhr				
Untoasted	2 tbsp (0.5 oz)	58	0	2
WHEY				
acid dry	1 tbsp (3 g)	10	tr	tr
acid fluid	1 cup (8 fl oz)	59	tr	tr
sweet dry	1 tbsp (8 g)	26	tr	tr
sweet fluid	1 cup (8 fl oz)	66	1	1
whey cheese	3.5 oz	440	18	27
WHIPPED TOPPINGS				
(see also CREAM)				
cream pressurized	1 cup (2.1 oz)	154	8	13
cream pressurized	1 tbsp (3 g)	8	tr	tr
nondairy frzn	1 tbsp	13	1	1
nondairy powdered as prep w/ whole milk	1 cup	151	9	10
nondairy powdered as prep w/ whole milk	1 tbsp (4 g)	8	tr	tr
nondairy pressurized	1 tbsp (4 g)	11	1	1
nondairy pressurized	1 cup	184	13	16
Cool Whip				
Extra Creamy	2 tbsp (0.3 oz)	25	2	2
Free	2 tbsp (0.3 oz)	15	0	0
Lite	2 tbsp (0.3 oz)	20	1	1
Original	2 tbsp (0.3 oz)	25	2	2
Dream Whip				
Mix as prep	2 tbsp (0.3 oz)	20	1	1
Estee				
Whipped Topping	1 serv	10	0	1
Hood				
Instant	2 tbsp	20	1	2
Light Instant	2 tbsp	15	0	1
Kraft				
Dairy Whip Light Cream	2 tbsp (0.2 oz)	10	1	1
Fat Free	1 tbsp (0.3 oz)	15	0	0
La Creme				
Topping	1 tbsp	16	—	1
Pet				
Whip	1 tbsp	14	—	1

FOOD	PORTION	CALS.	SAT. FAT	FAT
Reddiwip				
Lite	2 tbsp (8 g)	15	0	1
Non-Dairy	2 tbsp (8 g)	20	1	2
Real Whipped Heavy Cream	2 tbsp (8 g)	30	2	3
Real Whipped Light Cream	2 tbsp (8 g)	20	1	2
WHITE BEANS				
CANNED				
white beans	1 cup	306	tr	1
Goya				
Spanish Style	7.5 oz	130	—	1
Progresso				
Cannellini	½ cup (4.6 oz)	100	0	1
DRIED				
regular cooked	1 cup	249	tr	1
small cooked	1 cup	253	tr	1
WHITEFISH				
baked	3 oz	146	1	6
smoked	1 oz	39	tr	tr
smoked	3 oz	92	tr	1
WHITING				
cooked	3 oz	98	tr	1
raw	3 oz	77	tr	1
WILD RICE				
cooked	1 cup (5.7 oz)	166	tr	1
Haddon House				
Extra Fancy	¼ cup (1.6 oz)	170	0	1
WINE				
(see also CHAMPAGNE, WINE COOLERS)				
madeira	3.5 oz	169	—	0
port	3.5 oz	156	—	0
red	3.5 oz	74	0	0
rose	3.5 oz	73	0	0
sweet dessert	2 oz	90	0	0
white	3.5 oz	70	0	0
Boone's				
Country Kwencher	1 fl oz	24	0	0
Delicious Apple	1 fl oz	21	0	0
Sangria	1 fl oz	22	0	0
Snow Creek Berry	1 fl oz	18	0	0
Strawberry Hill	1 fl oz	22	0	0
Sun Peak Peach	1 fl oz	18	0	0
Wild Island	1 fl oz	18	0	0

FOOD	PORTION	CALS.	SAT. FAT	FAT
Carlo Rossi				
Blush	1 fl oz	21	0	0
Burgundy	1 fl oz	22	0	0
Chablis	1 fl oz	21	0	0
Paisano	1 fl oz	23	0	0
Red Sangria	1 fl oz	24	0	0
Rhine	1 fl oz	21	0	0
Vin Rose'	1 fl oz	21	0	0
White Grenache	1 fl oz	20	0	0
Fairbanks				
Cream Sherry	1 fl oz	42	0	0
Port	1 fl oz	44	0	0
Sherry	1 fl oz	34	0	0
White Port	1 fl oz	44	0	0
Gallo				
Blush Chablis	1 fl oz	22	0	0
Burgundy	1 fl oz	22	0	0
Cabernet Sauvignon	1 fl oz	22	0	0
Chablis Blanc	1 fl oz	20	0	0
Chardonnay	1 fl oz	23	0	0
Classic Burgundy	1 fl oz	21	0	0
French Colombard	1 fl oz	21	0	0
Hearty Burgundy	1 fl oz	22	0	0
Johannisbery Riesling '88	1 fl oz	20	0	0
Pink Chablis	1 fl oz	20	0	0
Red Rose'	1 fl oz	23	0	0
Rhine	1 fl oz	22	0	0
Sauvignon Blanc '90	1 fl oz	20	0	0
White Grenache '92	1 fl oz	20	0	0
White Grenache New Vintage	1 fl oz	20	0	0
White Zinfandel '91	1 fl oz	18	0	0
White Zinfandel New Vintage	1 fl oz	18	0	0
Zinfandel '87	1 fl oz	23	0	0
Sheffield Cellars				
Sherry	1 fl oz	44	0	0
Tawny Port	1 fl oz	45	0	0
Vermouth Extra Dry	1 fl oz	28	0	0
Vermouth Sweet	1 fl oz	43	0	0
Very Dry Sherry	1 fl oz	32	0	0

WINE COOLERS

Bartles & Jaymes

Berry	12 fl oz	210	0	0
Margarita	12 fl oz	260	0	0

FOOD	PORTION	CALS.	SAT. FAT	FAT
Bartles & Jaymes (CONT.)				
Original	12 fl oz	190	0	0
Peach	12 fl oz	210	0	0
Pina Colada	12 fl oz	280	0	0
Planter's Punch	12 fl oz	230	0	0
Strawberry	12 fl oz	210	0	0
Strawberry Daquiri	12 fl oz	230	0	0
Tropical	12 fl oz	230	0	0
WINGED BEANS				
dried cooked	1 cup	252	1	10
WOLFFISH				
atlantic baked	3 oz	105	tr	3
WRAPS				
(see BREAD)				
YAM				
(see also SWEET POTATO)				
CANNED				
Allen				
Cut	⅔ cup (5.8 oz)	160	0	1
Princella				
Cut	⅔ cup (5.8 oz)	160	0	1
Royal Prince				
Whole	4 pieces (5.9 oz)	200	0	1
Sugary Sam				
Cut	⅔ cup (5.8 oz)	160	0	1
Trappey				
Whole	4 pieces (5.9 oz)	200	0	1
FRESH				
mountain yam hawaii cooked	½ cup	59	tr	tr
yam cubed cooked	½ cup	79	tr	tr
YAMBEAN				
cooked	¾ cup	38	—	tr
YARDLONG BEANS				
dried cooked	1 cup	202	tr	1
YAUTIA (TANNIER)				
raw sliced	1 cup (4.7 oz)	132	—	1
root raw	1 (10.7 oz)	299	—	1
YEAST				
baker's compressed	1 cake (0.6 oz)	18	tr	tr
baker's dry	1 pkg (¼ oz)	21	tr	tr

FOOD	PORTION	CALS.	SAT. FAT	FAT
baker's dry	1 tbsp	35	tr	1
brewer's dry	1 tbsp	25	tr	tr
Fleischmann's				
Active Dry	1 pkg (7 g)	23	—	3
Bread Machine	1 pkg (7 g)	26	—	2
RapidRise	1 pkg (7 g)	26	—	2
Red Star				
Yeast	4 tbsp (0.5 oz)	47	0	tr
Yeast Flakes	3 tbsp (0.5 oz)	47	0	tr

YELLOW BEANS

FOOD	PORTION	CALS.	SAT. FAT	FAT
dried cooked	1 cup	254	tr	2
fresh cooked	½ cup	22	tr	tr
fresh raw	½ cup	17	tr	tr

YELLOWEYE BEANS

CANNED

B&M

FOOD	PORTION	CALS.	SAT. FAT	FAT
Baked	½ cup (4.6 oz)	170	1	2

DRIED

Bean Cuisine

FOOD	PORTION	CALS.	SAT. FAT	FAT
Dried	½ cup	115	—	1

YELLOWTAIL

FOOD	PORTION	CALS.	SAT. FAT	FAT
baked	3 oz	159	—	6

YOGURT

(see also YOGURT FROZEN)

FOOD	PORTION	CALS.	SAT. FAT	FAT
coffee lowfat	8 oz	194	2	3
fruit lowfat	8 oz	225	2	3
fruit lowfat	4 oz	113	1	1
plain	8 oz	139	5	7
plain lowfat	8 oz	144	2	4
plain no fat	8 oz	127	tr	tr
vanilla lowfat	8 oz	194	2	3
Breyers				
Blended Blueberry	4.4 oz	130	1	1
Blended Peach	4.4 oz	130	1	1
Blended Strawberry	4.4 oz	130	1	1
Light Nonfat Apple Pie A La Mode	8 oz	120	0	0
Light Nonfat Berry Banana Split	8 oz	120	0	0
Light Nonfat Black Cherry Jubilee	8 oz	120	0	0
Light Nonfat Blueberries N' Cream	8 oz	120	0	0

FOOD	PORTION	CALS.	SAT. FAT	FAT
Breyers (CONT.)				
Light Nonfat Cherry Bon-Bon	8 oz	120	0	0
Light Nonfat Cherry Vanilla Cream	8 oz	120	0	0
Light Nonfat Classic Strawberry	8 oz	120	0	0
Light Nonfat Key Lime Pie	8 oz	120	0	0
Light Nonfat Lemon Chiffon	8 oz	120	0	0
Light Nonfat Peaches N' Cream	8 oz	120	0	0
Light Nonfat Raspberries N' Cream	8 oz	120	0	0
Light Nonfat Strawberry Cheesecake	8 oz	120	0	0
Lowfat Black Cherry	8 oz	240	2	3
Lowfat Blueberry	8 oz	230	2	3
Lowfat Mixed Berry	8 oz	320	2	3
Lowfat Peach	8 oz	240	2	3
Lowfat Pineapple	8 oz	240	2	3
Lowfat Red Raspberry	8 oz	230	2	3
Lowfat Strawberry	8 oz	230	2	3
Lowfat Strawberry Banana	8 oz	240	2	3
Lowfat Vanilla	8 oz	220	2	3
Smooth & Creamy Apple Cobbler	8 oz	230	1	2
Smooth & Creamy Black Cherry Parfait	8 oz	240	1	2
Smooth & Creamy Black Cherry Parfait	4.4 oz	130	1	1
Smooth & Creamy Blueberries 'N Cream	8 oz	240	1	2
Smooth & Creamy Blueberries 'N Cream	4.4 oz	130	1	1
Smooth & Creamy Classic Strawberry	8 oz	230	1	2
Smooth & Creamy Classic Strawberry	4.4 oz	130	1	1
Smooth & Creamy Orange Vanilla Cream	8 oz	230	1	2
Smooth & Creamy Peaches 'N Cream	4.4 oz	130	1	1
Smooth & Creamy Peaches 'N Cream	8 oz	230	1	2
Smooth & Creamy Raspberries 'N Cream	8 oz	230	1	2

FOOD	PORTION	CALS.	SAT. FAT	FAT
Breyers (CONT.)				
Smooth & Creamy Strawberry Banana Split	8 oz	240	1	2
Smooth & Creamy Strawberry Cheesecake	8 oz	240	1	2
Cabot				
All Flavors	8 oz	220	2	3
Plain	8 oz	140	2	4
Colombo				
Banana Strawberry	8 oz	210	2	4
Black Cherry	8 oz	200	2	4
Blueberry	8 oz	200	2	4
Fat Free Apples 'n Spice	8 oz	190	0	0
Fat Free Apricot	8 oz	190	0	0
Fat Free Banana Strawberry	8 oz	200	0	0
Fat Free Blueberry	8 oz	190	0	0
Fat Free Cappuccino	8 oz	180	0	0
Fat Free Cherry	8 oz	190	0	0
Fat Free Cranberry Strawberry	8 oz	200	0	0
Fat Free French Roast	8 oz	180	0	0
Fat Free Fruit Cocktail	8 oz	190	0	0
Fat Free Lemon	8 oz	170	0	0
Fat Free Peach	8 oz	190	0	0
Fat Free Plain	8 oz	110	0	0
Fat Free Raspberry	8 oz	190	0	0
Fat Free Strawberry	8 oz	190	0	0
Fat Free Strawberry Pineapple Orange	8 oz	190	0	0
Fat Free Vanilla	8 oz	170	0	0
French Vanilla	8 oz	180	3	4
Light 100 Blueberry	8 oz	100	0	0
Light 100 Cherry Vanilla	8 oz	100	0	0
Light 100 Coffee & Cream	8 oz	100	0	0
Light 100 Creamy Vanilla	8 oz	100	0	0
Light 100 Fruit Medley	8 oz	100	0	0
Light 100 Juicy Peach	8 oz	100	0	0
Light 100 Lemon Creme	8 oz	100	0	0
Light 100 Mandarin Orange	8 oz	100	0	0
Light 100 Mixed Berries	8 oz	100	0	0
Light 100 Raspberry	8 oz	100	0	0
Light 100 Strawberry	8 oz	100	0	0
Peach Melba	8 oz	200	2	4
Plain	8 oz	120	3	5

FOOD	PORTION	CALS.	SAT. FAT	FAT
Colombo (CONT.)				
Raspberry	8 oz	200	2	4
Strawberry	8 oz	200	2	4
Dannon				
Chunky Fruit Nonfat Apple Cinnamon	6 oz	160	0	0
Chunky Fruit Nonfat Blueberry	6 oz	160	0	0
Chunky Fruit Nonfat Cherry Vanilla	6 oz	160	0	0
Chunky Fruit Nonfat Peach	6 oz	160	0	0
Chunky Fruit Nonfat Strawberry	6 oz	160	0	0
Chunky Fruit Nonfat Strawberry Banana	6 oz	160	0	0
Danimls Lowfat Tropical Punch	4.4 oz	130	1	1
Danimals Lowfat Blueberry	4.4 oz	130	1	1
Danimals Lowfat Grape Lemonade	4.4 oz	120	1	1
Danimals Lowfat Lemon Ice	4.4 oz	120	1	1
Danimals Lowfat Orange Banana	4.4 oz	130	1	1
Danimals Lowfat Strawberry	4.4 oz	130	1	1
Danimals Lowfat Vanilla	4.4 oz	120	1	1
Danimals Lowfat Wild Raspberry	4.4 oz	120	1	1
Double Delights Banana Creme Strawberry	6 oz	160	1	1
Double Delights Bavarian Creme Raspberry	6 oz	170	1	1
Double Delights Cheesecake Cherry	6 oz	170	1	1
Double Delights Cheesecake Strawberry	6 oz	170	1	1
Double Delights Chocolate Cheesecake	6 oz	220	1	1
Double Delights Chocolate Dipped Strawberry	6 oz	210	1	1
Double Delights Chocolate Eclair	6 oz	220	1	1
Double Delights Vanilla Strawberry	6 oz	170	1	1
Double Delights Vanilla Peach & Apricot	6 oz	170	1	1

FOOD	PORTION	CALS.	SAT. FAT	FAT
Dannon (CONT.)				
Fruit On The Bottom Lowfat Apple Cinnamon	8 oz	240	2	3
Fruit On The Bottom Lowfat Blueberry	8 oz	240	2	3
Fruit On The Bottom Lowfat Boysenberry	8 oz	240	2	3
Fruit On The Bottom Lowfat Cherry	8 oz	240	2	3
Fruit On The Bottom Lowfat Minipack Mixed Berry	4.4 oz	130	1	2
Fruit On The Bottom Lowfat Minipack Strawberry	4.4 oz	130	1	2
Fruit On The Bottom Lowfat Mixed Berries	8 oz	240	2	3
Fruit On The Bottom Lowfat Orange	8 oz	240	2	3
Fruit On The Bottom Lowfat Peach	8 oz	240	2	3
Fruit On The Bottom Lowfat Raspberry	8 oz	240	2	3
Fruit On The Bottom Lowfat Strawberry	8 oz	240	2	3
Fruit On The Bottom Lowfat Strawberry Banana	8 oz	240	2	3
Light 'N Crunchy Mint Chocolate Chip	8 oz	140	0	0
Light 'N Crunchy Nonfat Caramel Apple Crunch	8 oz	140	0	0
Light 'N Crunchy Nonfat Lemon Blueberry Cobbler	8 oz	140	0	0
Light 'N Crunchy Nonfat Mocha Cappuccino	8 oz	140	0	0
Light 'N Crunchy Nonfat Raspberry w/ Granola	8 oz	140	0	0
Light 'N Crunchy Nonfat Vanilla Chocolate Crunch	8 oz	130	0	0
Light Duets Cherry Cheesecake	6 oz	90	0	0
Light Duets Peaches N' Cream	6 oz	90	0	0
Light Duets Raspberry Royale	6 oz	90	0	0
Light Duets Strawberry Cheesecake	6 oz	90	0	0
Light Nonfat Banana Cream Pie	8 oz	100	0	0

FOOD	PORTION	CALS.	SAT. FAT	FAT
Dannon (CONT.)				
Light Nonfat Blueberry	8 oz	100	0	0
Light Nonfat Cappuccino	8 oz	100	0	0
Light Nonfat Cherry Vanilla	8 oz	100	0	0
Light Nonfat Coconut Cream Pie	8 oz	100	0	0
Light Nonfat Creme Caramel	8 oz	100	0	0
Light Nonfat Lemon Chiffon	8 oz	100	0	0
Light Nonfat Mint Chocolate Cream Pie	8 oz	100	0	0
Light Nonfat Peach	8 oz	100	0	0
Light Nonfat Raspberry	8 oz	100	0	0
Light Nonfat Strawberry	8 oz	100	0	0
Light Nonfat Strawberry Banana	8 oz	100	0	0
Light Nonfat Strawberry Kiwi	8 oz	100	0	0
Light Nonfat Tangerine Chiffon	8 oz	100	0	0
Light Nonfat Vanilla	8 oz	100	0	0
Lowfat Coffee	8 oz	210	2	3
Lowfat Cranberry Raspberry	8 oz	210	2	3
Lowfat Lemon	8 oz	210	2	3
Lowfat Vanilla	8 oz	210	2	3
Minipack Blended Nonfat Blueberry	4.4 oz	120	0	0
Minipack Blended Nonfat Cherry	4.4 oz	110	0	0
Minipack Blended Nonfat Peach	4.4 oz	120	0	0
Minipack Blended Nonfat Raspberry	4.4 oz	120	0	0
Minipack Blended Nonfat Strawberry	4.4 oz	120	0	0
Minipack Blended Nonfat Strawberry Banana	4.4 oz	120	0	0
Sprinkl'ins Cherry Vanilla	1 (4.1 oz)	130	1	2
Sprinkl'ins Strawberry	1 (4.1 oz)	130	1	2
Sprinkl'ins Strawberry Banana	1 (4.1 oz)	130	1	2
Sprinkl'ins Vanilla w/ Cherry Crystals	1 (4.1 oz)	110	1	1
Sprinkl'ins Vanilla w/ Orange Crystals	1 (4.1 oz)	110	1	1
Friendship				
Coffee	8 oz	210	2	3
Fruit Crunch Peach	6 oz	190	2	5

FOOD	PORTION	CALS.	SAT. FAT	FAT
Friendship (CONT.)				
Fruit Crunch Strawberry	6 oz	190	2	5
Fruit Crunch Strawberry Banana	6 oz	190	2	4
Plain	8 oz	150	2	3
Hood				
Fat Free Blueberry	1 (8 oz)	190	0	0
Fat Free Cherry	1 (8 oz)	190	0	0
Fat Free Peach	1 (8 oz)	190	0	0
Fat Free Plain	1 (8 oz)	130	0	0
Fat Free Raspberry	1 (8 oz)	190	0	0
Fat Free Strawberry	1 (8 oz)	190	0	0
Fat Free Strawberry Banana	1 (8 oz)	190	0	0
Fat Free Vanilla	1 (8 oz)	190	0	0
Fat Free Swiss Blueberry	1 (8 oz)	210	0	0
Fat Free Swiss Lemon	1 (8 oz)	210	0	0
Fat Free Swiss Raspberry	1 (8 oz)	210	0	0
Fat Free Swiss Strawberry	1 (8 oz)	210	0	0
Fat Free Swiss Strawberry Banana	1 (8 oz)	210	0	0
Fat Free Swiss Vanilla	1 (8 oz)	210	0	0
Jell-O				
Lowfat Cherry	4.4 oz	130	1	1
Lowfat Grape	4.4 oz	130	1	1
Lowfat Raspberry	4.4 oz	130	1	1
Lowfat Tropical Berry Twist	4.4 oz	130	1	1
Lowfat Tropical Punch	4.4 oz	130	1	1
Lowfat Watermelon	4.4 oz	130	1	1
Lowfat Wild Berry	4.4 oz	130	1	1
Lowfat Wild Strawberry	4.4 oz	130	1	1
La Yogurt				
French Style Banana	6 oz	180	2	3
French Style Blueberry	6 oz	180	2	3
French Style Cherry	6 oz	180	2	3
French Style Cherry Vanilla	6 oz	190	2	3
French Style Guava	6 oz	180	2	3
French Style Key Lime	6 oz	180	2	3
French Style Mango	6 oz	180	2	3
French Style Mixed Berry	6 oz	180	2	3
French Style Nonfat Blueberry	6 oz	70	0	0
French Style Nonfat Cherry	6 oz	75	0	0
French Style Nonfat Raspberry	6 oz	70	0	0

FOOD	PORTION	CALS.	SAT. FAT	FAT
La Yogurt (CONT.)				
French Style Nonfat Strawberry	6 oz	70	0	0
French Style Nonfat Strawberry Banana	6 oz	70	0	0
French Style Peach	6 oz	180	2	3
French Style Pina Colada	6 oz	180	2	3
French Style Raspberry	6 oz	180	2	3
French Style Strawberry	6 oz	180	2	3
French Style Strawberry Banana	6 oz	180	2	3
French Style Strawberry Fruit Cup	6 oz	180	2	3
French Style Tropical Orange	6 oz	180	2	4
French Style Vanilla	6 oz	170	2	3
Latin Style Banana	6 oz	190	2	3
Latin Style Guava	6 oz	190	2	3
Latin Style Mango	6 oz	190	2	3
Latin Style Papaya	6 oz	190	2	3
Latin Style Passion Fruit	6 oz	190	2	3
Latin Style Strawberry Kiwi	6 oz	180	2	3
Light N'Lively				
Free Blueberry	4.4 oz	70	0	0
Free Peach	4.4 oz	70	0	0
Free Strawberry	4.4 oz	70	0	0
Free Strawberry Banana Cream	4.4 oz	70	0	0
Free Strawberry Fruit Cup	4.4 oz	70	0	0
Lowfat Blueberry	4.4 oz	130	1	1
Lowfat Peach	4.4 oz	130	1	1
Lowfat Pineapple	4.4 oz	130	1	1
Lowfat Red Raspberry	4.4 oz	120	1	1
Lowfat Strawberry	4.4 oz	130	1	1
Lowfat Strawberry Banana Cream	4.4 oz	130	1	1
Lowfat Strawberry Fruit Cup	4.4 oz	130	1	1
Lite Line				
Swiss Style Cherry Vanilla	1 cup	240	—	2
Swiss Style Peach	1 cup	230	—	2
Swiss Style Plain	1 cup	140	—	2
Swiss Style Strawberry	1 cup	240	—	2
Meadow Gold				
Plain	1 cup	160	—	5
Sundae Style Raspberry	1 cup	250	—	4

FOOD	PORTION	CALS.	SAT. FAT	FAT
Mountain High				
Blueberry	1 cup	220	—	6
Plain	1 cup	200	—	9
Yoplait				
99% Fat Free Blueberry	6 oz	180	1	2
99% Fat Free Boysenberry	6 oz	180	1	2
99% Fat Free Cherry	6 oz	180	1	2
99% Fat Free Harvest Peach	6 oz	180	1	2
99% Fat Free Harvest Peach	6 oz	120	1	1
99% Fat Free Key Lime Pie	6 oz	180	1	2
99% Fat Free Lemon	6 oz	180	1	2
99% Fat Free Mixed Berry	6 oz	120	1	1
99% Fat Free Mixed Berry	6 oz	180	1	2
99% Fat Free Orange	6 oz	180	1	2
99% Fat Free Pina Colada	6 oz	180	1	2
99% Fat Free Pineapple	6 oz	180	1	2
99% Fat Free Raspberry	6 oz	180	1	2
99% Fat Free Strawberry	6 oz	180	1	2
99% Fat Free Strawberry	6 oz	120	1	1
99% Fat Free Strawberry Banana	6 oz	120	1	1
99% Fat Free Strawberry Banana	6 oz	180	1	2
99% Fat Free Strawberry Cheesecake	6 oz	180	1	2
Custard Style Banana	6 oz	190	2	4
Custard Style Banana	6 oz	190	—	4
Custard Style Blueberry	6 oz	190	2	4
Custard Style Cherry Vanilla	6 oz	190	2	4
Custard Style Key Lime Pie	6 oz	190	2	4
Custard Style Lemon	6 oz	190	2	4
Custard Style Peaches'n Cream	6 oz	190	2	4
Custard Style Raspberry	6 oz	190	2	4
Custard Style Raspberry Cheesecake	6 oz	190	2	4
Custard Style Strawberry	6 oz	190	2	4
Custard Style Strawberry Banana	6 oz	190	2	4
Custard Style Strawberry Vanilla	4 oz	120	2	2
Custard Style Vanilla	6 oz	190	2	4
Go-Gurt Strawberry Banana Burst	1 pkg (2.25 oz)	80	1	2
Go-Gurt Watermelon Meltdown	1 pkg (2.25 oz)	80	1	2

FOOD	PORTION	CALS.	SAT. FAT	FAT
Yoplait (CONT.)				
Light Amaretto Cheesecake	6 oz	90	0	0
Light Apricot Mango	6 oz	90	0	0
Light Banana Cream	6 oz	90	0	0
Light Blueberry	6 oz	90	0	0
Light Boston Cream Pie	6 oz	90	0	0
Light Caramel Apple	6 oz	90	0	0
Light Cherry	6 oz	90	0	0
Light Key Lime Pie	6 oz	90	0	0
Light Lemon Cream Pie	6 oz	90	0	0
Light Peach	6 oz	90	0	0
Light Peach Melba	6 oz	90	0	0
Light Raspberry	6 oz	90	0	0
Light Raspberry	6 oz	90	0	0
Light Strawberry	6 oz	90	0	0
Light Strawberry Banana	6 oz	90	0	0
Light White Chocolate Strawberry	6 oz	90	0	0
Original Cafe Au Lait	6 oz	170	1	2
Original Coconut Cream Pie	6 oz	200	3	4
Original French Vanilla	6 oz	180	1	2
Trix Rainbow Punch	6 oz	190	1	2
Trix Raspberry Rainbow	6 oz	190	1	2
Trix Strawberry Banana Bash	6 oz	190	1	2
Trix Strawberry Punch	4 oz	130	1	2
Trix Triple Cherry	6 oz	190	1	2
Trix Watermelon Burst	4 oz	130	1	2
Trix Wild Berry Blue	4 oz	130	1	2
YOGURT FROZEN				
chocolate soft serve	½ cup (4 fl oz)	115	3	4
vanilla soft serve	½ cup (4 fl oz)	114	2	4
Ben & Jerry's				
Cherry Garcia	½ cup	170	2	3
Chocolate Cherry Garcia	½ cup	190	3	4
Chocolate Chip Cookie Dough	½ cup	200	3	5
Chocolate Fudge Brownie	½ cup	190	1	3
Chocolate Heath Bar Crunch	½ cup	210	3	6
Chunky Monkey	½ cup	200	3	6
Pop Cherry Garcia	1	260	9	14
Breyers				
Chocolate	½ cup (2.6 oz)	130	2	3
Fat Free Chocolate	½ cup (2.6 oz)	100	0	0
Fat Free Cookies N Cream	½ cup (2.6 oz)	110	0	0
Fat Free Peach	½ cup (2.6 oz)	90	0	0

FOOD	PORTION	CALS.	SAT. FAT	FAT
Breyers (CONT.)				
Fat Free Strawberry	½ cup (2.6 oz)	100	0	0
Fat Free Take Two Vanilla Chocolate	½ cup (2.6 oz)	100	0	0
Fat Free Vanilla	½ cup (2.6 oz)	100	0	0
Fat Free Vanilla Fudge Twirl	½ cup (2.6 oz)	110	0	0
Vanilla	½ cup (2.6 oz)	120	2	3
Vanilla Chocolate Strawberry	½ cup (2.6 oz)	120	2	3
Dannon				
Light Cappuccino	½ cup (2.8 oz)	80	0	0
Light Cherry Vanilla Swirl	½ cup (2.8 oz)	90	0	0
Light Chocolate	½ cup (2.7 oz)	80	0	0
Light Mint Chocolate Fudge	½ cup (2.8 oz)	90	0	0
Light Peach Raspberry Melba	½ cup (2.8 oz)	90	0	0
Light Strawberry Cheesecake	½ cup (2.8 oz)	90	0	0
Light Vanilla	½ cup (2.8 oz)	80	0	0
Light 'N Crunchy Carmel Toffee Crunch	½ cup (2.8 oz)	110	1	1
Light 'N Crunchy Rocky Road	½ cup (2.8 oz)	110	0	1
Light 'N Crunchy Vanilla Streusel	½ cup (2.8 oz)	110	1	1
Light Duets Strawberry Sundae	6 oz	90	0	0
Light Nonfat Cappuccino	8 oz	100	0	0
Light'N Crunchy Banana Cream Pie	½ cup (2.8 oz)	110	0	1
Light'N Crunchy Mocha Chocolate Chunk	½ cup (2.8 oz)	110	1	1
Light'N Crunchy Peanut Chocolate Crunch	½ cup (2.8 oz)	110	1	1
Light'N Crunchy Triple Chocolate	½ cup (2.8 oz)	110	1	1
Edy's				
Banana Strawberry	3 oz	80	—	1
Blueberry	3 oz	80	—	1
Cherry	3 oz	80	—	1
Chocolate	3 oz	80	—	1
Chocolate Chip	3 oz	100	—	1
Citrus Heights	3 oz	80	—	1
Cookies'N'Cream	3 oz	100	—	1
Marble Fudge	3 oz	100	—	1
Perfectly Peach	3 oz	80	—	1
Raspberry	3 oz	80	—	1
Raspberry Vanilla Swirl	3 oz	80	—	1

FOOD	PORTION	CALS.	SAT. FAT	FAT
Edy's (CONT.)				
Strawberry	3 oz	80	—	1
Vanilla	3 oz	80	—	1
Elan				
Blueberry	4 oz	130	—	3
Caramel Almond Praline	4 oz	150	—	4
Chocolate	4 oz	130	—	3
Chocolate Almond	4 oz	160	—	6
Coffee	4 oz	130	—	3
Coffee Decaffeinated	4 oz	130	—	3
Peach	4 oz	130	—	3
Rum Raisin	4 oz	135	—	3
Strawberry	4 oz	125	—	3
Vanilla	4 oz	130	—	3
Fi-Bar				
Chocolate	1	190	—	7
Strawberry	1	190	—	7
Vanilla	1	190	—	7
Friendly's				
Apple Bettie	½ cup (2.6 oz)	140	2	3
Fabulous Fudge Swirl	½ cup (2.6 oz)	140	3	3
Fudge Berry Swirl	½ cup (2.6 oz)	150	3	4
Lowfat Perfectly Peach	½ cup (2.6 oz)	110	1	2
Lowfat Purely Chocolate	½ cup (2.6 oz)	120	2	3
Lowfat Raspberry Delight	½ cup (2.6 oz)	120	2	3
Lowfat Simply Vanilla	½ cup (2.6 oz)	120	2	3
Lowfat Strawberry Patch	½ cup (2.6 oz)	110	1	2
Mint Chocolate Chip	½ cup (2.6 oz)	130	2	4
Strawberry Cheesecake Blast	½ cup (2.6 oz)	140	2	4
Toffee Almond Crunch	½ cup (2.6 oz)	160	2	5
Good Humor				
Creamsicle Raspberry	1 (2.8 oz)	100	1	1
Frista Cup	1 (6.2 oz)	220	4	5
Haagen-Dazs				
Banana Nut Blast	½ cup (3.5 oz)	220	4	8
Bars Cherry Chocolate Fudge	1 (2.6 oz)	240	8	13
Bars Peach	1 (2.5 oz)	90	1	1
Bars Pina Colada	1 (2.5 oz)	100	1	1
Bars Raspberry & Vanilla	1 (2.5 oz)	90	0	1
Bars Strawberry Daiquiri	1 (2.5 oz)	90	1	1
Chocolate	½ cup (3.4 oz)	160	2	3
Coffee	½ cup (3.4 oz)	160	2	3

FOOD	PORTION	CALS.	SAT. FAT	FAT
Haagen-Dazs (CONT.)				
Fat Free Bar Raspberry & Vanilla	1 (2.5 oz)	90	—	0
Fat Free Cherry Vanilla	½ cup (3.3 oz)	140	—	0
Fat Free Chocolate	½ cup (3.3 oz)	140	—	0
Fat Free Coffee	½ cup (3.3 oz)	140	—	0
Fat Free Vanilla	½ cup (3.3 oz)	140	—	0
Fat Free Vanilla Fudge	½ cup (3.3 oz)	160	—	0
Orange Tango	½ cup (3.5 oz)	130	1	1
Pina Colada	½ cup (3.4 oz)	130	1	2
Raspberry Randevous	½ cup (3.5 oz)	130	1	2
Strawberry Cheesecake Craze	½ cup (3.6 oz)	220	4	8
Strawberry Duet	½ cup (3.4 oz)	130	1	2
Vanilla	½ cup (3.4 oz)	160	2	3
Hood				
Bavarian Truffle & Twist	½ cup (2.6 oz)	150	3	4
Coffee Toffee Chunk Sundae	½ cup (2.6 oz)	150	3	4
Combo Bars	1 (2.2 oz)	90	1	2
Cookies & Cream	½ cup (2.6 oz)	140	2	4
Grandma's Raisin Oatmeal Cookie Dough	½ cup (2.6 oz)	140	2	3
Mixed Berry Swirl	½ cup (2.6 oz)	120	2	2
Natural Strawberry	½ cup (2.6 oz)	110	2	3
Natural Strawberry Banana	½ cup (2.6 oz)	110	2	3
Natural Vanilla	½ cup (2.6 oz)	120	2	3
Nonfat Caramel & Brownie Sundae	½ cup (2.6 oz)	120	0	0
Nonfat Chocolate Marshmallow	½ cup (2.6 oz)	110	0	0
Nonfat Double Raspberry	½ cup (2.6 oz)	120	0	0
Nonfat Mocha Fudge	½ cup (2.6 oz)	120	0	0
Nonfat Olde Fashioned Vanilla	½ cup (2.6 oz)	110	0	0
Nonfat Peach Cobbler A La Mode	½ cup (2.6 oz)	110	0	0
Nonfat Strawberry	½ cup (2.6 oz)	100	0	0
Nonfat Vanilla Fudge	½ cup (2.6 oz)	120	0	0
Raspberry Swirl	½ cup (2.6 oz)	130	2	2
Sundae Cups Chocolate & Strawberry	1 (2.2 oz)	110	1	2
Vanilla Chocolate Strawberry	½ cup (2.6 oz)	120	2	3
Vanilla Swiss Almond Sundae	½ cup (2.6 oz)	150	2	4

FOOD	PORTION	CALS.	SAT. FAT	FAT
Sealtest				
Chocolate	½ cup (2.7 oz)	120	1	2
Mocha Fudge	½ cup (2.6 oz)	130	2	2
Vanilla	½ cup (2.6 oz)	120	1	2
Tofutti				
Better Than Yogurt Chocolate Fudge	4 fl oz	120	1	2
Better Than Yogurt Coffee Mashmallow Swirl	4 fl oz	100	0	1
Better Than Yogurt Passion Island Fruit	4 fl oz	100	0	1
Better Than Yogurt Peach Mango	4 fl oz	100	0	1
Better Than Yogurt Strawberry Banana	4 fl oz	100	0	1
Better Than Yogurt Vanilla Fudge	4 fl oz	120	0	2
Turkey Hill				
Chocolate Cherry Cordial	½ cup (2.6 oz)	130	2	3
Chocolate Chip Cookie Dough	½ cup (2.6 oz)	140	3	5
Death By Chocolate	½ cup (2.6 oz)	150	3	4
Nonfat Chocolate Cherry Cordial	½ cup (2.4 oz)	100	0	0
Nonfat Chocolate Marshmallow	½ cup (2.4 oz)	130	0	0
Nonfat Coffee Cappuccino	½ cup (2.4 oz)	110	0	0
Nonfat Mint Cookie 'N Cream	½ cup (2.4 oz)	110	0	0
Nonfat Neapolitan	½ cup (2.4 oz)	100	0	0
Nonfat Raspberry Chocolate Bliss	½ cup (2.4 oz)	110	0	0
Nonfat Southern Lemon Pie	½ cup (2.4 oz)	110	0	0
Nonfat Vanilla Fudge	½ cup (2.4 oz)	110	0	0
Peach Raspberry	½ cup (2.6 oz)	110	2	2
Strawberry	½ cup (2.6 oz)	110	2	2
Tin Roof Sundae	½ cup (2.6 oz)	140	3	5
Vanilla & Chocolate	½ cup (2.6 oz)	110	2	3
Vanilla Bean	½ cup (2.6 oz)	110	2	3

ZUCCHINI
CANNED

FOOD	PORTION	CALS.	SAT. FAT	FAT
italian style	½ cup	33	tr	tr
Del Monte				
With Italian Tomato Sauce	½ cup (4.2 oz)	30	0	0
Progresso				
Italian Style	½ cup (4.2 oz)	40	0	2

FOOD	PORTION	CALS.	SAT. FAT	FAT
FRESH				
baby raw	1 (0.5 oz)	3	tr	tr
raw sliced	½ cup	9	tr	tr
sliced cooked	½ cup	14	tr	tr
FROZEN				
cooked	½ cup	19	tr	tr
Big Valley				
Zucchini	¾ cup (3 oz)	10	0	0
Empire				
Breaded	1 (2.9 oz)	100	0	0
Southland				
Zucchini Sliced	3.2 oz	15	—	0
TAKE-OUT				
indian paalkora	1 serv	46	tr	2

PART · TWO

RESTAURANT CHAINS

FOOD	PORTION	CALS.	SAT. FAT	FAT
ARBY'S				
BEVERAGES				
Chocolate Shake	1 (12 oz)	451	3	12
Hot Chocolate	1 serv (8 oz)	110	1	1
Jamocha Shake	1 (12 oz)	384	3	10
Orange Juice	1 serv (6 oz)	82	0	0
Vanilla Shake	1 (12 oz)	360	4	12
BREAKFAST SELECTIONS				
Bacon	2 strips (0.53 oz)	90	3	7
Biscuit Plain	1 (2.9 oz)	280	3	15
Blueberry Muffin	1 (2.3 oz)	230	2	9
Cinnamon Nut Danish	1 (3.5 oz)	360	1	11
Croissant Plain	1 (2 oz)	220	7	12
Egg Portion	1 serv (1.6 oz)	95	2	8
Ham	1 serv (1.5 oz)	45	1	1
Sausage	1 (1.3 oz)	163	6	15
Swiss	1 serv (0.5 oz)	45	2	3
Table Syrup	1 serv (1 oz)	100	0	0
Toastix	6 pieces (4.4 oz)	430	5	21
DESSERTS				
Apple Turnover	1 (3.2 oz)	330	7	14
Cheesecake Plain	1 serv (3 oz)	320	14	23
Cherry Turnover	1 (3.2 oz)	320	5	13
Chocolate Chip Cookie	1 (1 oz)	125	2	6
Polar Swirl Butterfinger	1 (11.6 oz)	457	8	18
Polar Swirl Heath	1 (11.6 oz)	543	5	22
Polar Swirl Oreo	1 (11.6 oz)	329	10	22
Polar Swirl Peanut Butter Cup	1 (11.6 oz)	517	8	24
Polar Swirl Snickers	1 (11.6 oz)	511	7	19
MAIN MENU SELECTIONS				
Arby's Sauce	1 serv (0.5 oz)	15	0	tr
Baked Potato Broccoli'n Cheddar	1 (15.7 oz)	571	5	20
Baked Potato Deluxe	1 (15.3 oz)	736	16	36
Baked Potato Plain	1 (11.5 oz)	355	0	tr
Baked Potato w/ Margarine & Sour Cream	1 (14 oz)	578	9	24
Barbeque Sauce	1 serv (0.5 oz)	30	0	0
Beef Stock Au Jus	1 serv (2 oz)	10	0	0
Breaded Chicken Fillet	1 (7.2 oz)	536	5	28
Cheddar Cheese Sauce	1 serv (0.75 oz)	35	1	3
Cheddar Curly Fried	1 serv (4.25 oz)	333	4	18
Chicken Cordon Bleu	1 (8.5 oz)	623	8	33
Chicken Finger	2 (3.6 oz)	290	2	16

FOOD	PORTION	CALS.	SAT. FAT	FAT
Curly Fries	1 serv (3.5 oz)	300	3	15
Fish Fillet Sandwich	1 (7.7 oz)	529	7	27
French Fries	1 serv (2.5 oz)	246	3	13
Garden Salad	1 (11.9 oz)	61	0	1
Grilled Chicken BBQ	1 (7.1 oz)	388	3	13
Grilled Chicken Deluxe	1 (8.1 oz)	430	4	20
Ham 'n Cheese Sandwich	1 (5.9 oz)	359	5	14
Ham'n Cheese Melt	1 (4.9 oz)	329	4	13
Honey Mayonnaise Reduced Calorie	1 serv (0.5 oz)	70	1	7
Horsey Sauce	1 serv (0.5 oz)	60	1	5
Italian Sub	1 (10.1 oz)	675	13	36
Italian Sub Sauce	1 serv (0.5 oz)	70	1	7
Ketchup	1 serv (0.5 oz)	16	0	0
Light Roast Beef Deluxe	1 (6.4 oz)	296	3	10
Light Roast Chicken Deluxe	1 (6.8 oz)	276	2	6
Light Roast Chicken Salad	1 serv (14.4 oz)	149	1	2
Light Roast Turkey Deluxe	1 (6.8 oz)	260	2	7
Mayonnaise	1 serv (0.5 oz)	110	7	12
Mayonnaise Light Cholesterol Free	1 serv (0.25 oz)	12	0	1
Mustard German Style	1 serv (0.16 oz)	5	0	0
Parmesan Cheese Sauce	1 serv (0.5 oz)	70	1	7
Potato Cakes	2 (3 oz)	204	2	12
Roast Beef Arby's Melt w/ Cheddar	1 (5.2 oz)	368	6	18
Roast Beef Arby-Q	1 (6.4 oz)	431	6	18
Roast Beef Bac'n Cheddar Deluxe	1 (8.1 oz)	539	10	34
Roast Beef Beef'n Cheddar	1 (6.7 oz)	487	9	28
Roast Beef Gaint	1 (8.1 oz)	555	11	28
Roast Beef Junior	1 (4.4 oz)	324	5	14
Roast Beef Regular	1 (5.4 oz)	388	7	19
Roast Beef Sub	1 (10.8 oz)	700	14	42
Roast Beef Super	1 (8.7 oz)	523	9	27
Roast Chicken Club	1 (8.5 oz)	546	9	31
Roast Chicken Deluxe	1 (7.6 oz)	433	5	22
Roast Chicken Santa Fe	1 (6.4 oz)	436	6	22
Side Salad	1 (5 oz)	23	0	tr
Sub Roll French Dip	1 (6.8 oz)	475	8	22
Sub Roll Hot Ham 'n Swiss	1 (9.3 oz)	500	7	23
Sub Roll Pilly Beef'n Swiss	1 (10.4 oz)	755	15	47
Sub Roll Triple Cheese Melt	1 (8.4 oz)	720	16	45
Tartar Sauce	1 serv (1 oz)	140	2	15
Turkey Sub	1 (9.8 oz)	550	7	27

FOOD	PORTION	CALS.	SAT. FAT	FAT
SALAD DRESSINGS				
Buttermilk Ranch Reduced Calorie	1 serv (2 oz)	50	0	0
Honey French	1 serv (2 oz)	280	3	23
Italian Reduced Calorie	1 serv (2 oz)	20	0	1
Red Ranch	1 serv (0.5 oz)	75	1	6
Thousand Island	1 serv (2 oz)	260	4	26
SOUPS				
Boston Clam Chowder	1 serv (8 oz)	190	3	9
Cream of Broccoli	1 serv (8 oz)	160	4	8
Lumberjack Mixed Vegetable	1 serv (8 oz)	90	2	4
Old Fashioned Chicken Noodle	1 serv (8 oz)	80	0	2
Potato w/ Bacon	1 serv (8 oz)	170	3	7
Timberline Chili	1 serv (8 oz)	220	4	10
Wisconsin Cheese	1 serv (8 oz)	280	7	18
AU BON PAIN				
BAKED SELECTIONS				
Apple Coffee Cake	1 piece (4.6 oz)	480	12	24
Bagel Chocolate Chip	1 (5 oz)	380	4	7
Bagel Dutch Apple w/ Walnut Streussel	1 (5 oz)	360	0	5
Baguette Loaf	1 slice (1.8 oz)	140	0	5
Biscotti	1 (1.5 oz)	200	4	10
Biscotti Chocolate	1 (1.7 oz)	240	6	13
Braided Roll	1 (1.8 oz)	170	—	5
Cinnamon Roll	1 (7 oz)	710	10	26
Cookie Chocolate Chip	1 (2.1 oz)	280	8	13
Cookie Oatmeal Raisin	1 (2.1 oz)	250	4	10
Cookie Peanut Butter	1 (2.1 oz)	280	5	15
Cookie Shortbread	1 (2.4 oz)	390	15	25
Croissant Almond	1 (4.3 oz)	560	15	37
Croissant Apple	1 (3.4 oz)	280	6	10
Croissant Chocolate	1 (3.4 oz)	440	15	23
Croissant Cinnamon Raisin	1 (3.7 oz)	380	8	13
Croissant Plain	1 (2.1 oz)	270	9	15
Croissant Raspberry Cheese	1 (3.5 oz)	380	11	19
Croissant Sweet Cheese	1 (3.6 oz)	390	12	22
Danish Cheese Swirl	1 (3.8 oz)	450	14	28
Danish Lemon Swirl	1 (4 oz)	450	12	24
Danish Raspberry	1 (3.6 oz)	370	10	21
Danish Sweet Cheese	1 (3.6 oz)	420	13	26
Four Grain Loaf	1 slice (1.8 oz)	130	0	1
French Sandwich Roll	1 (1.8 oz)	120	0	5

FOOD	PORTION	CALS.	SAT. FAT	FAT
Hazelnut Fudge Brownie	1 (4 oz)	380	11	18
Holiday Cookie Cranberry Almond Macaroon	1 (1.5 oz)	160	5	8
Holiday Cookie Cranberry Almond Macaroon w/ Chocolate	1 (1.9 oz)	210	9	11
Holiday Cookie English Toffee	1 (1.8 oz)	220	7	12
Holiday Cookie Ginger Pecan	1 (2 oz)	260	6	15
Mochaccino Bar	1 (4 oz)	404	10	24
Muffin Blueberry	1 (4.5 oz)	410	3	15
Muffin Carrot	1 (5 oz)	480	5	23
Muffin Chocolate Chip	1 (4.5 oz)	490	7	20
Muffin Corn	1 (4.6 oz)	470	3	18
Muffin Pumpkin w/ Streusel Topping	1 (5.5 oz)	470	3	18
Muffin Low Fat Chocolate Cake	1 (4 oz)	290	1	3
Muffin Low Fat Triple Berry	1 (4.2 oz)	270	1	3
Multigrain Loaf	1 slice (1.8 oz)	130	0	1
Parisienne Loaf	1 slice (1.8 oz)	120	0	5
Pear Ginger Tea Cake	1 piece (4 oz)	380	3	20
Pecan Roll	1 (6.8 oz)	900	16	48
Roll 3 Seed Pecan Raisin	1 (2.7 oz)	250	1	6
Roll Hearth Sandwich	1 (2.8 oz)	220	0	2
Rolls Petit Pan	1 (2.5 oz)	200	0	1
Rye Loaf	1 slice (1.8 oz)	110	0	2
Scone Cinnamon	1 (4.1 oz)	520	14	28
Scone Current	1 (3.7 oz)	430	13	23
Scone Orange	1 (4.1 oz)	440	13	23
Sourdough Bagel Asiago Cheese	1 (4.2 oz)	380	4	6
Sourdough Bagel Cinnamon Raisin	1 (4.5 oz)	390	0	1
Sourdough Bagel Cranberry Walnut	1 (5 oz)	460	1	4
Sourdough Bagel Everything	1 (4.2 oz)	360	0	3
Sourdough Bagel Honey 8 Grain	1 (4.2 oz)	360	0	2
Sourdough Bagel Mocha Chip Swirl	1 (5 oz)	370	2	4
Sourdough Bagel Plain	1 (4 oz)	350	0	1
Sourdough Bagel Sesame	1 (4.2 oz)	380	1	4
Sourdough Bagel Wild Blueberry	1 (4.5 oz)	380	0	2
Valentine Cookie Chocolate Dipped Shortbread	1 (2.8 oz)	410	19	27
Valentine Cookie Red Sugar Shortbread Heart	1 (2.4 oz)	350	14	22
Valentine Cookie Shortbread	1 (2.4 oz)	340	14	22

FOOD	PORTION	CALS.	SAT. FAT	FAT
BEVERAGES				
Frozen Java Blast	1 serv (16 oz)	220	2	2
Frozen Mocha Blast	1 serv (16 oz)	320	2	3
Hot Apple Cider	1 med (16 oz)	310	0	0
Hot Apple Cider	1 sm (10 oz)	190	0	0
Hot Apple Cider	1 lg (20 oz)	350	0	0
Hot Hazelnut Blast	1 serv (16 oz)	310	4	6
Hot Mocha Blast	1 lg (17 oz)	310	5	8
Hot Mocha Blast	1 med (13 oz)	260	4	6
Hot Mocha Blast	1 sm (9 oz)	160	3	4
Hot Raspberry Mocha Blast	1 serv (16 oz)	300	4	6
Hot Raspberry Mocha Blast	1 serv (10 oz)	180	3	4
Hot Raspberry Mocha Blast	1 serv (20 oz)	350	5	8
Hot Strawberry Chocolate Blast	1 serv (16 oz)	330	4	6
Hot Vanilla Chocolate Blast	1 serv (16 oz)	310	4	6
Iced Caffee Latte	1 lg (20.5 oz)	270	6	10
Iced Caffee Latte	1 sm (9 oz)	130	3	5
Iced Caffee Latte	1 med (12 oz)	150	4	6
Iced Cappuccino	1 sm (9 oz)	110	3	4
Iced Cappuccino	1 lg (20.5 oz)	270	6	10
Iced Cappuccino	1 med (12 oz)	150	4	6
Iced Cocoa	1 lg (20.5 oz)	440	7	11
Iced Cocoa	1 sm (9 oz)	200	4	6
Iced Cocoa	1 med (12 oz)	280	4	6
Iced Hazelnut Blast	1 serv (16 oz)	310	4	6
Iced Mocha Blast	1 med (12 oz)	260	4	6
Iced Mocha Blast	1 lg (20.5 oz)	360	6	10
Iced Mocha Blast	1 sm (9 oz)	180	3	5
Iced Raspberry Mocha Blast	1 serv (24 oz)	330	4	7
Iced Raspberry Mocha Blast	1 serv (16 oz)	310	4	6
Iced Raspberry Mocha Blast	1 serv (12 oz)	160	2	4
Iced Strawberry Chocolate Blast	1 serv (16 oz)	310	4	6
Iced Vanilla Chocolate Blast	1 serv (16 oz)	310	4	6
Iced Tea Peach	1 med (12 oz)	130	0	0
Iced Tea Peach	1 sm (12 oz)	90	0	0
Iced Tea Peach	1 lg (16 oz)	170	0	0
Iced Tea Raspberry	1 lg (16 oz)	150	0	0
Iced Tea Raspberry	1 med (12 oz)	110	0	0
Iced Tea Raspberry	1 sm (8 oz)	80	0	0
Whipped Cream	1 serv (1.2 oz)	160	8	11
SALAD DRESSINGS				
Bleu Cheese	1 serv (3 oz)	370	8	41
Buttermilk Ranch	1 serv (3 oz)	310	4	32

FOOD	PORTION	CALS.	SAT. FAT	FAT
Caesar	1 serv (3 oz)	380	5	39
Fat Free Tomato Basil	1 serv (3 oz)	70	0	0
Greek	1 serv (3 oz)	440	7	50
Lemon Basil Vinaigrette	1 serv (3 oz)	330	2	32
Lite Honey Mustard	1 serv (3 oz)	280	3	17
Lite Italian	1 serv (3 oz)	230	2	20
Sesame French	1 serv (3 oz)	370	5	30
SALADS AND SALAD BARS				
Caesar	1 serv (8.9 oz)	270	6	10
Chicken Caesar	1 serv (11.4 oz)	360	6	11
Garden	1 sm (7.5 oz)	100	0	1
Garden	1 lg (10.6 oz)	160	0	2
Mozzarella & Roasted Pepper Salad	1 serv (13.7 oz)	340	10	18
Pesto Chicken Salad	1 serv (10.7 oz)	230	2	11
Tuna	1 serv (15 oz)	490	5	27
SANDWICHES AND FILLINGS				
Bagel Spreads Lite Strawberry	1 serv (2 oz)	150	7	11
Bagel Spreads Lite Vanilla Hazelnut	1 serv (2 oz)	150	7	11
Cheddar	½ serv (1.5 oz)	170	9	14
Chicken Tarragon	1 serv (4 oz)	240	3	17
Club Sandwich Hot Roasted Turkey	1 (14.9 oz)	950	16	50
Country Ham	1 serv (3.7 oz)	150	3	7
Cracked Pepper Chicken	1 serv (3.9 oz)	140	0	2
Cream Cheese Lite	1 serv (2 oz)	130	8	12
Cream Cheese Lite Honey Walnut	1 serv (2 oz)	260	5	12
Cream Cheese Lite Raspberry	1 serv (2 oz)	200	5	8
Cream Cheese Lite Sun-Dried Tomato	1 serv (2 oz)	130	8	11
Cream Cheese Plain	1 serv (2 oz)	190	12	18
Cream Cheese Veggie Lite	1 serv (2 oz)	100	5	10
Grilled Chicken	1 serv (3.9 oz)	140	0	2
Hot Croissant Ham & Cheese	1 (4.2 oz)	380	12	20
Hot Croissants Spinach & Cheese	1 (3.6 oz)	270	9	16
Provolone	½ serv (1.5 oz)	150	7	11
Roast Beef	1 serv (3.7 oz)	140	0	5
Sandwich Arizona Chicken	1 (12.7 oz)	720	12	33
Sandwich Buffalo Chicken	1 (13.7 oz)	640	4	19
Sandwich California Chicken	1 (13.2 oz)	820	12	44

FOOD	PORTION	CALS.	SAT. FAT	FAT
Sandwich Fresh Mozzarella Tomato & Pesto	1 (10.5 oz)	650	12	30
Sandwich Honey Dijon Chicken	1 (15.3 oz)	730	6	18
Sandwich Parmesan Chicken	1 (11.1 oz)	740	9	24
Sandwich Steak & Cheese Melt	1 (11.7 oz)	750	8	32
Sandwich Thai Chicken	1 (8.3 oz)	420	1	6
Swiss	½ serv (1.5 oz)	160	8	12
Tuna Salad	1 serv (4.5 oz)	360	5	29
Turkey Breast	1 serv (3.7 oz)	120	0	1
Wraps Chicken Caesar	1 (9.9 oz)	630	8	31
Wraps Southwestern Tuna	1 (14.4 oz)	950	17	64
Wraps Summer Turkey	1 (11.7 oz)	340	1	9
SOUPS				
Beef Barley	1 serv (12 oz)	112	1	3
Beef Barley	1 serv (16 oz)	150	2	4
Beef Barley	1 serv (8 oz)	75	1	2
Beef Stew	1 serv (8 oz)	140	3	7
Bohemian Cabbage	1 serv (8 oz)	70	1	3
Bohemian Cabbage	1 serv (12 oz)	110	2	5
Bohemian Cabbage	1 serv (16 oz)	140	2	6
Bread Bowl	1 (9 oz)	640	1	4
Broccoli & Cheddar	1 serv (8 oz)	260	11	22
Broccoli & Cheddar	1 serv (16 oz)	520	22	44
Broccoli & Cheddar	1 serv (12 oz)	390	17	33
Caribbean Black Bean	1 serv (16 oz)	250	0	2
Caribbean Black Bean	1 serv (12 oz)	180	0	2
Caribbean Black Bean	1 serv (8 oz)	120	0	1
Chicken Chili	1 serv (12 oz)	350	10	18
Chicken Chili	1 serv (8 oz)	240	7	12
Chicken Chili	1 serv (16 oz)	470	13	24
Chicken Noodle	1 serv (16 oz)	170	1	3
Chicken Noodle	1 serv (12 oz)	120	1	2
Chicken Noodle	1 serv (8 oz)	80	0	2
Chili	1 serv (12 oz)	340	6	14
Chili	1 serv (16 oz)	460	7	19
Chili	1 serv (8 oz)	230	4	10
Clam Chowder	1 serv (8 oz)	270	9	19
Clam Chowder	1 serv (16 oz)	540	18	39
Clam Chowder	1 serv (12 oz)	400	14	29
Corn Chowder	1 serv (16 oz)	530	19	33
Corn Chowder	1 serv (12 oz)	390	14	24
Corn Chowder	1 serv (8 oz)	260	10	16
Cream Of Broccoli	1 serv (16 oz)	440	17	37
Cream Of Broccoli	1 serv (12 oz)	330	13	28

FOOD	PORTION	CALS.	SAT. FAT	FAT
Cream Of Broccoli	1 serv (8 oz)	220	9	18
Cream Of Chicken With Wild Rice	1 serv (16 oz)	330	11	19
French Onion	1 serv (12 oz)	120	1	5
French Onion	1 serv (16 oz)	170	1	7
French Onion	1 serv (8 oz)	80	1	4
In A Bread Bowl Beef Barley	1 serv (21 oz)	760	2	7
In A Bread Bowl Carribean Black Bean	1 serv (21 oz)	830	1	5
In A Bread Bowl Chicken Chili	1 serv (21 oz)	990	11	22
In A Bread Bowl Chicken Noodle	1 serv (21 oz)	760	1	6
In A Bread Bowl Clam Chowder	1 serv (21 oz)	1050	15	32
In A Bread Bowl Cream of Broccoli	1 serv (21 oz)	970	15	31
In A Bread Bowl French Onion	1 serv (21 oz)	760	2	8
In A Bread Bowl New England Potato & Cheese w/ Ham	1 serv (21 oz)	860	9	15
In A Bread Bowl Tomato Florentine	1 serv (21 oz)	760	2	5
In A Bread Bowl Vegetarian Chili	1 serv (21 oz)	870	1	7
Louisiana Beans & Rice	1 serv (16 oz)	360	2	9
Louisiana Beans & Rice	1 serv (8 oz)	180	1	5
Louisiana Beans & Rice	1 serv (12 oz)	280	2	7
New England Potato & Cheese w/ Ham	1 serv (8 oz)	150	5	8
New England Potato & Cheese w/ Ham	1 serv (12 oz)	220	8	12
New England Potato & Cheese w/ Ham	1 serv (16 oz)	290	11	15
Potato Leek	1 serv (12 oz)	320	12	20
Potato Leek	1 serv (8 oz)	200	8	13
Potato Leek	1 serv (16 oz)	400	15	25
Sante Fe Chicken Tortilla	1 serv (16 oz)	300	4	13
Sante Fe Chicken Tortilla	1 serv (8 oz)	150	2	7
Sante Fe Chicken Tortilla	1 serv (12 oz)	230	3	10
Seafood Gumbo	1 serv (8 oz)	130	1	6
Seafood Gumbo	1 serv (12 oz)	190	1	9
Seafood Gumbo	1 serv (16 oz)	260	2	12
Tomato Florentine	1 serv (8 oz)	61	1	1
Tomato Florentine	1 serv (16 oz)	122	1	2
Tomato Florentine	1 serv (12 oz)	90	1	2
Tomato Tortellini	1 serv (12 oz)	90	1	2
Tomato Tortellini	1 serv (8 oz)	60	0	1
Tomato Tortellini	1 serv (16 oz)	110	1	2

FOOD	PORTION	CALS.	SAT. FAT	FAT
Vegetable Stew	1 serv (8 oz)	60	0	1
Vegetable Stew	1 serv (12 oz)	100	1	2
Vegetable Stew	1 serv (16 oz)	130	1	2
Vegetarian Lentil	1 serv (16 oz)	270	0	1
Vegetarian Lentil	1 serv (8 oz)	130	0	0
Vegetarian Lentil	1 serv (12 oz)	200	0	1
Vegetarian Chili	1 serv (16 oz)	278	1	5
Vegetarian Chili	1 serv (12 oz)	210	0	4
Vegetarian Chili	1 serv (8 oz)	139	0	3
Vegetarian Corn & Green Chili Bisque	1 serv (8 oz)	190	6	10
Vegetarian Corn & Green Chili Bisque	1 serv (16 oz)	380	12	20
Vegetarian Corn & Green Chili Bisque	1 serv (12 oz)	300	9	16
AUNTIE ANNE'S				
Caramel Dip	1 serv (1.5 oz)	135	2	3
Cheese Sauce	1 serv (1 oz)	70	4	5
Chocolate Dip	1 serv (1.25 oz)	130	2	4
Cream Cheese Light	1 serv (.75 oz)	45	3	4
Cream Cheese Pineapple	1 serv (.75 oz)	70	4	6
Cream Cheese Strawberry	1 serv (.75 oz)	70	4	6
Dutch Ice Kiwi Banana	1 (12 oz)	160	0	0
Dutch Ice Kiwi Banana	1 (18 oz)	250	0	0
Dutch Ice Lemonade	1 (12 oz)	270	0	0
Dutch Ice Lemonade	1 (18 oz)	405	0	0
Dutch Ice Mocha	1 (18 oz)	340	8	9
Dutch Ice Mocha	1 (18 oz)	500	12	14
Dutch Ice Orange Creme	1 (18 oz)	360	0	0
Dutch Ice Orange Creme	1 (12 oz)	240	0	0
Dutch Ice Raspberry	1 (18 oz)	220	0	0
Dutch Ice Raspberry	1 (12 oz)	150	0	0
Dutch Ice Strawberry	1 (18 oz)	280	0	0
Dutch Ice Strawberry	1 (12 oz)	190	0	0
Marinara Sauce	1 serv (1 oz)	10	0	0
Pretzel Almond w/ Butter	1	400	5	8
Pretzel Almond w/o Butter	1	350	1	2
Pretzel Cinnamon Raisin w/o Butter	1	350	0	2
Pretzel Cinnamon Sugar w/ Butter	1	450	5	9
Pretzel Garlic w/ Butter	1	350	3	5
Pretzel Garlic w/o Butter	1	320	0	1

FOOD	PORTION	CALS.	SAT. FAT	FAT
Pretzel Glazin' Raisin w/ Butter	1	510	2	4
Pretzel Glazin' Raisin w/o Butter	1	470	0	1
Pretzel Jalapeno w/ Butter	1	310	3	5
Pretzel Jalapeno w/o Butter	1	270	0	1
Pretzel Original w/ Butter	1	370	2	4
Pretzel Original w/o Butter	1	340	0	1
Pretzel Sesame w/ Butter	1	410	4	12
Pretzel Sesame w/o Butter	1	350	1	6
Pretzel Sour Cream & Onion w/ Butter	1	340	3	5
Pretzel Sour Cream & Onion w/o Butter	1	310	0	1
Pretzel Whole Wheat w/ Butter	1	370	2	5
Pretzel Whole Wheat w/o Butter	1	350	0	2
Sweet Mustard	1 serv (1 oz)	60	1	2

BASKIN-ROBBINS

FROZEN YOGURT

FOOD	PORTION	CALS.	SAT. FAT	FAT
Maui Brownie Madness	½ cup	140	1	3
Perils Of Pauline	½ cup	140	2	3

ICE CREAM

FOOD	PORTION	CALS.	SAT. FAT	FAT
Banana Strawberry	½ cup	130	5	7
Baseball Nut	½ cup	160	5	9
Black Walnut	½ cup	160	5	11
Cherries Jubilee	½ cup	140	5	7
Chocolate	½ cup	150	6	9
Chocolate Almond	½ cup	180	5	11
Chocolate Chip	½ cup	150	6	10
Chocolate Chip Cookie Dough	½ cup	170	6	9
Chocolate Fudge	½ cup	160	6	9
Chocolate Mousse Royale	½ cup	170	5	10
Chocolate Raspberry Truffle	½ cup	180	6	9
Chunky Heath Bar	½ cup	170	6	10
Cookies N Cream	½ cup	170	7	11
Dirt'N Worms	½ cup	160	5	8
Egg Nog	½ cup	150	5	8
Everybody's Favorite Candy Bar	½ cup	170	5	9
French Vanilla	½ cup	160	6	10
French Vanilla	½ cup	170	7	11
Fudge Brownie	½ cup	170	6	11
Fudge Brownie	½ cup	180	7	10
German Chocolate Cake	½ cup	180	6	10

FOOD	PORTION	CALS.	SAT. FAT	FAT
Gold Medal Ribbon	½ cup	150	5	8
Gold Medal Ribbon	½ cup	150	5	7
Jamoca	½ cup	140	5	9
Jamoca Almond Fudge	½ cup	150	5	8
Jomoca Almond Fudge	½ cup	140	5	9
Lemon Custard	½ cup	150	5	8
Lowfat Carmel Apple AlaMod	½ cup	100	1	2
Lowfat Espresso'N Cream	½ cup	100	1	3
Mint Chocolate Chip	½ cup	150	6	10
No Sugar Added Call Me Nuts	½ cup	110	1	2
No Sugar Added Cherry Cordial	½ cup	100	2	2
No Sugar Added Mad About Chocolate	½ cup	100	1	2
No Sugar Added Pineapple Coconut	½ cup	90	1	2
No Sugar Added Thin Mint	½ cup	100	2	3
Nonfat Berry Innocent Cheese	½ cup	110	0	0
Nonfat Check-It-Out Cherry	½ cup	100	0	0
Nonfat Jamoca Swirl	½ cup	110	0	0
Ocean Commotion	½ cup	150	5	7
Old Fashion Butter Pecan	½ cup	160	6	11
Oregon Blueberry	½ cup	140	5	8
Peanut Butter N Chocolate	½ cup	180	6	12
Pink Bubblegum	½ cup	150	5	8
Pistachio Almond	½ cup	170	5	12
Pralines N Cream	½ cup	160	5	9
Pumpkin Pie	½ cup	130	5	7
Quarterback Crunch	½ cup	160	7	10
Reeses Peanut Butter	½ cup	180	6	11
Rocky Road	½ cup	170	5	10
Rum Raisin	½ cup	140	5	7
Strawberry Cheesecake	½ cup	150	5	9
Triple Chocolate Passion	½ cup	180	7	11
Vanilla	½ cup	140	5	8
Very Berry Strawberry	½ cup	130	4	7
Winter White Chocolate	½ cup	150	6	9
World Class Chocolate	½ cup	160	5	9
ICES AND ICE POPS				
Daiquiri Ice	½ cup	110	0	0
Sherbet Blue Raspberry	½ cup	120	1	2
Sherbet Orange	½ cup	120	1	2
Sherbet Rainbow	½ cup	120	1	2
Sorbet Pink Raspberry Lemon	½ cup	120	0	0

FOOD	PORTION	CALS.	SAT. FAT	FAT
The Mask Ice	½ cup	120	0	0
Watermelon Ice	½ cup	110	0	0
Watermelon Ice	½ cup	110	0	0

BEN & JERRY'S

Sugar Cone	1	48	tr	tr
FROZEN YOGURT				
Cherry Garcia	½ cup (3.3 oz)	150	2	3
Chocolate Cherry Garcia	½ cup (3.3 oz)	170	3	4
Chocolate Fudge Brownie	½ cup (3.3 oz)	180	2	3
No Fat Black Raspberry	½ cup (3.4 oz)	140	0	0
No Fat Coffee Fudge	½ cup (3.4 oz)	140	0	0
No Fat Vanilla	½ cup (3.4 oz)	140	0	0
No Fat Vanilla Fudge Swirl	½ cup (3.4 oz)	130	0	0
ICE CREAM				
Bovinity Divinity	½ cup (3.1 oz)	240	10	14
Butter Pecan	½ cup (3.1 oz)	270	9	21
Cherry Garcia	½ cup (3.1 oz)	210	9	12
Chocolate Chip Cookie Dough	½ cup (3.1 oz)	180	8	11
Chocolate Fudge Brownie	½ cup (3.1 oz)	230	7	11
Chubby Hubby	½ cup (3.1 oz)	280	10	17
Chunky Monkey	½ cup (3.1 oz)	220	9	13
Coconut Almond Fudge Chip	½ cup (3.1 oz)	250	11	18
Coffee Coffee Buzz Buzz	½ cup (3.1 oz)	240	11	16
Coffee Ole	½ cup (3.1 oz)	200	9	13
Coffee w/ Heath Bar Crunch	½ cup (3.1 oz)	250	9	16
Deep Dark Chocolate	½ cup (3.1 oz)	210	8	12
Dilbert's World Totally Nuts	½ cup (3.1 oz)	260	9	18
Low Fat Blackberry Cobbler	½ cup (3.2 oz)	160	2	2
Low Fat Chocolate Comfort	½ cup (3.2 oz)	150	2	2
Low Fat Coconut Creme Pie	½ cup (3.2 oz)	160	2	3
Low Fat Mocha Latte	½ cup (3.2 oz)	150	2	2
Low Fat Rockin Road	½ cup (3.2 oz)	180	2	3
Low Fat Smore's	½ cup (3.2 oz)	180	1	2
Low Fat Vanilla & Chocolate Mint Patty	½ cup (3.2 oz)	170	2	3
Maple Walnut	½ cup (3.1 oz)	240	8	13
Mint Chocolate Chunk	½ cup (3.1 oz)	240	11	16
Mint Chocolate Cookie	½ cup (3.1 oz)	230	8	14
New York Super Fudge Chunk	½ cup (3.1 oz)	250	9	16
Peanut Butter Cup	½ cup (3.1 oz)	270	10	18
Phish Food	½ cup (3.1 oz)	230	8	12
Pistachio Pistachio	½ cup (3.1 oz)	190	8	13
Praline Pecan	½ cup (3.1 oz)	230	8	14

FOOD	PORTION	CALS.	SAT. FAT	FAT
Southern Pecan Pie	½ cup (3.1 oz)	240	9	16
Strawberry	½ cup (3.1 oz)	180	7	10
Sweet Cream Cookie	½ cup (3.1 oz)	230	8	14
Triple Caramel Chunk	½ cup (3.1 oz)	240	9	13
Vanilla Caramel Fudge	½ cup (3.1 oz)	230	8	13
Vanilla Chocolate Chunk	½ cup (3.1 oz)	240	11	16
Vanilla World's Best	½ cup (3.1 oz)	200	9	13
Vanilla w/ Heath Toffee Crunch	½ cup (3.1 oz)	250	9	16
Wavy Gravy	½ cup (3.1 oz)	260	8	17
White Russian	½ cup (3.1 oz)	200	9	13
SORBETS				
Doonesberry	½ cup (3.2 oz)	100	0	0
Lemon Swirl	½ cup (3.2 oz)	100	0	0
Purple Passion Fruit	½ cup (3.2 oz)	100	0	0
Strawberry Kiwi	½ cup (3.2 oz)	110	0	0
BIG BOY				
DESSERTS				
Frozen Yogurt Fat Free	1 serv	118	—	0
Frozen Yogurt Shake	1	156	—	1
MAIN MENU SELECTIONS				
Baked Cod w/ Salad Baked Potato Roll & Margarine	1 meal	744	—	21
Baked Potato	1	163	—	2
Breast of Chicken Pita w/ Mozzarella & Ranch Dressing	1	361	—	11
Breast of Chicken w/ Mozzarella Salad Baked Potato Roll & Margarine	1 meal	697	—	20
Cabbage Soup	1 bowl	40	—	5
Cabbage Soup	1 cup	34	—	4
Cajun Cod w/ Salad Baked Potato Roll & Margarine	1 meal	736	—	21
Chicken & Pasta Primavera w/ Salad Roll & Margarine	1 meal	676	—	14
Chicken 'n Vegetable Stir Fry w/ Salad Baked Potato Roll & Margarine	1 meal	795	—	18
Dinner Roll	1	210	—	5
Plain Egg Beaters Omelette w/ Whole Wheat Bread & Margarine	1 meal	305	—	10
Promise Margarine	1 pat	25	—	3
Rice Pilaf	1 serv	153	—	4

FOOD	PORTION	CALS.	SAT. FAT	FAT
Scrambled Egg Beaters w/ Whole Wheat Bread & Margarine	1 meal	305	—	10
Southwest Chicken w/ Salad Baked Potato Roll & Margarine	1 meal	702	—	18
Spaghetti Marinara w/ Salad Roll & Margarin	1 meal	754	—	11
Turkey Pita w/ Ranch Dressing	1	245	—	6
Vegetable Stir Fry w/ Salad Baked Potato Roll & Margarine	1 meal	616	—	14
Vegetarian Egg Beaters Omelette w/ Whole Wheat Bread & Margarine	1 meal	330	—	10
SALAD DRESSINGS				
Italian Fat Free	1 oz	11	—	0
Lo Cal Oriental	1 oz	20	—	2
Lo Cal Ranch	1 oz	41	—	3
SALADS AND SALAD BARS				
Chicken Breast Salad w/ Roll & Margarine	1 serv	523	—	16
Oriental Chicken Breast Salad w/ Dinner Roll & Margarine	1 serv	660	—	20
Tossed Salad	1	35	—	2

BLIMPIE
6 INCH SUB

FOOD	PORTION	CALS.	SAT. FAT	FAT
5 Meatball	1 (7.8 oz)	500	8	22
Blimpie Best	1 (8.5 oz)	410	5	13
Cheese Trio	1 (8.2 oz)	510	13	23
Club	1 (9.8 oz)	450	6	13
Grilled Chicken	1 (9.1 oz)	400	2	9
Ham & Swiss	1 (8.2 oz)	400	7	13
Ham Salami Provolone	1 (9.8 oz)	590	11	28
Roast Beef	1 (8.5 oz)	340	1	5
Steak & Cheese	1 (7.1 oz)	550	4	26
Tuna	1 (10.2 oz)	570	5	32
Turkey	1 (8.2 oz)	320	1	5
SALADS AND SALAD BARS				
Grilled Chicken Salad	1 serv (16.2 oz)	350	0	12

BOJANGLES
BAKED SELECTIONS

FOOD	PORTION	CALS.	SAT. FAT	FAT
Biscuit	1	243	3	12
Multi-Grain Roll	1	150	0	3
Sweet Biscuit Apple Cinnamon	1	330	3	13

FOOD	PORTION	CALS.	SAT. FAT	FAT
Sweet Biscuit Bo*Berry	1	220	3	10
Sweet Biscuit Cinnamon	1	320	4	18
MAIN MENU SELECTIONS				
Biscuit Sandwich Bacon	1	290	5	17
Biscuit Sandwich Bacon Egg & Cheese	1	550	14	42
Biscuit Sandwich Cajun Filet	1	454	6	21
Biscuit Sandwich Country Ham	1	270	4	15
Biscuit Sandwich Egg	1	400	6	30
Biscuit Sandwich Sausage	1	350	7	23
Biscuit Sandwich Smoked Sausage	1	380	9	26
Biscuit Sandwich Steak	1	649	13	49
Bo Rounds	1 serv	235	4	11
Buffalo Bites	1 serv	180	2	5
Cajun Pintos	1 serv	110	0	0
Cajun Roast Skinfree Breast	1 serv	143	—	5
Cajun Roast Skinfree Leg	1 serv	161	—	8
Cajun Roast Skinfree Thigh	1 serv	215	—	15
Cajun Roast Wing	1 serv	231	—	15
Cajun Spiced Breast	1 serv	278	—	17
Cajun Spiced Leg	1 serv	310	—	23
Cajun Spiced Thigh	1 serv	264	—	16
Cajun Spiced Wing	1 serv	355	—	25
Chicken Supremes	1 serv	337	6	16
Corn On The Cob	1 serv	140	0	2
Dirty Rice	1 serv	166	2	6
Green Beans	1 serv	25	0	0
Macaroni & Cheese	1 serv	198	5	14
Marinated Cole Slaw	1 serv	136	0	3
Potatoes w/o Gravy	1 serv	80	0	1
Sandwich Cajun Filet w/ Mayonnaise	1	437	7	22
Sandwich Cajun Steak w/ Horseradish Sauce & Pickles	1	434	8	26
Sandwich Cjun Filet w/o Mayonnaise	1	337	5	11
Sandwich Grilled Filet w/ Mayonnaise	1	335	5	16
Sandwich Grilled Filet w/o Mayonnaise	1 serv (5.2 oz)	329	—	7
Seasoned Fries	1 serv	344	5	19
Southern Style Breast	1 serv	261	—	16

FOOD	PORTION	CALS.	SAT. FAT	FAT
Southern Style Leg	1 serv	254	—	15
Southern Style Thigh	1 serv	308	—	21
Southern Style Wing	1 serv	337	—	21

BOSTON MARKET
BAKED SELECTIONS

Brownie	1 (3.3 oz)	450	7	27
Cookie Chocolate Chip	1 (2.8 oz)	340	6	17
Cookie Oatmeal Raisin	1 (2.8 oz)	320	3	13
Honey Wheat Roll	½ roll (2 oz)	150	0	2

MAIN MENU SELECTIONS

½ Chicken w/ Skin	1 serv (10 oz)	630	19	37
¼ Dark Meat Chicken No Skin	1 serv (3.6 oz)	210	3	10
¼ Dark Meat Chicken w/ Skin	1 serv (4.6 oz)	330	6	22
¼ White Meat Chicken No Skin Or Wing	1 serv (3.6 oz)	160	1	4
¼ White Meat Chicken w/ Skin	1 serv (5.4 oz)	330	5	18
BBQ Baked Beans	¾ cup (7.1 oz)	330	3	9
Butternut Squash Low Fat	¾ cup (6.8 oz)	160	4	6
Caesar Salad Entree	1 serv (10 oz)	520	12	43
Caesar Salad w/o Dressing	1 serv (8 oz)	240	7	13
Caesar Side Salad	1 (4 oz)	210	5	17
Chicken Caesar Salad	1 serv (13 oz)	670	13	47
Chicken Gravy	1 serv (1 oz)	15	0	1
Chicken Salad Sandwich	1 (10.7 oz)	680	5	30
Chicken Sandwich w/ Cheese & Sauce	1 (12.4 oz)	750	12	33
Chicken Sandwich w/o Cheese & Sauce Low Fat	1 (10 oz)	430	1	4
Chunky Chicken Salad	¾ cup (5.5 oz)	370	5	27
Cole Slaw	¾ cup (6.5 oz)	280	3	16
Corn Bread	1 (2.4 oz)	200	2	6
Cranberry Relish Low Fat	¾ cup (7.9 oz)	370	1	5
Creamed Spinach	¾ cup (6.4 oz)	280	13	21
Fruit Salad Low Fat	¾ cup (5.5 oz)	70	0	1
Green Bean Casserole	¾ cup (6 oz)	170	2	5
Ham & Turkey Club w/ Cheese & Sauce	1 (13.3 oz)	890	20	44
Ham & Turkey Club w/o Cheese & Sauce	1 (9.3 oz)	430	2	6
Ham Sandwich w/ Cheese & Sauce	1 (11.8 oz)	760	13	35
Ham Sandwich w/o Cheese & Sauce	1 (9.3 oz)	450	3	9

FOOD	PORTION	CALS.	SAT. FAT	FAT
Ham w/ Cinnamon Apples	1 serv (8 oz)	350	5	13
Homestyle Mashed Potatoes & Gravy	¾ cup (6.6 oz)	200	5	9
Hot Cinnamon Apples	¾ cup (6.4 oz)	250	1	5
Macaroni & Cheese	¾ cup (6.7 oz)	280	6	10
Mashed Potatoes	⅔ cup (5.6 oz)	180	5	8
Meat Loaf & Brown Gravy	1 serv (7 oz)	390	8	22
Meat Loaf & Chunky Tomato Sauce	1 serv (8 oz)	370	8	18
Meat Loaf Sandwich w/ Cheese	1 (13.8 oz)	860	16	33
Meat Loaf Sandwich w/o Cheese	1 (12.3 oz)	690	7	21
Mediterranean Pasta Salad	¾ cup (4.5 oz)	170	3	10
New Potatoes Low Fat	¾ cup (4.6 oz)	130	0	3
Original Chicken Pot Pie	1 serv (14.9 oz)	750	9	34
Rice Pilaf	⅔ cup (5.1 oz)	180	1	5
Rotisserie Turkey Breast Skinless Low Fat	1 serv (5 oz)	170	1	1
Steamed Vegetables Low Fat	⅔ cup (3.7 oz)	35	0	1
Stuffing	¾ cup (6.1 oz)	310	2	12
Tortellini Salad	¾ cup (5.6 oz)	380	5	24
Turkey Sandwich w/ Cheese & Sauce	1 (11.8 oz)	710	10	28
Turkey Sandwich w/o Cheese & Sauce	1 (9.3 oz)	400	1	4
Whole Kernel Corn Low Fat	¾ cup (5.8 oz)	180	1	4
Zucchini Marinara	¾ cup (6.6 oz)	80	1	4
SOUPS				
Chicken Low Fat	¾ cup (6.8 oz)	80	1	3
Chicken Tortilla	1 cup (8.4 oz)	220	4	11

BROWN'S CHICKEN

Breadsticks w/ Garlic Butter	1	199	—	4
Breast	3.5 oz	284	—	15
Coleslaw	3.5 oz	131	—	10
Corn Fritters	3.5 oz	415	—	25
Corn On Cob	1 ear (3 inch)	126	—	3
Fettucini Alfredo	1 serv (12 oz)	1507	—	64
French Fries	3.5 oz	503	—	22
Gizzard	3.5 oz	387	—	20
Leg	3.5 oz	287	—	16
Liver	3.5 oz	341	—	19
Mostaccioli w/ Meat	1 serv (12 oz)	835	—	14
Mostaccioli w/o Meat	1 serv (12 oz)	792	—	10
Mushrooms	3.5 oz	289	—	16

FOOD	PORTION	CALS.	SAT. FAT	FAT
Potato Salad	3.5 oz	94	—	4
Ravioli w/ Meat	1 serv (12 oz)	865	—	20
Ravioli w/o Meat	1 serv (12 oz)	822	—	16
Shrimp	3.5 oz	277	—	10
Thigh	3.5 oz	355	—	24
Wing	3.5 oz	385	—	25

BRUEGGER'S BAGELS

FOOD	PORTION	CALS.	SAT. FAT	FAT
Blueberry	1 (3.5 oz)	300	0	2
Cinnamon Raisin	1 (3.5 oz)	290	0	2
Egg	1 (3.5 oz)	280	1	1
Everything	1 (3.6 oz)	290	0	2
Garlic	1 (3.6 oz)	280	0	2
Honey Grain	1 (3.6 oz)	300	1	3
Onion	1 (3.6 oz)	280	0	2
Orange Cranberry	1 (3.5 oz)	290	0	1
Pesto	1 (3.5 oz)	280	0	2
Plain	1 (3.5 oz)	280	0	2
Poppy Seed	1 (3.6 oz)	280	0	2
Pumpernickel	1 (3.5 oz)	280	0	2
Salt	1 (3.6 oz)	270	0	2
Sesame	1 (3.6 oz)	290	1	3
Spinach	1 (3.5 oz)	280	0	1
Sun Dried Tomato	1 (3.5 oz)	280	0	2
Wheat Bran	1 (3.5 oz)	280	0	2

BURGER KING
BEVERAGES

FOOD	PORTION	CALS.	SAT. FAT	FAT
Shake Chocolate	1 med (10 oz)	320	4	7
Shake Vanilla	1 med (10 oz)	300	4	6
Tropicana Orange Juice	1 serv (11 oz)	140	0	0

BREAKFAST SELECTIONS

FOOD	PORTION	CALS.	SAT. FAT	FAT
AM Express Grape Jam	1 serv (0.4 oz)	30	0	0
AM Express Strawberry Jam	1 serv (0.4 oz)	30	0	0
AM Express Dip	1 serv (1 oz)	80	0	0
Biscuit	1 (3.3 oz)	330	4	18
Biscuit w/ Bacon Egg & Cheese	1 (6 oz)	510	10	31
Biscuit w/ Egg	1 (5.3 oz)	420	6	24
Biscuit w/ Sausage	1 (4.8 oz)	530	11	36
Cini-minis	4	550	7	26
Croissan'wich Sausage Egg & Cheese	1 (5.7 oz)	550	14	42
Croissan'wich w/ Sausage & Cheese	1 (3.7 oz)	450	12	35
French Toast Sticks	1 serv (4.9 oz)	500	7	27

FOOD	PORTION	CALS.	SAT. FAT	FAT
Hash Browns	1 sm (2.6 oz)	240	6	15
Land O'Lakes Whipped Classic Blend	1 serv (0.4 oz)	65	1	7
MAIN MENU SELECTIONS				
American Cheese	2 slices (0.9 oz)	90	5	8
BK Big Fish Sandwich	1 (8.8 oz)	720	9	43
BK Broiler Chicken Sandwich	1 (8.7 oz)	530	5	16
Bacon Bits	1 serv (3 g)	15	0	1
Big King Sandwich	1 (7.9 oz)	660	18	43
Broiled Chicken Salad w/o Dressing	1 serv (10.6 oz)	190	4	8
Bull's Eye Barbecue Sauce	1 serv (0.5 oz)	20	0	0
Cheeseburger	1 (5 oz)	380	9	19
Chicken Sandwich	1 (8 oz)	710	9	43
Chicken Tenders	8 pieces (4.3 oz)	350	7	22
Coated French Fries Salted	1 med (4.1 oz)	400	8	21
Croutons	1 serv (0.2 oz)	30	0	1
Dipping Sauce Barbecue	1 serv (1 oz)	35	0	0
Dipping Sauce Honey	1 serv (1 oz)	90	0	0
Dipping Sauce Ranch	1 serv (1 oz)	170	3	17
Dipping Sauce Sweet & Sour	1 serv (1 oz)	45	0	0
Double Cheeseburger	1 (7.5 oz)	600	17	36
Double Cheeseburger w/ Bacon	1 (7.6 oz)	640	18	39
Double Whopper	1 (12.3 oz)	870	19	56
Double Whopper w/ Cheese	1 (13.2 oz)	960	24	63
Dutch Apple Pie	1 serv (4 oz)	300	3	15
French Fries Salted	1 med (4.1 oz)	370	5	20
Garden Salad w/o Dressing	1 (7.5 oz)	100	3	5
Hamburger	1 (4.5 oz)	330	6	15
Ketchup	1 serv (0.5 oz)	15	0	0
King Sauce	1 serv (0.5 oz)	70	1	7
Lettuce	1 leaf (0.7 oz)	0	0	0
Mayonnaise	1 serv (1 oz)	210	3	23
Mustard	1 serv (3 g)	0	0	0
Onion	1 serv (0.5 oz)	5	0	0
Onion Rings	1 serv (4.4 oz)	310	2	14
Pickles	4 slices (0.5 oz)	0	0	0
Side Salad w/o Dressing	1 (4.7 oz)	60	2	3
Tartar Sauce	1 serv (1 oz)	180	3	19
Tomato	2 slices (1 oz)	5	0	0
Whopper	1 (9.5 oz)	640	11	39
Whopper Jr.	1 (5.9 oz)	420	8	24
Whopper Jr. w/ Cheese	1 (6.3 oz)	460	10	28
Whopper w/ Cheese	1 (10.3 oz)	730	16	46

FOOD	PORTION	CALS.	SAT. FAT	FAT
SALAD DRESSINGS				
Bleu Cheese	1 serv (1 oz)	160	4	16
French	1 serv (1 oz)	140	2	10
Ranch	1 serv (1 oz)	180	4	19
Reduced Calorie Light Italian	1 serv (1 oz)	15	0	1
Thousand Island	1 serv (1 oz)	140	3	12
CAPTAIN D'S				
DESSERTS				
Carrot Cake	1 piece (4 oz)	434	—	23
Cheesecake	1 piece (4 oz)	420	—	31
Chocolate Cake	1 piece (4 oz)	303	—	10
Lemon Pie	1 piece (4 oz)	351	—	10
Pecan Pie	1 piece (4 oz)	458	—	20
MAIN MENU SELECTIONS				
Baked Potato	1	278	0	0
Breadstick	1	113	0	4
Broiled Chicken Lunch	1 serv	503	2	9
Broiled Chicken Platter	1 serv	802	2	10
Broiled Chicken Sandwich	1 (8.2 oz)	451	—	19
Broiled Fish & Chicken Platter	1 serv	777	1	10
Broiled Fish & Chicken Lunch	1 serv	478	1	8
Broiled Fish Lunch	1 serv	435	1	7
Broiled Fish Platter	1 serv	734	1	7
Broiled Shrimp Lunch	1 serv	421	1	7
Broiled Shrimp Platter	1 serv	720	1	8
Cheese	1 slice (1 oz)	54	—	5
Cob Corn	1 serv (9.5 oz)	251	—	2
Cocktail Sauce	1 lg serv (1 fl oz)	34	—	tr
Cocktail Sauce	1 serv (1 fl oz)	137	—	tr
Cole Slaw	1 pt (16 oz)	633	—	47
Cole Slaw	1 serv (4 oz)	158	—	12
Crackers	4 (0.5 oz)	50	—	1
Cracklins	1 serv (1 oz)	218	—	17
Dinner Salad w/o Dressing	1 (2.5 oz)	27	—	1
French Fried Potatoes	1 serv (3.5 oz)	302	—	10
Fried Okra	1 serv (4 oz)	300	—	16
Green Beans Seasoned	1 serv (4 oz)	46	—	2
Hushpuppies	6 (6.7 oz)	756	—	25
Hushpuppy	1 (1.1 oz)	126	—	4
Imitation Sour Cream	1 serv	29	3	3
Margarine	1 serv	102	7	12
Non-Dairy Creamer	1 serv	14	—	1
Rice	1 serv (4 oz)	124	0	0
Stuffed Crab	1 serv	91	—	7

FOOD	PORTION	CALS.	SAT. FAT	FAT
Sugar	1 pkg	18	0	0
Sweet & Sour Sauce	1 serv (1.8 fl oz)	52	0	0
Sweet & Sour Sauce	1 lg serv (4 fl oz)	206	0	0
Tartar Sauce	1 lg serv (4 fl oz)	298	—	27
Tartar Sauce	1 serv (1 fl oz)	75	—	7
Vegetable Medley	1 serv	36	0	1
White Beans	1 serv (4 oz)	126	—	1
SALAD DRESSINGS				
Blue Cheese	1 pkg (1 fl oz)	105	—	12
French	1 pkg (1 fl oz)	111	—	11
Light Italian	1 serv	16	0	1
Ranch	1 pkg (1 fl oz)	92	—	10

CARL'S JR.
BAKED SELECTIONS

FOOD	PORTION	CALS.	SAT. FAT	FAT
Cheese Danish	1 (4.1 oz)	400	5	22
Cheesecake Strawberry Swirl	1 serv (3.5 oz)	300	9	17
Chocolate Cake	1 serv (3 oz)	300	3	10
Chocolate Chip Cookie	1 (2.5 oz)	370	8	19
Cinnamon Roll	1 (4.2 oz)	420	4	13
Muffin Blueberry	1 (4.2 oz)	340	2	14
Muffin Bran	1 (4.7 oz)	370	2	13
BEVERAGES				
Hot Chocolate	1 reg (12 oz)	110	0	1
Orange Juice	1 (6 fl oz)	90	0	0
Shake Chocolate	1 sm (13.5 oz)	390	5	7
Shake Strawberry	1 sm (13.5 oz)	400	5	7
Shake Vanilla	1 sm (13.5 fl oz)	330	5	8
BREAKFAST SELECTIONS				
Bacon	2 strips (0.3 oz)	40	2	4
Breakfast Burrito	1 (5.3 oz)	430	12	26
Breakfast Quesadilla Cheese	1 (5.2 oz)	300	6	14
English Muffin w/ Margarine	1 (2.6 oz)	230	2	10
French Toast Dips w/o Syrup	1 serv (3.7 oz)	410	6	25
Grape Jelly	1 serv (0.5 oz)	35	0	0
Hash Brown Nuggets	1 serv (3.3 oz)	270	4	17
Sausage	1 patty (1.8 oz)	200	7	18
Scrambed Eggs	1 serv (3.5 oz)	160	4	11
Strawberry Jam	1 serv (0.5 oz)	35	0	0
Sunrise Sandwich	1 (4.6 oz)	370	6	21
Table Syrup	1 serv (1 oz)	90	0	0
MAIN MENU SELECTIONS				
American Cheese	1 slice (0.5 oz)	60	3	5
BBQ Chicken Sandwich	1 (6.7 oz)	310	2	6
BBQ Sauce	1 serv (1.1 oz)	50	0	0

FOOD	PORTION	CALS.	SAT. FAT	FAT
Big Burger	1 (6.8 oz)	470	8	20
Breadstick	1 (0.3 oz)	35	0	1
Carl's Catch Fish Sandwich	1 (7.5 oz)	560	7	30
Chicken Club Sandwich	1 (8.8 oz)	550	8	29
Chicken Stars	6 pieces (3 oz)	230	3	14
CrissCut Fries	1 lg (5.7 oz)	550	9	34
Croutons	1 serv (7 g)	35	0	1
Double Western Bacon Cheeseburger	1 (11.5 oz)	970	27	57
Famous Big Star Hamburger	1 (8.6 oz)	610	11	38
French Fries	1 reg (4.4 oz)	370	7	20
Great Stuff Potato Bacon & Cheese	1 (14.2 oz)	630	7	29
Great Stuff Potato Broccoli & Cheese	1 (14.2 oz)	530	5	22
Great Stuff Potato Plain	1 (9.4 oz)	290	0	0
Great Stuff Potato Sour Cream & Chive	1 (10.9 oz)	430	3	14
Hamburger	1 (3.1 oz)	200	4	8
Honey Sauce	1 serv (1 oz)	90	0	0
Hot & Crispy Sandwich	1 (5 oz)	400	5	22
Mustard Sauce	1 serv (1 oz)	45	0	1
Onion Rings	1 serv (5.3 oz)	520	6	26
Salsa	1 serv (0.9 oz)	10	0	0
Sante Fe Chicken Sandwich	1 (7.9 oz)	530	7	30
Super Star Hamburger	1 (11.2 oz)	820	20	53
Sweet N'Sour Sauce	1 serv (1 oz)	50	0	0
Swiss Cheese	1 slice (0.5 oz)	45	3	4
Western Bacon Cheeseburger	1 (8.1 oz)	870	16	35
Zucchini	1 serv (5.9 oz)	380	6	23
SALAD DRESSINGS				
1000 Island	2 fl oz	250	4	24
Blue Cheese	2 fl oz	310	6	34
French Fat Free	2 fl oz	70	0	0
House	2 fl oz	220	4	22
Italian Fat Free	2 fl oz	15	0	0
SALADS AND SALAD BARS				
Salad-To-Go Charbroiled Chicken	1 serv (12 oz)	260	5	9
Salad-To-Go Garden	1 (4.8 oz)	50	2	3

CARVEL
FROZEN YOGURT

FOOD	PORTION	CALS.	SAT. FAT	FAT
Vanilla Low Fat No Sugar Added	4 fl oz	110	—	2

FOOD	PORTION	CALS.	SAT. FAT	FAT
ICE CREAM				
Brown Bonnet Cone	1 (4.7 oz)	380	15	21
Brown Bonnet Cone No Fat Vanilla	1 (4.7 oz)	300	9	11
Cake	1 pkg (7 oz)	450	15	23
Cake	1 pkg (4 oz)	270	9	14
Cake Cheesecake	1 serv (4 oz)	280	9	14
Cake Chocolate Vanilla Chocolate Crunchies	⅟₁₅ cake (3.4 oz)	230	8	12
Cake Cookies & Cream	1 serv (4 oz)	270	8	14
Cake Fudge Drizzle	⅛ cake (4 oz)	310	10	17
Cake Fudgie The Whale	⅟₁₄ cake (3.6 oz)	290	7	16
Cake Holiday	⅟₁₅ cake (3.4 oz)	240	8	12
Cake S'mores	1 serv (4 oz)	270	9	14
Cake Sinfully Chocolate	1 serv (4 oz)	280	9	14
Cake Strawberries & Cream	⅛ cake (3.8 oz)	240	8	12
Chocolate	4 fl oz	190	6	10
Chocolate No Fat	4 fl oz	120	0	0
Flying Saucer Chocolate	1 (4 oz)	230	5	9
Flying Saucer Chocolate w/ Sprinkles	1 (4 oz)	330	7	14
Flying Saucer Low Fat Chocolate	1 (4 oz)	190	1	3
Flying Saucer Low Fat Vanilla	1 (4 oz)	180	1	3
Flying Saucer Vanilla	1 (4 oz)	240	5	10
Flying Saucer Vanilla w/ Sprinkles	1 (4 oz)	340	7	14
Lil'Love Cake All Vanilla	1 piece (4.4 oz)	330	10	16
Lil'Love Cake Chocolate & Vanilla	1 piece (4 oz)	260	8	13
Nature's Crunch	1 (4.2 g)	450	14	25
Olde Fashion Sundae Butterscotch	1 (8 oz)	500	10	17
Olde Fashion Sundae Chocolate	1 (8 oz)	470	12	19
Olde Fashion Sundae Strawberry	1 (8 oz)	420	9	15
Sheet Cake Chocolate Vanilla Chocolate Crunchies	⅟₂₈ cake (3.3 oz)	230	8	12
Sinful Love Bar	1 (4.2 oz)	460	14	29
Thick Shake Chocolate	1 (16 oz)	719	18	31
Thick Shake Low Fat Chocolate	1 (16 oz)	490	1	1
Thick Shake Low Fat Strawberry	1 (16 oz)	460	1	1
Thick Shake Low Fat Vanilla	1 (16 oz)	460	1	1
Thick Shake No Fat Chocolate	1 (16 oz)	524	4	8
Thick Shake No Fat Strawberry	1 (16 oz)	453	4	7
Thick Shake No Fat Vanilla	1 (16 oz)	462	4	7
Thick Shake Strawberry	1 (16 oz)	648	18	30

FOOD	PORTION	CALS.	SAT. FAT	FAT
Thick Shake Vanilla	1 (16 oz)	657	18	30
Vanilla	4 fl oz	200	6	10
Vanilla No Fat	4 fl oz	120	0	0
SHERBET				
Black Raspberry	½ cup (3.4 oz)	150	1	1
Blueberry	½ cup (3.4 oz)	150	1	1
Lemon	½ cup (3.5 oz)	150	1	1
Lime	½ cup (3.5 oz)	150	1	1
Mango	½ cup (3.5 oz)	140	1	1
Orange	½ cup (3.5 oz)	150	1	1
Peach	½ cup (3.4 oz)	150	1	1
Pineapple	½ cup (3.5 oz)	150	1	1
Strawberry	½ cup (3.5 oz)	150	1	1

CHICK-FIL-A

DESSERTS

FOOD	PORTION	CALS.	SAT. FAT	FAT
Cheesecake	1 slice (3.1 oz)	270	9	21
Cheesecake w/ Blueberry Topping	1 slice (4.1 oz)	290	10	23
Cheesecake w/ Strawberry Topping	1 slice (4.1 oz)	290	10	23
Fudge Nut Brownie	1 (2.6 oz)	350	3	16
Icedream Cone	1 sm (4.5 oz)	140	1	4
Icedream Cup	1 sm (7.5 oz)	350	3	10
Lemon Pie	1 slice (4 oz)	320	5	16
MAIN MENU SELECTIONS				
Carrot & Raisin Salad	1 sm (2.7 oz)	150	0	2
Chargrilled Chicken Club Sandwich w/o Dressing	1 (8.2 oz)	390	5	12
Chargrilled Chicken Deluxe Sandwich	1 (7.4 oz)	290	1	3
Chargrilled Chicken Garden Salad	1 serv (14 oz)	170	1	3
Chargrilled Chicken Sandwich	1 (5.3 oz)	280	1	3
Chargrilled Chicken w/o Bun Or Pickles	1 piece (2.8 oz)	130	1	3
Chick-n-Strips	4 (4.2 oz)	230	2	8
Chick-n-Strips Salad	1 serv (15.9 oz)	290	2	9
Chicken Sandwich	1 (5.9 oz)	290	2	9
Chicken Deluxe Sandich	1 (8 oz)	300	2	9
Chicken Salad Plate	1 serv (16.5 oz)	290	0	21
Chicken Salad Sandwich On Whole Wheat	1 (5.9 oz)	320	2	5
Chicken w/o Bun Or Pickles	1 piece (3.7 oz)	160	2	8
Cole Slaw	1 sm (2.8 oz)	130	1	6

FOOD	PORTION	CALS.	SAT. FAT	FAT
Hearty Breast of Chicken Soup	1 cup (7.6 oz)	110	0	1
Nuggets	8 (3.9 oz)	290	3	14
Tossed Salad	1 serv (4.6 oz)	70	0	5
Waffle Potato Fries	1 sm (3 oz)	290	4	10
Waffle Potato Fries w/o Salt	1 sm (3 oz)	290	4	10

CHILI'S
DESSERTS

Diet By Chocolate Cake	1 serv	370	1	2
Diet By Chocolate Cake w/ Yogurt	1 serv	465	1	2
Diet By Chocolate Cake w/ Yogurt & Fudge Topping	1 serv	534	1	3

MAIN MENU SELECTIONS

Guiltless Grill Chicken Fijitas	1 serv	726	4	13
Guiltless Grill Chicken Platter	1 serv	563	3	7
Guiltless Grill Chicken Salad w/ Dressing	1 serv	254	1	3
Guiltless Grill Chicken Sandwich	1	527	2	7
Guiltless Grill Veggie Pasta	1 serv	590	3	11
Guiltless Grill Veggie Pasta w/ Chicken	1 serv	696	4	13

CHURCH'S CHICKEN

Apple Pie	1 serv (3.1 oz)	280	—	12
Biscuit	1 (2.1 oz)	250	—	16
Breast	1 serv (2.8 oz)	200	—	12
Cajun Rice	1 serv (3.1 oz)	130	—	7
Cole Slaw	1 serv (3 oz)	92	—	6
Corn On The Cob	1 serv (5.7 oz)	139	—	3
French Fries	1 serv (2.7 oz)	210	—	11
Leg	1 serv (2 oz)	140	—	9
Okra	1 serv (2.8 oz)	210	—	16
Potatoes & Gravy	1 serv (3.7 oz)	90	—	3
Tender Strip	1 (1.1 oz)	80	—	4
Thigh	1 serv (2.8 oz)	230	—	16
Wing	1 serv (3.1 oz)	250	—	16

COLOMBO FROZEN YOGURT

Alpine Strawberry Nonfat	4 fl oz	100	0	0
Banana Strawberry Nonfat	4 fl oz	50	0	0
Brazlian Banana Nonfat	4 fl oz	100	0	0
Butter Pecan Nonfat	4 fl oz	100	0	0
Cappuccino Nonfat	4 fl oz	100	0	0
Cherry Amaretto Nonfat	4 fl oz	50	0	0

FOOD	PORTION	CALS.	SAT. FAT	FAT
Cherry Vanilla Nonfat	4 fl oz	100	0	0
Chocolate Nonfat	4 fl oz	50	0	0
Coconut Cooler Nonfat	4 fl oz	100	0	0
Cool Berry Blue Nonfat	4 fl oz	100	0	0
Country Pumpkin Nonfat	4 fl oz	100	0	0
Double Dutch Chocolate Nonfat	4 fl oz	100	0	0
Egg Nog Nonfat	4 fl oz	100	0	0
French Vanilla Lowfat	4 fl oz	110	1	2
French Vanilla Nonfat	4 fl oz	100	0	0
Georgia Peach Nonfat	4 fl oz	100	0	0
German Fudge Chocolate Nonfat	4 fl oz	100	0	0
Hawaiian Pineapple Nonfat	4 fl oz	100	0	0
Hazelnut Amaretto Nonfat	4 fl oz	100	0	0
Honey Almond Nonfat	4 fl oz	100	0	0
Irish Cream Nonfat	4 fl oz	100	0	0
New York Cheesecake Nonfat	4 fl oz	100	0	0
Old World Chocolate Lowfat	4 fl oz	110	1	2
Orange Bavarian Creme Nonfat	4 fl oz	100	0	0
Peanut Butter Lowfat	4 fl oz	110	1	2
Pecan Praline Nonfat	4 fl oz	100	0	0
Pina Colada Nonfat	4 fl oz	100	0	0
Raspberry Nonfat	4 fl oz	50	0	0
Rockin' Raspberry Nonfat	4 fl oz	100	0	0
Simply Vanilla Lowfat	4 fl oz	110	1	2
Simply Vanilla Nonfat	4 fl oz	100	0	0
Strawberry Nonfat	4 fl oz	50	0	0
Tropical Tango Nonfat	4 fl oz	100	0	0
Vanilla Nonfat	4 fl oz	50	0	0
White Chocolate Almond Nonfat	4 fl oz	100	0	0
Wild Strawberry Lowfat	4 fl oz	110	1	2

DAIRY QUEEN
FOOD SELECTIONS

FOOD	PORTION	CALS.	SAT. FAT	FAT
Chicken Breast Fillet Sandwich	1 (6.7 oz)	430	4	20
Chicken Strip Basket	1 serv (14.5 oz)	1000	13	50
Chili 'n' Cheese Dog	1 (5 oz)	330	9	21
DQ Homestyle Bacon Double Cheeseburger	1 (8.9 oz)	610	18	36
DQ Homestyle Cheeseburger	1 (5.3 oz)	340	8	17
DQ Homestyle Double Cheeseburger	1 (7.7 oz)	540	16	31
DQ Homestyle Hamburger	1 (4.8 oz)	290	5	12
DQ Ultimate Burger	1 (9.4 oz)	670	19	43
French Fries	1 med (3.9 oz)	350	4	18

FOOD	PORTION	CALS.	SAT. FAT	FAT
French Fries	1 lg (4.9 oz)	440	5	23
Grilled Chicken Sandwich	1 (6.5 oz)	310	3	10
Hot Dog	1 (3.5 oz)	240	5	14
Onion Rings	1 serv (4 oz)	320	4	16
ICE CREAM				
Banana Split	1 (12.9 oz)	510	8	12
Blizzard Chocolate Sandwich Cookie	1 med (11.4 oz)	640	11	23
Blizzard Chocolate Sandwich Cookie	1 sm (12 oz)	520	9	18
Blizzard Chocolate Chip Cookie Dough	1 med (15.4 oz)	950	19	36
Blizzard Chocolate Chip Cookie Dough	1 sm (12 oz)	660	13	24
Breeze Heath	1 med (14.2 oz)	710	11	18
Breeze Heath	1 sm (10.2 oz)	470	6	10
Breeze Strawberry	1 sm (12 oz)	320	1	1
Breeze Strawberry	1 med (13.4 oz)	460	1	1
Buster Bar	1 (5.2 oz)	450	12	28
Chocolate Malt	1 med (19.9 oz)	880	14	22
Chocolate Malt	1 sm (14.7 oz)	650	10	16
Cone Chocolate	1 med (6.9 oz)	340	7	11
Cone Chocolate	1 sm (5 oz)	240	5	8
Cone Vanilla	1 sm (5 oz)	230	5	7
Cone Vanilla	1 med (6.9 oz)	330	6	9
Cone Vanilla	1 lg (8.9 oz)	410	8	12
Cone Yogurt	1 med (6.9 oz)	260	1	1
Cone Dipped	1 med (7.7 oz)	490	13	24
Cone Dipped	1 sm (5.5 oz)	340	9	17
Cup Of Yogurt	1 med (6.7 oz)	230	0	1
DQ 8 Inch Round Cake Undecorated	⅛ of cake (6.2 oz)	340	7	12
DQ Fudge Bar No Sugar Added	1 (2.3 oz)	50	0	0
DQ Lemon Freez'r	½ cup (3.2 oz)	80	0	0
DQ Nonfat Frozen Yogurt	½ cup (3 oz)	100	0	0
DQ Sandwich	1 (2.1 oz)	150	2	5
DQ Soft Serve Chocolate	½ cup (3.3 oz)	150	4	5
DQ Soft Serve Vanilla	½ cup (3.3 oz)	140	3	5
DQ Treatzza Pizza Heath	⅛ of pie (2.3 oz)	180	4	7
DQ Treatzza Pizza M&M	⅛ of pie (2.4 oz)	190	4	7
DQ Vanilla Orange Bar No Sugar Added	1 (2.3 oz)	60	0	0
Dilly Bar Chocolate	1 (3 oz)	210	7	13
Fudge Cake Supreme	1 serv (11.2 oz)	890	22	38

FOOD	PORTION	CALS.	SAT. FAT	FAT
Misty Slush	1 med (20.9 oz)	290	0	0
Misty Slush	1 sm (15.9 oz)	220	0	0
Peanut Buster Parfait	1 (10.7 oz)	730	17	31
Shake Chocolate	1 med (18.9 oz)	770	13	20
Shake Chocolate	1 sm (13.9 oz)	560	10	15
Starkiss	1 (3 oz)	80	—	0
Strawberry Shortcake	1 (8.5 oz)	430	9	14
Sundae Chocolate	1 med (8.2 oz)	400	6	10
Sundae Chocolate	1 sm (5.7 oz)	280	5	7
Yogurt Sundae Strawberry	1 med (8.2 oz)	280	0	1

D'ANGELO SANDWICH SHOPS
SALADS AND SALAD BARS

FOOD	PORTION	CALS.	SAT. FAT	FAT
Antipasto Salad w/o Dressing	1	420	—	14
Caesar Salad w/ Dressing	1	740	—	45
Caesar Salad w/o Dressing	1	490	—	20
Chicken Caesar Salad w/ Dressing	1	860	—	48
Chicken Caesar Salad w/o Dressing	1	600	—	23
Chicken Salad D'Lite	1	325	—	4
Chicken Salad w/o Dressing	1	390	—	5
D'Lite Turkey	1 serv	355	—	2
Greek Salad w/ Dressing	1	940	—	71
Greek Salad w/ Tuna & Dressing	1	1010	—	72
Greek Salad w/ Tuna w/o Dressing	1	490	—	15
Greek Salad w/o Dressing	1	420	—	15
Roast Beef Salad D'Lite	1	350	—	5
Roast Beef Salad w/o Dressing	1	400	—	6
Tossed Garden Salad w/o Dressing	1	270	—	2
Tuna Salad D'Lite	1	305	—	2
Tuna Salad w/o Dressing	1	330	—	3
Turkey Salad w/o Dressing	1	400	—	3
SANDWICHES				
BLT w/ Cheese	1	1170	—	62
BLT w/ Cheese Medium Sub	1	870	—	47
BLT w/ Cheese Pokket	1	570	—	31
BLT w/ Cheese Small Sub	1	600	—	33
Barbecue Curls	1	480	—	19
Buffalo Chicken Wrap w/ Blue Cheese Dressing	1	621	—	28
Buffalo Chicken Wrap w/o Dressing	1	417	—	13

FOOD	PORTION	CALS.	SAT. FAT	FAT
Caesar Salad w/ Dressing Pokket	1	590	—	26
Caesar Salad w/o Dressing Pokket	1	460	—	13
Caesar Salad w/ Chicken w/ Dressing Pokket	1	700	—	28
Caesar Salad w/ Chicken w/ Dressing Pokket	1	570	—	16
Caesar Wrap w/ Dressing	1	484	—	15
Caesar Wrap w/ Fat Free Dressing	1	484	—	15
Capicola Ham & Cheese Large Sub	1	740	—	23
Capicola Ham & Cheese Medium Sub	1	550	—	17
Capicola Ham & Cheese Pokket	1	350	—	11
Capicola Ham & Cheese Small Sub	1	390	—	13
Cheeseburger Large Sub	1	1060	—	49
Cheeseburger Medium Sub	1	780	—	37
Cheeseburger Pokket	1	490	—	23
Cheeseburger Small Sub	1	530	—	25
Chicken Salad Large Sub	1	1370	—	78
Chicken Salad Medium Sub	1	970	—	55
Chicken Salad Pokket	1	650	—	38
Chicken Salad Small Sub	1	690	—	39
Chicken Stir Fry D'Lite Pokket	1	360	—	5
Chicken Stir Fry D'Lite Sub	1	280	—	6
Chicken Stir Fry Large Sub	1	800	—	12
Chicken Stir Fry Medium Sub	1	560	—	9
Chicken Stir Fry Pokket	1	360	—	5
Chicken Stir Fry Small Sub	1	380	—	6
Classic Vegetable D'Lite Pokket	1	340	—	10
Classic Vegetable Large Sub	1	860	—	33
Classic Vegetable Medium Sub	1	610	—	23
Classic Vegetable Pokket	1	400	—	15
Classic Vegetable Small Sub	1	430	—	15
Crunchy Vegetable D'Lite Pokket	1	350	—	10
Crunchy Vegetable D'Lite Small Sub	1	385	—	11
Crunchy Vegetable Large Sub	1	880	—	33
Crunchy Vegetable Pokket	1	410	—	15
Crunchy Vegetables Medium Sub	1	620	—	23
Crunchy Vegetables Small Sub	1	440	—	16

FOOD	PORTION	CALS.	SAT. FAT	FAT
Ginger Chicken Stir Fry D'Lite Pokket	1	400	—	5
Greek Pokket	1	910	—	71
Grilled Spicy Steak D'Lite Pokket	1	425	—	11
Grilled Steak Cheese Large Sub	1	1160	—	54
Grilled Steak Cheese Medium Sub	1	820	—	38
Grilled Steak Cheese Pokket	1	550	—	26
Grilled Steak Cheese Small Sub	1	580	—	28
Grilled Steak Combo Large Sub	1	1170	—	54
Grilled Steak Combo Medium Sub	1	830	—	38
Grilled Steak Combo Pokket	1	550	—	26
Grilled Steak Combo Small Sub	1	590	—	28
Grilled Steak D'Lite Pokket	1	390	—	11
Grilled Steak Large Sub	1	990	—	40
Grilled Steak Medium Sub	1	680	—	27
Grilled Steak Mushrooms Large Sub	1	1000	—	40
Grilled Steak Mushrooms Medium Sub	1	690	—	27
Grilled Steak Mushrooms Pokket	1	450	—	18
Grilled Steak Mushrooms Small Sub	1	480	—	19
Grilled Steak Onion Large Sub	1	1000	—	40
Grilled Steak Onion Medium Sub	1	700	—	27
Grilled Steak Onion Small Sub	1	480	—	19
Grilled Steak Onions Pokket	1	450	—	17
Grilled Steak Peppers	1	690	—	27
Grilled Steak Peppers Large Sub	1	1000	—	40
Grilled Steak Peppers Pokket	1	540	—	17
Grilled Steak Pokket	1	440	—	17
Grilled Steak Small Sub	1	470	—	19
Ham & Cheese Large Sub	1	760	—	25
Ham & Cheese Medium Sub	1	550	—	19
Ham & Cheese Pokket	1	370	—	13
Ham & Cheese Small Sub	1	400	—	14
Ham Salami & Cheese Large Sub	1	870	—	36
Ham Salami & Cheese Medium Sub	1	630	—	27
Ham Salami & Cheese Pokket	1	420	—	18
Ham Salami & Cheese Small Sub	1	450	—	20
Hamburger Large Sub	1	920	—	38
Hamburger Medium Sub	1	680	—	28

FOOD	PORTION	CALS.	SAT. FAT	FAT
Hamburger Pokket	1	430	—	18
Hamburger Small Sub	1	460	—	19
Italian Cold Cut Large Sub	1	1130	—	61
Italian Cold Cut Medium Sub	1	820	—	44
Italian Cold Cut Pokket	1	550	—	30
Italian Cold Cut Small Sub	1	580	—	32
Meatball Large Sub	1	1010	—	42
Meatball Medium Sub	1	750	—	32
Meatball Pokket	1	480	—	20
Meatball Small Sub	1	520	—	21
Meatball w/ Cheese Large Sub	1	1170	—	54
Meatball w/ Cheese Medium Sub	1	880	—	41
Meatball w/ Cheese Pokket	1	580	—	28
Meatball w/ Cheese Small Sub	1	620	—	29
Pastrami Large Sub	1	1250	—	69
Pastrami Medium Sub	1	860	—	46
Pastrami Pokket	1	550	—	30
Pastrami Small Sub	1	580	—	31
Pastrami w/ Cheese Large Sub	1	1640	—	102
Pastrami w/ Cheese Medium Sub	1	1170	—	73
Pastrami w/ Cheese Pokket	1	780	—	49
Pastrami w/ Cheese Small Sub	1	820	—	51
Roast Beef D'Lite Pokket	1	330	—	6
Roast Beef D'Lite Small Sub	1	365	—	7
Roast Beef Large Sub	1	710	—	14
Roast Beef Medium Sub	1	520	—	10
Seafood Salad Large Sub	1	1210	—	68
Seafood Salad Medium Sub	1	860	—	48
Seafood Salad Pokket	1	570	—	33
Seafood Salad Small Sub	1	610	—	34
Stuffed Turkey D'Lite Pokket	1	510	—	8
Stuffed Turkey D'Lite Small Sub	1	545	—	9
Stuffed Turkey Large Sub	1	1070	—	19
Stuffed Turkey Medium Sub	1	790	—	14
Tuna Salad Large Sub	1	1510	—	102
Tuna Salad Medium Sub	1	1070	—	72
Tuna Salad Pokket	1	720	—	50
Turkey D'Lite Pokket	1	330	—	2
Turkey D'Lite Small Sub	1	365	—	4
Turkey Large Sub	1	710	—	7
Turkey Medium Sub	1	520	—	5
Turkey Club Large Sub	1	860	—	20
Turkey Club Medium Sub	1	630	—	15

FOOD	PORTION	CALS.	SAT. FAT	FAT
Turkey Club Pokket	1	400	—	9
Turkey Club Small Sub	1	430	—	10
DELTACO				
BEVERAGES				
M&M's Toppers	1 serv	256	4	8
Orange Juice	1 serv	83	0	tr
Oreos Toppers	1 serv	257	4	10
Shake Chocolate	1 sm	549	10	16
Shake Chocolate	1 med	755	14	22
Shake Orange	1 sm	609	10	16
Shake Orange	1 med	837	14	22
Shake Strawberry	1 sm	486	10	16
Shake Strawberry	1 med	668	14	22
Shake Vanilla	1 med	707	17	25
Shake Vanilla	1 sm	514	12	18
BREAKFAST SELECTIONS				
Burrito Beef And Egg	1	529	10	27
Burrito Breakfast	1	256	4	11
Burrito Egg And Cheese	1	443	8	22
Burrito Egg and Bean	1	470	8	22
Burrito Steak And Egg	1	500	9	25
CHILDREN'S MENU SELECTIONS				
Kid's Meal Hamburger	1 meal	617	7	20
Kid's Meal Taco	1 meal	532	6	17
MAIN MENU SELECTIONS				
American Cheese	1 slice	53	3	4
Beans And Cheese	1	122	2	3
Burrito Chicken	1	264	4	10
Burrito Combination	1	413	7	17
Burrito Del Beef	1	440	9	20
Burrito Deluxe Chicken	1	549	10	34
Burrito Deluxe Combo	1	453	9	20
Burrito Deluxe Del Beef	1	479	10	23
Burrito Green	1	229	3	8
Burrito Green Regular	1	330	5	11
Burrito Macho Beef	1	893	18	41
Burrito Macho Combo	1	774	15	31
Burrito Red	1	235	4	8
Burrito Red Regular	1	342	5	12
Burrito Spicy Chicken	1	392	3	11
Burrito The Works	1	448	6	18
Cheeseburger	1	284	6	13
Chicken Salad	1	254	6	19

FOOD	PORTION	CALS.	SAT. FAT	FAT
Chicken Salad Deluxe	1	716	15	47
Del Burger	1	385	6	20
Del Cheeseburger	1	439	9	25
Double Del Cheeseburger	1	618	16	39
French Fries	1 sm	242	4	11
French Fries	1 reg	404	6	19
French Fries	1 lg	566	9	26
Fries Chili Cheese	1 serv	562	13	30
Fries Deluxe Chili Cheese	1 serv	600	15	33
Fries Nacho	1 serv	669	11	34
Guacamole	1 oz	60	0	6
Hamburger	1	231	3	8
Hot Sauce	1 pkg	2	0	tr
Nacho Cheese Sauce	1 side order	100	2	8
Nachos	1 serv	390	4	32
Nachos Macho	1	1089	13	61
Quesadilla	1	257	6	12
Quesadilla Chicken	1	544	16	31
Quesadilla Regular	1	483	16	27
Quesadilla Spicy Jack	1	254	6	12
Quesadilla Spicy Jack Chicken	1	537	17	30
Quesadilla Spicy Jack Regular	1	476	16	27
Salsa	2 oz	14	0	tr
Salsa Dressing	1 oz	33	2	3
Soft Taco	1	146	3	6
Soft Taco Chicken	1	197	3	11
Soft Taco Deluxe Double Beef	1	211	5	11
Soft Taco Double Beef	1	178	3	8
Sour Cream	1 oz	60	4	6
Taco	1	140	3	8
Taco Chicken	1	186	3	13
Taco Deluxe Double Beef	1	205	5	13
Taco Double Beef	1	172	3	10
Taco Salad	1	235	6	19
Taco Salad Deluxe	1	741	16	49
Tostada	1	140	3	8

DENNY'S
BEVERAGES

FOOD	PORTION	CALS.	SAT. FAT	FAT
Chocolate Milk	1 serv (10 oz)	235	6	9
Coffee French Vanilla	1 serv (8 oz)	76	1	1
Coffee Hazelnut	1 serv (8 oz)	66	1	1
Coffee Irish Cream	1 serv (8 oz)	73	1	1
Grapefruit Juice	1 serv (10 oz)	115	0	0

FOOD	PORTION	CALS.	SAT. FAT	FAT
Hot Chocolate	1 serv (8 oz)	90	0	2
Orange Juice	1 serv (10 oz)	126	0	0
Tomato Juice	1 serv (10 oz)	56	0	0
BREAKFAST SELECTIONS				
All American Slam	1 serv (15 oz)	1028	21	87
Applesauce	1 serv (3 oz)	60	0	0
Bacon	4 strips (1 oz)	162	5	18
Bagel Dry	1 (3 oz)	235	0	1
Banana	1 (4 oz)	110	0	0
Banana Strawberry Medley	1 serv (4 oz)	108	0	1
Biscuit Plain	1 (3 oz)	375	5	22
Biscuit w/ Sausage Gravy	1 serv (7 oz)	570	10	38
Blueberry Topping	1 serv (3 oz)	106	0	0
Canadian Bacon	1 serv (3 oz)	110	2	5
Cantaloup	1 serv (3 oz)	32	0	0
Cheddar Cheese Omelette	1 serv (13 oz)	770	20	62
Cherry Topping	1 serv (3 oz)	86	0	0
Chicken Fried Steak & Eggs	1 serv (14 oz)	723	18	56
Country Scramble	1 serv (16 oz)	795	11	50
Cream Cheese	1 oz	100	6	10
Egg	1 (2 oz)	134	3	12
Egg Beaters	1 serv (2.3 oz)	71	1	5
Eggs Benedict	1 serv (19 oz)	860	23	56
English Muffin Dry	1 (4 oz)	125	0	1
Farmer's Omelette	1 serv (18 oz)	912	19	69
French Slam	1 serv (14 oz)	1029	20	71
French Toast	2 pieces (8 oz)	510	6	25
Fresh Fruit Mix	1 serv (3 oz)	36	0	0
Grapefruit	½ (5 oz)	60	0	0
Grapes	1 serv (3 oz)	55	0	1
Grits	1 serv (4 oz)	80	0	0
Ham	1 serv (3 oz)	94	1	3
Ham'n'Cheddar Omelette	1 serv (14 oz)	743	10	55
Hashed Browns	1 serv (4 oz)	218	2	14
Hashed Browns Covered	1 serv (6 oz)	318	7	23
Hashed Browns Covered & Smothered	1 serv (8 oz)	359	7	26
Honeydew	1 serv (3 oz)	31	0	0
Junior Meals Basic Breakfast	1 serv (9 oz)	558	9	39
Junior Meals Junior French Slam	1 serv (7 oz)	461	10	35
Junior Meals Junior Grand Slam	1 serv (5 oz)	397	7	25
Junior Meals Junior Waffle Supreme	1 serv (4 oz)	190	2	11
Meat Lover's Sampler	1 serv (14 oz)	806	17	62

FOOD	PORTION	CALS.	SAT. FAT	FAT
Moon Over My Hammy	1 serv (12 oz)	807	8	48
Muffin Blueberry	1 (3 oz)	309	0	14
Oatmeal	1 serv (4 oz)	100	0	2
Original Grand Slam	1 serv (10 oz)	795	14	50
Pancakes	3 (5 oz)	491	1	7
Pork Chop & Eggs	1 serv (12 oz)	555	9	36
Porterhouse Steak & Eggs	1 serv (18 oz)	1223	32	95
Ready To Eat Cereal	1 serv (1 oz)	100	0	0
Sausage	4 links (3 oz)	354	2	32
Sausage Cheddar Omelette	1 serv (16 oz)	1036	29	86
Scram Slam	1 serv (18 oz)	974	23	80
Senior Belgian Waffle Slam	1 serv (6 oz)	399	8	33
Senior Omelette	1 serv (12 oz)	623	10	47
Senior Starter	1 serv (7 oz)	336	5	24
Senior Triple Play	1 serv (8 oz)	537	6	25
Sirloin Steak & Eggs	1 serv (13 oz)	808	18	64
Slim Slam	1 serv (14 oz)	638	3	12
Southern Slam	1 serv (13 oz)	1065	23	84
Strawberries w/ Sugar	1 serv (3 oz)	115	0	1
Strawberry Topping	1 serv (3 oz)	115	0	1
Sunshine Slam	1 serv (8 oz)	537	6	25
Super Play It Again Slam	1 serv (15 oz)	1192	21	75
Syrup	3 tbsp (1.5 oz)	143	0	0
Syrup Reduced Calorie	1 serv (1.5 oz)	25	0	0
T-Bone Steak & Eggs	1 serv (16 oz)	1045	26	82
Toast Dry	1 slice (1 oz)	92	0	1
Ultimate Omelette	1 serv (17 oz)	780	14	62
Veggie Cheese Omelette	1 serv (16 oz)	714	10	53
Waffle	1 (6 oz)	304	3	21
Whipped Margarine	1 serv (0.5 oz)	87	2	10
Whipped Cream	1 serv (2 oz)	23	0	2
DESSERTS				
Apple Pie	1 serv (7 oz)	430	5	20
Apple Pie w/ Equal	1 serv (7 oz)	370	5	20
Banana Split	1 serv (19 oz)	894	19	43
Blueberry Topping	1 serv (3 oz)	106	0	0
Cheesecake Pie	1 serv (4 oz)	470	13	27
Cherry Topping	1 serv (3 oz)	86	0	0
Cherry Pie	1 serv (7 oz)	540	5	21
Chocolate Topping	1 serv (2 oz)	317	0	25
Chocolate Cake	1 serv (4 oz)	370	4	17
Chocolate Pecan Pie	1 serv (6 oz)	790	9	37
Chocolate Shake	1 serv (10 oz)	579	17	27
Coconut Cream Pie	1 serv (7 oz)	480	16	26

FOOD	PORTION	CALS.	SAT. FAT	FAT
Double Scoop Sundae	1 serv (6 oz)	375	12	27
Dutch Apple Pie	1 serv (7 oz)	440	5	19
French Silk Pie	1 serv (6 oz)	650	26	43
Fudge Topping	1 serv (2 oz)	201	7	10
German Chocolate Pie	1 serv (7 oz)	580	18	33
Hot Fudge Cake Sundae	1 serv (8 oz)	687	11	38
Ice Cream Float	1 serv (12 oz)	280	6	10
Key Lime Pie	1 serv (6 oz)	600	15	27
Lemon Meringue Pie	1 serv (7 oz)	460	4	17
Pecan Pie	1 serv (6 oz)	600	4	28
Single Scoop Sundae	1 serv (3 oz)	188	6	14
Strawberry Topping	1 serv (3 oz)	115	0	1
Vanilla Shake	1 serv (11 oz)	581	17	27
MAIN MENU SELECTIONS				
BBQ Sauce	1 serv (1.5 oz)	47	0	1
Bacon Cheddar Burger	1 (14 oz)	935	25	63
Bacon Lettuce & Tomato Sandwich	1 (6 oz)	634	8	46
Baked Potato Plain	1 (6 oz)	186	0	0
Battered Cod Dinner w/ Tartar Sauce	1 serv (9 oz)	732	7	47
Broccoli In Butter Sauce	2 serv (4 oz)	50	2	2
Brown Gravy	1 serv (1 oz)	13	0	0
Buffalo Chicken Strips	1 serv (10 oz)	734	4	42
Buffalo Wings	12 pieces (15 oz)	856	17	54
Carrots In Honey Glaze	2 serv (4 oz)	80	1	3
Charleston Chicken Sandwich	1 (11 oz)	632	7	32
Chicken Quesadilla	1 serv (16 oz)	827	23	55
Chicken Fried Chicken	1 serv (6 oz)	327	4	18
Chicken Fried Steak w/ Gravy	1 serv (4 oz)	265	8	17
Chicken Gravy	1 serv (1 oz)	14	0	1
Chicken Melt Sandwich	1 (7 oz)	520	5	29
Chicken Strip w/ Dressing	1 serv (10 oz)	635	1	25
Chicken Strips	5 pieces (10 oz)	720	4	33
Classic Burger	1 (11 oz)	673	15	40
Classic Burger w/ Cheese	1 (13 oz)	836	19	53
Club Sandwich	1	485	6	35
Corn In Butter Sauce	2 serv (4 oz)	120	2	4
Cornbread Stuffing Plain	1 serv (2 oz)	182	0	9
Cottage Cheese	1 serv (3 oz)	72	2	3
Country Gravy	1 serv (1 oz)	17	0	1
Delidinger Sandwich	1 (14 oz)	852	6	45
Deluxe Grilled Cheese Sandwich	1 (7 oz)	482	2	26
Dinner Roll	1 (1.5 oz)	132	0	2

FOOD	PORTION	CALS.	SAT. FAT	FAT
French Fries Unsalted	1 serv (4 oz)	323	3	14
Fried Fish Sandwich	1 (11 oz)	905	8	56
Gardenburger Patty	1 patty (3.4 oz)	160	0	3
Gardenburger Patty w/ Bun & Fat Free Honey Mustard Dressing	1 serv (11.1 oz)	653	6	32
Green Beans w/ Bacon	2 serv (4 oz)	60	2	4
Green Peas In Butter Sauce	2 serv (4 oz)	100	2	2
Grilled Mushrooms	1 serv (2 oz)	14	0	0
Grilled Alaskan Salmon	1 serv (7 oz)	296	2	14
Grilled Chicken Breast	1 serv (4 oz)	130	1	4
Grilled Chicken Dinner	1 serv (4 oz)	130	1	4
Grilled Chicken Sandwich	1 (11 oz)	509	5	19
Grilled Chopped Steak w/ Gravy	1 serv (10 oz)	400	11	26
Ham & Swiss On Rye	1 (9 oz)	533	4	31
Hashed Browns	1 serv (4 oz)	218	2	14
Herb Toast	1 serv (2 oz)	200	2	11
Horseradish Sauce	1 serv (1.5 oz)	170	3	20
Junior Meals Junior Burger	1 serv (3 oz)	261	4	15
Junior Meals Junior Chicken Strips	1 serv (5 oz)	318	1	12
Junior Meals Junior Fried Fish	1 serv (5 oz)	465	5	34
Junior Meals Junior Grilled Cheese	1 serv (4 oz)	375	3	22
Junior Meals Junior Shrimp Basket	1 serv (4 oz)	291	3	16
Lunch Basket Charleston Chicken Ranch Melt	1 serv (14 oz)	975	10	59
Lunch Basket Chicken Strips	1 serv (8 oz)	568	4	26
Lunch Basket Classic Burger	1 serv (12 oz)	674	13	39
Lunch Basket Delidinger	1 serv (14 oz)	852	6	45
Lunch Basket Five Star Philly	1 serv (10 oz)	657	8	29
Lunch Basket Patty Melt	1 serv (8 oz)	696	12	42
Mashed Potatoes Plain	1 serv (6 oz)	105	0	1
Mayonnaise	2 tbsp (1 oz)	200	3	22
Mozzarella Sticks w/ Sauce	8 pieces (10 oz)	756	24	43
Onion Ring Basket	1 serv (5 oz)	439	7	27
Onion Rings	1 serv (3 oz)	264	4	16
Patty Melt Sandwich	1 (8 oz)	695	13	44
Pork Chop Dinner w/ Gravy	1 serv (8 oz)	386	8	24
Porterhouse Steak	1 (14 oz)	708	24	54
Pot Roast Dinner w/ Gravy	1 serv (7 oz)	260	4	11
Rice Pilaf	1 serv (3 oz)	112	0	2
Roast Turkey & Stuffing	1 serv (12 oz)	701	1	27
Sampler	1 serv (15 oz)	1120	19	59

FOOD	PORTION	CALS.	SAT. FAT	FAT
Seasoned Fries	1 serv (4 oz)	261	3	12
Senior Battered Cod	1 serv (5 oz)	465	5	34
Senior Chicken Fried Steak	1 serv (8 oz)	341	8	18
Senior Grilled Cheese Sandwich	1 serv	360	10	25
Senior Grilled Chicken Breast	1 serv (6 oz)	219	1	6
Senior Liver w/ Bacon & Onions	1 serv (8 oz)	322	5	19
Senior Pork Chop	1 serv (4 oz)	193	4	12
Senior Pot Roast	1 serv (5 oz)	149	2	6
Senior Roast Turkey & Stuffing	1 serv (8 oz)	596	1	25
Senior Turkey Sandwich	1	340	3	27
Senior Sandwich Ham & Swiss	1 serv (9 oz)	497	4	30
Shrimp Dinner	1 serv (8 oz)	558	6	32
Sirloin Steak Dinner	1 serv (5.5 oz)	271	9	21
Sliced Tomatoes	3 slices (2 oz)	13	0	0
Sour Cream	1 serv (1.5 oz)	91	6	9
Steak & Shrimp Dinner w/ Gravy	1 serv (9 oz)	645	14	42
Super Bird Sandwich	1 (9 oz)	620	5	32
T-Bone Steak Dinner	1 serv (10 oz)	530	18	40
Turkey Breast On Multigrain	1 (9 oz)	476	3	26
SALAD DRESSINGS				
Bleu Cheese	1 oz	124	4	12
Caesar	1 oz	142	2	15
Creamy Italian	1 oz	106	2	10
Fat Free Honey Mustard	1 oz	38	0	0
French	1 oz	106	2	10
Oriental Peanut Dressing	1 serv (1 oz)	106	1	8
Ranch	1 oz	101	2	11
Reduced Calorie French	1 oz	76	1	5
Reduced Calorie Italian	1 oz	32	0	1
Thousand Island	1 oz	104	2	10
SALADS AND SALAD BARS				
Buffalo Chicken Salad	1 serv (17 oz)	615	8	37
Fried Chicken Salad	1 serv (13 oz)	506	8	31
Garden Chicken Delight Salad	1 serv (16 oz)	277	1	5
Grilled Chicken Caesar Salad w/ Dressing	1 serv (13 oz)	655	9	47
Oriental Chicken Salad w/ Dressing	1 serv (20 oz)	568	5	26
Side Caesar w/ Dressing	1 serv (6 oz)	338	5	25
Side Garden Salad w/ Dressing	1 serv (7 oz)	113	1	4
SOUPS				
Cheese	1 serv (8 oz)	293	13	23
Chicken Noodle	1 serv (8 oz)	60	0	2
Clam Chowder	1 serv (8 oz)	214	9	11

FOOD	PORTION	CALS.	SAT. FAT	FAT
Cream Of Broccoli	1 serv (8 oz)	193	9	12
Cream of Potato	1 serv (8 oz)	222	9	12
Split Pea	1 serv (8 oz)	146	2	6
Vegetable Beef	1 serv (8 oz)	79	1	1

DOMINO'S PIZZA

12 INCH MEDIUM PIZZAS

FOOD	PORTION	CALS.	SAT. FAT	FAT
Add A Topping Anchovies	1 topping serv	23	tr	1
Add A Topping Bacon	1 topping serv	81	2	7
Add A Topping Banana Peppers	1 topping serv	3	—	tr
Add A Topping Canned Mushrooms	1 topping serv	4	tr	tr
Add A Topping Cheddar Cheese	1 topping serv	57	3	5
Add A Topping Cooked Beef	1 topping serv	56	2	5
Add A Topping Extra Cheese	1 topping serv	48	2	4
Add A Topping Fresh Mushrooms	1 topping serv	4	tr	tr
Add A Topping Green Olives	1 topping serv	12	tr	1
Add A Topping Green Peppers	1 topping serv	3	—	tr
Add A Topping Ham	1 topping serv	18	tr	1
Add A Topping Italian Sausage	1 topping serv	55	2	4
Add A Topping Onion	1 topping serv	4	—	tr
Add A Topping Pepperoni	1 topping serv	62	2	6
Add A Topping Pineapple Tidbits	1 topping serv	10	0	0
Add A Topping Ripe Olives	1 topping serv	14	tr	1
Deep Dish Cheese	2 slices (6.3 oz)	477	8	22
Hand Tossed Cheese	2 slices (5.2 oz)	347	5	11
Thin Crust Cheese	¼ pie (3.7 oz)	271	5	12

14 INCH LARGE PIZZAS

FOOD	PORTION	CALS.	SAT. FAT	FAT
Add A Topping Anchovies	1 topping serv	23	tr	1
Add A Topping Bacon	1 topping serv	75	2	6
Add A Topping Banana Peppers	1 topping serv	3	—	tr
Add A Topping Canned Mushrooms	1 topping serv	3	tr	tr
Add A Topping Cheddar Cheese	1 topping serv	48	2	4
Add A Topping Cooked Beef	1 topping serv	44	2	4
Add A Topping Extra Cheese	1 topping serv	45	2	4
Add A Topping Fresh Mushrooms	1 topping serv	3	tr	tr
Add A Topping Green Olives	1 topping serv	11	tr	1
Add A Topping Green Peppers	1 topping serv	2	—	tr
Add A Topping Ham	1 topping serv	17	tr	1
Add A Topping Italian Sausage	1 topping serv	44	1	3
Add A Topping Onion	1 topping serv	3	—	tr
Add A Topping Pepperoni	1 topping serv	55	2	5
Add A Topping Pineapple Tidbits	1 topping serv	8	0	0

FOOD	PORTION	CALS.	SAT. FAT	FAT
Add A Topping Ripe Olives	1 topping serv	12	tr	1
Deep Dish Cheese	2 slices (6.1 oz)	455	8	20
Hand-Tossed Cheese	2 slices (4.8 oz)	317	5	10
Thin Crust Cheese	⅛ pie (3.5 oz)	253	5	11
6 INCH DEEP DISH PIZZAS				
Add A Topping Anchovies	1 topping serv	45	tr	2
Add A Topping Bacon	1 topping serv	82	2	7
Add A Topping Banana Peppers	1 topping serv	3	—	tr
Add A Topping Canned Mushrooms	1 topping serv	2	0	tr
Add A Topping Cheddar Cheese	1 topping serv	86	4	7
Add A Topping Cooked Beef	1 topping serv	44	2	4
Add A Topping Extra Cheese	1 topping serv	57	3	5
Add A Topping Fresh Mushrooms	1 topping serv	2	0	tr
Add A Topping Green Olives	1 topping serv	10	tr	1
Add A Topping Green Peppers	1 topping serv	2	—	tr
Add A Topping Ham	1 topping serv	17	tr	1
Add A Topping Italian Sausage	1 topping serv	44	1	3
Add A Topping Onion	1 topping serv	3	—	tr
Add A Topping Pepperoni	1 topping serv	50	2	5
Add A Topping Pineapple Tidbits	1 topping serv	5	0	0
Add A Topping Ripe Olives	1 topping serv	11	tr	1
Cheese	1 pie (7.6 oz)	595	11	27
MAIN MENU SELECTIONS				
Breadstick	1 (0.8 oz)	78	1	3
Buffalo Wings Barbeque	1 piece (0.9 oz)	50	1	2
Buffalo Wings Hot	1 piece (0.9 oz)	45	1	2
Cheesy Bread	1 piece (1 oz)	103	2	5
Garden Salad	1 sm (4.3 oz)	22	tr	tr
Garden Salad	1 lg (7.7 oz)	39	tr	tr
SALAD DRESSINGS				
Marzetti Blue Cheese	1 serv (1.5 oz)	220	4	24
Marzetti Creamy Caesar	1 serv (1.5 oz)	200	3	22
Marzetti Fat Free Ranch	1 serv (1.5 oz)	40	0	0
Marzetti Honey French	1 serv (1.5 oz)	210	3	18
Marzetti House Italian	1 serv (1.5 oz)	220	3	24
Marzetti Light Italian	1 serv (1.5 oz)	20	0	1
Marzetti Ranch	1 serv (1.5 oz)	260	4	29
Marzetti Thousand Island	1 serv (1.5 oz)	200	3	20

DUNKIN' DONUTS
BAGELS AND CREAM CHEESE

FOOD	PORTION	CALS.	SAT. FAT	FAT
Bagel Blueberry	1 (4.4 oz)	330	0	1
Bagel Cinnamon Raisin	1 (4.4 oz)	340	0	1

FOOD	PORTION	CALS.	SAT. FAT	FAT
Bagel Egg	1 (4.4 oz)	340	0	2
Bagel Everything	1 (4.4 oz)	340	0	2
Bagel Garlic	1 (4.4 oz)	330	0	1
Bagel Onion	1 (4.4 oz)	320	0	1
Bagel Plain	1 (4.4 oz)	330	0	1
Bagel Plain	1 (3 oz)	200	0	1
Bagel Poppy	1 (4.4 oz)	340	0	3
Bagel Pumpernickel	1 (4.4 oz)	340	0	2
Bagel Salt	1 (4.4 oz)	320	0	1
Bagel Sesame	1 (4.4 oz)	350	0	4
Bagel Whole Wheat	1 (4.4 oz)	320	0	2
Bagel Sticks Cinnamon Sugar	1 (2.9 oz)	210	0	1
Bagel Sticks Jalapeno Cheddar	1 (2.9 oz)	210	0	1
Bagel Sticks Santa Fe Ranch	1 (2.9 oz)	210	0	1
Bagel Sticks Spinach Romano	1 (2.9 oz)	210	0	1
Cream Cheese Classic Lite	2 tbsp (1 oz)	60	3	5
Cream Cheese Classic Plain	2 tbsp (1 oz)	100	6	10
Cream Cheese Garden Veggie	2 tbsp (1 oz)	90	5	9
Cream Cheese Honey Walnut	2 tbsp (1 oz)	100	5	9
Cream Cheese Savory Chive	2 tbsp (1 oz)	100	6	10
Cream Cheese Smoked Salmon	2 tbsp (1 oz)	100	5	9
Cream Cheese Strawberry	2 tbsp (1 oz)	100	5	9
Super Bagel Glazed Apple Cinnamon	1 (4.6 oz)	350	0	1
BAKED SELECTIONS				
Bismark	1 (2.8 oz)	310	4	14
Bow Tie	1 (2.5 oz)	250	3	10
Brownie Blondie w/ Chocolate Chips	1 (2.4 oz)	300	3	13
Brownie Fudge	1 (2.4 oz)	290	3	13
Brownie Peanut Butter Blondie	1 (2.4 oz)	330	4	18
Cake Donut Blueberry	1 (2.4 oz)	230	3	10
Cake Donut Blueberry Crumb	1 (2.6 oz)	260	3	11
Cake Donut Butternut	1 (2.6 oz)	340	5	20
Cake Donut Chocolate	1 (2.1 oz)	210	3	14
Cake Donut Chocolate Coconut	1 (2.4 oz)	250	5	15
Cake Donut Chocolate Glazed	1 (2.5 oz)	250	3	14
Cake Donut Cinnamon	1 (2.3 oz)	300	4	19
Cake Donut Coconut	1 (2.5 oz)	320	5	20
Cake Donut Double Chocolate	1 (2.6 oz)	260	3	14
Cake Donut Old Fashioned	1 (2.1 oz)	280	4	19
Cake Donut Peanut	1 (2.6 oz)	340	4	22
Cake Donut Powdered	1 (2.4 oz)	310	4	19
Cake Donut Sugared	1 (2.4 oz)	310	4	20

FOOD	PORTION	CALS.	SAT. FAT	FAT
Cake Donut Toasted Coconut	1 (2.5 oz)	320	5	19
Cake Donut Whole Wheat Glazed	1 (2.7 oz)	230	3	11
Coffee Roll	1 (2.6 oz)	280	3	13
Coffee Roll Chocolate Frosted	1 (2.7 oz)	290	3	14
Coffee Roll Cinnamon Raisin	1 (3.1 oz)	330	3	13
Coffee Roll Maple Frosted	1 (2.7 oz)	300	3	13
Coffee Roll Vanilla Frosted	1 (2.7 oz)	300	3	13
Cookie Chocolate Chocolate Chunk	1 (1.5 oz)	200	6	11
Cookie Chocolate Chunk	1 (1.5 oz)	200	6	10
Cookie Chocolate Chunk w/ Nut	1 (1.5 oz)	200	6	11
Cookie Chocolate White Chocolate Chunk	1 (1.5 oz)	200	6	11
Cookie Oatmeal Raisin Pecan	1 (1.5 oz)	190	5	9
Cookie Peanut Butter Chocolate Chunk w/ Nuts	1 (1.5 oz)	210	6	13
Cookie Peanut Butter Chocolate Chunk w/ Peanuts	1 (1.5 oz)	210	5	12
Croissant Almond	1 (2.7 oz)	360	5	21
Croissant Cheese	1 (2.5 oz)	240	3	15
Croissant Chocolate	1 (2.5 oz)	370	8	23
Croissant Plain	1 (2.1 oz)	270	4	17
Crullers/Sticks Dunkin' Donut	1 (2.1 oz)	240	3	14
Crullers/Sticks Glazed	1 (3 oz)	340	3	14
Crullers/Sticks Glazed Chocolate	1 (3.2 oz)	410	6	24
Crullers/Sticks Jelly	1 (3.2 oz)	330	3	14
Crullers/Sticks Plain	1 (2.1 oz)	260	3	14
Crullers/Sticks Powdered	1 (2.3 oz)	290	4	14
Crullers/Sticks Sugar	1 (2.2 oz)	270	3	14
Eclair	1 (3.2 oz)	290	3	12
English Muffin	1 (2 oz)	130	1	1
French Roll	1 (2.1 oz)	140	0	1
Fritter Apple	1 (3.3 oz)	300	3	13
Fritter Glazed	1 (2.7 oz)	290	3	13
Muffin Banana Nut	1 (3.3 oz)	340	3	12
Muffin Blueberry	1 (3.3 oz)	310	2	10
Muffin Cherry	1 (3.3 oz)	330	3	11
Muffin Chocolate Chip	1 (3.3 oz)	400	6	16
Muffin Corn	1 (3.3 oz)	350	1	14
Muffin Cranberry Orange Nut	1 (3.5 oz)	310	3	11
Muffin Honey Raisin Bran	1 (3.3 oz)	330	0	10
Muffin Lemon Poppy Seed	1 (3.3 oz)	360	3	13
Muffin Oat Bran	1 (3.2 oz)	290	1	11

FOOD	PORTION	CALS.	SAT. FAT	FAT
Muffin Lowfat Apple n' Spice	1 (3.3 oz)	220	0	2
Muffin Lowfat Banana	1 (3.3 oz)	240	0	2
Muffin Lowfat Blueberry	1 (3.3 oz)	230	0	2
Muffin Lowfat Bran	1 (3.3 oz)	260	0	2
Muffin Lowfat Cherry	1 (3.3 oz)	230	0	2
Muffin Lowfat Corn	1 (3.3 oz)	250	0	2
Muffin Lowfat Cranberry Orange	1 (3.3 oz)	230	0	2
Munchkins Butternut	3 (2 oz)	230	4	11
Munchkins Chocolate Glazed	3 (2 oz)	180	2	10
Munchkins Cinnamon	4 (2 oz)	240	3	13
Munchkins Coconut	3 (1.7 oz)	200	4	11
Munchkins Glazed Cake	3 (2.1 oz)	220	2	9
Munchkins Glazed Raised	4 (2.1 oz)	210	2	7
Munchkins Jelly	3 (1.9 oz)	170	1	5
Munchkins Lemon	3 (2 oz)	160	1	6
Munchkins Plain	4 (1.8 oz)	200	3	12
Munchkins Powdered Sugar	4 (2 oz)	240	3	13
Munchkins Sugar Raised	6 (1.9 oz)	210	3	10
Munchkins Toasted Coconut	3 (1.8 oz)	210	3	11
Tart Apple	1 (3.4 oz)	310	3	10
Tart Blueberry	1 (3.4 oz)	300	3	10
Tart Lemon	1 (3.4 oz)	280	3	11
Tart Raspberry	1 (3.4 oz)	310	3	10
Tart Strawberry	1 (3.4 oz)	310	3	10
Turnover Apple	1 (3.8 oz)	350	4	15
Turnover Blueberry	1 (3.8 oz)	370	4	15
Turnover Lemon	1 (3.8 oz)	350	4	15
Turnover Raspberry	1 (3.8 oz)	380	4	15
Turnover Strawberry	1 (3.8 oz)	380	4	15
Yeast Donut Apple Crumb	1 (2.6 oz)	250	3	11
Yeast Donut Apple n' Spice	1 (2.5 oz)	230	3	10
Yeast Donut Bavarian Kreme	1 (2.5 oz)	250	3	11
Yeast Donut Black Raspberry	1 (2.4 oz)	240	3	10
Yeast Donut Boston Kreme	1 (2.8 oz)	270	3	11
Yeast Donut Chocolate Kreme Filled	1 (2.6 oz)	320	4	16
Yeast Donut Chocolate Frosted	1 (2.1 oz)	210	2	8
Yeast Donut Glazed	1 (1.6 oz)	160	2	7
Yeast Donut Jelly Filled	1 (2.4 oz)	240	3	10
Yeast Donut Lemon	1 (2.5 oz)	240	3	11
Yeast Donut Maple Frosted	1 (2.1 oz)	210	2	8
Yeast Donut Marble Frosted	1 (2.1 oz)	210	2	8
Yeast Donut Strawberry	1 (2.4 oz)	240	3	10

FOOD	PORTION	CALS.	SAT. FAT	FAT
Yeast Donut Strawberry Frosted	1 (2.1 oz)	220	2	8
Yeast Donut Sugar Raised	1 (1.6 oz)	170	2	7
Yeast Donut Vanilla Frosted	1 (2.1 oz)	220	2	8
BEVERAGES				
Coffee Coolatta w/ 2% Milk	1 (15.7 oz)	210	2	2
Coffee Coolatta w/ Cream	1 (15.7 oz)	370	14	22
Coffee Coolatta w/ Skim Milk	1 (15.7 oz)	190	0	0
Coffee Coolatta w/ Whole Milk	1 (15.7 oz)	230	3	4
Cream	1 serv (1 oz)	60	3	5
Dark Roast	1 serv (10 oz)	5	0	0
Decaf	1 serv (10 oz)	0	0	0
French Vanilla	1 serv (10 oz)	5	0	0
Hazelnut	1 serv (10 oz)	5	0	0
Hazelnut Coolatta w/ 2% Milk	1 (15.7 oz)	210	2	2
Hazelnut Coolatta w/ Cream	1 (15.7 oz)	370	13	22
Hazelnut Coolatta w/ Skim Milk	1 (15.7 oz)	200	0	0
Hazelnut Coolatta w/ Whole Milk	1 (15.7 oz)	230	3	4
Mocha Coolatta w/ 2% Milk	1 (15.7 oz)	220	2	2
Mocha Coolatta w/ Cream	1 (15.7 oz)	380	13	22
Mocha Coolatta w/ Skim Milk	1 (15.7 oz)	200	0	0
Mocha Coolatta w/ Whole Milk	1 (15.7 oz)	230	3	4
Regular	1 serv (10 oz)	5	0	0
Vanilla Coolatta w/ 2% Milk	1 (15.7 oz)	220	2	2
Vanilla Coolatta w/ Cream	1 (15.7 oz)	380	13	22
Vanilla Coolatta w/ Skim Milk	1 (15.7 oz)	200	0	0
Vanilla Coolatta w/ Whole Milk	1 (15.7 oz)	230	3	4
SANDWICHES				
Croissant Sandwich Broccoli & Cheese	1 (6.1 oz)	370	6	21
Croissant Sandwich Chicken Salad	1 (7.6 oz)	540	7	31
Croissant Sandwich Egg & Cheese	1 (5 oz)	430	9	27
Croissant Sandwich Egg Bacon & Cheese	1 (5.4 oz)	500	12	34
Croissant Sandwich Egg Ham & Cheese	1 (6 oz)	530	9	29
Croissant Sandwich Egg Sausage & Cheese	1 (6.9 oz)	630	15	49
Croissant Sandwich Ham & Cheese	1 (6.7 oz)	710	13	32
Croissant Sandwich Roast Beef & Cheese	1 (6 oz)	490	8	27

FOOD	PORTION	CALS.	SAT. FAT	FAT
Croissant Sandwich Seafood Salad	1 (7.6 oz)	480	6	26
Croissant Sandwich Tuna Salad	1 (7.5 oz)	540	6	30
SOUPS				
Beef Barley	1 serv (8 oz)	90	0	1
Beef Noodle	1 serv (8 oz)	90	0	1
Chicken Noodle	1 serv (8 oz)	80	1	2
Chili	1 serv (8 oz)	170	3	6
Chili Con Carne w/ Beans	1 serv (8 oz)	300	0	15
Cream Of Broccoli	1 serv (8 oz)	200	6	11
Cream Of Potato	1 serv (8 oz)	190	5	10
Harvest Vegetable	1 serv (8 oz)	80	0	2
Manhattan Clam Chowder	1 serv (8 oz)	70	0	1
Minestrone	1 serv (8 oz)	100	0	1
New England Clam Chowder	1 serv (8 oz)	200	3	10
Split Pea w/ Ham	1 serv (8 oz)	190	3	9

EINSTEIN BROS. BAGELS
BAGELS

FOOD	PORTION	CALS.	SAT. FAT	FAT
Bagel Chips Cinnamon Raisin Swirl	1 serv (1 oz)	90	0	1
Bagel Chips Plain	1 serv (1 oz)	90	0	0
Bagel Chips Sourdough Dill	1 serv (1 oz)	90	0	1
Bagel Chips Sun Dried Tomato	1 serv (1 oz)	90	0	1
Bagel Chips Sunflower	1 serv (1 oz)	100	0	2
Bagel Chips Wild Blueberry	1 serv (1 oz)	90	0	1
Chocolate Chip	1 (4 oz)	380	2	3
Chopped Garlic	1 (4.2 oz)	377	1	4
Chopped Onion	1 (4 oz)	340	1	3
Cinnamon Raisin Swirl	1 (4 oz)	360	0	1
Cinnamon Sugar	1	330	0	0
Dark Pumpernickel	1 (3.8 oz)	330	0	1
Everything	1 (4 oz)	342	0	2
Honey 8 Grain	1 (4 oz)	320	0	1
Nutty Banana	1 (4 oz)	370	1	3
Plain	1 (3.7 oz)	330	0	1
Poppy Dip'd	1 (3.9 oz)	346	0	2
Salt	1 (3.9 oz)	330	0	1
Sesame Dip'd	1 (4.1 oz)	381	1	5
Spinach Herb	1 (3.8 oz)	320	0	1
Sun Dried Tomato	1 (3.8 oz)	320	0	1
Veggie Confetti	1 (3.8 oz)	330	0	1
Wild Blueberry	1 (4 oz)	360	0	1

FOOD	PORTION	CALS.	SAT. FAT	FAT
SANDWICHES AND FILLINGS				
Butter & Margarine Blend	1 serv (0.4 oz)	60	2	7
Capers	1 tbsp	0	0	0
Cheddar Cheese	1 serv (0.75 oz)	110	5	9
Classic New York Lox & Bagel	1 (11.4 oz)	560	13	24
Cream Cheese Cheddarpeno	1 serv (1 oz)	90	5	8
Cream Cheese Chive	1 serv (1 oz)	90	6	9
Cream Cheese Maple Walnut Raisin	1 serv (1 oz)	100	5	8
Cream Cheese Plain	1 serv (1 oz)	100	6	9
Cream Cheese Smoked Salmon	1 serv (1 oz)	90	5	8
Cream Cheese Strawberry	1 serv (1 oz)	90	5	8
Cream Cheese Sun Dried Tomato	1 serv (1 oz)	90	5	8
Cucumbers	1 serv (1 oz)	0	0	0
Fruit Spreads	1 tbsp	40	0	0
Ham	1 serv (2.5 oz)	75	1	2
Ham & Cheese Sandwich	1 (9.9 oz)	520	6	15
Honey	1 tbsp	64	0	0
Hummus	2 tbsp	60	0	3
Hummus Sandwich	1 (6 oz)	440	0	7
Lettuce	1 leaf	0	0	0
Lite Cream Cheese Plain	1 serv (1 oz)	60	3	5
Lite Cream Cheese Spinach Dill	1 serv (1 oz)	60	3	5
Lite Cream Cheese Veggie	1 serv (1 oz)	60	3	5
Lite Cream Cheese Wildberry	1 serv (1 oz)	70	3	4
Lowfat Chicken Salad Sandwich	1 (11.6 oz)	440	2	9
Lowfat Tuna Salad Sandwich	1 (11.6 oz)	440	2	8
Marshall's Loz	1 serv (2 oz)	90	2	4
Mayonnaise Lite Reduced Calorie	1 serv (0.5 oz)	50	1	5
Peanut Butter	1 serv (1.1 oz)	190	2	16
Peanut Butter & Jelly Sandwich	1 (6 oz)	595	2	17
Scrambled Egg Sandwich	1 (7.7 oz)	480	7	17
Scrambled Egg Sandwich w/ Meat & Cheese	1 (8.9 oz)	520	18	31
Smoked Turkey	1 serv (2.5 oz)	75	0	1
Smoked Turkey Sandwich	1 (9.9 oz)	480	5	14
Spouts Alfalfa	1 serv (0.5 oz)	0	0	0
Sweet Onions	1 serv (1 oz)	0	0	0
Swiss Cheese	1 serv (0.75 oz)	100	5	8
Tasty Turkey Sandwich	1 (10 oz)	530	12	22
Tomato	1 serv (1.5 oz)	0	0	0
Turkey Pastrami 99% Fat Free	1 serv (2.5 oz)	75	1	6
Turkey Pastrami Sandwich	1 (9.7 oz)	460	5	12

FOOD	PORTION	CALS.	SAT. FAT	FAT
Veg Out Sandwich	1 (8.9 oz)	350	6	17
Whitefish Salad Sandwich	1 (9.2 oz)	630	4	23

EL POLLO LOCO
MAIN MENU SELECTIONS

FOOD	PORTION	CALS.	SAT. FAT	FAT
Broccoli Slaw	1 serv (5 oz)	203	0	17
Burrito BRC	1 (9.3 oz)	482	5	15
Burrito Classic Chicken	1 (9.3 oz)	556	7	22
Burrito Grilled Steak	1 (11.3 oz)	705	13	32
Burrito Loco Grande	1 (13.1 oz)	632	7	26
Burrito Smokey Black Bean	1 (9.3 oz)	566	8	22
Burrito Spicy Hot Chicken	1 (9.8 oz)	559	7	22
Burrito Whole Wheat Chicken	1 (10.8 oz)	592	9	26
Chicken Breast	1 piece (3 oz)	160	2	6
Chicken Leg	1 piece (1.75 oz)	90	2	5
Chicken Soft Taco	1 (4 oz)	224	4	12
Chicken Thigh	1 piece (2 oz)	180	4	12
Chicken Wing	1 (1.5 oz)	110	2	6
Chicken Tamale	1 (3.5 oz)	190	2	8
Cole Slaw	1 serv (5 oz)	206	3	16
Corn-On-Cob	1 ear (5.5 oz)	146	0	2
Cornbread Stuffing	1 serv (6 oz)	281	2	12
Crispy Green Beans	1 serv (5 oz)	41	1	2
Cucumber Salad	1 serv (4.2 oz)	34	0	0
Fiesta Corn	1 serv (5 oz)	152	1	6
Flame Broiled Chicken Salad	1 serv (14.9 oz)	167	0	5
French Fries	1 serv (4.4 oz)	323	3	14
Garden Salad	1 serv (6.4 oz)	29	0	0
Gravy	1 serv (1 oz)	14	0	0
Honey Glazed Carrots	1 serv (5 oz)	104	1	6
Lime Parfait	1 serv (5 oz)	125	3	3
Macaroni & Cheese	1 serv (6 oz)	238	5	12
Mashed Potatoes	1 serv (5 oz)	97	0	1
Pinto Beans	1 serv (6 oz)	185	0	4
Polo Bowl	1 serv (19 oz)	504	2	13
Potato Salad	1 serv (6 oz)	256	2	14
Rainbow Pasta Salad	1 serv (5 oz)	157	0	1
Salad Shell	1 (5.6 oz)	440	4	27
Smokey Black Beans	1 serv (5 oz)	255	5	13
Southwest Cole Slaw	1 serv (5 oz)	178	2	13
Spanish Rice	1 serv (4 oz)	130	1	3
Spiced Apples	1 serv (5 oz)	146	0	0
Steak Bowl	1 serv (15.2 oz)	616	10	26

FOOD	PORTION	CALS.	SAT. FAT	FAT
Taco Al Carbon Chicken	1 serv (4.4 oz)	265	2	12
Taco Al Carbon Steak	1 (4.4 oz)	394	7	22
Taquito	1 serv (5 oz)	370	4	17
Tortilla Corn	1 (1.1 oz)	70	0	1
Tortilla Flour	1 (1 oz)	90	0	3
Tortilla Wrap Chicken Caesar	1 (10.47 oz)	518	3	19
Tortilla Wrap Southwest	1 (11.97 oz)	632	4	27
Tostada Salad Chicken	1 serv (14.7 oz)	332	5	14
Tostado Salad Steak	1 serv (13.2 oz)	525	14	31
SALAD DRESSINGS				
Blue Cheese	1 serv (2 oz)	300	6	32
Light Italian	1 serv (2 oz)	25	1	1
Ranch	1 serv (2 oz)	350	6	39
Thousand Island	1 serv (2 oz)	270	4	27

FOSTERS FREEZE
Soft Serve Vanilla	1 serv (4 oz)	152	—	4

FRIENDLY'S
FROZEN YOGURT

Apple Bettie	½ cup (2.6 oz)	140	2	3
Chocolate Fudge Brownie	½ cup (2.6 oz)	160	3	5
Fabulous Fudge Swirl	½ cup (2.6 oz)	140	3	3
Fudge Berry Swirl	½ cup (2.6 oz)	150	3	4
Lowfat Perfectly Peach	½ cup (2.6 oz)	110	1	2
Lowfat Purely Chocolate	½ cup (2.6 oz)	120	2	3
Lowfat Raspberry Delight	½ cup (2.6 oz)	120	2	3
Lowfat Simply Vanilla	½ cup (2.6 oz)	120	2	3
Lowfat Strawberry Patch	½ cup (2.6 oz)	110	1	2
Mint Chocolate Chip	½ cup (2.6 oz)	130	2	4
Strawberry Cheesecake Blast	½ cup (2.6 oz)	140	2	4
Toffee Almond Crunch	½ cup (2.6 oz)	160	2	5
ICE CREAM				
Black Raspberry	½ cup	150	5	7
Chocolate Almond Chip	½ cup	170	6	10
Forbidden Chocolate	½ cup	150	5	9
Fudge Nut Brownie	½ cup	200	7	11
Heath English Toffee	½ cup (2.7 oz)	190	6	10
Purely Pistachio	½ cup	160	6	10
Vanilla	½ cup	150	5	8
Vienna Mocha Chunk	½ cup	180	7	11

FRULLATI CAFE
BAKED SELECTIONS

Muffin Banana Nut	1 (4 oz)	394	3	15

FOOD	PORTION	CALS.	SAT. FAT	FAT
Muffin Cranberry Orange	1 (4 oz)	357	3	12
Muffin Fat Free Apple Streusel	1 (4 oz)	260	0	0
Muffin Fat Free Chocolate	1 (4 oz)	260	0	0
Muffin Fat Free Very Berry	1 (4 oz)	260	0	0
Muffin Sugar Free Blueberry	1 (4 oz)	308	1	9
Muffin Wild Blueberry	1 (4 oz)	344	3	11
BEVERAGES				
Apple Juice	1 serv (12 oz)	131	0	tr
Carrot Juice	1 serv (12 oz)	111	tr	tr
Celery Juice	1 serv (12 oz)	22	tr	tr
Lemondae	1 serv	209	0	tr
Lemondae Apple	1 serv	245	tr	tr
Lemondae Cherry	1 serv	237	tr	tr
Lemondae Orange	1 serv	270	tr	tr
Lemondae Strawberry	1 serv	234	0	tr
Orange Banana Juice	1 serv (12 oz)	150	tr	tr
Orange Juice	1 serv (12 oz)	126	0	tr
Smoothie A La Frullati	1 sm	275	6	9
Smoothie A La Frullati	1 lg	426	12	16
Smoothie Affinity	1 lg	378	12	16
Smoothie Affinity	1 sm	226	6	8
Smoothie Fiesta	1 lg	257	tr	1
Smoothie Fiesta	1 sm	234	tr	1
Smoothie Peach Banana	1 sm	266	tr	1
Smoothie Peach Banana	1 lg	289	tr	1
Smoothie Pina Colada	1 sm	236	6	8
Smoothie Pina Colada	1 lg	387	12	16
Smoothie Strawberry Banana	1 sm	165	tr	1
Smoothie Strawberry Banana	1 lg	188	tr	1
Smoothie Strawberry Blueberry	1 sm	90	0	1
Smoothie Strawberry Blueberry	1 lg	113	0	1
Smoothie Strawberry Fruit	1 lg	101	0	1
Smoothie Strawberry Fruit	1 sm	79	0	1
Smoothie Strawberry Watermelon	1 lg	123	0	1
Smoothie Strawberry Watermelon	1 sm	100	0	1
DESSERTS				
Frozen Yogurt	1 reg	205	tr	tr
Frozen Yogurt	1 lg	263	tr	tr
Frozen Yogurt	1 sm	146	tr	tr
Yogurt Smoothie Cappuccino	1 serv	472	2	3
Yogurt Smoothie Chocolate Fudge	1 serv	555	2	4
Yogurt Smoothie Fiesta	1 serv	432	2	4
Yogurt Smoothie Oreo Cookie	1 serv	566	4	8

FOOD	PORTION	CALS.	SAT. FAT	FAT
Yogurt Smoothie Peach	1 serv	486	2	4
Yogurt Smoothie Peach Banana	1 serv	519	2	4
Yogurt Smoothie Peanut Butter	1 serv	630	5	18
Yogurt Smoothie Pina Colada	1 serv	519	tr	1
Yogurt Smoothie Strawberry Banana	1 serv	514	2	4
Yogurt Smoothie Strawberry Fruit	1 serv	487	2	4
Yogurt Smoothie Strawberry Vanilla	1 serv	462	2	4
Yogurt Smoothie Strawberry Watermelon	1 serv	503	2	4
SALADS AND SALAD BARS				
Fruit Salad	1 lg	148	tr	1
Fruit Salad	1 sm	99	0	1
Garden Salad	1 sm	56	tr	1
Garden Salad w/ Italian Fat Free Dressing	1 lg	72	tr	2
Pasta Salad	1 lg	256	tr	2
Pasta Salad	1 sm	179	tr	2
SANDWICHES				
Chicken On Croissant	1	481	12	24
Chicken On Honey Wheat	1	297	2	8
Chicken On Jewish Rye	1	261	1	7
Chicken On Pita	1	281	1	6
Chicken On White	1	291	2	7
Ham & Cheese On Croissant	1	797	22	50
Ham & Cheese On Honey Wheat	1	613	11	34
Ham & Cheese On Jewish Rye	1	577	11	32
Ham & Cheese On Pita	1	597	11	32
Ham & Cheese On White	1	607	11	33
Roast Beef On Croissant	1	631	15	36
Roast Beef On Honey Wheat	1	348	2	8
Roast Beef On Jewish Rye	1	312	2	7
Roast Beef On Pita	1	332	2	7
Roast Beef On White	1	342	2	8
Tuna On Croissant	1	480	12	23
Tuna On Honey Wheat	1	295	1	6
Tuna On Jewish Rye	1	259	1	5
Tuna On Pita	1	280	1	5
Tuna On White	1	289	1	6
Turkey On Croissant	1	566	14	33
Turkey On Honey Wheat	1	342	3	9
Turkey On Jewish Rye	1	306	3	8

FOOD	PORTION	CALS.	SAT. FAT	FAT
Turkey On Pita	1	326	3	7
Turkey On White	1	338	3	9
Veggie On Croissant	1	510	14	35
Veggie On Honey Wheat	1	227	1	7
Veggie On Jewish Rye	1	191	1	6
Veggie On Pita	1	211	1	5
Veggie On White	1	221	1	7

GODFATHER'S PIZZA

FOOD	PORTION	CALS.	SAT. FAT	FAT
Golden Crust Cheese	1/10 lg (3.5 oz)	242	—	9
Golden Crust Cheese	1/8 med (3.1 oz)	212	—	8
Golden Crust Combo	1/8 med (4.4 oz)	271	—	12
Golden Crust Combo	1/10 lg (4.9 oz)	305	—	14
Original Crust Cheese	1/10 jumbo (5.8 oz)	382	—	9
Original Crust Cheese	1/4 mini (1.9 oz)	131	—	3
Original Crust Cheese	1/8 med (3.5 oz)	231	—	5
Original Crust Cheese	1/10 lg (4 oz)	258	—	6
Original Crust Combo	1/10 lg (5.6 oz)	338	—	12
Original Crust Combo	1/8 med (5.1 oz)	306	—	11
Original Crust Combo	1/10 jumbo (8.3 oz)	503	—	18
Original Crust Combo	1/4 mini (2.9 oz)	176	—	7

GODIVA

FOOD	PORTION	CALS.	SAT. FAT	FAT
Almond Butter Dome	3 pieces (1.5 oz)	240	6	17
Bouchee Au Chocolat	1 piece (1.5 oz)	210	6	11
Bouchee Ivory Raspberry	1 pieces (1 oz)	160	3	9
Gold Ballotin	3 pieces (1.5 oz)	210	4	10
Truffle Amaretto Di Saronno	2 pieces (1.5 oz)	210	6	12
Truffle Deluxe Liqueur	2 pieces (1.5 oz)	210	6	13

HAAGEN-DAZS

FROZEN YOGURT

FOOD	PORTION	CALS.	SAT. FAT	FAT
Brownie Nut Blast	1/2 cup (3.5 oz)	215	3	8
Chocolate	1/2 cup (3.4 oz)	160	1	3
Coffee	1/2 cup (3.4 oz)	161	1	3
Orange Tango	1/2 cup (3.5 oz)	132	1	1
Pina Colada	1/2 cup (3.4 oz)	139	1	2
Raspberry Randezvous	1/2 cup (3.5 oz)	132	1	1
Soft Serve Coffee	1/2 cup (3.3 oz)	145	3	4
Soft Serve Nonfat Chocolate	1/2 cup (3.3 oz)	116	tr	tr
Soft Serve Nonfat Chocolate Mousse	1/2 cup (3.3 oz)	86	tr	tr
Soft Serve Nonfat Vanilla	1/2 cup (3.3 oz)	114	tr	tr
Soft Serve Nonfat Vanilla Mousse	1/2 cup (3.3 oz)	78	tr	tr

FOOD	PORTION	CALS.	SAT. FAT	FAT
Strawberry Cheesecake Craze	½ cup (3.6 oz)	213	4	7
Strawberry Duet	½ cup (3.4 oz)	135	1	2
Vanilla	½ cup (3.4 oz)	162	1	3
Vanilla Almond Crunch	½ cup (3.4 oz)	198	2	5
ICE CREAM				
Bar Chocolate	1 (2.7 oz)	247	10	17
Bar Coffee	1 (2.7 oz)	249	10	17
Bar Vanilla	1 (2.7 oz)	251	10	17
Belgian Chocolate Chocolate	½ cup (3.6 oz)	315	12	21
Brownies A La Mode	½ cup (3.5 oz)	284	11	18
Butter Pecan	½ cup (3.7 oz)	304	10	23
Cappuccino Commotion	½ cup (3.6 oz)	305	12	21
Caramel Cone Explosion	½ cup (3.6 oz)	298	12	20
Chocolate	½ cup (3.7 oz)	249	10	17
Chocolate Chocolate Chip	½ cup (3.7 oz)	282	11	19
Chocolate Chocolate Mint	½ cup (3.6 oz)	285	11	20
Coffee	½ cup (3.7 oz)	251	10	17
Coffee Chip	½ cup (3.6 oz)	285	11	19
Cookie Dough Dynamo	½ cup (3.6 oz)	298	11	19
Cookies & Cream	½ cup (3.6 oz)	264	10	17
Deep Chocolate Peanut Butter	½ cup (3.7 oz)	339	11	23
Macadamia Brittle	½ cup (3.7 oz)	282	11	19
Macadamia Nut	½ cup (3.6 oz)	309	11	24
Midnight Cookies & Cream	½ cup (3.6 oz)	285	11	18
Peanut Butter Burst	½ cup (2.6 oz)	314	11	21
Pralines & Cream	½ cup (3.6 oz)	278	9	17
Rum Raisin	½ cup (3.7 oz)	256	10	16
Strawberry	½ cup (3.7 oz)	242	9	16
Strawberry Cheesecake Craze	½ cup (3.7 oz)	273	10	17
Swiss Chocolate Almond	½ cup (3.6 oz)	288	11	20
Triple Brownie Overload	½ cup (3.5 oz)	298	11	20
Vanilla	½ cup (3.7 oz)	252	10	17
Vanilla Chip	½ cup (3.6 oz)	286	12	19
Vanilla Fudge	½ cup (3.7 oz)	268	11	17
Vanilla Swiss Almond	½ cup (3.7 oz)	288	11	20
SORBET				
Mango	½ cup (4 oz)	107	0	tr
Raspberry	½ cup (4 oz)	110	0	tr
Soft Serve Lemonade	½ cup (3.3 oz)	113	0	0
Soft Serve Mango	½ cup (3.3 oz)	107	0	tr
Soft Serve Raspberry	½ cup (3.3 oz)	108	0	tr
Strawberry	½ cup (4 oz)	118	0	tr
Zesty Lemon	½ cup (4 oz)	111	0	0

FOOD	PORTION	CALS.	SAT. FAT	FAT
HARDEE'S				
BEVERAGES				
Orange Juice	1 serv (11 oz)	140	tr	tr
Shake Chocolate	1 (12.2 oz)	370	3	5
Shake Peach	1 (12.1 oz)	390	3	4
Shake Strawberry	1 (12.7 oz)	420	3	4
Shake Vanilla	1 (12.2 oz)	350	3	5
BREAKFAST SELECTIONS				
Apple Cinnamon 'N' Raisin Biscuit	1 (2.18 oz)	200	2	8
Bacon & Egg Biscuit	1 (5.5 oz)	570	11	33
Bacon Egg & Cheese Biscuit	1 (5.9 oz)	610	13	37
Big Country Breakfast Bacon	1 serv (9.4 oz)	820	15	49
Big Country Breakfast Sausage	1 serv (11.4 oz)	1000	38	66
Biscuit 'N' Gravy	1 (7.8 oz)	510	9	28
Country Ham Biscuit	1 (3.8 oz)	430	5	22
Frisco Breakfast Sandwich Ham	1 (7.4 oz)	500	9	25
Ham Biscuit	1 (4 oz)	400	6	20
Ham Egg & Cheese Biscuit	1 (6.5 oz)	540	11	30
Hash Rounds	1 serv (2.8 oz)	230	3	14
Jelly Biscuit	1 (3.5 oz)	440	6	21
Rise 'N' Shine Biscuit	1 (2.9 oz)	390	6	21
Sausage Biscuit	1 (4.1 oz)	510	10	31
Sausage & Egg Biscuit	1 (6.3 oz)	630	22	40
Three Pancakes	1 serv (4.8 oz)	280	1	2
Ultimate Omelet Biscuit	1 (5.8 oz)	570	12	33
DESSERTS				
Big Cookie	1 (2.0 oz)	280	4	12
Cone Chocolate	1 (4.1 oz)	180	1	2
Cone Vanilla	1 (4.1 oz)	170	1	2
Cool Twist Cone Vanilla/ Chocolate	1 (4.1 oz)	180	1	2
Peach Cobbler	1 serv (6 oz)	310	1	7
Sundae Hot Fudge	1 (5.5 oz)	290	3	6
Sundae Strawberry	1 (5.8 oz)	210	1	2
MAIN MENU SELECTIONS				
Baked Beans	1 serv (5 oz)	170	0	1
Big Roast Beef Sandwich	1 (6.5 oz)	460	9	24
Cheeseburger	1 (4.3 oz)	310	6	14
Chicken Fillet Sandwich	1 (7.5 oz)	480	3	18
Cole Slaw	1 serv (4 oz)	240	3	20
Cravin' Bacon Cheeseburger	1 (8.1 oz)	690	15	46
Fisherman's Fillet	1 (8.3 oz)	560	7	27
French Fries	1 med (5 oz)	350	4	15

FOOD	PORTION	CALS.	SAT. FAT	FAT
French Fries	1 lg (6 oz)	430	5	18
French Fries	1 sm (3.4 oz)	240	3	10
Fried Chicken Breast	1 piece (5.2 oz)	370	4	15
Fried Chicken Leg	1 piece (2.4 oz)	170	2	7
Fried Chicken Thigh	1 piece (4.2 oz)	330	4	15
Fried Chicken Wing	1 piece (2.3 oz)	200	2	8
Frisco Burger	1 (8.1 oz)	720	16	46
Gravy	1 serv (1.5 oz)	20	tr	tr
Grilled Chicken Sandwich	1 (7.1 oz)	350	2	11
Hamburger	1 (3.9 oz)	270	3	11
Hot Ham 'N' Cheese	1 (5.1 oz)	310	6	12
Mashed Potatoes	1 serv (4 oz)	70	tr	tr
Mesquite Bacon Cheeseburger	1 (4.5 oz)	370	7	18
Mushroom 'N' Swiss Burger	1 (6.8 oz)	490	12	25
Quarter Pound Double Cheeseburger	1 (6 oz)	470	11	27
Regular Roast Beef	1 (4.3 oz)	320	6	16
The Boss	1 (7 oz)	570	12	33
The Works Burger	1 (8.1 oz)	530	12	30
SALAD DRESSINGS				
Fat Free French	1 serv (2 oz)	70	0	0
Ranch	1 serv (2 oz)	290	4	29
Thousand Island	1 serv (2 oz)	250	3	23
SALADS AND SALAD BARS				
Garden Salad	1 (10.2 oz)	220	9	13
Grilled Chicken Salad	1 (11.5 oz)	150	1	3
Side Salad	1 (4.6 oz)	25	tr	tr

H.SALT SEAFOOD

FOOD	PORTION	CALS.	SAT. FAT	FAT
Chicken	3 oz	108	—	6
Cod	3 oz	62	—	2
Hamburger	3 oz	228	—	18
Pork Loin	3 oz	254	—	21
Sirloin Steak	3 oz	239	—	20

IHOP

FOOD	PORTION	CALS.	SAT. FAT	FAT
Pancake Buckwheat	1 (2.5 oz)	134	1	5
Pancake Buttermilk	1 (2 oz)	108	1	3
Pancake Country Griddle	1 (2.25 oz)	134	1	4
Pancake Egg	1 (2 oz)	102	1	5
Pancake Harvest Grain 'N Nut	1 (2.25 oz)	160	1	8
Waffle	1 (4 oz)	305	3	15
Waffle Belgian	1 (6 oz)	408	11	20
Waffle Belgian Harvest Grain 'N Nut	1 (6 oz)	445	12	28

FOOD	PORTION	CALS.	SAT. FAT	FAT
JACK IN THE BOX				
BEVERAGES				
Classic Ice Cream Shake Chocolate	1 reg (11 fl oz)	630	16	27
Classic Ice Cream Shake Oreo Cookie	1 reg (12 oz)	740	19	36
Classic Ice Cream Shake Strawberry	1 reg (10 fl oz)	640	15	28
Classic Ice Cream Shake Vanilla	1 reg (11 oz)	610	18	31
Classice Ice Cream Shake Cappuccino	1 reg (11 oz)	630	17	29
BREAKFAST SELECTIONS				
Breakfast Jack	1 (4.2 oz)	300	5	12
Country Crock Spread	1 pat (5 g)	25	1	3
Grape Jelly	1 serv (0.5 oz)	40	0	0
Hash Browns	1 serv (2 oz)	160	11	11
Pancake Syrup	1 serv (1.5 oz)	120	0	0
Pancakes w/ Bacon	1 serv (5.6 oz)	400	3	12
Sausage Croissant	1 (6.4 oz)	670	19	48
Sourdough Breakfast Sandwich	1 (5.2 oz)	380	8	21
Supreme Croissant	1 (6 oz)	570	7	20
Ultimate Breakfast Sandwich	1 (8.5 oz)	620	15	36
DESSERTS				
Carrot Cake	1 serv (3.5 oz)	370	3	16
Cheesecake	1 serv (3.5 oz)	310	9	18
Double Fudge Cake	1 serv (3 oz)	300	3	10
Hot Apple Turnover	1 (3.8 oz)	340	4	18
MAIN MENU SELECTIONS				
¼ lb Burger	1 (6 oz)	510	10	27
American Cheese	1 slice (0.4 oz)	45	3	4
Bacon & Cheddar Potato Wedges	1 serv (9.3 oz)	800	16	58
Bacon Ultimate Cheeseburger	1 (10.4 oz)	1150	30	89
Barbeque Dipping Sauce	1 serv (1 fl oz)	45	0	0
Cheeseburger	1 (4 oz)	330	6	15
Chicken & Fries	1 serv (9.3 oz)	730	7	34
Chicken Caesar Sandwich	1 (8.3 oz)	520	6	26
Chicken Fajita Pita	1 (6.6 oz)	280	4	9
Chicken Sandwich	1 (5.9 oz)	450	5	26
Chicken Strips Breaded	5 pieces (5.3 oz)	360	3	17
Chicken Supreme Sandwich	1 (8.2 oz)	680	11	45
Chili Cheese Curly Fries	1 serv (8.1 oz)	650	12	41
Double Cheeseburger	1 (5.3 oz)	450	12	24
Egg Rolls	3 pieces (6 oz)	440	6	24

FOOD	PORTION	CALS.	SAT. FAT	FAT
Egg Rolls	5 pieces (10 oz)	730	10	41
Fish & Chips	1 serv (9 oz)	720	8	35
French Fries	1 reg (4.1 oz)	360	4	17
Grilled Chicken Fillet Sandwich	1 (8.1 oz)	520	6	26
Hamburger	1 (3.6 oz)	280	4	12
Jumbo Fries	1 serv (5 oz)	430	5	20
Jumbo Jack	1 (7.8 oz)	560	12	36
Jumbo Jack w/ Cheese	1 (8.6 oz)	650	16	43
Ketchup	1 pkg (0.3 oz)	10	0	0
Monster Taco	1 (4 oz)	290	6	18
Onion Rings	1 serv (4.2 oz)	460	5	25
Pilly Cheesesteak Sandwich	1 (7.6 oz)	520	9	25
Salsa	1 serv (1 oz)	10	0	0
Seasoned Curly Fries	1 serv (4.5 oz)	420	5	24
Sour Cream	1 serv (1 oz)	60	4	6
Sourdough Jack	1 (7.8 oz)	670	16	43
Soy Sauce	1 serv (0.3 oz)	5	0	0
Spicy Crispy Chicken Sandwich	1 (7.9 oz)	560	5	27
Stuffed Jalapenos	10 pieces (7.6 oz)	680	15	40
Stuffed Jalapenos	7 pieces (5.3 oz)	470	11	28
Super Scoop French Fries	1 serv (7 oz)	610	6	28
Sweet & Sour Dipping Sauce	1 serv (1 oz)	40	0	0
Swiss-Style Cheese	1 slice (0.4 oz)	40	2	3
Taco	1 (2.7 oz)	190	4	11
Tartar Dipping Sauce	1 pkg (1.5 oz)	220	4	23
Teriyaki Bowl Chicken	1 serv (17.6 oz)	670	1	4
Ultimate Cheeseburger	1 (9.8 oz)	1030	26	79
SALAD DRESSINGS				
Blue Cheese	1 serv (2 fl oz)	210	4	18
Buttermilk House	1 serv (2 fl oz)	290	11	30
Buttermilk House Dipping Sauce	1 serv (0.9 oz)	130	5	13
Low Calorie Italian	1 serv (2 fl oz)	25	0	2
Thousand Island	1 serv (2 fl oz)	250	4	24
SALADS AND SALAD BARS				
Croutons	1 serv (0.4 oz)	50	1	2
Garden Chicken Salad	1 serv (8.9 oz)	200	4	9
Side Salad	1 (3 oz)	50	2	3

JAMBA JUICE

Jambolas Honey Nut Energy	1 serv	192	—	1
Jambolas Mighty Multi Grain	1 serv	208	—	3
Jambolas Mind Over Blueberry	1 serv	170	—	1
Jambolas Pizza Protein	1 serv	199	—	3

FOOD	PORTION	CALS.	SAT. FAT	FAT
KENNY ROGERS ROASTERS				
MAIN MENU SELECTIONS				
½ Chicken w/ Skin	1 serv (9.06 oz)	515	7	28
½ Chicken w/o Skin & Wing	1 serv (7.03 oz)	313	3	10
¼ Chicken Dark Meat w/ Skin	1 serv (4.35 oz)	271	4	17
¼ Chicken Dark Meat w/o Skin & Wing	1 serv (3.29 oz)	169	2	7
¼ Chicken White Meat w/ Skin	1 serv (4.71 oz)	244	3	11
¼ Chicken White Meat w/o Skin & Wing	1 serv (3.74 oz)	144	1	2
Baked Sweet Potato	1 (9 oz)	263	0	tr
Chicken Caesar Salad	1 serv (9.4 oz)	285	3	9
Cinnamon Apples	1 serv (5.27 oz)	199	3	5
Cole Slaw	1 serv (5.05 oz)	225	3	16
Corn Muffin	1 (2 oz)	175	2	8
Corn On The Cob	1 (2.25 oz)	68	tr	1
Corn Stuffing	1 serv (7.1 oz)	326	3	19
Creamy Parmesan Spinach	1 serv (5.3 oz)	119	3	69
Garlic Parsley Potatoes	1 serv (6.5 oz)	259	5	12
Honey Baked Beans	1 serv (5 oz)	148	tr	1
Italian Green Beans	1 serv (6.1 oz)	116	1	8
Macaroni & Cheese	1 serv (5.51 oz)	197	3	6
Pasta Salad	1 serv (5 oz)	236	2	12
Pita BBQ Chicken	1 (7.33 oz)	401	1	7
Pita Chicken Caesar	1 (9.2 oz)	606	3	35
Pita Roasted Chicken	1 (10.8 oz)	685	3	35
Pot Pie Chicken	1 (12 oz)	708	11	33
Potato Salad	1 serv (7.01 oz)	390	3	27
Real Mashed Potatoes	1 serv (8 oz)	295	3	14
Rice Pilaf	1 serv (5 oz)	173	1	5
Roasted Chicken Salad	1 serv (16.9 oz)	292	2	10
Sandwich Turkey	1 (9.2 oz)	385	2	12
Side Salad	1 serv (4.73 oz)	23	0	1
Sour Cream & Dill Pasta Salad	1 serv (5 oz)	233	3	16
Steamed Vegetables	1 serv (4.25 oz)	48	0	tr
Sweet Corn Niblets	1 serv (5 oz)	112	tr	1
Tomato Cucumber Salad	1 serv (6 oz)	123	1	2
Turkey Sliced Breast	1 serv (4.5 oz)	158	1	2
Zucchini & Squash Santa Fe	1 serv (5 oz)	70	1	5
SALAD DRESSINGS				
Blue Cheese	1 serv (2.47 oz)	370	7	39
Buttermilk Ranch	1 serv (2.47 oz)	430	7	48
Caesar	1 serv (2.47 oz)	340	5	36

FOOD	PORTION	CALS.	SAT. FAT	FAT
Honey French	1 serv (2.47 oz)	350	4	29
Honey Mustard	1 serv (2.47 oz)	320	4	28
Italian Fat Free	1 serv (2.47 oz)	35	0	0
Thousand Island	1 serv (2.47 oz)	330	5	33
SOUPS				
Chicken Noodle	1 bowl (10 oz)	91	tr	2
Chicken Noodle	1 cup (6 oz)	55	tr	1
KFC				
BBQ Baked Beans	1 serv (5.5 oz)	190	1	3
Biscuit	1 (2 oz)	180	3	10
Chicken Pot Pie	1 (13 oz)	770	13	42
Chicken Twister	1 (8.7 oz)	550	7	32
Cole Slaw	1 serv (5 oz)	180	2	9
Corn On The Cob	1 ear (5.7 oz)	150	0	2
Cornbread	1 (2 oz)	228	2	13
Crispy Strips Colonel's	3 (3.25 oz)	261	4	16
Crispy Strips Spicy Buffalo	3 (4.2 oz)	350	4	19
Extra Tasty Crispy Breast	1 (5.9 oz)	470	7	28
Extra Tasty Crispy Drumstick	1 (2.4 oz)	190	3	11
Extra Tasty Crispy Thigh	1 (4.2 oz)	370	6	25
Extra Tasty Crispy Whole Wing	1 (1.9 oz)	200	4	13
Green Beans	1 serv (4.7 oz)	45	1	2
Hot & Spicy Breast	1 (6.5 oz)	530	8	35
Hot & Spicy Drumstick	1 (2.3 oz)	190	3	11
Hot & Spicy Thigh	1 (3.8 oz)	370	7	27
Hot & Spicy Whole Wing	1 (1.9 oz)	210	4	15
Hot Wings	6 (4.8 oz)	471	8	33
Macaroni & Cheese	1 serv (5.4 oz)	180	3	8
Mashed Potatoes With Gravy	1 serv (4.8 oz)	120	1	6
Mean Greens	1 serv (5.4 oz)	70	1	3
Original Recipe Breast	1 (5.4 oz)	400	6	24
Original Recipe Chicken Sandwich	1 (7.3 oz)	497	5	22
Original Recipe Drumstick	1 (2.2 oz)	140	2	9
Original Recipe Thigh	1 (3.2 oz)	250	5	18
Original Recipe Whole Wing	1 (1.6 oz)	140	3	10
Potato Salad	1 serv (5.6 oz)	230	2	14
Potato Wedges	1 serv (4.8 oz)	280	4	13
Tender Roast Breast w/ Skin	1 (4.9 oz)	251	3	11
Tender Roast Breast w/o Skin	1 (4.2 oz)	169	1	4
Tender Roast Drumstick w/ Skin	1 (1.9 oz)	97	1	4
Tender Roast Drumstick w/o Skin	1 (1.2 oz)	67	1	2

FOOD	PORTION	CALS.	SAT. FAT	FAT
Tender Roast Thigh w/ Skin	1 (3.2 oz)	207	4	12
Tender Roast Thigh w/o Skin	1 (2.1 oz)	106	2	6
Tender Roast Wing w/ Skin	1 (1.8 oz)	121	2	8
Value BBQ Chicken Sandwich	1 (5.3 oz)	256	1	8
KRISPY KREME				
Chocolate Iced	1 (2 oz)	260	5	14
Chocolate Iced Cake	1 (2 oz)	230	3	12
Chocolate Iced Creme Filled	1 (2.3 oz)	270	3	14
Chocolate Iced Cruller	1 (1.7 oz)	240	4	14
Chocolate Iced Custard Filled	1 (2.7 oz)	250	3	9
Chocolated Iced w/ Sprinkles	1 (2 oz)	220	3	10
Cinnamon Apple Filled	1 (2.3 oz)	210	3	9
Cinnamon Bun	1 (2.1 oz)	220	3	11
Glazed Blueberry	1 (2.4 oz)	300	3	15
Glazed Creme Filled	1 (2.3 oz)	270	3	14
Glazed Cruller	1 (1.5 oz)	220	3	14
Glazed Devil's Food	1 (1.9 oz)	240	3	13
Lemon Filled	1 (2.2 oz)	210	3	10
Maple Iced	1 (1.8 oz)	200	3	9
Original Glazed	1 (1.3 oz)	180	3	10
Powdered Blueberry Filled	1 (2.1 oz)	200	3	9
Powdered Cake	1 (1.8 oz)	220	3	11
Raspberry Filled	1 (2 oz)	210	3	10
Traditional Cake	1 (1.7 oz)	200	3	11
KRYSTAL				
BEVERAGES				
Chocolate Shake	1 (16 fl oz)	275	5	10
BREAKFAST SELECTIONS				
Biscuit	1 (2.5 oz)	244	2	12
Biscuit Bacon	1 (2.9 oz)	306	5	17
Biscuit Bacon, Egg & Cheese	1 (4.7 oz)	421	8	26
Biscuit Country Ham	1 (3.7 oz)	334	4	17
Biscuit Egg	1 (4 oz)	327	4	19
Biscuit Gravy	1 (7.5 oz)	419	7	26
Biscuit Sausage	1 (4.1 oz)	437	8	30
Sunriser	1 (3.8 oz)	259	5	17
DESSERTS				
Apple Pie	1 serv (4.5 oz)	300	4	10
Donut Plain	1 (1.3 oz)	150	2	9
Donut w/ Chocolate Icing	1 (1.8 oz)	212	3	11
Donut w/ Vanilla Icing	1 (1.8 oz)	198	2	9
Lemon Meringue Pie	1 serv (4 oz)	340	3	9
Pecan Pie	1 serv (4 oz)	450	6	23

FOOD	PORTION	CALS.	SAT. FAT	FAT
MAIN MENU SELECTIONS				
Bacon Cheeseburger	1 (7.4 oz)	521	14	34
Big K	1 (8 oz)	540	14	35
Burger Plus	1 (6.5 oz)	415	10	26
Burger Plus w/ Cheese	1 (7.1 oz)	473	13	31
Cheese Krystal	1 (2.5 oz)	187	4	10
Chili	1 lg (12 oz)	327	5	12
Chili	1 reg (8 oz)	218	3	8
Chili Cheese Pup	1 (2.7 oz)	211	7	13
Chili Pup	1 (2.5 oz)	182	6	10
Corn Pup	1 (2.3 oz)	214	6	14
Crispy Crunchy Chicken Sandwich	1 (5.75 oz)	467	7	24
Double Cheese Krystal	1 (4.5 oz)	337	8	19
Double Krystal	1 (4 oz)	277	4	14
Fries	1 reg (4.1 oz)	358	6	18
Fries	1 sm (3 oz)	262	5	13
Fries	1 lg (5.3 oz)	463	8	23
Krys Kross Fries	1 serv (4.3 oz)	486	11	29
Krys Kross Fries Chili Cheese	1 serv (6.8 oz)	625	16	39
Krys Kross Fries w/ Cheese	1 serv (5.3 oz)	515	12	31
Krystal	1 (2.2 oz)	158	2	7
Plain Pup	1 (1.9 oz)	160	5	9

LITTLE CAESARS
MAIN MENU SELECTIONS

FOOD	PORTION	CALS.	SAT. FAT	FAT
Crazy Bread	1 piece (1.4 oz)	106	1	3
Crazy Sauce	1 serv (6 oz)	170	0	tr
Deli-Style Sandwich Ham & Cheese	1 (11.6 oz)	728	13	35
Deli-Style Sandwich Italian	1 (11.9 oz)	740	12	37
Deli-Style Sandwich Veggie	1 (11.9 oz)	647	9	29
Hot Oven-Baked Sandwich Cheeser	1 (12.1 oz)	822	20	39
Hot Oven-Baked Sandwich Meatsa	1 (15 oz)	1036	24	56
Hot Oven-Baked Sandwich Pepperoni	1 (11.2 oz)	899	23	47
Hot Oven-Baked Sandwich Supreme	1 (13.1 oz)	894	21	46
Hot Oven-Baked Sandwich Veggie	1 (13.7 oz)	669	14	23
PIZZA				
Baby Pan!Pan!	1 serv (8.4 oz)	616	12	24

FOOD	PORTION	CALS.	SAT. FAT	FAT
Pan!Pan! Cheese	1 med slice (2.9 oz)	181	3	6
Pan!Pan! Pepperoni	1 med slice (3 oz)	199	4	8
Pizza!Pizza! Cheese	1 med slice (3.2 oz)	201	4	7
Pizza!Pizza! Pepperoni	1 med slice (3.3 oz)	220	4	9
SALAD DRESSINGS				
1000 Island	1 serv (1.5 oz)	183	3	17
Blue Cheese	1 serv (1.5 oz)	160	2	14
Caesar	1 serv (1.5 oz)	255	4	27
French	1 serv (1.5 oz)	166	2	16
Greek	1 serv (1.5 oz)	268	8	30
Italian	1 serv (1.5 oz)	200	3	21
Italian Fat Free	1 serv (1.5 oz)	15	0	0
Ranch	1 serv (1.5 oz)	221	3	22
SALADS AND SALAD BARS				
Antipasto Salad	1 serv (8.4 oz)	176	2	12
Caesar Salad	1 serv (5 oz)	140	3	5
Greek Salad	1 serv (10.3 oz)	168	tr	10
Tossed Salad	1 serv (8.5 oz)	116	tr	3

LONG JOHN SILVER'S
MAIN MENU SELECTIONS

FOOD	PORTION	CALS.	SAT. FAT	FAT
Batter-Dipped Chicken	1 piece (2 oz)	120	2	6
Batter-Dipped Fish	1 piece (3 oz)	170	3	11
Batter-Dipped Shrimp	1 piece (0.4 oz)	35	1	3
Breaded Chicken Strips	1 piece (1.15 oz)	100	1	5
Breaded Clams	1 serv (3 oz)	300	4	17
Breaded Fish	1 piece (1.6 oz)	110	1	5
Cheese Sticks	1 serv (1.6 oz)	160	4	9
Chicken Salsa	1 reg (11 oz)	690	7	32
Corn Cobbette w/ Butter	1 piece (3.3 oz)	140	2	8
Corn Cobbette w/o Butter	1 (3.1 oz)	80	0	1
Fish Cajun	1 lg (23 oz)	1450	15	70
Flavorbaked Chicken	1 piece (2.6 oz)	110	1	3
Flavorbaked Fish	1 piece (2.3 oz)	90	1	3
Fries	1 reg (3 oz)	250	3	15
Fries	1 lg (5 oz)	420	4	24
Honey Mustard Sauce	1 serv (0.4 oz)	20	0	0
Hushpuppy	1 (0.8 oz)	60	0	3
Ketchup	1 serv (.32 oz)	10	0	0
Popcorn Chicken Munchers	1 serv (4 oz)	380	4	23
Popcorn Fish Munchers	1 serv (4 oz)	300	3	14
Popcorn Shrimp Munchers	1 serv (4 oz)	320	3	15
Rice	1 serv (3 oz)	140	1	3

FOOD	PORTION	CALS.	SAT. FAT	FAT
Sandwich Batter Dipped Fish No Sauce	1 (5.4 oz)	320	4	13
Sandwich Flavorbaked Chicken	1 (5.8 oz)	290	2	10
Sandwich Flavorbaked Fish	1 (6 oz)	320	7	14
Sandwich Ultimate Fish	1 (6.4 oz)	430	7	21
Shrimp Sauce	1 serv (0.4 oz)	15	0	0
Side Salad	1 (4.3 oz)	25	0	0
Slaw	1 serv (3.4 oz)	140	—	6
Sweet'N'Sour Sauce	1 serv (0.4 oz)	20	0	0
Tartar Sauce	1 serv (0.4 oz)	35	—	2
Wraps Chicken Cajun	1 reg (11 oz)	720	7	35
Wraps Chicken Cajun	1 lg (22 oz)	1440	14	71
Wraps Chicken Ranch	1 reg (11 oz)	730	7	36
Wraps Chicken Ranch	1 lg (22 oz)	1450	14	72
Wraps Chicken Salsa	1 lg (22 oz)	1370	13	64
Wraps Chicken Tartar	1 lg (22 oz)	1450	14	72
Wraps Chicken Tartar	1 reg (11 oz)	730	7	36
Wraps Fish Cajun	1 reg (11.5 oz)	730	8	35
Wraps Fish Ranch	1 reg (11.5 oz)	730	8	36
Wraps Fish Ranch	1 lg (23 oz)	1460	15	72
Wraps Fish Salsa	1 lg (23 oz)	1380	14	64
Wraps Fish Salsa	1 reg (11.5 oz)	690	7	32
Wraps Fish Tartar	1 reg (11.5 oz)	730	8	36
Wraps Fish Tartar	1 lg (23 oz)	1470	15	72
Wraps Popcorn Shrimp Cajun	1 lg (22 oz)	1450	18	71
Wraps Popcorn Shrimp Cajun	1 reg (11 oz)	720	9	35
Wraps Popcorn Shrimp Ranch	1 lg (22 oz)	1460	18	72
Wraps Popcorn Shrimp Ranch	1 reg (11 oz)	720	9	35
Wraps Popcorn Shrimp Salsa	1 lg (22 oz)	1380	17	64
Wraps Popcorn Shrimp Salsa	1 reg (11 oz)	690	9	32
Wraps Popcorn Shrimp Tartar	1 reg (11 oz)	730	9	36
Wraps Popcorn Shrimp Tartar	1 lg (22 oz)	1460	18	72
SALAD DRESSINGS				
Fat-Free French	1 serv (1.5 oz)	50	0	0
Fat-Free Ranch	1 serv (1.5 oz)	50	0	0
Italian	1 serv (1 oz)	130	2	14
Malt Vinegar	1 serv (0.3 oz)	0	0	0
Ranch Dressing	1 serv (1 oz)	170	3	18
Thousand Island	1 serv (1 oz)	110	2	10

LYONS RESTAURANTS
MAIN MENU SELECTIONS

Light & Healthy Halibut Brochette	1 serv	502	—	7

FOOD	PORTION	CALS.	SAT. FAT	FAT
Light & Healthy Lime & Cilantro Chicken	1 serv	511	—	9

MACHEEZMO MOUSE
CHILDREN'S MENU SELECTIONS

FOOD	PORTION	CALS.	SAT. FAT	FAT
Quesadilla Kid Cheese	1 serv (5 oz)	360	—	13
Quesadilla Kid Chicken	1 serv (7 oz)	430	—	15

MAIN MENU SELECTIONS

FOOD	PORTION	CALS.	SAT. FAT	FAT
Broccoli	1 oz	4	—	0
Burrito Vegetarian	1 (14 oz)	655	—	8
Dinner Rice, Beans, Broccoli	1 serv (10 oz)	328	—	tr
Dinner Rice, Beans, Salad	1 serv (12 oz)	344	—	tr
Green Sauce	1 oz	5	—	0
Snack Famouse #5	1 serv (14 oz)	585	—	5
Snack Tacos Chicken	1 serv (6 oz)	290	—	8
Snack Tacos Veggie	1 serv (6 oz)	290	—	6

MANHATTAN BAGEL

FOOD	PORTION	CALS.	SAT. FAT	FAT
Blueberry	1 (4 oz)	260	0	tr
Cheddar Cheese	1 (4 oz)	270	2	4
Chocolate Chip	1 (4 oz)	290	2	3
Cinnamon Raisin	1 (4 oz)	280	0	tr
Egg	1 (4 oz)	270	0	2
Everything	1 (4 oz)	290	0	3
Garlic	1 (4 oz)	270	0	tr
Jalapeno Cheddar	1 (4 oz)	260	0	2
Marble	1 (4 oz)	260	0	tr
Oat Bran	1 (4 oz)	260	0	1
Oat Bran Raisin Walnut	1 (4 oz)	270	0	3
Onion	1 (4 oz)	270	0	tr
Plain	1 (4 oz)	260	0	tr
Poppy	1 (4 oz)	300	1	4
Pumpernickel	1 (4 oz)	250	0	1
Rye	1 (4 oz)	260	0	1
Salt	1 (4 oz)	260	0	tr
Sesame	1 (4 oz)	310	1	5
Spinach	1 (4 oz)	270	0	tr
Sun-Dried Tomato	1 (4 oz)	260	0	1
Whole Wheat	1 (4 oz)	260	0	tr

MAX & IRMA'S

FOOD	PORTION	CALS.	SAT. FAT	FAT
Black Bean Roll Up	1 serv	401	3	8
Fat Free French	2 tbsp	126	0	tr
Fat Free Honey Mustard	2 tbsp	60	0	0
Fruit Smoothie	1 serv	114	tr	tr

FOOD	PORTION	CALS.	SAT. FAT	FAT
Garden Grill	1 serv	467	3	7
Garlic Breadstick	1	156	0	6
Gourmet Garden Grill	1 serv	484	3	8
Grilled Zucchini & Mushroom Pasta	1 serv	448	4	10
Grilled Zucchini & Mushroom Pasta w/ Chicken	1 serv	621	6	18
Hula Bowl w/ Fat Free Honey Mustard Dressing	1 serv	526	1	8
Lo-Cal Ranch	2 tbsp	54	1	6
Tijuana Tortilla Wrap	1	692	3	15

MCDONALD'S

BAKED SELECTIONS

FOOD	PORTION	CALS.	SAT. FAT	FAT
Apple Pie Baked	1 (2.7 oz)	260	4	13
Chocolate Chip Cookie	1 (1.2 oz)	170	6	10
Cinnamon Roll	1 (3.3 oz)	400	5	20
Danish Apple	1 (3.7 oz)	360	5	16
Danish Cheese	1 (3.7 oz)	410	8	22
Lowfat Muffin Apple Bran	1 (4 oz)	300	1	3
McDonaldland Cookies	1 pkg (1.5 oz)	180	1	5

BEVERAGES

FOOD	PORTION	CALS.	SAT. FAT	FAT
Orange Juice	1 serv (6 oz)	80	0	0
Shake Chocolate	1 sm (14.5 oz)	360	6	9
Shake Strawberry	1 sm (14.5 oz)	360	6	9
Shake Vanilla	1 sm (14.5 oz)	360	6	9

BREAKFAST SELECTIONS

FOOD	PORTION	CALS.	SAT. FAT	FAT
Bacon Egg & Cheese Biscuit	1 (5.5 oz)	470	8	25
Biscuit	1 (2.9 oz)	290	3	15
Breakfast Burrito	1 (4.1 oz)	320	7	19
Egg McMuffin	1 (4.8 oz)	290	5	14
English Muffin	1 (1.9 oz)	140	0	2
Hash Browns	1 serv (1.9 oz)	130	2	8
Hotcakes Margarine & Syrup	2 serv (7.8 oz)	570	3	16
Hotcakes Plain	1 serv (5.3 oz)	310	2	7
Sausage	1 (1.5 oz)	170	5	16
Sausage Biscuit	1 (4.5 oz)	470	9	31
Sausage Biscuit With Egg	1 (6.2 oz)	550	10	37
Sausage McMuffin	1 (3.9 oz)	360	8	23
Sausage McMuffin With Egg	1 (5.7 oz)	440	10	28
Scrambled Eggs	2 (3.6 oz)	160	4	11

DESSERTS

FOOD	PORTION	CALS.	SAT. FAT	FAT
Nuts For Sundaes	1 serv (7 g)	40	0	4

FOOD	PORTION	CALS.	SAT. FAT	FAT
Reduced Fat Ice Cream Cone Vanilla	1 (3.2 oz)	150	3	5
Sundae Hot Caramel	1 (6.4 oz)	360	6	10
Sundae Hot Fudge	1 (6.3 oz)	340	9	12
Sundae Strawberry	1 (6.2 oz)	290	5	7
MAIN MENU SELECTIONS				
Arch Deluxe	1 (8.4 oz)	550	11	31
Arch Deluxe With Bacon	1 (8.7 oz)	590	12	34
Barbeque Sauce	1 pkg (1 oz)	45	0	0
Big Mac	1 (7.5 oz)	560	10	31
Cheeseburger	1 (4.2 oz)	320	6	13
Chicken McNuggets	6 pieces (3.7 oz)	290	4	17
Chicken McNuggets	4 pieces (2.5 oz)	190	3	11
Chicken McNuggets	9 pieces (5.6 oz)	430	5	26
Crispy Chicken Deluxe	1 (7.8 oz)	500	4	25
Fish Filet Deluxe	1 (8 oz)	560	6	28
French Fries	1 sm (2.4 oz)	210	2	10
French Fries	1 lg (5.2 oz)	450	4	22
French Fries	1 super (6.2 oz)	540	5	26
Grilled Chicken Deluxe	1 (7.8 oz)	440	3	20
Grilled Chicken Deluxe Plain w/o Mayonnaise	1 (7.2 oz)	300	1	5
Grilled Chicken Salad Deluxe	1 serv (9 oz)	120	0	2
Hamburger	1 (3.7 oz)	260	4	9
Honey	1 pkg (0.5 oz)	45	0	0
Honey Mustard	1 pkg (0.5 oz)	40	1	5
Hot Mustard	1 pkg (1 oz)	60	0	4
Light Mayonnaise	1 pkg (0.4 oz)	40	1	4
Quarter Pounder	1 (6 oz)	420	8	21
Quarter Pounder With Cheese	1 (7 oz)	530	13	30
Sweet 'N Sour Sauce	1 pkg (1 oz)	50	0	0
SALAD DRESSINGS				
Caesar	1 pkg (2.1 oz)	160	3	14
Fat Free Herb Vinaigrette	1 pkg (2.1 oz)	50	0	0
Ranch	1 pkg (2.1 oz)	230	3	21
Reduced Calorie Red French	1 pkg (2.1 oz)	160	1	8
SALADS AND SALAD BARS				
Croutons	1 pkg (0.4 oz)	50	0	2
Garden Salad	1 serv (6.2 oz)	35	0	0

MORRISON'S
DESSERTS

FOOD	PORTION	CALS.	SAT. FAT	FAT
Boston Cream Cake	1 slice	218	—	4

FOOD	PORTION	CALS.	SAT. FAT	FAT
MAIN MENU SELECTIONS				
Baked Potato	1	220	—	tr
Broccoli	1 serv (4 oz)	37	—	2
Cabbage	1 serv (4 oz)	36	—	tr
Cantaloupe Compote	1 serv (4 oz)	130	—	1
Cauliflower	1 serv (4 oz)	68	—	5
Chicken Stew & Dumplings	1 serv (7 oz)	362	—	14
Chicken Teriyaki	1 serv (5.5 oz)	232	—	10
French Bread	1 slice	207	—	2
Grilled Chicken Pecan Salad	1 serv (6 oz)	298	—	8
Lima Beans	1 serv (4 oz)	170	—	4
Okra & Tomatoes	1 serv (5 oz)	40	—	2
Pinto Beans	1 serv (4 oz)	105	—	4
Plain Jello	1 serv (3 oz)	131	—	tr
Rutabagas	1 serv (4 oz)	33	—	1
Sliced Tomato	4 slices	40	—	1
Soft Roll	1 (2 oz)	170	—	4
Strawberries & Banana Bowl	1 serv (6 oz)	203	—	1
Strawberries Peaches & Bananas	1 serv (6 oz)	203	—	1
Turnip Greens	1 serv (4 oz)	30	—	2
Watermelon	1 serv (6 oz)	102	—	1
Yellow Squash	1 serv (4 oz)	22	—	1
SALADS AND SALAD BARS				
Garden Salad	1 serv (2.5 oz)	75	—	2
Tossed Salad	1 serv (3 oz)	30	—	tr
MRS. FIELDS				
Brownie Double Fudge	1 (3.1 oz)	420	11	20
Brownie Fudge Walnut	1 (3.4 oz)	500	10	29
Brownie Pecan Fudge	1 (2.8 oz)	390	9	21
Brownie Pecan Pie	1 (3 oz)	400	7	21
Cookie Chewy Fudge	1 (1.7 oz)	230	7	12
Cookie Coconut Macadamia	1 (1.7 oz)	250	7	15
Cookie Milk Chocolate Chip	1 (1.7 oz)	240	7	12
Cookie Milk Chocolate Macadamia	1 (1.7 oz)	250	7	14
Cookie Milk Chocolate w/ Walnuts	1 (1.7 oz)	250	7	13
Cookie Oatmeal Raisin	1 (1.7 oz)	220	5	10
Cookie Peanut Butter	1 (1.7 oz)	240	6	13
Cookie Semi-Sweet Chocolate	1 (1.7 oz)	230	7	12
Cookie Semi-Sweet Chocolate w/ Walnuts	1 (1.8 oz)	240	7	13
Cookie Triple Chocolate	1 (1.7 oz)	230	7	12

FOOD	PORTION	CALS.	SAT. FAT	FAT
Cookie White Chunk Macadamia	1 (1.7 oz)	260	7	15
Muffin Banana Walnut	1 (3.9 oz)	460	5	24
Muffin Blueberry	1 (4 oz)	390	6	15
Muffin Chocolate Chip	1 (4 oz)	450	8	19
Muffin Mandarin Orange	1 (4 oz)	420	7	17
Peanut Butter Dream Bar	1 (5 oz)	750	18	40
PRETZELS				
Hot Sam Bavarian	1 reg (2.5 oz)	200	0	0
Hot Sam Bavarian	1 lg (5.1 oz)	390	0	0
Hot Sam Bavarian Stix	10 (5 oz)	390	0	0
Hot Sam Sweet Dough	1 (4.5 oz)	360	1	3
Hot Sam Sweet Dough Blueberry	1 (4.5 oz)	400	2	4
MY FAVORITE MUFFIN				
Basic Muffin	⅓ muffin	220	2	10
Double Chocolate	⅓ muffin	190	2	8
Fat Free Bavarian	⅓ muffin	100	0	0
Fat Free Bavarian Chocolate	⅓ muffin	130	0	0
NATHAN'S				
BEVERAGES				
Lemonade	22 fl oz	260	—	0
Lemonade	32 fl oz	378	—	0
Lemonade	16 fl oz	189	—	0
MAIN MENU SELECTIONS				
Breaded Chicken Sandwich	1 (7.2 oz)	510	4	25
Charbroiled Chicken Sandwich	1 (4.5 oz)	288	1	5
Cheese Steak Sandwich	1 (6.1 oz)	485	10	26
Chicken 2 Pieces	1 serv (7.1 oz)	693	9	44
Chicken 4 Pieces	1 serv (14.2 oz)	1382	18	88
Chicken Platter 2 Pieces	1 serv (14.8 oz)	1096	14	66
Chicken Platter 4 Pieces	1 serv (21.9 oz)	1788	23	109
Chicken Salad	1 serv (12.7 oz)	154	1	4
Double Burger	1 (7.3 oz)	671	18	41
Filet of Fish Platter	1 serv (22 oz)	1455	10	74
Filet of Fish Sandwich	1 (5.2 oz)	403	2	15
Frank Nuggets	11 pieces (5.1 oz)	563	10	38
Frank Nuggets	15 pieces (6.9 oz)	764	13	52
Frank Nuggets	7 pieces (3.2 oz)	357	6	24
Frankfurter	1 (3.2 oz)	310	8	19
French Fries	1 serv (8.6 oz)	514	4	26
Fried Clam Platter	1 serv (13.1 oz)	1024	7	51
Fried Clam Sandwich	1 (5.4 oz)	620	4	29
Fried Shrimp	1 serv (4.4 oz)	348	2	11
Fried Shrimp Platter	1 serv (12.6 oz)	796	5	34

FOOD	PORTION	CALS.	SAT. FAT	FAT
Hamburger	1 (4.7 oz)	434	10	23
Knish	1 (5.9 oz)	318	2	7
Pastrami Sandwich	1 (4.1 oz)	325	4	12
Sauteed Onions	1 serv (3.5 oz)	39	0	1
Super Burger	1 (7.6 oz)	533	9	32
Turkey Sandwich	1 (4.9 oz)	270	0	2
SALADS AND SALAD BARS				
Garden Salad	1 serv (10.9 oz)	193	7	13

NEWPORT CREAMERY
ICE CREAM

FOOD	PORTION	CALS.	SAT. FAT	FAT
Reduced Fat No Sugar Added Chocolate	½ cup (2.6 oz)	110	2	3
Reduced Fat No Sugar Added Coffee	½ cup (2.6 oz)	100	2	4
Soft Serve Nonfat Frozen Yogurt Cone or Dish	1 reg (5 oz)	125	0	0
SALAD DRESSINGS				
Corn Oil & Vinegar	1 tbsp	45	0	6
Fat Free Ranch	1.5 oz	48	0	0
Low-Cal French	1.5 oz	48	0	0
SALADS AND SALAD BARS				
Chef's Salad	1 serv	215	—	8
Chicken Fajita	1 serv	295	—	20
Grilled Chicken	1 serv	247	—	13
SANDWICHES				
Lite Chicken Salad	1	379	—	19
Lite Grilled Cheese	1	274	—	17
Lite Grilled Chicken Breast Pocket	1	327	—	12
Lite Sliced Turkey	1	288	—	12
Lite Tuna Salad	1	358	—	21
Lite Vegetarian Pocket Broccoli Mushrooms Onions Peppers Cheese	1	211	—	5
Lite Vegetarian Pocket Broccoli Cheese	1	214	—	5
Lite Vegetarian Pocket Peppers Onions Mushrooms Cheese	1	230	—	6
Low Fat Cheese	1 slice	73	—	4
Mayonnaise	2 tsp	71	—	8
Smart Sides Broccoli	1 serv	23	—	tr
Smart Sides Cottage Cheese	1 serv	90	—	4
Smart Sides Side Salad	1 serv	30	0	0

FOOD	PORTION	CALS.	SAT. FAT	FAT
OLIVE GARDEN				
Garden Fare Apple Carmellina	1 serv (12.2 oz)	560	1	2
Garden Fare Dinner Capellini Pomodoro	1 serv (21.1 oz)	610	3	16
Garden Fare Dinner Capellini Primavera	1 serv (20.1 oz)	400	4	7
Garden Fare Dinner Capellini Primavera w/ Chicken	1 serv (23.8 oz)	560	5	10
Garden Fare Dinner Chicken Giardino	1 serv (20.6 oz)	550	4	11
Garden Fare Dinner Linguine Alla Marinara	1 serv (16.3 oz)	500	2	9
Garden Fare Dinner Penne Fra Diavolo	1 serv (14.3 oz)	420	3	7
Garden Fare Dinner Shrimp Primavera	1 serv (28.4 oz)	740	5	15
Garden Fare Lunch Capellini Pamodoro	1 serv (11.7 oz)	360	2	9
Garden Fare Lunch Capellini Primavera	1 serv (11.2 oz)	260	3	5
Garden Fare Lunch Capellini Primavera w/ Chicken	1 serv (14.9 oz)	420	4	8
Garden Fare Lunch Chicken Giardino	1 serv (12.8 oz)	360	4	9
Garden Fare Lunch Linguine Alla Marinara	1 serv (10.2 oz)	310	1	6
Garden Fare Lunch Penne Fra Diavolo	1 serv (10.2 oz)	300	2	5
Garden Fare Lunch Shrimp Primavera	1 serv (15.2 oz)	410	3	8
Minestrone Soup	1 serv (6 oz)	80	0	1
PERKINS				
Low Fat Brownie	1 (5.4 oz)	260	—	1
Low Fat Muffin Banana	1 (5.8 oz)	330	—	3
Low Fat Muffin Blueberry	1 (5.8 oz)	270	—	3
Low Fat Muffin Honey Bran	1 (5.8 oz)	270	—	3
Low Fat Muffin Plain	1 (5.8 oz)	300	—	3
PICCADILLY CAFETERIA				
BAKED SELECTIONS				
Corn Sticks	1 (2 oz)	165	—	10
French Bread	1 slice	132	—	2
Garlic Bread	1 serv (15.8 oz)	1154	—	24
Mexican Corn Bread	1 piece	220	—	14

FOOD	PORTION	CALS.	SAT. FAT	FAT
Roll	1 (2 oz)	130	—	2
Roll Whole Wheat	1 (1.7 oz)	117	—	1
Texas Toast	1 serv (15.5 oz)	1088	—	17
BEVERAGES				
Punch	1 serv (9 oz)	133	—	0
DESSERTS				
Apple Pie	1 slice (7.2 oz)	439	—	19
Cantaloupe	1 serv (9 oz)	89	—	1
Cantaloupe	1 serv (5.5 oz)	55	—	tr
Chocolate Cream Pie	1 slice (7.5 oz)	512	—	25
Custard	1 cup (5.4 oz)	183	—	1
Custard Pie	1 slice (6.2 oz)	412	—	18
Dole Whip Topping	1 serv (3 oz)	68	—	1
Fresh Fruit Plate	1 serv (21.1 oz)	389	—	5
Gelatin	1 serv (4.75 oz)	128	—	4
Honeydew Melon	1 serv (5.5 oz)	55	—	tr
Honeydew Melon	1 serv (9 oz)	89	—	tr
Lemon Chiffon Pie	1 slice (6.3 oz)	481	—	20
Pound Cake	1 slice (3.8 oz)	371	—	17
Watermelon	1 serv (11 oz)	100	—	1
MAIN MENU SELECTIONS				
Au Jus	1 serv (3 oz)	5	—	tr
Baby Lima Beans	1 serv (4.5 oz)	151	—	6
Baked Potato	1	218	—	tr
Baked Potato w/ Topping	1	350	—	15
Beef Chopped Steak Fried	1 serv (4 oz)	311	—	23
Beef Leg Roast	1 serv (4 oz)	311	—	18
Beef Liver Fried	1 serv (4.5 oz)	430	—	29
Beef Tips Braised	1 serv (10 oz)	470	—	26
Black-eyed Peas w/ Pork Jowls	1 serv (4 oz)	108	—	6
Broccoli Buttered	1 serv (4 oz)	77	—	6
Broccoli & Rice Au Gratin	½ cup	184	—	9
Carrots Young Buttered	½ cup	90	—	6
Cauliflower Buttered	1 serv	80	—	6
Chicken Baked w/o Skin	¼ chicken	352	—	11
Chicken Teriyaki	1 serv (4 oz)	445	—	22
Chicken Teriyaki Polynesian	1 serv (4 oz)	537	—	27
Corn	1 serv (4.5 oz)	128	—	7
Cornbread Stuffing	1 serv (4.5 oz)	164	—	9
Crackers	4 (0.4 oz)	51	—	1
Cranberry Sauce	1 serv (1.5 oz)	64	—	tr
Eggplant Escalloped	½ cup	180	—	10
Fish Baked	1 serv (7 oz)	195	—	10

FOOD	PORTION	CALS.	SAT. FAT	FAT
Green Beans	1 serv (4.5 oz)	77	—	6
Ham Baked	1 serv (4 oz)	224	—	10
Macaroni & Cheese	½ cup	317	—	11
Mashed Potatoes	1 serv (4.8 oz)	120	—	3
Meatballs Baked & Spaghetti	1 serv (11.5 oz)	108	—	5
New Potatoes Boiled	½ cup	148	—	12
Okra Smothered	1 serv (4 oz)	121	—	10
Onion Sauce	1 serv (4 oz)	152	—	7
Rice	½ cup	99	—	tr
Rice Polynesian	1 serv (4 oz)	140	—	6
Spaghetti Baked	1 serv (9.5 oz)	256	—	10
Squash Baked Italian	1 serv (4.75 oz)	73	—	3
Squash Mixed Yellow & Zucchini	1 serv (4 oz)	72	—	5
Squash Yellow Baked French Style	⅓ cup	86	—	5
Turkey Breast	1 serv (3 oz)	99	—	2
Vegetables Unseasoned	1 serv (5 oz)	29	—	tr
SALADS AND SALAD BARS				
Broccoli Salad	1 serv (4 oz)	202	—	20
Cabbage Combination Salad	1 serv (4.5 oz)	50	—	tr
Carrot & Raisin Salad	1 serv (4.5 oz)	321	—	23
Cole Slaw w/ Cream	1 serv (4 oz)	182	—	18
Cucumber & Celery Salad	1 serv (4 oz)	82	—	6
Fruit Salad	1 serv (6 oz)	59	—	1
Neptune Salad	1 serv	361	—	34
Spinach Tossed Salad	1 serv (4 oz)	88	—	6
Spring Salad Bowl	1 serv (4 oz)	22	—	tr
SOUPS				
Gumbo Chicken	1 serv (8 oz)	92	—	2
Gumbo Seafood	1 serv (8 oz)	98	—	2
Vegetable	1 serv (8 oz)	49	—	tr

PIZZA HUT
MAIN MENU SELECTIONS

FOOD	PORTION	CALS.	SAT. FAT	FAT
Bread Stick	1 (1.3 oz)	130	1	4
Bread Stick Dipping Sauce	1 serv (1.2 oz)	30	0	1
Cavatini Pasta	1 serv (12.5 oz)	480	6	14
Cavatini Supreme Pasta	1 serv (13.9 oz)	560	8	19
Garlic Bread	1 slice (1.3 oz)	150	2	8
Ham & Cheese Sandwich	1 (9.7 oz)	550	7	21
Hot Buffalo Wings	4 pieces (2.1 oz)	210	3	12
Spaghetti Marinara	1 serv (16.6 oz)	490	1	6
Spaghetti Meat Sauce	1 serv (16.4 oz)	600	5	13

FOOD	PORTION	CALS.	SAT. FAT	FAT
Spaghetti Meatballs	1 serv (18.8 oz)	850	10	24
Supreme Sandwich	1 (10.2 oz)	640	10	28
Wild Buffalo Wings	5 pieces (2.9 oz)	200	4	12
PIZZA				
Beef Topping Hand Tossed	1 slice (3.9 oz)	280	5	10
Beef Topping Pan	1 slice (3.9 oz)	310	5	14
Beef Topping Stuffed Crust	1 slice (5.6 oz)	410	6	14
Beef Topping Thin 'N Crispy	1 slice (3.1 oz)	240	5	11
Cheese Hand Tossed	1 slice (3.9 oz)	280	5	10
Cheese Pan	1 slice (3.9 oz)	300	6	14
Cheese Stuffed Crust	1 slice (5.4 oz)	380	5	11
Cheese Thin'N Crispy	1 slice (2.6oz)	210	5	9
Chicken Supreme Pan	1 slice (4.1 oz)	280	4	11
Chicken Supreme Stuffed Crust	1 slice (6.4 oz)	390	6	13
Chicken Supreme Thin 'N Crispy	1 slice (4.2 oz)	240	3	6
Dessert Apple	1 slice (2.8 oz)	250	1	5
Dessert Cherry	1 slice (2.8 oz)	250	1	5
Ham Hand Tossed	1 slice (3.4 oz)	230	3	6
Ham Pan	1 slice (3.4 oz)	250	4	9
Ham Stuffed Crust	1 slice (5.4 oz)	380	6	14
Ham Thin 'N Crispy	1 slice (2.4 oz)	190	3	6
Italian Sausage Hand Tossed	1 slice (4 oz)	300	5	12
Italian Sausage Pan	1 slice (4.3 oz)	350	6	18
Italian Sausage Stuffed Crust	1 slice (5.7 oz)	430	8	19
Italian Sausage Thin 'N Crispy	1 slice (3.4 oz)	300	6	16
Meat Lover's Hand Tossed	1 slice (3.9 oz)	290	5	11
Meat Lover's Pan	1 slice (4.4 oz)	360	6	19
Meat Lover's Stuffed Crust	1 slice (6.6 oz)	500	10	23
Meat Lover's Thin 'N Crispy	1 slice (3.7 oz)	310	7	16
Pepperoni Hand Tossed	1 slice (3.4 oz)	260	4	9
Pepperoni Lover's Hand Tossed	1 slice (4 oz)	320	6	13
Pepperoni Lover's Pan	1 slice (4.1 oz)	350	8	17
Pepperoni Lover's Stuffed Crust	1 slice (6.1 oz)	480	9	22
Pepperoni Lover's Thin 'N Crispy	1 slice (3.1 oz)	270	6	12
Pepperoni Pan	1 slice (3.4 oz)	280	5	12
Pepperoni Stuffed Crust	1 slice (5.3 oz)	410	7	17
Pepperoni Thin 'N Crispy	1 slice (2.3 oz)	220	4	9
Personal Pan Cheese	1 pie (8.1 oz)	630	11	24
Personal Pan Pepperoni	1 pie (8.1 oz)	670	12	29
Personal Pan Supreme	1 pie (9.5 oz)	710	13	31
Pork Topping Hand Tossed	1 slice (3.9 oz)	290	5	11
Pork Topping Pan	1 slice (3.6 oz)	300	5	13
Pork Topping Stuffed Crust	1 slice (5.6 oz)	420	7	16
Pork Topping Thin 'N Crispy	1 slice (3.2 oz)	270	6	13

FOOD	PORTION	CALS.	SAT. FAT	FAT
Super Supreme Hand Tossed	1 slice (4.7 oz)	290	5	10
Super Supreme Pan	1 slice (4.6 oz)	340	5	16
Super Supreme Stuffed Crust	1 slice (7.2 oz)	470	8	20
Super Supreme Thin 'N Crispy	1 slice (4 oz)	280	5	13
Supreme Hand Tossed	1 slice (3.9 oz)	270	5	9
Supreme Pan	1 slice (4 oz)	300	5	13
Supreme Stuffed Crust	1 slice (6.4 oz)	440	7	16
Supreme Thin 'N Crispy	1 slice (3.4 oz)	250	5	11
Veggie Lover's Hand Tossed	1 slice (4 oz)	240	3	7
Veggie Lover's Pan	1 slice (3.9 oz)	240	4	9
Veggie Lover's Stuffed Crust	1 slice (5.9 oz)	390	6	14
Veggie Lover's Thin 'N Crispy	1 slice (2.6 oz)	170	2	6

POLLO TROPICALE
(see TROPIGRILL)

POPEYE'S

FOOD	PORTION	CALS.	SAT. FAT	FAT
Apple Pie	1 serv (3.1 oz)	290	—	16
Biscuit	1 serv (2.3 oz)	250	—	15
Breast Mild	1 (3.7 oz)	270	—	16
Breast Spicy	1 (3.7 oz)	270	—	16
Cajun Rice	1 serv (3.9 oz)	150	—	5
Cole Slaw	1 serv (4 oz)	149	—	11
Corn On The Cob	1 serv (5.2 oz)	127	—	3
French Fries	1 serv (3 oz)	240	—	12
Leg Mild	1 (1.7 oz)	120	—	7
Leg Spicy	1 (1.7 oz)	120	—	7
Nuggets	1 serv (4.2 oz)	410	—	32
Nuggets Mild Tender	1 (1.2 oz)	110	—	7
Nuggets Spicy Tender	1 (1.2 oz)	110	—	7
Onion Rings	1 serv (3.1 oz)	310	—	19
Potatoes & Gravy	1 serv (3.8 oz)	100	—	6
Red Beans & Rice	1 serv (5.9 oz)	270	—	17
Shrimp	1 serv (2.8 oz)	250	—	16
Thigh Mild	1 (3.1 oz)	300	—	23
Thigh Spicy	1 (3.1 oz)	300	—	23
Wing Mild	1 (1.6 oz)	160	—	11
Wing Spicy	1 (1.6 oz)	160	—	11

PUDGIE'S FAMOUS CHICKEN

FOOD	PORTION	CALS.	SAT. FAT	FAT
Fried Chicken	3.5 oz	233	3	13

QUINCY'S
BAKED SELECTIONS

FOOD	PORTION	CALS.	SAT. FAT	FAT
Banana Nut Bread	1 serv (2 oz)	165	1	7
Biscuit	1 (2.5 oz)	270	4	15

FOOD	PORTION	CALS.	SAT. FAT	FAT
Cornbread	1 serv (2 oz)	140	1	5
Yeast Roll	1 (2 oz)	160	tr	4
BREAKFAST SELECTIONS				
Bacon	1 serv (0.25 oz)	35	1	3
Corned Beef Hash	1 serv (4.5 oz)	210	8	15
Country Ham	1 serv (1.5 oz)	90	2	6
Escalloped Apples	1 serv (3.5 oz)	120	0	2
Oatmeal	1 serv (1 oz)	175	0	2
Pancakes	1 (1.5 oz)	95	1	3
Sausage Gravy	1 serv (4 oz)	70	2	6
Sausage Links	1 (2 oz)	225	8	22
Sausage Patties	1 (2 oz)	230	9	23
Scrambled Eggs	1 serv (2 oz)	95	2	7
Steak Fingers	1 serv (3.5 oz)	360	11	25
Syrup	1 oz	75	0	0
DESSERTS				
Banana Pudding	1 serv (5 oz)	240	9	12
Brownie Pudding Cake	1 serv (4 oz)	310	tr	5
Caramel Topping	1 serv (1 oz)	105	tr	1
Chocolate Chip Cookies	1 (0.5 oz)	60	1	8
Cobbler Apple	1 serv (6 oz)	255	2	8
Cobbler Cherry	1 serv (6 oz)	410	2	8
Cobbler Peach	1 serv (6 oz)	305	2	8
Frozen Yogurt	1 serv (4 oz)	135	1	2
Fudge Topping	1 serv (1 oz)	105	1	4
Sugar Cookie	1 (0.5 oz)	60	1	3
MAIN MENU SELECTIONS				
⅓ Pound Hamburger	1 serv (8 oz)	565	16	33
BBQ Beans	1 serv (4 oz)	114	1	1
Bacon Cheese Burger	1 (9 oz)	663	17	41
Baked Potato	1 (6 oz)	115	0	0
Broccoli	1 serv (4 oz)	34	0	0
Cheese Sauce	1 serv (1 oz)	58	2	5
Chopped Steak Steak	1 serv (8 oz)	499	20	42
Cinnamon Apples	1 serv (4 oz)	172	1	5
Corn	1 serv (4 oz)	96	0	1
Country Steak w/ Gravy	1 serv (8 oz)	530	7	25
Cowboy Steak	1 serv (14 oz)	580	15	33
Filet w/ Bacon	1 serv (8 oz)	340	7	17
Green Beans	1 serv (4 oz)	61	1	4
Grilled Chicken	1 reg serv (5 oz)	120	0	2
Grilled Chicken Sandwich	1 (9 oz)	324	1	4
Grilled Salmon	1 serv (7 oz)	228	1	4

FOOD	PORTION	CALS.	SAT. FAT	FAT
Homestyle Chicken Fillet	1 serv (3 oz)	217	2	9
Junior Sirloin Steak	1 serv (5.5 oz)	194	5	10
Large Sirloin Steak	1 serv (10 oz)	368	9	20
Mashed Potatoes	1 serv (4 oz)	54	1	6
NY Strip Steak	1 serv (10 oz)	450	13	26
Philly Cheese Steak	1 serv (11 oz)	588	11	30
Porterhouse Steak	1 serv (17 oz)	683	23	46
Regular Sirloin Steak	1 serv (8 oz)	285	7	16
Ribeye Steak	1 serv (10 oz)	452	13	29
Rice Pilaf	1 serv (4 oz)	119	0	2
Roasted BBQ Chicken	1 serv (14 oz)	941	17	65
Roasted Herb Chicken	1 serv (14 oz)	875	17	65
Sirloin Tips w/ Mushroom Gravy	1 serv (6 oz)	196	3	7
Sirloin Tips w/ Peppers & Onions	1 serv (5 oz)	203	3	8
Smothered Steak Sandwich	1 (9 oz)	429	6	15
Smothered Strip Steak	1 serv (10 oz)	622	16	41
Southern Breaded Shrimp	1 serv (7 oz)	546	6	31
Spicy BBQ Chicken Sandwich	1 (10 oz)	368	1	1
Steak & Shrimp	1 serv (9 oz)	677	12	39
Steak Fries	1 serv (4 oz)	358	6	19
T-Bone Steak	1 serv (13 oz)	521	18	35
SALAD DRESSINGS				
Blue Cheese	1 serv (1 oz)	155	3	16
French	1 serv (1 oz)	125	1	12
Honey Mustard	1 serv (1 oz)	100	tr	6
Italian	1 serv (1 oz)	135	2	14
Light Creamy Italian	1 serv (1 oz)	65	0	4
Light French	1 serv (1 oz)	85	0	4
Light Italian	1 serv (1 oz)	20	0	2
Light Thousand Island	1 serv (1 oz)	65	0	4
Parmesan Peppercorn	1 serv (1 oz)	150	0	14
Ranch	1 serv (1 oz)	110	2	11
SOUPS				
Chili With Beans	1 serv (6 oz)	235	2	11
Clam Chowder	1 serv (6 oz)	180	1	9
Cream Of Broccoli	1 serv (6 oz)	170	1	10
Vegetable Beef	1 serv (6 oz)	90	1	2

RALLY'S
BEVERAGES

FOOD	PORTION	CALS.	SAT. FAT	FAT
Shake Banana	1 serv	399	—	11
Shake Chocolate	1 serv	411	—	12

FOOD	PORTION	CALS.	SAT. FAT	FAT
Shake Strawberry	1 serv	399	—	11
Shake Vanilla	1 serv	320	—	11
MAIN MENU SELECTIONS				
Big Buford	1	743	—	46
Chicken Fillet Sandwich	1	399	—	15
Chili w/ Cheese & Onion	1 serv (13 oz)	669	—	41
Chili w/ Cheese & Onion	1 serv (7 oz)	360	—	22
French Fries	1 reg (4 oz)	211	—	11
French Fries	1 lg (6 oz)	317	—	16
French Fries	1 extra lg (8 oz)	423	—	21
Onion Rings	1 serv	210	—	2
Rallyburger	1	433	—	22
Rallyburger w/ Cheese	1	488	—	35
Spicy Chicken Sandwich	1	437	—	18
Super Barbecue Bacon	1	593	—	31
Super Double Cheeseburger	1	762	—	48

RAX

BEVERAGES

FOOD	PORTION	CALS.	SAT. FAT	FAT
Chocolate Shake	1 (11 fl oz)	445	8	12
DESSERTS				
Chocolate Chip Cookie	1 (2 oz)	262	4	12
MAIN MENU SELECTIONS				
Bacon	1 slice (0.1 oz)	14	tr	1
Baked Potato	1 (10 oz)	264	0	0
Baked Potato w/ 1 Tbsp Margarine	1 (10.5 oz)	364	2	11
Barbecue Sauce	1 pkg (0.4 oz)	11	0	0
Beef Bacon 'N Cheddar	1 (6.7 oz)	523	8	32
Cheddar Cheese Sauce	1 fl oz	29	0	tr
Country Fried Chicken Breast Sandwich	1 (7.4 oz)	618	15	29
Deluxe Roast Beef	1 (7.9 oz)	498	7	30
French Fries	1 serv (3.25 oz)	282	4	14
Grilled Chicken Breast Sandwich	1 (6.9 oz)	402	4	23
Grilled Chicken Garden Salad w/ French Dressing	1 serv (12.7 oz)	477	6	31
Grilled Chicken Garden Salad w/ Lite Italian Dressing	1 serv (12.7 oz)	264	3	12
Mushroom Sauce	1 fl oz	16	0	tr
Philly Melt	1 (8.2 oz)	396	7	16
Regular Rax	1 (4.7 oz)	262	4	10
Swiss Slice	1 slice (0.4 oz)	42	3	3

FOOD	PORTION	CALS.	SAT. FAT	FAT
SALAD DRESSINGS				
French	2 fl oz	275	3	22
Lite Italian	2 fl oz	63	0	3
SALADS AND SALAD BARS				
Gourmet Garden Salad w/ French Dressing	1 serv (10.7 oz)	409	5	29
Gourmet Garden Salad w/ Lite Italian Dressing	1 serv (10.7 oz)	305	2	10
Gourmet Garden Salad w/o Dressing	1 serv (8.7 oz)	134	2	6
Grilled Chicken Garden Salad w/o Dressing	1 serv (10.7 oz)	202	2	9
RED LOBSTER				
CHILDREN'S MENU SELECTIONS				
Cheeseburger	1 serv	1040	18	56
Fried Chicken Fingers	1 serv	680	6	33
Fried Shrimp	1 serv	650	6	33
Grilled Chicken Teneders	1 serv	580	4	24
Hamburger	1 serv	920	12	47
Popcorn Shrimp	1 serv	650	6	35
Popcorn Shrimp & Cheesesticks	1 serv	750	9	41
Spaghetti & Cheesesticks	1 serv	830	6	39
DESSERTS				
Carrot Cake	1 serv (6.5 oz)	730	—	31
Cheesecake	1 serv (5.5 oz)	530	—	41
Fudge Overboard	1 serv	620	12	23
Ice Cream	1 serv (4.5 oz)	140	5	7
Key Lime Pie	1 serv (5 oz)	450	—	15
Raspberry Cobbler	1 serv (3 oz)	530	—	33
Sensational 7	1 serv	790	19	41
MAIN MENU SELECTIONS				
Admiral's Feast	1 serv	1060	12	52
Appetizer Calamari	1 serv	350	6	22
Appetizer Chicken Fingers	1 serv	390	4	18
Appetizer Chilled Shrimp In The Shell	1 serv (6 oz)	110	0	2
Appetizer Crab & Shrimp Cakes	1 serv	480	6	24
Appetizer Crab Add-On	1 serv	60	0	1
Appetizer Fresh Fried Mushrooms	1 serv	790	13	51
Appetizer Lobster Quesadilla	1 serv	760	24	47
Appetizer Lobster Stuffed Mushroom	1 serv	400	13	26

FOOD	PORTION	CALS.	SAT. FAT	FAT
Appetizer Mozzarella Cheesesticks	1 serv	730	20	46
Appetizer Parmesan Zucchini	1 serv	620	11	40
Appetizer Shrimp Cocktail	1 serv	50	0	1
Appetizer Stuffed Mushrooms	1 serv	420	13	27
Applesauce	1 serv (4 oz)	90	0	0
Atlantic Cod	1 serv (8 oz)	200	0	2
Atlantic Cod	1 lunch serv (5 oz)	110	0	1
Atlantic Salmon	1 lunch serv (5 oz)	200	2	9
Atlantic Salmon	1 serv (8 oz)	340	3	15
Baked Atlantic Cod	1 serv	220	1	6
Baked Atlantic Haddock	1 serv	220	1	6
Baked Flounder	1 lunch serv	190	1	7
Baked Potato	1 (8 oz)	130	0	0
Broccoli	1 serv (3 oz)	25	0	0
Broiled Fisherman's Platter	1 serv	600	4	23
Broiled Rock Lobster Tail	1 tail	190	1	6
Broiled Seafarer's Platter	1 serv	450	2	19
Caesar Salad w/ Dressing	1 serv	240	4	21
Catfish	1 serv (8 oz)	220	1	3
Catfish	1 lunch serv (5 oz)	130	0	2
Catfish Santa Fe	1 serv	340	2	9
Catfish Sante Fe	1 lunch serv	180	1	6
Chicken Fingers	1 lunch serv	390	4	18
Chicken Fresco	1 serv	1320	33	73
Chicken Fresco	1 lunch serv	660	17	36
Clam Strips	1 serv	720	9	39
Clam Strips	1 lunch serv	360	5	19
Cocktail Sauce	1 oz	30	0	0
Cole Slaw	1 serv (4 oz)	190	2	16
Crab Alfredo	1 serv	1170	35	66
Crab Alfredo	1 lunch serv	590	17	33
Fish & Shrimp Combo	1 serv	730	9	35
Fish Nuggets	1 lunch serv	320	4	14
Fish Seasoning Add On For Blackened Dinner	1 serv	70	1	5
Fish Seasoning Add On For Blackened Lunch	1 serv	50	1	4
Fish Seasoning Add On For Broiled Dinner	1 serv	45	1	5
Fish Seasoning Add On For Broiled Lunch	1 serv	35	1	4
Fish Seasoning Add On For Grilled Dinner	1 serv	35	1	4

FOOD	PORTION	CALS.	SAT. FAT	FAT
Fish Seasoning Add On For Grilled Lunch	1 serv	25	1	3
Fish Seasoning Add On For Lemon Pepper Dinner	1 serv	35	1	4
Fish Seasoning Add On For Lemon Pepper Lunch	1 serv	30	1	3
Fish Seasoning Add On For Sante Fe Style Dinner	1 serv	60	1	4
Fish Seasoning Add On For Sante Fe Style Lunch	1 serv	40	1	3
Flounder	1 lunch serv (5 oz)	130	2	2
Flounder	1 serv (8 oz)	220	1	3
French Fries	1 serv (4 oz)	350	3	22
Fried Flounder	1 lunch serv	230	3	10
Fried Shrimp	1 lunch serv	270	4	15
Fried Shrimp	12 lg	500	7	27
Garden Salad w/o Dressing	1 serv	50	0	1
Garlic Cheese Biscuit	1	140	3	8
Grilled Cheeseburger	1	580	15	34
Grilled Chicken Breasts	1 serv	230	2	7
Grilled Chicken Salad w/o Dressing	1 serv	320	2	10
Grouper	1 lunch serv (5 oz)	130	0	2
Grouper	1 serv (8 oz)	220	1	3
Haddock	1 serv (8 oz)	210	0	2
Haddock	1 lunch serv (5 oz)	120	0	1
Halibut	1 lunch serv (5 oz)	150	0	4
Halibut	1 serv (8 oz)	260	1	6
King Salmon	1 lunch serv (5 oz)	250	4	15
King Salmon	1 serv (8 oz)	420	6	25
Lake Trout	1 lunch serv (5 oz)	200	2	9
Lake Trout	1 serv (8 oz)	340	3	16
Lemon Pepper Grilled Maki Mahi	1 serv	240	1	7
Lobster Shrimp & Scallop Scampi	1 lunch serv	430	3	16
Lobster Shrimp & Scallop Scampi	1 serv	870	5	33
Mahi Mahi	1 lunch serv (5 oz)	130	0	2
Mahi Mahi	1 serv (8 oz)	220	1	3
Maine Lobster Steamed	1 serv (1.25 lb)	160	0	1
Maine Lobster Stuffed	1 serv (2 lb)	430	2	10
Marinara Sauce	1 serv	50	0	4
Melted Butter	1 oz	200	14	22
Neptune's Feast	1 serv	1210	14	62
New York Strip Steak	1 serv	560	13	34
Perch	1 serv (8 oz)	220	1	3
Perch	1 lunch serv (5 oz)	130	0	2

FOOD	PORTION	CALS.	SAT. FAT	FAT
Pollack	1 lunch serv (5 oz)	120	0	2
Pollock	1 serv (8 oz)	120	0	2
Popcorn Shrimp	1 lunch serv	380	6	24
Popcorn Shrimp	1 serv	580	9	37
Red Rockfish	1 lunch serv (5 oz)	130	1	2
Red Rockfish	1 serv (8 oz)	230	1	4
Red Snapper	1 lunch serv (5 oz)	140	0	2
Red Snapper	1 serv (8 oz)	240	1	3
Rice Pilaf	1 serv (4 oz)	180	0	2
Roasted Vegetables	1 serv (6 oz)	120	1	4
Roasted Vegetables	1 lunch serv (4 oz)	80	1	3
Sailor's Platter	1 lunch serv	250	2	12
Sandwich Blackened Catfish	1	340	2	9
Sandwich Broiled Fish	1	300	2	8
Sandwich Cajun Grilled Chicken	1	370	3	14
Sandwich Classic Fish	1	520	9	23
Sandwich Grilled Chicken	1	290	2	7
Sassy Sauce	1 oz	80	1	6
Seafood Broil	1 lunch serv	310	2	14
Shrimp & Chicken	1 serv	340	4	15
Shrimp Caesar Salad w/o Dressing	1 serv	240	4	11
Shrimp Carbonara	1 serv	1290	38	76
Shrimp Carbonara	1 lunch serv	650	19	38
Shrimp Combo	1 serv	380	5	23
Shrimp Feast	1 serv	470	5	24
Shrimp Milano	1 serv	1190	35	65
Shrimp Milano	1 lunch serv	590	17	33
Shrimp Scampi	1 lunch serv	110	1	7
Smothered Chicken	1 serv	530	15	31
Snow Crab Legs	1 serv	110	0	2
Sockeye Salmon	1 lunch serv (5 oz)	240	2	12
Sockeye Salmon	1 serv (8 oz)	410	4	21
Sole	1 serv (8 oz)	220	1	3
Sole	1 lunch serv (5 oz)	130	0	2
Soup Bread Salad w/o Dressing	1 lunch serv	430	7	18
Steak & Fried Shrimp	1 serv	780	15	46
Steak & Rock Lobster Tail	1 serv	570	11	31
Swordfish	1 serv (6 oz)	290	3	10
Swordfish	1 lunch serv (5 oz)	170	2	6
Tartar Sauce	1 oz	160	3	17
Teriyaki Grilled Chicken Breast	1 serv	240	2	7
Twice Baked Potato	1	430	14	23
Walleye	1 serv (8 oz)	210	1	3

FOOD	PORTION	CALS.	SAT. FAT	FAT
Walleye	1 lunch serv (5 oz)	120	0	2
Yellow Lake Perch	1 serv (8 oz)	220	1	3
Yellow Lake Perch	1 lunch serv (5 oz)	130	0	2
SALAD DRESSINGS				
Blue Cheese	1 serv	170	3	18
Buttermilk Ranch	1 serv	110	2	11
Caesar	1 serv	170	3	18
Dijon Honey Mustard	1 serv	140	2	13
Fat Free Ranch	1 serv	50	0	0
Lite Red Wine Vinaigrette	1 serv	50	0	3
SOUPS				
Bayou Style Gumbo	1 serv (6 oz)	120	1	4
Broccoli Cheese	1 serv	160	6	9
Clam Chowder	1 serv (6 oz)	130	3	5

ROY ROGERS

BEVERAGES

FOOD	PORTION	CALS.	SAT. FAT	FAT
Orange Juice	11 fl oz	140	tr	tr
BREAKFAST SELECTIONS				
3 Pancakes	1 serv (4.8 oz)	280	1	2
3 Pancakes w/ 1 Sausage	1 serv (6.2 oz)	430	6	16
3 Pancakes w/ 2 Bacon	1 serv (5.3 oz)	350	3	9
Bagel Cinnamon Raisin	1 (4 oz)	300	tr	1
Bagel Plain	1 (4 oz)	300	tr	2
Big Country Platters w/ Bacon	1 serv (7.6 oz)	740	13	43
Big Country Platters w/ Ham	1 serv (9.4 oz)	710	11	39
Big Country Platters w/ Sausage	1 serv (9.6 oz)	920	19	60
Biscuit	1 (2.9 oz)	390	6	21
Biscuit Bacon	1 (3.1 oz)	420	7	23
Biscuit Bacon & Egg	1 (4.2 oz)	470	8	26
Biscuit Cinnamon 'N' Raisin	1 (2.8 oz)	370	5	18
Biscuit Ham & Cheese	1 (4.5 oz)	450	8	24
Biscuit Ham & Egg	1 (5.1 oz)	460	7	23
Biscuit Ham, Egg & Cheese	1 (5.6 oz)	500	10	27
Biscuit Sausage	1 (4.1 oz)	510	10	31
Biscuit Sausage & Egg	1 (5.2 oz)	560	11	35
Hashrounds	1 serv (2.8 oz)	230	3	14
Sourdough Ham, Egg & Cheese	1 (6.8 oz)	480	9	24
DESSERTS				
Strawberry Shortcake	1 serv (6.6 oz)	480	5	21
ICE CREAM				
Ice Cream Cone	1 (4.1 oz)	180	3	4
Sundae Hot Fudge	1 (6 oz)	320	5	10
Sundae Strawberry	1 (5.5 oz)	260	3	6

FOOD	PORTION	CALS.	SAT. FAT	FAT
MAIN MENU SELECTIONS				
¼ Cheeseburger	1 (6 oz)	510	—	26
¼ Hamburger	1 (5.5 oz)	460	—	22
¼ Roaster Dark Meat	7.4 oz	490	10	34
¼ Roaster Dark Meat w/ Skin Off	4 oz	190	3	10
¼ Roaster White Meat	8.6 oz	500	9	29
¼ Roaster White Meat w/ Skin Off	4.7 oz	190	2	6
Bacon Cheeseburger	1 (5.9 oz)	520	—	31
Baked Beans	1 serv (5 oz)	160	1	2
Baked Potato	1 (3.9 oz)	130	0	1
Baked Potato w/ Margarine	1 (4.4 oz)	240	2	13
Baked Potato w/ Margarine & Sour Cream	1 (5.4 oz)	300	6	19
Cheeseburger	1 (4.2 oz)	300	7	13
Chicken Fillet Sandwich	1 (8.3 oz)	500	5	24
Cole Slaw	1 serv (5 oz)	295	4	25
Cornbread	1 serv (2.7 oz)	310	3	17
Fisherman's Fillet	1 (6.5 oz)	490	5	21
Fried Chicken Breast	1 (5.2 oz)	370	4	15
Fried Chicken Leg	1 (2.4 oz)	170	2	7
Fried Chicken Thigh	1 (4.2 oz)	330	4	15
Fried Chicken Wing	1 (2.3 oz)	200	2	8
Fry	1 lg (6.1 oz)	430	5	18
Fry	1 reg (5 oz)	350	4	15
Gravy	1 serv (1.5 fl oz)	20	tr	tr
Grilled Chicken Sandwich	1 (8.3 oz)	340	2	11
Hamburger	1 (3.8 oz)	260	4	9
Mashed Potatoes	1 serv (5 oz)	92	tr	tr
Nuggets	6 (4 oz)	290	4	18
Nuggets	9 (6.2 oz)	460	6	29
Pizza	1 serv (4.75 oz)	282	3	6
Roast Beef Sandwich	1 (5.7 oz)	260	1	4
Sourdough Bacon Cheeseburger	1 (9.1 oz)	770	—	50
Sourdough Grilled Chicken	1 (10.1 oz)	500	6	21
SALADS AND SALAD BARS				
Garden Salad	1 (9.3 oz)	190	9	14
Grilled Chicken Salad	1 serv (9.8 oz)	120	1	4
Side Salad	1 (4.9 oz)	20	tr	tr

SCHLOTZSKY'S DELI
PIZZA

FOOD	PORTION	CALS.	SAT. FAT	FAT
Chicken & Pesto	1	634	—	18
Onion & Mushroom	1	577	—	20
Smoked Turkey & Jalapeno	1	589	—	13
Vegetarian	1	555	—	17

FOOD	PORTION	CALS.	SAT. FAT	FAT
SALAD AND SALAD BARS				
Chicken Chef	1 serv	192	—	8
Turkey Club	1 serv	233	—	10
SANDWICHES				
Chicken Breast	1 sm	514	—	22
Dijon Chicken Breast	1 sm	469	—	16
Smoked Turkey	1 sm	510	—	22
The Original	1 sm	598	—	33
SOUPS				
Creole Vegetable	1 serv (8 fl oz)	120	—	3
Red Bean	1 serv (8 fl oz)	110	—	2
Shrimp & Okra	1 serv (8 fl oz)	100	—	3
Spicy Chicken	1 serv (8 fl oz)	120	—	3
SHAKEY'S				
MAIN MENU SELECTIONS				
3 Piece Fried Chicken And Potatoes	1 serv	947	—	56
5 Piece Fried Chicken And Potatoes	1 serv	1700	—	90
Hot Ham And Cheese	1	550	—	21
Potatoes	15 pieces	950	—	36
Spaghetti With Meat Sauce And Garlic Bread	1 serv	940	—	33
PIZZA				
Thick Crust Cheese	1 slice	170	—	5
Thick Crust Green Pepper, Black Olives, Mushrooms	1 slice	162	—	4
Thick Crust Pepperoni	1 slice	185	—	6
Thick Crust Sausage, Mushrooms	1 slice	179	—	6
Thick Crust Sausage, Pepperoni	1 slice	177	—	8
Thick Crust Shakey's Special	1 slice	208	—	8
Thin Crust Cheese	1 slice	133	—	5
Thin Crust Onion, Green Pepper, Black Olives, Mushrooms	1 slice	125	—	5
Thin Crust Pepperoni	1 slice	148	—	7
Thin Crust Sausage, Mushroom	1 slice	141	—	6
Thin Crust Sausage, Pepperoni	1 slice	166	—	8
Thin Crust Shakey's Special	1 slice	171	—	9
SHONEY'S				
BEVERAGES				
Hot Chocolate	1 cup	110	—	2
Orange Juice	4 oz	54	—	tr

FOOD	PORTION	CALS.	SAT. FAT	FAT
BREAKFAST SELECTIONS				
100% Natural	½ cup	244	—	11
Ambrosia Salad	¼ cup	75	—	3
Apple	1	81	—	1
Apple Butter	1 tbsp	37	—	tr
Apple Grape Surprise	¼ cup	19	0	0
Apple Ring	1	15	0	0
Apple sliced	1 slice	13	—	tr
Bacon	1 strip	36	—	3
Beef Stick	1	43	—	1
Biscuit	1	170	—	8
Blueberries	¼ cup	21	—	tr
Blueberry Muffin	1	107	—	4
Bread Pudding	1 sq	305	—	11
Breakfast Ham	1 slice	26	—	1
Brunch Cake Apple	1 sq	160	—	8
Brunch Cake Banana	1 sq	152	—	7
Brunch Cake Carrot	1 sq	150	—	7
Brunch Cake Pineapple	1 sq	147	—	7
Brunch Cake Sour Cream	1 sq	160	—	8
Buttered Toast	2 slices	163	—	5
Cantaloupe Sliced	1 slice	8	—	tr
Cantaloupe diced	½ cup	28	—	tr
Captain Crunch Berry	½ cup	73	—	2
Cheese Sauce	1 ladle	26	—	2
Chicken Pieces	1 piece	40	—	2
Chocolate Pudding	¼ cup	81	—	2
Cinnamon Honey Bun	1	344	—	12
Cottage Cheese	1 tbsp	12	—	tr
Cottage Fries	¼ cup	62	—	2
Country Gravy	¼ cup	82	—	7
Croissant	1	260	—	16
Donut Mini Cinnamon	1 (14 g)	56	—	3
DoughNugget	1	157	—	10
Egg Fried	1	159	—	15
Egg Scrambled	¼ cup	95	—	7
English Muffin w/ margarine	1	140	—	2
Fluff	¼ cup	16	0	0
French Toast	1 slice	69	—	3
Fruit Delight	¼ cup	54	—	2
Fruit Topping All Flavors	1 tbsp	24	0	0
Glaced Fruit	¼ cup	51	—	tr
Golden Pound Cake	1 slice	134	—	5
Grape Jelly	1 tbsp	60	0	0

FOOD	PORTION	CALS.	SAT. FAT	FAT
Grapefruit Canned	¼ cup	24	—	tr
Grapes	25	57	—	1
Grits	¼ cup	57	—	3
Hashbrowns	¼ cup	43	—	2
Home Fries	¼ cup	53	—	2
Honey Bun	1	265	—	14
Honeydew Sliced	1 slice	13	0	0
Jelly Packet	1	40	0	0
Jr. Bun Chocolate	1	141	—	5
Jr. Bun Honey	1	141	—	5
Jr. Bun Maple	1	141	—	5
Kiwi Sliced	1 slice	11	—	tr
Marble Cake w/ Icing	1 slice	136	—	5
Mixed Fruit	¼ cup	37	—	tr
Mushroom Topping	1 oz	25	—	2
Oleo Whipped	1 tbsp	70	—	8
Omelette Topping	1 spoonful	23	—	2
Orange	1 med	65	—	tr
Orange Sections	1 section	7	0	0
Oriental Salad	¼ cup	79	—	3
Pancake	1	41	—	tr
Pear	1	98	—	1
Pineapple Bits	1 tbsp	9	0	0
Pineapple Fresh Sliced	1 slice	10	—	tr
Pistachio Pineapple Salad	¼ cup	98	—	0
Prunes	1 tbsp	19	0	0
Raisin Bran	½ cup	87	—	1
Raisin English Muffin w/ Margarine	1	158	—	4
Sausage Link	1	91	—	9
Sausage Patty	1	136	—	13
Sausage Rice	¼ cup	110	—	6
Shortcake	1	60	—	2
Sirloin Steak Charbroiled	6 oz	357	—	25
Smoked Sausage	1	103	—	10
Snow Salad	¼ cup	72	—	4
Strawberries	5	23	—	tr
Syrup Light	1 ladle	60	0	0
Syrup Low-Cal	2.2 oz	98	0	0
Tangerine	1	37	—	tr
Trix	½ cup	54	—	tr
Waldorf Salad	¼ cup	81	—	5
Watermelon Diced	½ cup	50	—	1

FOOD	PORTION	CALS.	SAT. FAT	FAT
Watermelon Sliced	1 slice	9	—	tr
Whipped Topping	1 scoop	10	—	1
CHILDREN'S MENU SELECTIONS				
Jr. Burger All-American	1 serv	234	—	11
Kid's Chicken Dinner (fried)	1 serv	244	—	13
Kid's Fish N' Chips (includes fries)	1 serv	337	—	17
Kid's Fried Shrimp	1 serv	194	—	12
Kid's Spaghetti	1 serv	247	—	8
DESSERTS				
Apple Pie A La Mode	1 slice	492	—	23
Carrot Cake	1 slice	500	—	26
Strawberry Pie	1 slice	332	—	17
Walnut Brownie A La Mode	1	576	—	34
ICE CREAM				
Hot Fudge Cake	1 slice	522	—	20
Hot Fudge Sundae	1	451	—	22
Strawberry Sundae	1	380	—	19
MAIN MENU SELECTIONS				
All-American Burger	1	501	—	33
BBQ Sauce	1 souffle cup	41	—	1
Bacon Burger	1	591	—	40
Baked Fish	1 serv	170	—	1
Baked Fish Light	1 serv	170	—	1
Baked Ham Sandwich	1	290	—	10
Baked Potato	10 oz	264	—	tr
Beef Patty Light	1 serv	289	—	23
Charbroiled Chicken	1 serv	239	—	7
Charbroiled Chicken Sandwich	1	451	—	17
Chicken Fillet Sandwich	1	464	—	21
Chicken Tenders	1 serv	388	—	20
Cocktail Sauce	1 souffle cup	36	—	tr
Country Fried Sandwich	1	588	—	26
Country Fried Steak	1 serv	449	—	27
Fish N' Chips (includes fries)	1 serv	639	—	35
Fish N' Shrimp	1 serv	487	—	26
Fish Sandwich	1	323	—	13
French Fries	4 oz	252	—	10
French Fries	3 oz	189	—	8
Fried Fish Light	1 serv	297	—	14
Grecian Bread	1 slice	80	—	2
Grilled Bacon & Cheese Sandwich	1	440	—	28
Grilled Cheese Sandwich	1	302	—	17

FOOD	PORTION	CALS.	SAT. FAT	FAT
Half O'Pound	1 serv	435	—	34
Ham Club On Whole Wheat	1	642	—	36
Hawaiian Chicken	1 serv	262	—	7
Italian Feast	1 serv	500	—	20
Lasagna	1 serv	297	—	10
Liver N' Onions	1 serv	411	—	23
Mushroom Swiss Burger	1	616	—	42
Old-Fashioned Burger	1	470	—	28
Onion Rings	1	52	—	3
Patty Melt	1	640	—	42
Philly Steak Sandwich	1	673	—	44
Reuben Sandwich	1	596	—	35
Ribeye	6 oz	605	—	51
Rice	3.5 oz	137	—	4
Sauteed Mushrooms	3 oz	75	—	7
Sauteed Onions	2.5 oz	37	—	2
Seafood Platter	1 serv	566	—	28
Shoney Burger	1	498	—	36
Shrimp Bite-Size	1 serv	387	—	25
Shrimp Broiled	1 serv	93	—	18
Shrimp Charbroiled	1 serv	138	—	3
Shrimp Sampler	1 serv	412	—	23
Shrimper's Feast	1 serv	383	—	22
Shrimper's Feast Large	1 serv	575	—	33
Sirloin	6 oz	357	—	25
Slim Jim Sandwich	1	484	—	24
Spaghetti	1 serv	496	—	16
Steak N' Shrimp (charbroiled shrimp)	1 serv	361	—	23
Steak N' Shrimp (fried shrimp)	1 serv	507	—	33
Sweet N' Sour Sauce	1 souffle cup	58	0	0
Tartar Sauce	1 souffle cup	84	—	8
Turkey Club On Whole Wheat	1	635	—	33
SALAD DRESSINGS				
Biscayne Lo-Cal	2 tbsp	62	—	1
Blue Cheese	2 tbsp	113	—	13
Creamy Italian	2 tbsp	135	—	15
French	2 tbsp	124	—	12
Golden Italian	2 tbsp	141	—	15
Honey Mustard	2 tbsp	165	—	17
Ranch	2 tbsp	95	—	10
Rue French	2 tbsp	122	—	10
Thousand Island	2 tbsp	130	—	13
W.W. Italian	2 tbsp	10	—	0

FOOD	PORTION	CALS.	SAT. FAT	FAT
SALADS AND SALAD BARS				
Ambrosia Salad	¼ cup	75	—	3
Apple Grape Surprise	¼ cup	19	—	0
Apple Ring	1	15	—	0
Bacon Bits	1 spoonful	15	—	1
Beet Onion Salad	¼ cup	25	—	1
Broccoli	¼ cup	4	—	tr
Broccoli Cauliflower Carrot Salad	¼ cup	53	—	4
Broccoli Cauliflower Ranch	¼ cup	65	—	6
Broccoli & Cauliflower	¼ cup	98	—	9
Carrot	¼ cup	10	—	tr
Carrot Apple Salad	¼ cup	99	—	9
Cauliflower	¼ cup	8	—	tr
Celery	1 tbsp	5	—	0
Cheese Shredded	1 tbsp	21	—	2
Chocolate Pudding	¼ cup	81	—	2
Chow Mein Noodles	1 spoonful	13	—	1
Cole Slaw	¼ cup	69	—	5
Cottage Cheese	1 tbsp	12	—	tr
Croutons	1 spoonful	13	—	tr
Cucumber	1 tbsp	1	—	0
Cucumber Lite	¼ cup	12	—	tr
Don's Pasta	¼ cup	82	—	5
Egg Diced	1 tbsp	15	—	1
Fruit Delight	¼ cup	54	—	2
Fruit Topping All Flavors	¼ cup	64	—	tr
Glaced Fruit	¼ cup	51	—	tr
Granola	1 spoonful	25	—	1
Grapefruit	¼ cup	24	—	tr
Green Pepper	1 tbsp	1	—	0
Italian Vegetable	¼ cup	11	—	tr
Jello	¼ cup	40	—	0
Jello Fluff	¼ cup	16	—	tr
Kidney Bean Salad	¼ cup	55	—	2
Lettuce	1.8 oz	7	—	tr
Macaroni Salad	¼ cup	207	—	14
Margarine Whipped	1 tsp	23	—	3
Melba Toast	2	20	—	0
Mixed Fruit Salad	¼ cup	37	—	tr
Mixed Squash	¼ cup	49	—	4
Mushrooms	1 tbsp	1	—	0
Oil	1 tsp	45	—	5
Olives Black	2	10	—	1

FOOD	PORTION	CALS.	SAT. FAT	FAT
Olives Green	2	8	—	1
Onion Sliced	1 tbsp	1	—	0
Oriental Salad	¼ cup	79	—	3
Pea Salad	¼ cup	73	—	6
Pepperoni	1 tbsp	30	—	3
Pickle Chips	1 slice	5	—	0
Pickle Spear	1 spear	2	—	0
Pineapple Bits	1 tbsp	9	—	0
Pistachio Pineapple Salad	¼ cup	98	—	3
Prunes	1 tbsp	19	—	0
Radish	1 tbsp	1	—	0
Raisins	1 spoonful	26	—	0
Rotelli Pasta	¼ cup	78	—	4
Seign Salad	¼ cup	72	—	4
Snow Delight	¼ cup	72	—	4
Spaghetti Salad	¼ cup	81	—	5
Spinach	¼ cup	1	—	0
Spring Pasta	¼ cup	38	—	3
Summer Salad	¼ cup	114	—	12
Sunflower Seeds	1 spoonful	40	—	3
Three Bean Salad	¼ cup	96	—	5
Trail Mix	1 spoonful	30	—	0
Turkey Ham	1 tbsp	12	—	1
Waldorf	¼ cup	81	—	5
Wheat Bread	1 slice	71	—	1
SOUPS				
Bean	6 fl oz	63	—	1
Beef Cabbage	6 fl oz	86	—	3
Broccoli Cauliflower	6 fl oz	124	—	9
Cheddar Chowder	6 fl oz	91	—	2
Cheese Florentine Ham	6 fl oz	110	—	8
Chicken Gumbo	6 fl oz	60	—	2
Chicken Noodle	6 fl oz	62	—	1
Chicken Rice	6 fl oz	72	—	1
Clam Chowder	6 fl oz	94	—	5
Corn Chowder	6 fl oz	148	—	5
Cream Of Broccoli	6 fl oz	75	—	5
Cream Of Chicken	6 fl oz	136	—	9
Cream Of Chicken Vegetable	6 fl oz	79	—	1
Onion	6 fl oz	29	—	2
Potato	6 fl oz	102	—	3
Tomato Florentine	6 fl oz	63	—	1
Tomato Vegetable	6 fl oz	46	—	tr
Vegetable Beef	6 fl oz	82	—	2

FOOD	PORTION	CALS.	SAT. FAT	FAT
SIZZLER				
DESSERTS				
Chocolate & Vanilla Soft Serve	4 oz	136	4	4
Chocolate Syrup	1 oz	90	0	0
Strawberry Topping	1 oz	70	0	0
Whipped Topping	1 tbsp	12	1	1
HOT BUFFET				
Broccoli Cheese Soup	1 serv (4 oz)	139	2	9
Chicken Noodle Soup	1 serv (4 oz)	31	0	1
Chicken Wings	1 oz	73	1	4
Clam Chowder	1 serv (4 oz)	118	0	6
Fettucine	2 oz	80	0	1
Focaccia Bread	2 pieces	108	1	7
Marinara Sauce	1 oz	13	0	0
Meatballs	4	157	5	11
Minestrone Soup	1 serv (4 oz)	36	0	0
Nacho Cheese Soup	1 serv (4 oz)	120	5	10
Potato Skins	2 oz	160	1	8
Refried Beans	¼ cup	62	2	1
Saltine Crackers	2	25	0	1
Spaghetti	2 oz	80	0	0
Taco Filling	2 oz	103	4	9
Taco Shells	1	50	0	2
Vegetable Sirloin Soup	1 serv (4 oz)	60	1	2
MAIN MENU SELECTIONS				
Buttery Dipping Sauce	1 serv (1.5 oz)	330	7	37
Cheese Toast	1 piece	273	5	21
Cocktail Sauce	1 serv (1.5 oz)	40	0	0
Dakota Ranch Steak	1 (6 oz)	316	8	20
Dakota Ranch Steak	1 (8 oz)	421	11	27
Dakota Ranch Steak	1 (9.5 oz)	500	13	32
French Fries	1 serv (4 oz)	358	6	12
Hamburger	1	626	12	33
Hibachi Chicken Breast w/ Pineapple	5 oz	193	1	3
Hibachi Sauce	1 serv (1.5 oz)	57	0	0
Lemon Herb Chicken Breast	5 oz	140	1	3
Malibu Chicken Patty	1	310	3	19
Malibu Sauce	1 serv (1.5 oz)	283	6	31
Margarine Whipped	1½ tbsp	105	2	12
Potato Baked Plain	1 (4 oz)	105	0	0
Rice Pilaf	1 serv (6 oz)	256	1	5
Salmon	8 oz	110	2	12

FOOD	PORTION	CALS.	SAT. FAT	FAT
Sante Fe Chicken Breast	5 oz	150	1	3
Shrimp Broiled	5 oz	150	1	6
Shrimp Fried	4 pieces	223	0	2
Shrimp Mini	4 oz	152	0	1
Shrimp Scampi	5 oz	143	1	3
Sour Dressing	2 tbsp	60	5	6
Swordfish	8 oz	315	3	14
Tartar Sauce	1 serv (1.5 oz)	170	3	17
SALAD DRESSINGS				
Blue Cheese	1 oz	111	4	12
Honey Mustard	1 oz	160	2	16
Italian Lite	1 oz	14	0	0
Japanese Rice Vinegar Fat Free	1 oz	10	0	0
Parmesan Italian	1 oz	100	2	10
Ranch	1 oz	120	2	12
Ranch Reduced Calorie	1 oz	90	2	8
Thousand Island	1 oz	143	2	15
SALADS AND SALAD BARS				
Alfafa Sprouts	¼ cup	2	0	0
Avocado	½	153	2	15
Bean Sprouts	¼ cup	8	0	0
Beets	¼ cup	13	0	0
Bell Peppers	2 oz	8	0	0
Broccoli	½ cup	12	0	0
Cabbage Red	¼ cup	5	0	0
Cantoupe	½ cup	28	0	0
Carrot & Raisin Salad	2 oz	130	2	10
Carrots	¼ cup	12	0	0
Chinese Chicken Salad	2 oz	54	0	2
Chives	1 oz	62	1	6
Cottage Cheese	2 oz	51	1	1
Cucumber	2 oz	7	0	0
Eggs	1 oz	44	1	3
Garbanzo Beans	¼ cup	63	1	1
Grapes	½ cup	29	0	0
Guacamole	1 oz	42	1	4
Honeydew Melon	½ cup	30	0	0
Iceberg Lettuce	1 cup	7	0	0
Jicama	2 oz	13	0	0
Kidney Beans	¼ cup	52	0	0
Kiwifruit	2 oz	35	0	0
Mediterranean Minted Fruit Salad	2 oz	29	0	0
Mexican Fiesta Salad	2 oz	54	0	1

FOOD	PORTION	CALS.	SAT. FAT	FAT
Mushrooms	¼ cup	4	0	0
Old Fashioned Potato Salad	2 oz	84	1	5
Onions Red	2 tbsp	8	0	0
Peaches	¼ cup	34	0	0
Peas	¼ cup	31	0	0
Pineapple	½ cup	38	0	0
Real Bacon Bits	1 tbsp	27	0	2
Red Herb Potato Salad	2 oz	121	1	9
Romaine Lettuce	1 cup	9	0	0
Salsa	1 oz	7	0	0
Seafood Louis Pasta Salad	2 oz	64	0	2
Seafood Salad	2 oz	56	1	3
Spicy Jicama Salad	2 oz	16	0	0
Spinach	½ cup	6	0	0
Strawberries	½ cup	22	0	0
Teriyaki Beef Salad	2 oz	49	1	2
Tomatoes Cherry	¼ cup	12	0	0
Tuna Pasta Salad	2 oz	133	7	10
Turkey Ham	1 oz	62	2	5
Watermelon	½ cup	26	0	0
Zucchini	¼ cup	5	0	0

SKIPPER'S

BEVERAGES

Root Beer Float	1 (12 oz)	302	—	10

DESSERTS

Jell-O	1 serv (2.75 oz)	55	0	0

MAIN MENU SELECTIONS

Baked Fish With Margarine & Seas	1 serv (4.4 oz)	147	—	3
Baked Potato	1 (6 oz)	145	0	0
Captain's Cut	1 piece (2.6 oz)	160	—	7
Cocktail Sauce	1 tbsp	20	0	0
Coleslaw	1 serv (5 oz)	289	—	27
Corn Muffin	1 (2 oz)	91	—	5
English Style Fish	1 piece (2.4 oz)	187	—	12
French Fries	1 serv (3.5 oz)	239	—	12
Green Salad (no dressing)	1 serv (4 oz)	24	0	0
Ketchup	1 tbsp	17	0	0
Margarine	1 serv (0.5 oz)	50	—	6
Shrimp Fried Cajun	1 serv (4 oz)	342	—	21
Shrimp Fried Jumbo	1 piece (.65 oz)	51	—	2
Shrimp Fried Original	1 serv (4 oz)	266	—	13
Tartar Original	1 tbsp	65	—	7

FOOD	PORTION	CALS.	SAT. FAT	FAT
SOUPS				
Clam Chowder	1 pint (12 fl oz)	200	—	7
Clam Chowder	1 cup (6 fl oz)	100	—	4
SMOOTHIE KING				
Activator Banana	1 (20 oz)	429	tr	1
Activator Chocolate	1 (20 oz)	429	tr	1
Activator Strawberry	1 (20 oz)	559	tr	1
Activator Vanilla	1 (20 oz)	429	tr	1
Angel Food	1 (20 oz)	330	tr	1
Blackberry Dream	1 (20 oz)	343	tr	tr
Caribbean Way	1 (20 oz)	392	tr	tr
Celestial Cherry High	1 (20 oz)	285	tr	tr
Coconut Surprise	1 (20 oz)	457	2	6
Cranberry Supreme	1 (20 oz)	577	tr	1
Cranberry Cooler	1 (20 oz)	538	tr	tr
GoGuava	1 (20 oz)	300	0	0
Grape Expectations	1 (20 oz)	399	tr	tr
Grape Expectations II	1 (20 oz)	529	tr	tr
Hawaiian Cafe Au Lei	1 (20 oz)	286	tr	tr
High Protein Almond Mocha	1 (20 oz)	402	2	13
High Protein Banana	1 (20 oz)	412	2	14
High Protein Chocolate	1 (20 oz)	401	2	13
High Protein Lemon	1 (20 oz)	390	2	13
High Protein Pineapple	1 (20 oz)	380	2	13
Hulk Chocolate	1 (20 oz)	846	17	29
Hulk Strawberry	1 (20 oz)	953	16	29
Hulk Vanilla	1 (20 oz)	846	16	29
Immune Builder	1 (20 oz)	333	tr	1
Instant Vigor	1 (20 oz)	359	tr	1
Island Treat	1 (20 oz)	334	tr	1
Lemon Twist Banana	1 (20 oz)	339	tr	tr
Lemon Twist Strawberry	1 (20 oz)	399	tr	tr
Light & Fluffy	1 (20 oz)	389	tr	tr
Malt	1 (20 oz)	887	26	41
Mangofest	1 (20 oz)	320	0	0
Mo'cuccino	1 (20 oz)	440	7	12
Muscle Punch	1 (20 oz)	339	tr	1
Muscle Punch Plus	1 (20 oz)	340	tr	1
Peach Slice	1 (20 oz)	341	tr	tr
Peach Slice Plus	1 (20 oz)	471	tr	tr
Peanut Power	1 (20 oz)	502	4	21
Peanut Power Plus Grape	1 (20 oz)	703	4	21
Peanut Power Plus Strawberry	1 (20 oz)	632	4	21

FOOD	PORTION	CALS.	SAT. FAT	FAT
Pep Upper	1 (20 oz)	334	tr	1
Pineapple Pleasure	1 (20 oz)	313	tr	tr
Power Punch	1 (20 oz)	430	tr	1
Power Punch Plus	1 (20 oz)	499	tr	2
Raspberry Sunrise	1 (20 oz)	335	tr	1
Shake	1 (20 oz)	875	25	41
Slim & Trim Chocolate	1 (20 oz)	270	1	2
Slim & Trim Strawberry	1 (20 oz)	357	tr	1
Slim & Trim Vanilla	1 (20 oz)	227	tr	1
Super Punch	1 (20 oz)	425	tr	tr
Super Punch Plus	1 (20 oz)	516	tr	tr
Yogurt D'Lite	1 (20 oz)	341	2	4
Youth Fountain	1 (20 oz)	267	tr	tr

SONIC DRIVE-IN

FOOD	PORTION	CALS.	SAT. FAT	FAT
#1 Hamburger	1 (6.6 oz)	409	—	27
#2 Hamburger	1 (6.6 oz)	323	—	16
B-L-T Sandwich	1 (6.1 oz)	327	—	19
Bacon Cheeseburger	1 (7.2 oz)	548	—	39
Chicken Sandwich Breaded	1 (7.4 oz)	455	—	25
Chili Pie	1 (3.7 oz)	327	—	23
Corn Dog	1 (3 oz)	280	—	15
Extra Long Cheese Coney	1 (8.9 oz)	635	—	39
Extra Long Cheese Coney w/ Onions	1 (9.4 oz)	640	—	39
Fish Sandwich	1 (6.1 oz)	277	—	7
French Fries	1 lg (6.7 oz)	315	—	11
French Fries	1 reg (5 oz)	233	—	8
French Fries w/ Cheese	1 lg (7.7 oz)	219	—	20
Grilled Cheese Sandwich	1 (2.8 oz)	288	—	17
Grilled Chicken Sandwich w/o Dressing	1 (6.4 oz)	215	—	4
Hickory Burger	1 (5.1 oz)	314	—	16
Jalapeno Burger Double Meat & Cheese	1 (9.1 oz)	638	—	41
Mini Burger	1 (3.5 oz)	246	—	1
Mini Cheeseburger	1 (3.9 oz)	281	—	14
Onion Rings	1 reg (3.5 oz)	404	—	27
Onion Rings	1 lg (5 oz)	577	—	38
Regular Cheese Coney	1 (5 oz)	358	—	15
Regular Cheese Coney w/ Onions	1 (5.3 oz)	361	—	23
Regular Hot Dog	1 (3.5 oz)	258	—	15
Steak Sandwich Breaded	1 (3.9 oz)	631	—	42
Super Sonic Burger w/ Mustard Double Meat & Cheese	1 (10.1 oz)	644	—	41

FOOD	PORTION	CALS.	SAT. FAT	FAT
Super Sonic Burger w/ Mayo Double Meat & Cheese	1 (10.1 oz)	730	—	52
Tater Tots	1 serv (3 oz)	150	—	7
Tater Tots w/ Cheese	1 serv (3.6 oz)	220	—	13

STARBUCKS
BEVERAGES

FOOD	PORTION	CALS.	SAT. FAT	FAT
Americano Grande	1 serv	10	0	0
Americano Short	1 serv	5	0	0
Americano Tall	1 serv	5	0	0
Cappuccino Grande Lowfat Milk	1 serv	110	3	4
Cappuccino Grande Nonfat Milk	1 serv	80	0	0
Cappuccino Grande Whole Milk	1 serv	140	5	7
Cappuccino Short Lowfat Milk	1 serv	60	1	2
Cappuccino Short Nonfat Milk	1 serv	40	0	0
Cappuccino Short Whole Milk	1 serv	70	2	4
Cappuccino Tall Lowfat Milk	1 serv	80	2	3
Cappuccino Tall Nonfat Milk	1 serv	60	0	0
Cappuccino Tall Whole Milk	1 serv	110	4	6
Cocoa w/ Whipping Cream Grande Lowfat Milk	1 serv	350	12	20
Cocoa w/ Whipping Cream Grande Nonfat Milk	1 serv	310	9	15
Cocoa w/ Whipping Cream Grande Whole Milk	1 serv	400	16	26
Cocoa w/ Whipping Cream Short Lowfat Milk	1 serv	180	7	11
Cocoa w/ Whipping Cream Short Nonfat Milk	1 serv	160	5	8
Cocoa w/ Whipping Cream Short Whole Milk	1 serv	210	8	14
Cocoa w/ Whipping Cream Tall Lowfat Milk	1 serv	270	9	15
Cocoa w/ Whipping Cream Tall Nonfat Milk	1 serv	230	7	11
Cocoa w/ Whipping Cream Tall Whole Milk	1 serv	300	12	19
Drip Coffee Grande	1 serv	10	0	0
Drip Coffee Short	1 serv	5	0	0
Drip Coffee Tall	1 serv	10	0	0
Espresso Doppio	1 serv	5	0	0
Espresso Macchiato Doppio Lowfat Milk	1 serv	15	0	0
Espresso Macchiato Doppio Nonfat Milk	1 serv	15	0	0

FOOD	PORTION	CALS.	SAT. FAT	FAT
Espresso Macchiato Doppio Whole Milk	1 serv	15	0	1
Espresso Macchiato Solo Lowfat Milk	1 serv	10	0	0
Espresso Macchiato Solo Nonfat Milk	1 serv	10	0	0
Espresso Macchiato Solo Whole Milk	1 serv	15	0	1
Espresso Solo	1 serv	5	0	0
Espresso Con Panna Doppio	1 serv	45	3	4
Espresso Con Panna Solo	1 serv	40	3	4
Latte Grande Lowfat Milk	1 serv	170	4	6
Latte Grande Nonfat Milk	1 serv	130	0	1
Latte Grande Whole Milk	1 serv	220	7	11
Latte Short Lowfat Milk	1 serv	80	2	3
Latte Short Nonfat Milk	1 serv	60	0	0
Latte Short Whole Milk	1 serv	100	3	5
Latte Tall Lowfat Milk	1 serv	140	3	5
Latte Tall Nonfat Milk	1 serv	110	0	1
Latte Tall Whole Milk	1 serv	180	6	10
Latte Iced Grande Lowfat Milk	1 serv	170	4	6
Latte Iced Grande Nonfat Milk	1 serv	130	0	1
Latte Iced Grande Whole Milk	1 serv	210	7	11
Latte Iced Short Lowfat Milk	1 serv	90	2	3
Latte Iced Short Nonfat Milk	1 serv	70	0	0
Latte Iced Short Whole Milk	1 serv	120	4	6
Latte Iced Tall Lowfat Milk	1 serv	120	3	5
Latte Iced Tall Nonfat Milk	1 serv	90	0	0
Latte Iced Tall Whole Milk	1 serv	150	5	8
Mocha w/ Whipping Cream Grande Lowfat Milk	1 serv	350	12	20
Mocha w/ Whipping Cream Grande Nonfat Milk	1 serv	310	9	15
Mocha w/ Whipping Cream Grande Whole Milk	1 serv	390	15	25
Mocha w/ Whipping Cream Short Lowfat Milk	1 serv	170	6	10
Mocha w/ Whipping Cream Short Nonfat Milk	1 serv	150	5	8
Mocha w/ Whipping Cream Short Whole Milk	1 serv	180	8	12
Mocha w/ Whipping Cream Tall Lowfat Milk	1 serv	260	9	15

FOOD	PORTION	CALS.	SAT. FAT	FAT
Mocha w/ Whipping Cream Tall Nonfat Milk	1 serv	230	7	11
Mocha w/ Whipping Cream Tall Whole Milk	1 serv	290	11	18
Mocha w/o Whipping Cream Grande Lowfat Milk	1 serv	230	5	7
Mocha w/o Whipping Cream Grande Nonfat Milk	1 serv	190	2	3
Mocha w/o Whipping Cream Grande Whole Milk	1 serv	260	12	7
Mocha w/o Whipping Cream Short Lowfat Milk	1 serv	120	3	4
Mocha w/o Whipping Cream Short Nonfat Milk	1 serv	100	1	2
Mocha w/o Whipping Cream Short Whole Milk	1 serv	150	4	7
Mocha w/o Whipping Cream Tall Lowfat Milk	1 serv	170	4	5
Mocha w/o Whipping Cream Tall Nonfat Milk	1 serv	140	2	2
Mocha w/o Whipping Cream Tall Whole Milk	1 serv	190	5	9
Mocha Syrup Grande	1 serv (2 oz)	80	2	3
Mocha Syrup Short	1 serv (1 oz)	40	1	1
Mocha Syrup Tall	1 serv (1.5 oz)	60	1	2
Steamed Lowfat Milk Grande	1 serv	180	4	7
Steamed Lowfat Milk Short	1 serv	90	2	3
Steamed Lowfat Milk Tall	1 serv	140	3	5
Steamed Nonfat Milk Grande	1 serv	130	0	1
Steamed Nonfat Milk Short	1 serv	60	0	0
Steamed Nonfat Milk Tall	1 serv	100	0	1
Steamed Whole Milk Grande	1 serv	230	8	13
Steamed Whole Milk Short	1 serv	110	4	6
Steamed Whole Milk Tall	1 serv	180	6	10
Whipping Cream Grande	1 serv (1.1 oz)	110	7	12
Whipping Cream Short	1 serv (0.7 oz)	70	5	7
Whipping Cream Tall	1 serv (0.8 oz)	80	5	9
ICE CREAM				
Biscotte Bliss	½ cup	240	7	12
Caffe Almond Fudge	½ cup	260	7	13
Caffe Almond Roast	1 bar	280	9	18
Dark Roast Expresso Swirl	½ cup	220	6	10
Frappuccino Coffee	1 bar	110	1	2

FOOD	PORTION	CALS.	SAT. FAT	FAT
Italian Roast Coffee	½ cup	230	7	12
Javachip	½ cup	250	8	13
Low Fat Latte	½ cup	170	2	3
Low Fat Mocha Mambo	½ cup	170	2	3
Vanilla Mochachip	½ cup	270	10	16
SNACKS				
Crunchy Honey Bar	1 (1.06 oz)	150	3	7
Lively Lemon Bar	1 (1.23 oz)	140	1	4
Tangy Apple Bar	1 (1.23 oz)	140	1	4
STUFF'N TURKEY				
Chef's Salad	1 serv	288	3	9
Grilled Turkey Breast	1 serv	244	1	3
Homemade Turkey Salad	1 serv	651	5	29
Real Fresh Roasted Turkey Breast	1 serv	384	1	5
Rotisserie Turkey Breast	1 serv	251	1	3
Thanksgiving Dinner On A Sandwich	1 serv	605	4	16
Turkey Barbecue	1 serv	478	1	6
Turkey Powerhouse	1 serv	482	5	11
SUBWAY				
COOKIES				
Chocolate Chip	1	210	—	10
Chocolate Chip M&M	1	210	—	10
Chocolate Chunk	1	210	—	10
Double Chocolate Brazil Nut	1	230	—	12
Oatmeal Raisin	1	200	—	8
Peanut Butter	1	220	—	12
Sugar	1	230	—	12
White Chocolate Macadamia Nut	1	230	—	12
SALAD DRESSINGS				
Creamy Italian	1 tbsp	65	—	6
Fat Free French	1 tbsp	15	—	0
Fat Free Italian	1 tbsp	5	—	0
Fat Free Ranch	1 tbsp	12	—	0
French	1 tbsp	65	—	5
Ranch	1 tbsp	87	—	9
Thousand Island	1 tbsp	65	—	6
SALADS AND SALAD BARS				
B.L.T.	1 serv	140	—	8
Bread Bowl	1 serv	330	—	4
Chicken Taco	1 serv	250	—	14
Classic Italian B.M.T.	1 serv	274	—	20

FOOD	PORTION	CALS.	SAT. FAT	FAT
Cold Cut Trio	1 serv	191	—	11
Ham	1 serv	116	—	3
Meatball	1 serv	233	—	14
Pizza	1 serv	277	—	20
Roast Beef	1 serv	117	—	3
Roasted Chicken Breast	1 serv	162	—	4
Steak & Cheese	1 serv	212	—	8
Subway Club	1 serv	126	—	3
Subway Melt	1 serv	195	—	10
Subway Seafood & Crab	1 serv	244	—	17
Subway Seafood & Crab w/ Light Mayonnaise	1 serv	161	—	8
Tuna	1 serv	356	—	30
Tuna w/ Light Mayonnaise	1 serv	205	—	13
Turkey Breast	1 serv	102	—	2
Turkey Breast & Ham	1 serv	109	—	3
Veggie Delight	1 serv	51	—	1
SANDWICHES				
6 Inch Cold Ham	1	302	—	5
6 Inch Cold Tuna w/ Light Mayonnaise	1	391	—	15
6 Inch Cold Sub B.L.T.	1	327	—	10
6 Inch Cold Sub Classic Italian B.M.T.	1	460	—	22
6 Inch Cold Sub Cold Cut Trio	1	378	—	13
6 Inch Cold Sub Roast Beef	1	303	—	5
6 Inch Cold Sub Subway Club	1	312	—	5
6 Inch Cold Sub Subway Seafood & Crab	1	430	—	19
6 Inch Cold Sub Subway Seafood & Crab w/ Light Mayonniase	1	347	—	10
6 Inch Cold Sub Tuna	1	542	—	32
6 Inch Cold Sub Turkey Breast	1	289	—	4
6 Inch Cold Sub Turkey Breast & Ham	1	295	—	5
6 Inch Cold Sub Veggie Delight	1	237	—	3
6 Inch Hot Subway Melt	1	382	—	12
6 Inch Hot Sub Chicken Taco Sub	1	436	—	16
6 Inch Hot Sub Meatball	1	419	—	16
6 Inch Hot Sub Pizza Sub	1	464	—	22
6 Inch Hot Sub Roasted Chicken Breast	1	348	—	6
6 Inch Hot Sub Steak & Cheese	1	398	—	10
Bacon	2 strips	45	—	4

FOOD	PORTION	CALS.	SAT. FAT	FAT
Cheese	2 triangles	41	—	3
Deli Sandwich Bologna	1	292	—	12
Deli Sandwich Ham	1	234	—	4
Deli Sandwich Roast Beef	1	245	—	4
Deli Sandwich Tuna	1	354	—	18
Deli Sandwich Tuna w/ Light Mayonnaise	1	279	—	9
Deli Sandwich Turkey Breast	1	235	—	4
Light Mayonnaise	1 tsp	18	—	2
Mayonnaise	1 tsp	37	—	4
Mustard	2 tsp	8	—	0
Olive Oil Blend	1 tsp	45	—	5
Vinegar	1 tsp	1	—	0

TACO BELL
BEVERAGES

FOOD	PORTION	CALS.	SAT. FAT	FAT
Orange Juice	1 serv (6 oz)	80	0	0

BREAKFAST MENU SELECTIONS

FOOD	PORTION	CALS.	SAT. FAT	FAT
Breakfast Quesadilla Cheese	1 (5.5 oz)	380	9	21
Breakfast Quesadilla w/ Bacon	1 (6 oz)	450	11	27
Breakfast Quesadilla w/ Sausage	1 (6 oz)	430	10	25
Country Breakfast Burrito	1 (4 oz)	270	5	14
Double Bacon & Egg Burrito	1 (6.25 oz)	480	9	27
Fiesta Breakfast Burrito	1 (3.5 oz)	280	6	16
Grande Breakfast Burrito	1 (6.25 oz)	420	7	22
Hash Brown Nuggets	1 serv (3.5 oz)	280	5	18

MAIN MENU SELECTIONS

FOOD	PORTION	CALS.	SAT. FAT	FAT
7-Layer Burrito	1 (10 oz)	530	7	23
BLT Soft Taco	1 (4.5 oz)	340	8	23
Bacon Cheeseburger Burrito	1 (8.5 oz)	570	12	31
Bean Burrito	1 (7 oz)	380	4	12
Big Beef Burrito Supreme	1 (10.5 oz)	520	10	23
Big Beef MexiMelt	1 (4.75 oz)	290	7	15
Big Chicken Burrito Supreme	1 (9 oz)	510	7	24
Border Sauce Fire	1 serv (0.3 oz)	0	0	0
Border Sauce Hot	1 serv (0.3 oz)	0	0	0
Border Sauce Mild	1 serv (0.3 oz)	0	0	0
Burger Sauce	1 serv (0.5 oz)	60	1	5
Burrito Supreme	1 (9 oz)	440	8	19
Cheddar Cheese	1 serv (0.25 oz)	30	2	2
Cheese Quesadilla	1 (4.25 oz)	350	9	18
Chicken Fajita Wrap	1 (8 oz)	470	6	22
Chicken Fajita Wrap Supreme	1 (9 oz)	520	8	25
Chicken Quesadilla	1 (6 oz)	410	10	21

FOOD	PORTION	CALS.	SAT. FAT	FAT
Chicken Club Burrito	1 (8 oz)	540	10	32
Chili Cheese Burrito	1 (5 oz)	330	6	13
Choco Taco Ice Cream Dessert	1 serv (4 oz)	310	10	17
Cinnamon Twists	1 serv (1 oz)	140	0	6
Club Sauce	1 serv (0.5 oz)	80	1	8
Double Decker Taco	1 (5.75 oz)	340	5	15
Double Decker Taco Supreme	1 (7 oz)	390	8	19
Fajita Sauce	1 serv (0.5 oz)	70	1	7
Green Sauce	1 serv (1 oz)	5	0	0
Grilled Chicken Burrito	1 (7 oz)	410	5	15
Grilled Chicken Soft Taco	1 (4.5 oz)	240	4	12
Grilled Steak Soft Taco	1 (4.5 oz)	230	3	10
Grilled Steak Soft Taco Supreme	1 (5.75 oz)	290	5	14
Guacamole	1 serv (0.75 oz)	35	0	3
Mexican Pizza	1 serv (7.75 oz)	570	10	35
Mexican Rice	1 serv (4.75 oz)	190	4	9
Nacho Cheese Sauce	2 serv (2 oz)	120	3	10
Nachos	1 serv (3.5 oz)	320	4	18
Nachos Beef Beef Supreme	1 serv (7 oz)	450	8	24
Nachos Bellgrande	1 serv (11 oz)	770	11	39
Picante Sauce	1 serv (0.3 oz)	0	0	0
Pico De Gallo	1 serv (0.75 oz)	5	0	0
Pintos 'n Cheese	1 serv (4.5 oz)	190	4	9
Red Sauce	1 serv (1 oz)	10	0	0
Soft Taco	1 (3.5 oz)	220	5	10
Soft Taco Supreme	1 (5 oz)	260	7	14
Sour Cream	1 serv (0.75 oz)	40	3	4
Steak Fajita Wrap	1 (8 oz)	470	6	21
Steak Fajita Wrap Supreme	1 (9 oz)	510	8	25
Taco	1 (2.75 oz)	180	4	10
Taco Supreme	1 (4 oz)	220	7	14
Taco Salad w/ Salsa	1 (19 oz)	850	15	52
Taco Salad w/ Salsa w/o Shell	1 (16.5 oz)	420	11	22
Three Cheese Blend	1 serv (0.25 oz)	25	1	2
Tostada	1 (6.25 oz)	300	5	15
Veggie Fajita Wrap	1 (8 oz)	420	5	19
Veggie Fajita Wrap Supreme	1 (9 oz)	470	7	22

TACO JOHN'S
CHILDREN'S MENU SELECTIONS

Kid's Meal Softshell Taco	1 serv (8.5 oz)	617	10	33
Kids's Meal Crispy Taco	1 serv (8 oz)	579	10	34
DESSERTS				
Choco Taco	1 serv (3.5 oz)	320	11	17

FOOD	PORTION	CALS.	SAT. FAT	FAT
Churro	1 serv (1.5 oz)	147	2	8
Flauta Apple	1 serv (2 oz)	84	tr	1
Flauta Cherry	1 serv (2 oz)	143	1	4
Flauta Cream Cheese	1 serv (2 oz)	181	3	8
Italian Ice	1 serv (4 oz)	80	0	0
MAIN MENU SELECTIONS				
Bean Burrito	1 (6.5 oz)	387	5	11
Beans Refried	1 serv (9.5 oz)	357	2	9
Beef Burrito	1 (6.5 oz)	449	9	20
Chicken Fajita Burrito	1 (6.25)	370	5	12
Chicken Fajita Salad w/o Dressing	1 serv (12.25 oz)	557	9	33
Chicken Fajita Softshell	1 (4.5 oz)	200	3	7
Chili	1 serv (9.25 oz)	350	10	21
Chimichanga Platter	1 serv (18 oz)	979	15	38
Combination Burrito	1 (6.5 oz)	418	7	16
Crispy Tacos	1 serv (3.25 oz)	182	4	11
Double Enchilada Platter	1 serv (18.25 oz)	967	16	42
Meat & Potato Burrito	1 (7.75 oz)	503	7	24
Mexi Rolls w/ Nacho Cheese	1 serv (9.75 oz)	863	11	48
Mexican Rice	1 serv (8 oz)	567	5	18
Nacho Cheese	1 serv (2 oz)	300	0	10
Nachos	1 serv (3.5 oz)	333	2	21
Potato Oles	1 serv (4.63 oz)	363	5	23
Potato Oles	1 lg serv (6.12 oz)	484	7	30
Potato Oles Bravo	1 serv (8.88 oz)	579	7	38
Potato Oles w/ Nacho Cheese	1 serv (6.63 oz)	483	5	33
Ranch Burrito	1 (7 oz)	447	8	23
Sampler Platter	1 serv (25.5 oz)	1406	24	61
Sierra Chicken Fillet Sandwich	1 (8.5 oz)	534	8	29
Smothered Burrito Platter	1 serv (19.5 oz)	1031	16	40
Softshell Tacos	1 serv (4.25 oz)	230	4	10
Sour Cream	1 oz	60	—	5
Super Burrito	1 (8.5 oz)	465	9	19
Super Nachos	1 serv (13 oz)	919	13	56
Taco Bravo	1 serv (6.25 oz)	346	5	14
Taco Burger	1 (5 oz)	280	5	12
Taco Salad w/o Dressing	1 (12.4 oz)	584	11	38
TACOTIME				
Casita Burrito Meat	1 serv (12 oz)	647	15	31
Cheddar Cheese	1 serv (0.75 oz)	86	4	7
Chicken	1 serv (2.5 oz)	109	2	6
Chips	1 serv (2 oz)	266	3	12

FOOD	PORTION	CALS.	SAT. FAT	FAT
Crisp Burriot Chicken	1 (4.75 oz)	422	8	25
Crisp Burrito Bean	1 (5.25 oz)	427	5	18
Crisp Burrito Meat	1 (5.25 oz)	552	10	30
Crisp Taco	1 (4 oz)	295	7	17
Crustos	1 serv (3.5 oz)	373	—	15
Double Soft Bean Burrito	1 (9.5 oz)	506	6	12
Double Soft Combination Burrito	1 (9.5 oz)	617	10	23
Double Soft Meat Burrito	1 serv (6.5 oz)	726	14	33
Empanada Cherry	1 (4 oz)	250	—	9
Enchilada Sauce	1 serv (1 oz)	12	0	0
Flour Tortilla 10 in	1 (2.75 oz)	213	1	4
Flour Tortilla 7 in	1 (1.75 oz)	88	0	1
Flour Tortilla 8 in	1 (1.25 oz)	107	1	3
Fried Flour Tortilla 10 in	1 (2.75 oz)	318	4	16
Fried Flour Tortilla 8 in	1 (1.35 oz)	205	2	11
Guacamole	1 serv (1 oz)	29	0	2
Hot Sauce	1 serv (1 oz)	10	0	0
Lettuce	1 serv (0.5 oz)	2	0	0
Mexi Fries	1 lg (8 oz)	532	—	34
Mexi Fries	1 reg (4 oz)	266	—	17
Mexican Dressing No Fat	1 serv (2 oz)	20	—	0
Mexican Rice	1 serv (4 oz)	159	1	2
Nachos	1 serv (10.5 oz)	680	19	38
Nachos Deluxe	1 serv (15.25 oz)	1048	23	57
Natural Super Taco Meat	1 (11.25 oz)	627	13	27
Olives	1 serv (0.50 oz)	16	0	2
Quesadilla Cheese	1 serv (3.25 oz)	205	6	11
Ranchero Salsa	1 serv (2 oz)	21	0	1
Refritos	1 serv (2.5 oz)	97	0	0
Refritos	1 serv (7 oz)	326	5	10
Rolled Soft Flour Taco	1 (7 oz)	512	10	23
Shredded Beef	1 serv (2.5 oz)	70	—	7
Soft Taco Chicken	1 (7 oz)	387	6	16
Sour Cream	1 serv (1 oz)	55	3	5
Sour Cream Dressing	1 serv (1.5 oz)	137	5	14
Super Shredded Beef Soft Taco	1 (8 oz)	368	6	11
Taco Cheeseburger	1 (7.5 oz)	633	10	36
Taco Meat	1 serv (2.5 oz)	208	4	11
Taco Salad Chicken w/o Dressing	1 serv (9 oz)	370	7	21
Taco Salad w/o Dressing	1 serv (7.75 oz)	479	11	28
Taco Shell 6 in	1 (1.25 oz)	110	1	6
Thousand Island Dressing	1 serv (1 oz)	160	2	16
Tomato	1 serv (0.5 oz)	3	0	0
Tostada Delight Salad Meat	1 (9.75 oz)	628	14	33

FOOD	PORTION	CALS.	SAT. FAT	FAT
Value Soft Bean Burrito	1 (6.75 oz)	380	4	10
Value Soft Meat Burrito	1 (6.75 oz)	491	8	21
Value Soft Taco	1 (5.25 oz)	316	7	15
Veggie Burrito	1 (11 oz)	491	6	16
Wheat Tortilla 11 in	1 (3.5 oz)	175	1	3
TCBY				
Hand Dipped All Flavors 96% Fat Free	½ cup (3 oz)	140	2	3
Hand Dipped All Flavors Nonfat	½ cup (2.9 oz)	120	0	0
Lowfat Ice Cream All Flavors No Sugar Added	½ cup (2.6 oz)	110	2	3
Nonfat Ice Cream All Flavors	½ cup (2.9 oz)	120	0	0
Soft Serve All Flavors 96% Fat Free	½ cup (3.4 fl oz)	140	2	3
Soft Serve All Flavors No Sugar Added Nonfat	½ cup (2.8 oz)	80	0	0
Soft Serve All Flavors Nonfat	½ cup (3.4 oz)	110	0	0
Sorbet All Flavors Nonfat & Nondairy	½ cup (3.4 oz)	100	0	0
TGI FRIDAY'S				
Corn Salsa	1 serv	175	—	3
Fresh Vegetable Medley w/ Potato	1 serv	470	—	8
Fresh Vegetable Medley w/ Rice	1 serv	407	—	8
Friday's Gardenburger	1	445	—	9
Garden Dagwood Sandwich	1 serv	375	—	11
Pacific Coast Chicken	1 serv	415	—	8
Pacific Coast Tuna	1 serv	410	—	8
Pea Salsa	1 serv (6.4 oz)	175	—	3
Plum Sauce	1 serv	105	0	0
Salad & Baked Potato	1 serv	250	—	5
Turkey Burger	1 (9.8 oz)	410	—	19
TJ CINNAMONS				
Doughnuts Cake	2	454	—	22
Doughnuts Raised	2	352	—	22
Mini-Cinn Plain	1	75	—	5
Mini-Cinn With Icing	1	80	—	5
Original Gourmet Cinnamon Roll Plain	1	630	—	34
Original Gourmet Cinnamon Roll With Icing	1	686	—	34
Petite Cinnamon Roll Plain	1	185	—	10
Petite Cinnamon Roll With Icing	1	202	—	10

FOOD	PORTION	CALS.	SAT. FAT	FAT
Sticky Bun Cinnamon Pecan	1	607	—	35
Sticky Bun Petite Cinnamon Pecan	1	255	—	15
Triple Chocolate Classic Roll Plain	1	412	—	28
Triple Chocolate Classic Roll With Icing	1	462	—	31

TROPIGRILL

(RESTAURANTS IN THIS CHAIN MAY ALSO BE CALLED POLLO TROPICAL. MENU ITEMS ARE THE SAME FOR BOTH.)

FOOD	PORTION	CALS.	SAT. FAT	FAT
Banana Tropical	1 serv (7.55 oz)	498	—	14
Black Beans (combo meal portion)	1 serv (4.78 oz)	153	—	2
Black Beans (side)	1 serv (8.39 oz)	269	—	4
Boiled Yuca	1 serv (12 oz)	334	—	0
Boneless Breast	1 serv (3.14 oz)	140	—	4
Cheese Potatoes	1 serv (7.42 oz)	177	—	6
Chicken ¼ Dark Meat	1 serv (4.52 oz)	298	—	18
Chicken ¼ Dark Meat w/o Skin	1 serv (3.42 oz)	170	—	7
Chicken ¼ White Meat	1 serv (5.09 oz)	295	—	14
Chicken ¼ White Meat w/o Skin	1 serv (3.82 oz)	167	—	3
Chicken Caesar Sandwich	1 (6.4 oz)	457	—	20
Chicken Sandwich	1 (7.92 oz)	442	—	19
Congri	1 serv (7.08 oz)	439	—	13
Vegetable Kabob	1 (3.07 oz)	106	—	1
White Rice	1 serv (6.82 oz)	341	—	6
Yellow Rice	1 serv (7 oz)	294	—	5
Yucatan Fries	1 serv (5.3 oz)	440	—	24

UNO RESTAURANT

FOOD	PORTION	CALS.	SAT. FAT	FAT
DeepDish Pizza	1 serv	770	13	38

VILLAGE INN

FOOD	PORTION	CALS.	SAT. FAT	FAT
French Toast Cinnamon Raisin	1 serv	809	4	16
Fruit & Nut Pancakes Low Cholesterol	1 serv	936	2	19
Omelette Chcken & Cheese	1 serv	721	4	19
Omelette Fresh Veggie	1 serv	704	4	18
Omelette Mushroom & Cheese	1 serv	680	4	18
Turkey & Vegetable Scrambled Sensation	1 serv	726	4	19

WENDY'S

BEVERAGES

FOOD	PORTION	CALS.	SAT. FAT	FAT
Hot Chocolate	1 cup (6 fl oz)	80	0	3

FOOD	PORTION	CALS.	SAT. FAT	FAT
CHILDREN'S MENU SELECTIONS				
Kid's Meal Cheeseburger	1 (4.3 oz)	320	6	13
Kid's Meal Hamburger	1 (3.9 oz)	270	4	10
Kids'Meal Chicken Nuggets	4 pieces (2.1 oz)	190	3	13
DESSERTS				
Chocolate Chip Cookie	1 (2 oz)	270	6	13
Frosty Dairy Dessert	1 sm (12 oz)	330	5	8
Frosty Dairy Dessert	1 med (16 fl oz)	440	7	11
Frosty Dairy Dessert	1 lg (20 fl oz)	540	9	14
MAIN MENU SELECTIONS				
¼ lb Hamburger Patty	1 (2.6 oz)	200	6	14
2 oz Hamburger Patty	1 (1.3 oz)	100	3	7
American Cheese	1 slice (0.6 oz)	70	4	5
American Cheese Jr.	1 slice (0.4 oz)	45	3	4
Bacon	1 strip (4 g)	20	1	2
Baked Potato Bacon & Cheese	1 (13.3 oz)	530	4	18
Baked Potato Broccoli & Cheese	1 (14.4 oz)	470	3	14
Baked Potato Cheese	1 (13.4 oz)	570	8	23
Baked Potato Chili & Cheese	1 (15.4 oz)	630	9	24
Baked Potato Plain	1 (10 oz)	310	0	0
Baked Potato Sour Cream & Chives	1 (11 oz)	380	4	6
Big Bacon Classic	1 (9.9 oz)	580	12	30
Breaded Chicken Fillet	1 (3.5 oz)	230	3	12
Breaded Chicken Sandwich	1 (7.3 oz)	440	4	18
Cheddar Cheese Shredded	2 tbsp (0.6 oz)	70	4	6
Chicken Club Sandwich	1 (7.6 oz)	470	4	20
Chicken Nuggets	5 pieces (2.6 oz)	230	3	16
Chili	1 lg (12 oz)	310	4	10
Chili	1 sm (8 oz)	210	3	7
French Fries	1 Great Biggie (6.7 oz)	570	4	27
French Fries	1 sm (3.2 oz)	270	2	13
French Fries	1 Biggie (5.6 oz)	470	4	23
French Fries	1 med (4.6 oz)	390	3	19
Grilled Chicken Fillet	1 (2.9 oz)	110	1	3
Grilled Chicken Sandwich	1 (6.6 oz)	310	2	8
Honey Mustard Reduced Calorie	1 tsp (7 g)	25	0	2
Jr. Bacon Cheeseburger	1 (5.8 oz)	380	7	19
Jr. Cheeseburger	1 (4.6 oz)	320	6	13
Jr. Cheeseburger Deluxe	1 (6.3 oz)	360	6	17
Jr. Hamburger	1 (4.1 oz)	270	4	10
Kaiser Bun	1 (2.4 oz)	190	1	3
Ketchup	1 tsp (7 g)	10	0	0

FOOD	PORTION	CALS.	SAT. FAT	FAT
Lettuce	1 leaf (0.5 oz)	0	0	0
Mayonnaise	1½ tsp (9 g)	30	0	3
Mustard	½ tsp (5 g)	5	0	0
Nuggets Sauce Barbeque	1 pkg (1 oz)	45	0	0
Nuggets Sauce Honey Mustard	1 pkg (1 oz)	130	2	12
Nuggets Sauce Sweet & Sour	1 pkg (1 oz)	50	0	0
Onion	4 rings (0.5 oz)	5	0	0
Pickles	4 slices (0.4 oz)	0	0	0
Pita Dressing Caesar Vinaigrette Reduced Fat Reduced Calorie	1 tbsp (0.6 oz)	70	1	7
Pita Dressing Garden Ranch Sauce Reduced Fat Reduced Calorie	1 tbsp (0.6 oz)	50	1	5
Plain Single	1 (4.7 oz)	360	6	16
Saltines	2 (0.2 oz)	25	0	1
Sandwich Bun	1 (2 oz)	160	1	3
Single With Everything	1 (7.7 oz)	420	6	20
Sour Cream	1 pkt (1 oz)	60	4	6
Spicy Buffalo Wing Sauce	1 pkg (1 oz)	25	0	1
Spicy Chicken Fillet	1 (3.6 oz)	210	2	9
Spicy Chicken Sandwich	1 (7.5 oz)	410	3	15
Stuffed Pita Chicken Caesar w/Dressing	1 (8.3 oz)	490	5	18
Stuffed Pita Classic Greek w/Dressing	1 (8.2 oz)	440	8	20
Stuffed Pita Garden Ranch Chicken w/ Dressing	1 (9.9 oz)	480	4	18
Stuffed Pita Garden Veggie w/ Dressing	1 (9 oz)	400	4	17
Tomatoes	1 slice (0.9 oz)	5	0	0
Whipped Margarine	1 pkg (0.5 oz)	60	2	7
SALAD DRESSINGS				
Blue Cheese	2 tbsp (1 oz)	180	4	19
French	2 tbsp (1 oz)	120	2	10
French Fat Free	2 tbsp (1 oz)	35	0	0
Hidden Valley Ranch	2 tbsp (1 oz)	90	2	10
Hidden Valley Ranch Reduced Fat Reduced Calorie	2 tbsp (1 oz)	60	1	5
Italian Reduced Fat Reduced Calorie	2 tbsp (1 oz)	40	0	3
Italian Caesar	2 tbsp (1 oz)	150	3	16
Salad Oil	1 tbsp (0.5 oz)	120	2	14
Thousand Island	2 tbsp (1 oz)	90	2	8
Wine Vinegar	1 tbsp (0.5 oz)	0	0	0

FOOD	PORTION	CALS.	SAT. FAT	FAT
SALADS AND SALAD BARS				
Applesauce	2 tbsp (1.4 oz)	30	0	0
Bacon Bits	2 tbsp (0.5 oz)	45	1	2
Bananas & Strawberry Glaze	¼ cup (1.6 oz)	30	0	0
Broccoli	¼ cup (0.5 oz)	0	0	0
Cantaloupe Sliced	1 piece (1.6 oz)	15	0	0
Carrots	¼ cup (0.6 oz)	5	0	0
Cauliflower	¼ cup (0.6 g)	0	0	0
Ceasar Side Salad w/o Dressing	1 (3.1 oz)	100	2	4
Cheese Shredded Imitation	2 tbsp (0.6 oz)	50	1	4
Chicken Salad	2 tbsp (1.2 oz)	70	1	5
Cottage Cheese	2 tbsp (1.1 oz)	30	1	2
Croutons	2 tbsp (0.2 oz)	25	0	1
Cucumbers	2 slices (0.5 oz)	0	0	0
Deluxe Garden Salad w/o Dressing	1 (9.5 oz)	110	1	6
Eggs Hard Cooked	2 tbsp (0.9 oz)	40	1	3
Green Peas	2 tbsp (0.7 oz)	15	0	0
Green Peppers	2 pieces (0.3 oz)	0	0	0
Grilled Chicken Caesar Salad w/o Dressing	1 (9.2 oz)	260	3	9
Grilled Chicken Salad w/o Dressing	1 (11.9 oz)	200	2	8
Lettuce Iceberg/Romaine	1 cup (2.6 oz)	10	0	0
Mushrooms	¼ cup (0.5 oz)	0	0	0
Orange Sliced	2 slices (1.1 oz)	15	0	0
Parmesan Blend Grated	2 tbsp (0.5 oz)	70	2	4
Pasta Salad	2 tbsp (1.2 oz)	35	0	2
Peaches Sliced	1 piece (1 oz)	15	0	0
Pepperoni Sliced	6 slices (0.2 oz)	30	1	3
Potato Salad	2 tbsp (1.3 oz)	80	3	7
Pudding Chocolate	¼ cup (1.8 oz)	70	1	3
Red Onions	3 rings (0.5 oz)	0	0	0
Side Salad w/o Dressing	1 (5.4 oz)	60	0	3
Soft Breadstick	1 (1.5 oz)	130	1	3
Sunflower Seeds & Raisins	2 tbsp (0.5 oz)	80	1	5
Taco Chips	15 (1.5 oz)	210	2	11
Taco Salad w/o Dressing	1 (16.4 oz)	380	10	19
Tomatoes Wedged	1 piece (0.9 oz)	5	0	0
Turkey Ham Diced	2 tbsp (0.8 oz)	50	1	4
Watermelon Wedged	1 piece (2.2 oz)	20	0	0
WHATABURGER				
BAKED SELECTIONS				
Biscuit	1	280	—	13

FOOD	PORTION	CALS.	SAT. FAT	FAT
Blueberry Muffin	1	239	—	8
Cinnamon Roll	1	320	—	16
Cookie Chocolate Chunk	1	247	—	16
Cookie White Chocolate Macadamia Nut	1	269	—	16
Fried Apple Turnover	1	215	—	11
BEVERAGES				
Orange Juice	1 serv (10 oz)	140	0	0
Shake Chocolate	1 junior	364	—	9
Shake Strawberry	1 junior	352	—	9
Shake Vanilla	1 junior	325	—	10
BREAKFAST SELECTIONS				
Biscuit w/ Bacon	1	359	—	20
Biscuit w/ Bacon Egg & Cheese	1	511	—	33
Biscuit w/ Egg & Cheese	1	434	—	26
Biscuit w/ Sausage	1	446	—	29
Biscuit w/ Sausage Egg & Cheese	1	601	—	42
Biscuit w/ Sausage Gravy	1	479	—	27
Breakfast Platter w/ Bacon	1 serv	695	—	44
Breakfast Platter w/ Sausage	1 serv	785	—	53
Breakfast On A Bun w/ Bacon	1	365	—	19
Breakfast On A Bun w/ Sausage	1	455	—	28
Butter	1 pkg	36	—	4
Egg Omelette Sandwich	1	288	—	13
Grape Jelly	1 pkg	45	0	0
Hashbrown	1 serv	150	—	9
Honey	1 pkg	25	0	0
Margarine	1 pkg	25	—	3
Pancake Syrup	1 pkg	180	0	0
Pancakes	3	259	—	6
Pancakes w/ Bacon	1 serv	335	—	12
Pancakes w/ Sausage	1 serv	426	—	21
Srambled Eggs	2	189	—	15
Strawberry Jam	1 pkg	40	0	0
Taquito Bacon & Egg	1	335	—	16
MAIN MENU SELECTIONS				
Bacon	1 slice	38	—	3
Cheese Slice	1 lg	89	—	7
Cheese Slice	1 sm	46	—	4
Chicken Strips	2	120	—	5
Club Crackers	1 pkg	30	—	2
Croutons	1 pkg	30	—	1
Fajita Beef	1	326	—	12
Fajita Grilled Chicken	1	272	—	7

FOOD	PORTION	CALS.	SAT. FAT	FAT
French Fries	1 junior	221	—	12
French Fries	1 reg	332	—	18
French Fries	1 lg	442	—	24
Garden Salad	1	56	—	1
Grilled Chicken Salad	1 serv	150	—	1
Grilled Chicken Sandwich	1	442	—	14
Grilled Chicken Sandwich w/o Bun Oil w/ Mustard	1	300	—	3
Grilled Chicken Sandwich w/o Bun Oil & Dressing	1	358	—	6
Grilled Chicken Sandwich w/o Dressing	1	385	—	9
Jalapeno Pepper	1	3	—	tr
Justaburger	1	276	—	11
Ketchup	1 pkg	30	0	0
Onion Rings	1 lg	493	—	29
Onion Rings	1 reg	329	—	19
Peppered Gravy	1 serv (3 oz)	75	—	5
Picante Sauce	1 pkg	5	—	0
Taquito Potato & Egg	1	446	—	22
Taquito Sausage & Egg	1	443	—	26
Texas Toast	1 slice	147	—	5
Whataburger	1	598	—	26
Whataburger Double Meat	1	823	—	42
Whataburger Jr.	1	300	—	12
Whataburger w/o bun oil	1	407	—	19
Whatacatch Sandwich	1	467	—	25
Whatachick'n Sandwich	1	501	—	23
SALAD DRESSINGS				
Low Fat Ranch	1 pkg	66	—	3
Low Fat Vinaigrette	1 pkg	37	—	2
Ranch	1 pkg	320	—	33
Thousand Island	1 pkg	160	—	12
WHITE CASTLE				
Bun Only	1	74	—	tr
Cheese Only	0.3 oz	31	—	2
Cheeseburger	2 (3.6 oz)	310	9	17
Fish w/o Tarter Sandwich	1	155	—	5
French Fries	1 reg	301	—	15
Grilled Chicken Sandwich	2 (4 oz)	250	3	9
Grilled Chicken Sandwich w/ Sauce	2 (4.8 oz)	290	3	9
Hamburger	2 (3.2 oz)	270	6	14

FOOD	PORTION	CALS.	SAT. FAT	FAT
Onion Rings	1 reg	245	—	13
Sausage Sandwich	1	196	—	12
Sausage & Egg Sandwich	1	322	—	22

WINCHELL'S DONUTS

FOOD	PORTION	CALS.	SAT. FAT	FAT
Apple Fritter	1 (4.25 oz)	580	—	37
Cinnamon Crumb	1 (2 oz)	240	—	11
Cinnamon Roll	1 (3 oz)	360	—	21
Glazed Jelly	1 (3 oz)	300	—	13
Glazed Round	1 (1.75 oz)	210	—	12
Glazed Twist	1 (1.75 oz)	210	—	11
Iced Chocolate Bar	1 (2 oz)	220	—	11
Iced Chocolate Cake	1 (2 oz)	230	—	10
Iced Chocolate Devil's Food	1 (2 oz)	240	—	12
Iced Chocolate French	1 (1.89 oz)	220	—	13
Iced Chocolate Raised	1 (1.75 oz)	210	—	10
Plain	1 (1.58 oz)	200	—	11
Plain Donut Hole	1 (0.4 oz)	50	—	3

ZUZU

FOOD	PORTION	CALS.	SAT. FAT	FAT
Bean & Cheese Burrito Platter	1 serv	475	—	15
Beans	1 cup	210	—	6
Cheese Enchilada Platter	1 serv	395	—	13
Chicken Burrito Platter	1 serv	580	—	19
Chicken Taco Platter	1 serv	440	—	13
Chicken Taco w/o Mexican Cream	1	125	—	4
Frozen Yogurt	1 serv	200	0	0
Green Salad w/o Dressing or Avocado	1	20	0	0
Grilled Chicken Salad w/o Dressing	1 serv	305	—	10
Rice	1 cup	150	—	2
Salsa Roja Epazote	¼ cup	8	0	0
Tortilla Corn	1	35	0	0
Tortilla Flour	1	60	—	2

Visit

❖ **Pocket Books** ❖

online at

....

www.SimonSays.com

....

Keep up on the latest new
releases from your favorite
authors, as well as author
appearances, news, chats,
special offers and more.

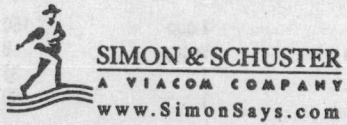
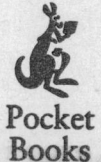